Anesthesia:
A Comprehensive Review

Anesthesia:
A Comprehensive Review

4th Edition

Brian A. Hall, M.D.

Assistant Professor of Anesthesiology
College of Medicine, Mayo Clinic
Rochester, Minnesota

Robert C. Chantigian, M.D.

Associate Professor of Anesthesiology
College of Medicine, Mayo Clinic
Rochester, Minnesota

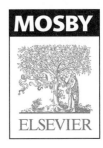

MOSBY

ELSEVIER

3251 Riverport Lane
Maryland Heights, Missouri 63043

ANESTHESIA: A COMPREHENSIVE REVIEW
Fourth Edition

Previous editions copyrighted 1997, 1992

Library of Congress Cataloging-in-Publication Data
Hall, Brian A.
    Anesthesia: a comprehensive review / Brian A. Hall, Robert C. Chantigian.—4th ed.
        p. ; cm.
    Includes bibliographical references and index.
    ISBN 978-0-323-06857-4
    1. Anesthesiology—Examinations, questions, etc. 2. Anesthesiology—Outlines, syllabi,
etc. I. Chantigian, Robert C. II. Mayo Foundation for Medical Education and Research. III. Title.
    [DNLM: 1. Anesthesia—Examination Questions. WO 218.2 H174a 2009]
RD82.3 .H35 2009
617.9'6076—dc22   2009039292

Editor: Natasha Andjelkovic
Editorial Assistant: Bradley McIlwain
Publishing Services Manager: Anitha Rajarathnam
Project Manager: Mahalakshmi Nithyanand
Design Direction: Louis Forgione

ISBN: 978-0-323-06857-4

Printed in Canada

Last digit is the print number: 9 8 7 6 5 4 3 2 1

Work started on the first edition of this book more than 20 years ago. Over the ensuing years and with each edition, changes in medicine and anesthesiology have occurred at an astounding rate. Several drugs were discovered and marketed and have since been withdrawn or replaced with better drugs. Some procedures and techniques, once very popular, have been relegated to historic significance only.

Although these advances and improvements in anesthesiology have been reflected in each subsequent edition, the fourth edition has unquestionably seen the greatest number of changes in both content and testing format.

Questions have been carefully reviewed. Those of dubious merit have been replaced. The format of the entire book has been changed to include type A (single answer) questions exclusively. All K-type (multiple true/false) questions have been eliminated because these are no longer used in the certification process.

This book, like its predecessors, is intended as a guide to aid learners in identifying areas of weakness. It was written to solidify the readers' knowledge and point out topics and concepts requiring further study. The questions range from very basic to complex and are useful for individuals just entering the field as well as for experienced practitioners preparing for recertification.

BRIAN A. HALL, M.D.
ROBERT C. CHANTIGIAN, M.D.

Contributors

Dorothee H. Bremerich, M.D.
   Professor and Chairman
   Department of Anesthesiology
   and Intensive Care Medicine
   St. Vincenz Hospital
   Limburg, Germany

Dawit T. Haile, M.D.
   Instructor of Anesthesiology
   College of Medicine, Mayo Clinic
   Rochester, Minnesota

Keith A. Jones, M.D.
   Professor and Chairman
   Department of Anesthesiology
   University of Alabama School of Medicine
   Birmingham, Alabama

C. Thomas Wass, M.D.
   Associate Professor of Anesthesiology
   College of Medicine, Mayo Clinic
   Rochester, Minnesota

Francis X. Whalen, M.D.
   Assistant Professor
   Department of Anesthesiology
   and Critical Care Medicine
   College of Medicine, Mayo Clinic
   Rochester, Minnesota

The following figures and tables are reprinted from other sources:

Figure on page 6
From van Genderingen HR, Gravenstein N, et al: Computer-assisted capnogram analysis. J Clin Monit 3:198, 1987, with kind permission of Kluwer Academic Publishers.

Figure on page 12
Modified from Willis BA, Pender JW, Mapleson WW: Rebreathing in a T-piece: Volunteer and theoretical studies of Jackson-Rees modification of Ayre's T-piece during spontaneous respiration. Br J Anaesth 47:1239-1246, 1975. © The Board of Management and Trustees of the British Journal of Anaesthesia. Reproduced by permission of Oxford University Press/British Journal of Anaesthesia.

Tables on pages 15, 67, 150 and 171
From Stoelting RK, Miller RD: Basics of Anesthesia, ed 4. New York, Churchill Livingstone, 2000.

Figure on page 15
Based on Check-out: A Guide for Preoperative Inspection of an Anesthesia Machine/1987 of the American Society of Anesthesiologists. A copy of the full text can be obtained from ASA, 520 N. Northwest Highway, Park Ridge, Illinois 60068-2573.

Figure on page 18
From Andrews JJ: Understanding your anesthesia machine and ventilator. In International Anesthesia Research Society (ed): 1989 Review Course Lectures. Cleveland, Ohio, 1989, p 59.

Figure on page 23
Courtesy of Draeger Medical, Inc., Telford, Pa

Figure on page 24
From Azar I, Eisenkraft JB: Waste anesthetic gas spillage and scavenging systems. In Ehrenwerth J, Eisenkraft JB (eds): Anesthesia Equipment: Principles and Applications. St. Louis, Mosby, 1993, p 128.

Figures on pages 41 and 108; Tables on pages 41, 65, 67, 68, 69 and 74
From Stoelting RK: Pharmacology and Physiology in Anesthetic Practice, ed 3. Philadelphia, Lippincott Williams & Wilkins, 1999.

Figure on page 44
From Stoelting RK, Dierdorf SF: Anesthesia and Co-existing Disease, ed 4. New York, Churchill Livingstone, 2002.

Table on page 78
Modified from Miller RD (ed): Anesthesia, ed 5. New York, Churchill Livingstone, 2000, p 1794.

Figure on page 160
From Avery ME: Lung and Its Disorders in the Newborn, ed 3. Philadelphia, WB Saunders, 1974, p 134.

Figure on page 173
From Moore KL (ed): Clinically Oriented Anatomy. Baltimore, Williams & Wilkins, 1980, p 653.

Figure on page 179
From Coté CJ, Todres ID: The pediatric airway. In Coté CJ, Ryan JF, Todres ID, et al (eds): A Practice of Anesthesia for Infants and Children. Philadelphia, WB Saunders, 1992, p 55.

Figure on page 199
From Benedetti TJ: Obstetric hemorrhage. In Gabbe SG, Niebyl JR, Simpson JL (eds): Obstetrics: Normal and Problem Pregnancies, ed 3. New York, Churchill Livingstone, 1996, p 511.

Figure on page 209
From Miller RD (ed): Anesthesia, ed 3. New York, Churchill Livingstone, 1990, p 1745.

Tables on page 217
From Darby JM, Stein K, Grenvik A, et al: Approach to management of the heart beating "brain dead" organ donor. JAMA 261: 2222, 1989. Copyrighted 1989, American Medical Association.

Figure on page 218
From Cucchiara RJ, Black S, Steinkeler JA: Anesthesia for intracranial procedures. In Barash PG, Cullen BF, Stoelting RK (eds): Clinical Anesthesia. Philadelphia, JB Lippincott, 1989, p 849.

Figure on page 243
By permission of Mayo Foundation for Medical Education and Research

Figure on page 244
From Raj PP: Practical Management of Pain, ed 2. St. Louis, Mosby-Year Book, 1992, p 785.

Figure on page 250
From Cousins MJ, Bridenbaugh PO (eds): Neural Blockade in Clinical Anesthesia and Management of Pain, ed 2. Philadelphia, JB Lippincott, 1988, pp 255-263.

Figure on page 261
From Mark JB: Atlas of Cardiovascular Monitoring. New York, Churchill Livingstone, 1998.

Figure on page 262
From Jackson JM, Thomas SJ, Lowenstein E: Anesthetic Management of Patients with Valvular Heart Disease. Semin Anesth 1:244, 1982.

Figure on page 264, question 961
From Morgan GE, Mikhail MS: Clinical Anesthesiology. East Norwalk, Appleton & Lange, 1992, p 301.

Figure on page 264, question 962
From Spiess BD, Ivankovich AD: Thromboelastography: A coagulation-monitoring technique applied to cardiopulmonary bypass. In Effective Hemostasis in Cardiac Surgery. Philadelphia, WB Saunders, 1988, p 165.

Acknowledgements

The practice of anesthesiology has become increasingly subspecialized and technical. The authors and co-authors are indebted to a multitude of other contributors. The combined efforts of all these individuals in proofreading, examining, and critiquing the questions and explanations have resulted in a very useful and technically accurate work. The authors wish to thank the anesthesia residents who checked the references for all questions taken from the third edition and updated them: Drs. Fawn Atchison, Ann Baetzel, Eric Deutsch, Andrea Dutoit, Tara Frost, Kendra Grim, Adam Niesen, Eduardo Rodrigues, William Shakespeare, Brandon Sloop, and Peter Stiles. Each chapter underwent a final proofreading before production; the authors are very appreciative of the efforts of Drs. Eric Deutsch, Joel Farmer, Antolin Flores, Ryan Gassin, Kendra Grim, Erin Grund, Rebecca Johnson, Westley Manske, David Prybilla, Troy Russon, and Hans Sviggum.

Several anesthesia staff members from the Mayo Clinic and other institutions were very helpful with development of many of the new questions. The authors wish to express their gratitude to Drs. Martin Abel, Thomas Comfere, Tim Curry, Niki Dietz, Robert Friedhoff, Tracy Harrison, James Hebl, Jeff Jensen, D.J. Kor, William Lanier, James Lynch, David Martin, Linda Mason, William Mauermann, Brian McGlinch, James Munis, Michael Johnson, Joseph Neal, Jeff Pasternak, William Perkins, Kent Rehfeldt, Greg Schears, David Warner, Denise Wedel, Margaret Weglinski, and Roger White.

The authors also thank Tara Hall, RRT; Robin Hardt, CRNA; and Natalie Johnson, CRNA, for help with proofreading and suggestions for question topics.

Work for the first edition of this book began in 1987, but the formation of the early manuscript into an organized book did not occur until 1989 at the suggestion of and with strong encouragement from Drs. Michael J. Joyner, Ronald A. MacKenzie, and Kenneth P. Scott.

The chairman of our department, Bradly J. Narr, was very supportive of our efforts in producing this book, and we wish to thank him. Lastly, our friends at Elsevier Medical Publishers, Dr. Natasha Andjelkovic, Angela Norton, Mahalakshmi Nithyanand, and Virgina Wilson were very patient, helpful, and supportive in the preparation of this manuscript. We are very appreciative of their benevolence.

BRIAN A. HALL, M.D.

ROBERT C. CHANTIGIAN, M.D.

Contents

Basic Sciences PART 1

Chapter 1

Anesthesia Equipment and Physics

1. A 58-year-old patient has severe shortness of breath and "wheezing." On examination, it is found that the patient has inspiratory and expiratory stridor. Further evaluation reveals marked extrinsic compression of the midtrachea by a tumor. The type of airflow at the point of obstruction within the trachea is
   - **A.** Laminar flow
   - **B.** Orifice flow
   - **C.** Undulant flow
   - **D.** Stenotic flow
   - **E.** None of the above

2. Concerning the patient in question 1, administration of 70% helium in O_2 instead of 100% O_2 will decrease the resistance to airflow through the stenotic region within the trachea because
   - **A.** Helium decreases the viscosity of the gas mixture
   - **B.** Helium decreases the friction coefficient of the gas mixture
   - **C.** Helium decreases the density of the gas mixture
   - **D.** Helium increases the Reynolds number of the gas mixture
   - **E.** None of the above

3. A 56-year-old patient is brought to the operating room (OR) for elective replacement of a stenotic aortic valve. An awake 20-gauge arterial catheter is placed into the right radial artery and is then connected to a transducer located at the same level as the patient's left ventricle. The entire system is zeroed at the transducer. Several seconds later, the patient raises both arms into the air such that his right wrist is 20 cm above his heart. As he is doing this, the blood pressure (BP) on the monitor reads 120/80. What would this patient's true BP be at this time?
   - **A.** 140/100 mm Hg
   - **B.** 135/95 mm Hg
   - **C.** 120/80 mm Hg
   - **D.** 105/65 mm Hg
   - **E.** 100/60 mm Hg

4. An admixture of room air in the waste gas disposal system during an appendectomy in a paralyzed, mechanically ventilated patient under general volatile anesthesia can best be explained by which mechanism of entry?
    A. Venous air embolism
    B. Positive pressure relief valve
    C. Negative pressure relief valve
    D. Soda lime canister
    E. Ventilator bellows

5. The relationship between intra-alveolar pressure, surface tension, and the radius of an alveolus is described by
    A. Graham's law
    B. Beer's law
    C. Newton's law
    D. Laplace's law
    E. Bernoulli's law

6. A size "E" compressed-gas cylinder completely filled with N_2O contains how many liters?
    A. 1160 L
    B. 1470 L
    C. 1590 L
    D. 1640 L
    E. 1750 L

7. Which of the following methods can be used to detect all leaks in the low-pressure circuit of any contemporary anesthesia machine?
    A. Oxygen flush test
    B. Common gas outlet occlusion test
    C. Traditional positive-pressure leak test
    D. Negative-pressure leak test
    E. No test can verify the integrity of all contemporary anesthesia machines

8. Which of the following valves prevents transfilling between compressed-gas cylinders?
    A. Fail-safe valve
    B. Pop-off valve
    C. Pressure-sensor shutoff valve
    D. Adjustable pressure-limiting valve
    E. Check valve

9. The expression that for a fixed mass of gas at constant temperature, the product of pressure and volume is constant is known as
    A. Graham's law
    B. Bernoulli's law
    C. Boyle's law
    D. Dalton's law
    E. Charles' law

10. The pressure gauge on a size "E" compressed-gas cylinder containing O_2 reads 1600 psi. How long could O_2 be delivered from this cylinder at a rate of 2 L/min?
    A. 90 minutes
    B. 140 minutes
    C. 250 minutes
    D. 320 minutes
    E. Cannot be calculated

11.   A 25-year-old healthy patient is anesthetized for a femoral hernia repair. Anesthesia is maintained with isoflurane and N_2O 50% in O_2 and the patient's lungs are mechanically ventilated. Suddenly, the "low-arterial saturation" warning signal on the pulse oximeter alarms. After the patient is disconnected from the anesthesia machine, he is ventilated with an Ambu bag with 100% O_2 without difficulty and the arterial saturation quickly improves. During inspection of your anesthesia equipment, you notice that the bobbin in the O_2 rotameter is not rotating. This most likely indicates
       A. The flow of N_2O through the O_2 rotameter
       B. No flow of O_2 through the O_2 rotameter
       C. A flow of O_2 through the O_2 rotameter that is markedly lower than indicated
       D. A leak in the O_2 rotameter above the bobbin
       E. A leak in the O_2 rotameter below the bobbin

12.   The O_2 pressure-sensor shutoff valve requires what O_2 pressure to remain open and allow N_2O to flow into the N_2O rotameter?
       A. 10 psi
       B. 25 psi
       C. 50 psi
       D. 100 psi
       E. 600 psi

13.   A 78-year-old patient is anesthetized for resection of a liver tumor. After induction and tracheal intubation, a 20-gauge arterial line is placed and connected to a transducer that is located 20 cm below the level of the heart. The system is zeroed at the stopcock located at the wrist while the patient's arm is stretched out on an arm board. How will the arterial line pressure compare with the true BP?
       A. It will be 20 mm Hg higher
       B. It will be 15 mm Hg higher
       C. It will be the same
       D. It will be 15 mm Hg lower
       E. It will be 20 mm Hg lower

14.   The second-stage O_2 pressure regulator delivers a constant O_2 pressure to the rotameters of
       A. 4 psi
       B. 8 psi
       C. 16 psi
       D. 32 psi
       E. 64 psi

15.   The highest trace concentration of N_2O allowed in the OR atmosphere by the National Institute for Occupational Safety and Health (NIOSH) is
       A. 1 part per million (ppm)
       B. 5 ppm
       C. 25 ppm
       D. 50 ppm
       E. 100 ppm

16.   A sevoflurane vaporizer will deliver an accurate concentration of an unknown volatile anesthetic if the latter shares which property with sevoflurane?
       A. Molecular weight
       B. Viscosity
       C. Vapor pressure
       D. Blood/gas partition coefficient
       E. Oil/gas partition coefficient

17. The portion of the ventilator (Ohmeda 7000, 7810, and 7900) on the anesthesia machine that compresses the bellows is driven by
    A. Compressed oxygen
    B. Compressed air
    C. Electricity alone
    D. Electricity and compressed oxygen
    E. Electricity and compressed air

18. Which of the following rotameter flow indicators is read in the middle of the dial?
    A. Bobbin
    B. "H" float
    C. Ball float
    D. Skirted float
    E. Nonrotating float

19. When the pressure gauge on a size "E" compressed-gas cylinder containing N_2O begins to fall from its previous constant pressure of 750 psi, approximately how many liters of gas will remain in the cylinder?
    A. 200 L
    B. 400 L
    C. 600 L
    D. 800 L
    E. Cannot be calculated

20. A 3-year-old child with severe congenital facial anomalies is anesthetized for extensive facial reconstruction. After inhalation induction with sevoflurane and oral tracheal intubation, a 22-gauge arterial line is placed in the right radial artery. The arterial cannula is then connected to a transducer that is located 10 cm below the patient's heart. After zeroing the arterial line at the transducer, how will the given pressure compare with the true arterial pressure?
    A. It will be 10 mm Hg higher
    B. It will be 7.5 mm Hg higher
    C. It will be the same
    D. It will be 7.5 mm Hg lower
    E. It will be 10 mm Hg lower

21. If the internal diameter of an intravenous catheter were doubled, flow through the catheter would be
    A. Decreased by a factor of 2
    B. Decreased by a factor of 4
    C. Increased by a factor of 8
    D. Increased by a factor of 16
    E. Increased by a factor of 32

22. Of the following statements concerning the safe storage of compressed-gas cylinders, choose the one that is **FALSE.**
    A. Should not be handled with oily hands
    B. Should not be stored near flammable material
    C. Should not be stored in extreme heat or cold
    D. Paper or plastic covers should not be removed from the cylinders before storage
    E. All of the above statements are true

23. For any given concentration of volatile anesthetic, the splitting ratio is dependent on which of the following characteristics of that volatile anesthetic?
    A. Vapor pressure
    B. Barometric pressure
    C. Molecular weight
    D. Specific heat
    E. Minimum alveolar concentration (MAC) at 1 atmosphere

24. A mechanical ventilator (e.g., Ohmeda 7000) is set to deliver a tidal volume (V_T) of 500 mL at a rate of 10 breaths/min and an inspiratory-to-expiratory (I:E) ratio of 1:2. The fresh gas flow into the breathing circuit is 6 L/min. In a patient with normal total pulmonary compliance, the actual V_T delivered to the patient would be
    A. 400 mL
    B. 500 mL
    C. 600 mL
    D. 700 mL
    E. 800 mL

25. In reference to question 24, if the ventilator rate were decreased from 10 to 6 breaths/min, the approximate V_T delivered to the patient would be
    A. 600 mL
    B. 700 mL
    C. 800 mL
    D. 900 mL
    E. 1000 mL

26. Vaporizers for which of the following volatile anesthetics could be used interchangeably with accurate delivery of the concentration of anesthetic set on the vaporizer dial?
    A. Halothane, sevoflurane, and isoflurane
    B. Sevoflurane and isoflurane
    C. Halothane and sevoflurane
    D. Halothane and isoflurane
    E. Sevoflurane and desflurane

27. If the anesthesia machine is discovered Monday morning having run with 5 L/min of oxygen all weekend long, the most reasonable course of action to take before administering the next anesthetic would be
    A. Turn machine off for 30 minutes before induction
    B. Place humidifier in line with the expiratory limb
    C. Avoid use of sevoflurane
    D. Change the CO_2 absorbent
    E. Administer 100% oxygen for the first hour of the next case

28. According to NIOSH regulations, the highest concentration of volatile anesthetic contamination allowed in the OR atmosphere when administered in conjunction with N_2O is
    A. 0.5 ppm
    B. 2 ppm
    C. 5 ppm
    D. 25 ppm
    E. 50 ppm

29. The device on anesthesia machines that most reliably detects delivery of hypoxic gas mixtures is the
    A. Fail-safe valve
    B. O_2 analyzer
    C. Second-stage O_2 pressure regulator
    D. Proportion-limiting control system
    E. Diameter-index safety system

30. A ventilator pressure-relief valve stuck in the closed position can result in
    A. Barotrauma
    B. Hypoventilation
    C. Hypoxia
    D. Hyperventilation
    E. Low breathing circuit pressure

31. A mixture of 1% isoflurane, 70% N_2O, and 30% O_2 is administered to a patient for 30 minutes. The expired isoflurane concentration measured is 1%. N_2O is shut off and a mixture of 30% O_2, 70% N_2 with 1% isoflurane is administered. The expired isoflurane concentration measured one minute after the start of this new mixture is 2.3%. The best explanation for this observation is
   A. Intermittent back pressure (pumping effect)
   B. Diffusion hypoxia
   C. Concentration effect
   D. Effect of N_2O solubility in isoflurane
   E. Effect of similar mass-to-charge ratios of N_2O and CO_2

32.

The mass spectrometer waveform above represents which of the following situations?
   A. Cardiac oscillations
   B. Kinked endotracheal tube
   C. Bronchospasm
   D. Incompetent inspiratory valve
   E. Incompetent expiratory valve

33. Select the **FALSE** statement.
   A. If a Magill forceps is used for a nasotracheal intubation, the right nares is preferable for insertion of the nasotracheal tube.
   B. Extension of the neck can convert an endotracheal intubation to an endobronchial intubation.
   C. Bucking signifies the return of the coughing reflex.
   D. Postintubation pharyngitis is more likely to occur in females.
   E. Stenosis becomes symptomatic when the adult tracheal lumen is reduced to less than 5 mm.

34. Gas from an N_2O compressed-gas cylinder enters the anesthesia machine through a pressure regulator that reduces the pressure to
   A. 60 psi
   B. 45 psi
   C. 30 psi
   D. 15 psi
   E. 10 psi

35. Which of the following factors is **LEAST** responsible for killing bacteria in anesthesia machines?
   A. Metallic ions
   B. High O_2 concentration
   C. Anesthetic gases (at clinical concentrations)
   D. Shifts in humidity
   E. Shifts in temperature

36. Which of the following systems prevents attachment of gas-administering equipment to the wrong type of gas line?
   A. Pin-index safety system
   B. Diameter-index safety system
   C. Fail-safe system
   D. Proportion-limiting control system
   E. None of the above

37. A volatile anesthetic has a saturated vapor pressure of 360 mm Hg at room temperature. At what flow would this agent be delivered from a bubble-through vaporizer if the carrier-gas flow through the vaporizing chamber is 100 mL/min?
    A. 30 mL/min
    B. 60 mL/min
    C. 90 mL/min
    D. 120 mL/min
    E. 150 mL/min

38. The dial of an isoflurane-specific, variable bypass, temperature-compensated, flowover, out-of-circuit vaporizer (i.e., modern vaporizer) is set on 2% and the mass spectrometer measures 2% isoflurane vapor from the common gas outlet. The flowmeter is set at a rate of 700 mL/min during this measurement. The output measurements are repeated with the flowmeter set at 100 mL/min and 15 L/min (vapor dial still set on 2%). How will these two measurements compare with the first measurement taken?
    A. Output will be less than 2% in both cases
    B. Output will be greater than 2% in both cases
    C. Output will be 2% at 100 mL/min O_2 flow and less than 2% at 15 L/min flow
    D. Output will be 2% in both cases
    E. Output will be less than 2% at 100 mL/min and 2% at 15 L/min

39. Which of the following would result in the greatest decrease in the arterial hemoglobin saturation (Spo_2) value measured by the dual-wavelength pulse oximeter?
    A. Intravenous injection of indigo carmine
    B. Intravenous injection of indocyanine green
    C. Intravenous injection of methylene blue
    D. Presence of elevated bilirubin
    E. Presence of fetal hemoglobin

40. A 75-year-old patient with chronic obstructive pulmonary disease is ventilated with a mixture of 50% oxygen with 50% helium. Isoflurane 2% is added to this mixture. What effect will helium have on the mass spectrometer reading of the isoflurane concentration?
    A. The mass spectrometer will give a slightly increased false value
    B. The mass spectrometer will give a false value equal to double the isoflurane concentration
    C. The mass spectrometer will give the correct value
    D. The mass spectrometer will give a wrong value equal to half the isoflurane concentration
    E. The mass spectrometer will give an erroneous value slightly less than the correct value of isoflurane

41. Which of the following combinations would result in delivery of a higher-than-expected concentration of volatile anesthetic to the patient?
    A. Halothane vaporizer filled with sevoflurane
    B. Halothane vaporizer filled with isoflurane
    C. Isoflurane vaporizer filled with halothane
    D. Isoflurane vaporizer filled with sevoflurane
    E. Sevoflurane vaporizer filled with halothane

42. At high altitudes, the flow of a gas through a rotameter will be
    A. Greater than expected
    B. Less than expected
    C. Greater than expected at high flows but less than expected at low flows
    D. Less than expected at high flows but greater than expected at low flows
    E. Greater than expected at high flows but accurate at low flows

43. A patient presents for knee arthroscopy and tells his anesthesiologist that he has a VDD pacemaker. Select the true statement regarding this pacemaker.
    A. It senses only the ventricle
    B. It paces only the ventricle
    C. Its response to a sensed event is always inhibition
    D. Its response to a sensed event is always a triggered pulse
    E. It is not useful in a patient with AV nodal block

44. All of the following would result in less trace gas pollution of the OR atmosphere **EXCEPT**
    A. Using a high gas flow in a circular system
    B. Tight mask seal during mask induction
    C. Use of a scavenging system
    D. Periodic maintenance of the anesthesia machine
    E. Allow patient to breath 100% O_2 as long as possible before extubation

45. The greatest source for contamination of the OR atmosphere is leakage of volatile anesthetics
    A. Around the anesthesia mask
    B. At the vaporizer
    C. At the rotameter
    D. At the CO_2 absorber
    E. At the endotracheal tube

46. Uptake of sevoflurane from the lungs during the first minute of general anesthesia is 50 mL. How much sevoflurane would be taken up from the lungs between the 16th and 36th minutes?
    A. 25 mL
    B. 50 mL
    C. 100 mL
    D. 200 mL
    E. 500 mL

47. Which of the drugs below would have the **LEAST** impact on somatosensory evoked potentials (SSEP) monitoring in a 15-year-old patient undergoing scoliosis surgery?
    A. Midazolam
    B. Fentanyl
    C. Thiopental
    D. Isoflurane
    E. Vecuronium

48. Select the **FALSE** statement regarding iatrogenic bacterial infections from anesthetic equipment.
    A. Even low concentrations of O_2 are lethal to airborne bacteria
    B. Bacteria released from the airway during violent exhalation originate almost exclusively from the anterior oropharynx
    C. Of all the bacterial forms, acid-fast bacteria are the most resistant to destruction
    D. Shifts in temperature and humidity are probably the most important factors responsible for bacterial killing
    E. Bacterial filters in the anesthesia breathing system lower the incidence of postoperative pulmonary infections

49. Frost develops on the outside of an N_2O compressed-gas cylinder during general anesthesia. This phenomenon indicates that
    A. The saturated vapor pressure of N_2O within the cylinder is rapidly increasing
    B. The cylinder is almost empty
    C. There is a rapid transfer of heat to the cylinder
    D. The flow of N_2O from the cylinder into the anesthesia machine is rapid
    E. None of the above

50. The **LEAST** reliable site for central temperature monitoring is the
    A. Pulmonary artery
    B. Skin on forehead
    C. Distal third of the esophagus
    D. Nasopharynx
    E. Tympanic membrane

51. Each of the following statements concerning rotameters is true **EXCEPT**
    A. Rotation of the bobbin within the Thorpe tube is important for accurate function
    B. The Thorpe tube increases in diameter from bottom to top
    C. Its accuracy is affected by changes in temperature and atmospheric pressure
    D. The rotameter for N_2O and CO_2 are interchangeable
    E. The rotameter for O_2 should be the last in the series

52. The reason a 40:60 mixture of helium and O_2 is more desirable than a 40:60 mixture of nitrogen and O_2 for a spontaneously breathing patient with tracheal stenosis is
    A. Helium has a lower density than nitrogen
    B. Helium is a smaller molecule than O_2
    C. Absorption atelectasis decreased
    D. Helium has a lower critical velocity for turbulent flow than does O_2
    E. Helium is toxic to most microorganisms

53. The maximum F_{IO_2} that can be delivered by a nasal cannula is
    A. 0.25
    B. 0.30
    C. 0.35
    D. 0.40
    E. 0.45

54. General anesthesia is administered to an otherwise healthy 38-year-old patient undergoing repair of a right inguinal hernia. During mechanical ventilation, the anesthesiologist notices that the scavenging system reservoir bag is distended during inspiration. The most likely cause of this is
    A. An incompetent pressure-relief valve in the mechanical ventilator
    B. An incompetent pressure-relief valve in the patient breathing circuit
    C. An incompetent inspiratory unidirectional valve in the patient breathing circuit
    D. An incompetent expiratory unidirectional valve in the patient breathing circuit
    E. None of the above; the scavenging system reservoir bag is supposed to distend during inspiration

55. Which color of nail polish would have the greatest effect on the accuracy of dual-wavelength pulse oximeters?
    A. Red
    B. Yellow
    C. Blue
    D. Green
    E. White

56. The minimum macroshock current required to elicit ventricular fibrillation is
    A. 1 mA
    B. 10 mA
    C. 100 mA
    D. 500 mA
    E. 5000 mA

57. The line isolation monitor
    A. Prevents microshock
    B. Prevents macroshock
    C. Provides electrical isolation in the OR
    D. Sounds an alarm when grounding occurs in the OR
    E. Provides a safe electrical ground

58. Kinking or occlusion of the transfer tubing from the patient breathing circuit to the closed scavenging system interface can result in
    A. Barotrauma
    B. Hypoventilation
    C. Hypoxia
    D. Hyperventilation
    E. None of the above

59. If the isoflurane vaporizer dial of an older (non- pressure compensating) machine is set to deliver 1.15% in Denver, Colo. (barometric pressure 630 mm Hg), how many MAC will the patient receive?
     A. About 20% more than 1 MAC
     B. About 10% more than 1 MAC
     C. One MAC
     D. About 10% less than 1 MAC
     E. About 20% less than 1 MAC

60. Select the **FALSE** statement regarding noninvasive arterial BP monitoring devices.
     A. If the width of the BP cuff is too narrow, the measured BP will be falsely lowered
     B. The width of the BP cuff should be 40% of the circumference of the patient's arm
     C. If the BP cuff is wrapped around the arm too loosely, the measured BP will be falsely elevated
     D. Oscillometric BP measurements are accurate in neonates
     E. Frequent cycling of automated BP monitoring devices can result in edema distal to the cuff

61. An incompetent ventilator pressure-relief valve can result in
     A. Hypoxia
     B. Barotrauma
     C. A low-circuit-pressure signal
     D. Hypoventilation
     E. Hyperventilation

62. The pressure gauge of a size "E" compressed-gas cylinder containing air shows a pressure of 1000 psi. Approximately how long could air be delivered from this cylinder at the rate of 10 L/min?
     A. 10 minutes
     B. 20 minutes
     C. 30 minutes
     D. 40 minutes
     E. 50 minutes

63. The most frequent cause of mechanical failure of the anesthesia delivery system to deliver adequate O_2 to the patient is
     A. Attachment of the wrong compressed-gas cylinder to the O_2 yoke
     B. Crossing of pipelines during construction of the OR
     C. Improperly assembled O_2 rotameter
     D. Fresh-gas line disconnection from the anesthesia machine to the in-line hosing
     E. Disconnection of the O_2 supply system from the patient

64. The esophageal detector device
     A. Uses a negative pressure bulb
     B. Is especially useful in children younger than 1 year of age
     C. Requires a cardiac output to function appropriately
     D. Is reliable in morbidly obese patients and parturients
     E. Is contraindicated if there is blood in the airway

65. The reason CO_2 measured by capnometer is less than the arterial $Paco_2$ value measure simultaneously is?
     A. Use of ion specific electrode for blood gas determination
     B. Alveolar capillary gradient
     C. One way values
     D. Alveolar dead space
     E. Intrapulmonary shunt

66. Which of the following arrangements of rotameters on the anesthesia machine manifold is safest with left to right gas flow?
     A. O_2, CO_2, N_2O, air
     B. CO_2, O_2, N_2O, air
     C. N_2O, O_2, CO_2, air
     D. Air, CO_2, O_2, N_2O
     E. Air, CO_2, N_2O, O_2

67. A Datex Ohmeda Sevotec 5 vaporizer is tipped over while being attached to the anesthesia machine, but is placed upright and installed. The soonest it can be safely used is
   A. After 30 minutes of flushing with dial set to "off"
   B. After 6 hours of flushing with dial to "off"
   C. After 24 hours of flushing with dial set to "off"
   D. After 30 minutes with dial set at low concentration
   E. After 12 hours with dial set to low concentration

68 In the event of misfilling, what percent sevoflurane would be delivered from an isoflurane vaporizer set at 1%?
   A. 0.6%
   B. 0.8%
   C. 1.0%
   D. 1.2%
   E. 1.4%

69. How long would a vaporizer (filled with 150 mL volatile) deliver 2% isoflurane if total flow set at 4.0 L/minute?
   A. 2 hours
   B. 4 hours
   C. 6 hours
   D. 8 hours
   E. 10 hours

70. Raising the frequency of an ultrasound transducer used for line placement or regional anesthesia, e.g., from 3 MHz to 10 MHz, will result in
   A. Higher penetration of tissue with lower resolution
   B. Higher penetration of tissue with higher resolution
   C. Lower penetration of tissue with higher resolution
   D. Higher resolution with no change in tissue penetration
   E. Higher penetration with no change in resolution

71. The fundamental difference between microshock and macroshock is related to
   A. Location of shock
   B. Duration
   C. Voltage
   D. Capacitance
   E. Lethality

72. Intraoperative awareness under general anesthesia can be eliminated by closely monitoring
   A. EEG
   B. BP/heart rate
   C. Bispectral index (BIS)
   D. End tidal volatile
   E. None of the above

73. A mechanically ventilated patient is transported from the OR to the intensive care unit (ICU) using a portable ventilator that consumes 2 L/min of oxygen to run the mechanically controlled valves and drive the ventilator. The transport cart is equipped with an "E" cylinder with a gauge pressure of 2000 psi. The patient receives a V_T of 500 mL at a rate of 10 breaths/minute. If the ventilator requires 200 psi to operate, how long could the patient be mechanically ventilated?
   A. 20 min
   B. 40 min
   C. 60 min
   D. 80 min
   E. 100 min

74. A 135 Kg man is ventilated at a rate of 14 breaths/minute with a V_T of 600 mL and positive end-expiratory pressure (PEEP) of 5 cm H_2O during a laparoscopic banding procedure. Peak airway pressure is 50 cm H_2O and the patient is fully relaxed with a non-depolarizing neuromuscular blocking agent. How can peak airway pressure be reduced without a loss of alveolar ventilation?
    A. Increase the inspiratory flow rate
    B. Take off PEEP
    C. Reduce the I:E ratio (e.g., change from 1:3 to 1:2)
    D. Decrease V_T to 300 and increase rate to 28
    E. None of the above

75. The pressure and volume per minute delivered from the central hospital oxygen supply are:
    A. 2100 psi and 650 L/minute
    B. 1600 psi and 100 L/minute
    C. 75 psi and 100 L/minute
    D. 50 psi and 50 L/minute
    E. 30 psi and 25 L/minute

76. During normal laminar airflow, resistance is dependent upon which characteristic of oxygen?
    A. Density
    B. Viscosity
    C. Molecular weight
    D. Vapor pressure
    E. Temperature

77. If the oxygen cylinder is being used as the source of oxygen at a remote anesthetizing location and the oxygen flush valve on an anesthesia machine were pressed and held down, as during an emergency situation, each of the items below would be bypassed during 100% oxygen delivery **EXCEPT:**
    A. O_2 flowmeter
    B. First stage regulator
    C. Vaporizer check valve
    D. Vaporizers
    E. Second stage regulator

78. After induction and intubation with confirmation of tracheal placement, the O_2 saturation begins to fall. The O_2 analyzer as well as mass spectrometer show 4% inspired oxygen. The oxygen line pressure is 65 psi. The O_2 tank on the back of anesthesia machine has a pressure of 2100 psi and is turned on. The oxygen saturation continues to fall. The next step should be
    A. Exchange the tank
    B. Switch the O_2 line with N_2O line
    C. Disconnect the O_2 line from hospital source
    D. Extubate and start mask ventilation
    E. Replace pulse oximeter probe

79. The correct location for placement of the V5 lead is
    A. Midclavicular line third intercostal space
    B. Anterior axillary line fourth intercostal space
    C. Midclavicular line fifth intercostal space
    D. Anterior axillary line fifth intercostal space.
    E. Any position on precordium

80. The Diameter Index Safety System (DISS) refers to the interface between
    A. Pipeline source and anesthesia machine
    B. Gas cylinders and anesthesia machine
    C. Vaporizers and refilling connectors attached to bottles of volatile anesthetics
    D. Float and tapered flow tube on machine manifold
    E. Both pipeline and gas cylinders interfaces with anesthesia machine

81. Each of the following is cited as an advantage of calcium hydroxide lime (Amsorb Plus, Drägersorb) over soda lime **EXCEPT:**
     A. Compound A is not formed
     B. Carbon monoxide is not formed
     C. More absorptive capacity per 100 g of granules
     D. Indicator dye once changed does not revert to normal
     E. It does not contain NaOH or KOH

82.

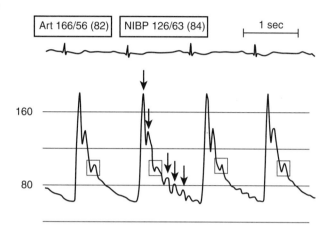

The arrows in the figure above indicate
     A. Respiratory variation
     B. An underdamped signal
     C. An overdamped signal
     D. Atrial fibrillation
     E. Aortic regurgitation

83. During a laparoscopic cholecystectomy exhaled CO_2 is 6%, but inhaled CO_2 is 1%. Which explanation could **NOT** account for rebreathing CO_2?
     A. Channeling through soda lime
     B. Faulty expiratory valve
     C. Exhausted soda lime
     D. Faulty inspiratory valve
     E. Absorption of CO_2 through peritoneum

DIRECTIONS (Question 84 though 86): Please match the color of the compressed gas cylinder with the appropriate gas.

84. Helium

85. Nitrogen

86. Carbon dioxide
     A. Black
     B. Brown
     C. Blue
     D. Gray
     E. Orange

DIRECTIONS (Questions 87 through 90): Match the figures below with the correct numbered statement. Each lettered figure may be selected once, more than once, or not at all.

87.   Best for spontaneous ventilation

88.   Best for controlled ventilation

89.   Bain system

90.   Jackson-Rees system

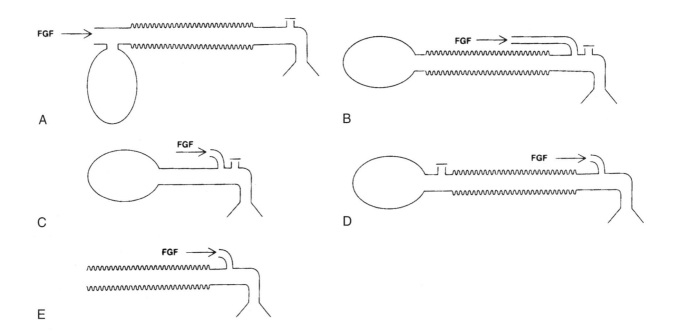

Anesthesia Equipment and Physics

Answers, References, and Explanations

1. **(B)** Orifice flow occurs when gas flows through a region of severe constriction such as described in this question. Laminar flow occurs when gas flows down parallel-sided tubes at a rate less than critical velocity. When the gas flow exceeds the critical velocity, it becomes turbulent *(Miller: Anesthesia, ed 6, pp 690-691; Ehrenwerth: Anesthesia Equipment: Principles and Applications, pp 224-225).*

2. **(C)** During orifice flow, the resistance to gas flow is directly proportional to the density of the gas mixture. Substituting helium for nitrogen will decrease the density of the gas mixture, thereby decreasing the resistance to gas flow (as much as threefold) through the region of constriction *(Ehrenwerth: Anesthesia Equipment: Principles and Applications, pp 224-225; Miller: Anesthesia, ed 6, pp 690-691, 2539).*

3. **(C)** Modern electronic blood pressure (BP) monitors are designed to interface with electromechanical transducer systems. These systems do not require extensive technical skill on the part of the anesthesia provider for accurate usage. A static zeroing of the system is built into most modern electronic monitors. Thus, after the zeroing procedure is accomplished, the system is ready for operation. The system should be zeroed with the reference point of the transducer at the approximate level of the aortic root, eliminating the effect of the fluid column of the system on arterial BP readings *(Ehrenwerth: Anesthesia Equipment: Principles and Applications, pp 275-278).*

4. **(C)** Waste gas disposal systems, also called scavenging systems, are designed to decrease pollution of the OR by anesthetic gases. These scavenging systems can be passive (waste gases flow from the anesthesia machine to a ventilation system on their own) or active (anesthesia machine connected to a vacuum system then to the ventilation system). The amount of air from a venous gas embolism would not be enough to be detected in the disposal system. Positive pressure relief valves open if there is an obstruction between the anesthesia machine and the disposal system, which would then leak the gas into the OR. A leak in the soda lime canisters would also vent to the OR. Since most ventilator bellows are powered by oxygen, a leak in the bellows would not add air to the evacuation system. The negative pressure relief valve is used in active systems and will entrap room air if the pressure in the system is less than -0.5 cm H_2O. *(Miller: Anesthesia, 6th ed. pp 303-307; Stoelting: Basics of Anesthesia, ed 5, pp 198-199).*

5. **(D)** The relationship between intra-alveolar pressure, surface tension, and the radius of alveoli is described by Laplace's law for a sphere, which states that the surface tension of the sphere is directly proportional to the radius of the sphere and pressure within the sphere. With regard to pulmonary alveoli, the mathematical expression of Laplace's law is as follows:

$$T = \frac{1}{2}PR$$

   where T is the surface tension, P is the intra-alveolar pressure, and R is the radius of the alveolus. In pulmonary alveoli, surface tension is produced by a liquid film lining the alveoli. This occurs because the attractive forces between the molecules of the liquid film are much greater than the attractive forces between the liquid film and gas. Thus, the surface area of the liquid tends to become as small as possible, which could collapse the alveoli *(Miller: Anesthesia, ed 6, pp 689-690).*

6. **(C)** The World Health Organization requires that compressed-gas cylinders containing N_2O for medical use be painted blue. Size "E" compressed-gas cylinders completely filled with N_2O contain approximately 1590 L of gas *(Stoelting: Basics of Anesthesia, ed 5, p 188).*

7. (D) Many anesthesia machines have a check valve downstream from the rotameters and vaporizers but upstream from the oxygen flush valve. When the oxygen flush valve button is depressed and the Y-piece (which would be connected to the endotracheal tube [ETT] or the anesthesia mask) is occluded, the circuit will be filled and the needle on the airway pressure gauge will indicate positive pressure. The positive pressure reading will not fall, however, even in the presence of a leak in the low-pressure circuit of the anesthesia machine. If a check valve is present on the common gas outlet, the positive-pressure leak test can be dangerous and misleading. In 1993, the United States Food and Drug Administration (FDA) established the FDA Universal Negative Pressure Leak Test. With the machine master switch, the flow control valves and the vaporizers turned off, a suction bulb is attached to the common gas outlet and compressed until it is fully collapsed. If a leak is present the suction bulb will inflate. It was so named because it can be used to check all anesthesia machines regardless of whether they contain a check valve in the fresh gas outlet *(Miller: Anesthesia, ed 6, pp 309-310).*

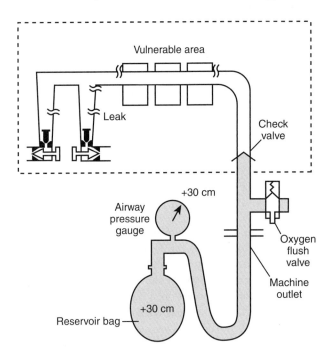

8. (E) Check valves permit only unidirectional flow of gases. These valves prevent retrograde flow of gases from the anesthesia machine or the transfer of gas from a compressed-gas cylinder at high pressure into a container at a lower pressure. Thus, these unidirectional valves will allow an empty compressed-gas cylinder to be exchanged for a full one during operation of the anesthesia machine with minimal loss of gas. The adjustable pressure-limiting valve is a synonym for a pop-off valve. A fail-safe valve is a synonym for a pressure-sensor shutoff valve. The purpose of a fail-safe valve is to discontinue the flow of N_2O if the O_2 pressure within the anesthesia machine falls below 25 psi *(Ehrenwerth: Anesthesia Equipment: Principles and Applications, pp 46-47; Miller: Anesthesia, ed 6, p 276.)*

9. (C) Boyle's law states that for a fixed mass of gas at constant temperature, the product of pressure and volume is constant. This concept can be used to estimate the volume of gas remaining in a compressed-gas cylinder by measuring the pressure within the cylinder *(Ehrenwerth: Anesthesia Equipment: Principles and Applications, p 224).*

10. (C) United States manufacturers require that all compressed-gas cylinders containing O_2 for medical use be painted green. A compressed-gas cylinder completely filled with O_2 has a pressure of approximately 2000 psi and contains approximately 625 L of gas. According to Boyle's law (see explanation to question 9) the volume of gas remaining in a closed container can be estimated by measuring the pressure within the container. Therefore, when the pressure gauge on a compressed-gas cylinder containing O_2 shows a pressure of 1600 psi, the cylinder contains 500 L of O_2. At a gas flow of 2 L/min, O_2 could be delivered from the cylinder for approximately 250 minutes *(Stoelting: Basics of Anesthesia ed 5, p 188).*

CHARACTERISTICS OF COMPRESSED GASES STORED IN "E" SIZE CYLINDERS THAT MAY BE ATTACHED TO THE ANESTHESIA MACHINE

Characteristics	Oxygen	Nitrous Oxide	Carbon Dioxide	Air
Cylinder color	Green*	Blue	Gray	Yellow*
Physical state in cylinder	Gas	Liquid and gas	Liquid and gas	Gas
Cylinder contents (L)	625	1590	1590	625
Cylinder weight empty (kg)	5.90	5.90	5.90	5.90
Cylinder weight full (kg)	6.76	8.80	8.90	
Cylinder pressure full (psi)	2000	750	838	1800

*The World Health Organization specifies that cylinders containing oxygen for medial use be painted white, but manufacturers in the United States use green. Likewise, the international color for air is white and black, whereas cylinders in the United States are color-coded yellow.
* (Stoelting: Basics of Anesthesia, ed 5, p 188.)

11. **(B)** All of the choices listed in this question can potentially result in inadequate flow of O_2 to the patient; however, given the description of the problem, no flow of O_2 through the O_2 rotameter is the correct choice. In a normally functioning rotameter, gas flows between the rim of the bobbin and the wall of the Thorpe tube, causing the bobbin to rotate. If the bobbin is rotating you can be certain that gas is flowing through the rotameter and that the bobbin is not stuck (Ehrenwerth: Anesthesia Equipment: Principles and Applications, pp 40-42).

12. **(B)**

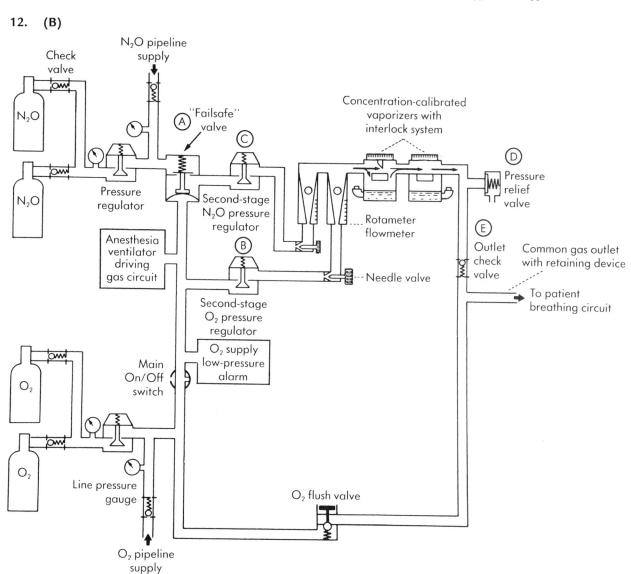

Fail-safe valve is a synonym for pressure-sensor shutoff valve. The purpose of the fail-safe valve is to prevent delivery of hypoxic gas mixtures from the anesthesia machine to the patient due to failure of the O_2 supply. When the O_2 pressure within the anesthesia machine decreases below 25 psi, this valve discontinues the flow of N_2O or proportionally decreases the flow of all gases. It is important to realize that this valve will not prevent delivery of hypoxic gas mixtures or pure N_2O when the O_2 rotameter is off, but the O_2 pressure within the circuits of the anesthesia machine is maintained by an open O_2 compressed-gas cylinder or central supply source. Under these circumstances, an O_2 analyzer would be needed to detect delivery of a hypoxic gas mixture *(Ehrenwerth: Anesthesia Equipment: Principles and Applications, pp 37-38).*

13. (C)   It is important to zero the electromechanical transducer system with the reference point at the approximate level of the heart. This will eliminate the effect of the fluid column of the transducer system on the arterial BP reading of the system. In this question, the system was zeroed at the stopcock, which was located at the patient's wrist (approximate level of the ventricle). Blood pressure expressed by the arterial line will, therefore, be accurate, provided the distance between the patient's wrist and the stopcock remains 20 cm. Also see explanation to question 3 *(Ehrenwerth: Anesthesia Equipment: Principles and Applications, p 276).*

14. (C) O_2 and N_2O enter the anesthesia machine from a central supply source or compressed-gas cylinders at pressures as high as 2200 psi (oxygen) and 750 psi (N_2O). First-stage pressure regulators reduce these pressures to approximately 45 psi. Before entering the rotameters, second-stage O_2 pressure regulators further reduce the pressure to approximately 14 to 16 psi (see figure with answer to question 12) *(Miller: Anesthesia, ed 6, pp 274-275).*

15. (C)   NIOSH sets guidelines and issues recommendations concerning the control of waste anesthetic gases. NIOSH mandates that the highest trace concentration of N_2O contamination of the OR atmosphere should be less than 25 ppm. In dental facilities where N_2O is used without volatile anesthetics, NIOSH permits up to 50 ppm *(Miller: Anesthesia, ed 6, pp 303-304).*

16. (C)   Agent-specific vaporizers, such as the Sevotec (sevoflurane) vaporizer, are designed for each volatile anesthetic. However, volatile anesthetics with identical saturated vapor pressures could be used interchangeably with accurate delivery of the volatile anesthetic.

VAPOR PRESSURES

Agent	Vapor Pressure mm Hg at 20° C
Halothane	243
Enflurane	172
Sevoflurane	160
Isoflurane	240
Desflurane	669

(Ehrenwerth: Anesthesia Equipment: Principles and Applications, pp 60-63; Stoelting: Basics of Anesthesia, ed 5, p 79.)

17. (A)   The control mechanism of standard anesthesia ventilators, such as the Ohmeda 7000, uses compressed oxygen (100%) to compress the ventilator bellows and electrical power for the timing circuits *(Miller: Anesthesia, ed 6, p 298).*

18. (C)   Five types of rotameter indicators are commonly used to indicate the flow of gases delivered from the anesthesia machine. As with all anesthesia equipment, proper understanding of their function is necessary for safe and proper use. All rotameter flow indicators should be read at the upper rim except ball floats, which should be read in the middle *(Ehrenwerth: Anesthesia Equipment: Principles and Applications, pp 40-43).*

19. (B)   The pressure gauge on a size "E" compressed-gas cylinder containing N_2O shows 750 psi when it is full and will continue to register 750 psi until approximately three-fourths of the gas has left the cylinder. A full cylinder of N_2O contains 1590 L. Therefore, when 400 L of gas remain in the cylinder, the pressure within the cylinder will begin to fall *(Stoelting: Basics of Anesthesia, ed 5, p 188).*

20. (B) In this question the reference point is the transducer, which is located 10 cm below the level of the patient's heart. Thus, there is an approximate 10 cm H_2O fluid column from the level of the patient's heart to the transducer. This will cause the pressure reading from the transducer system to read approximately 7.5 mm Hg higher than a true arterial pressure of the patient. A 20-cm column of H_2O will exert a pressure equal to 14.7 mm Hg. Also see explanations to questions 3 and 13 *(Ehrenwerth: Anesthesia Equipment: Principles and Applications, p 275).*

21. (D) Factors that influence the rate of laminar flow of a substance through a tube is described by the Hagen-Poiseuille law of friction. The mathematical expression of the Hagen-Poiseuille law of friction is as follows:

$$\dot{V} = \frac{\pi r^4 (\Delta P)}{8\,L\mu}$$

where $\dot{V}$ is the flow of the substance, r is the radius of the tube, ΔP is the pressure gradient down the tube, L is the length of the tube, and μ is the viscosity of the substance. Note that the rate of laminar flow is proportional to the radius of the tube to the fourth power. If the diameter of an intravenous catheter is doubled, flow would increase by a factor of 2 raised to the fourth power (i.e., a factor of 16) *(Ehrenwerth: Anesthesia Equipment: Principles and Applications, p 225).*

22. (D) The safe storage and handling of compressed-gas cylinders is of vital importance. Compressed-gas cylinders should not be stored in extremes of heat or cold, and they should be unwrapped when stored or when in use. Flames should not be used to detect the presence of a gas. Oily hands can lead to difficulty in handling of the cylinder, which can result in dropping the cylinder. This can cause damage to or rupture of the cylinder, which can lead to an explosion *(Ehrenwerth: Anesthesia Equipment: Principles and Applications, pp 8-11).*

23. (A) Vaporizers can be categorized into variable-bypass and measured-flow vaporizers. Measured-flow vaporizers (nonconcentration calibrated vaporizers) include the copper kettle and Vernitrol vaporizer. With measured-flow vaporizers, the flow of oxygen is selected on a separate flowmeter to pass into the vaporizing chamber from which the anesthetic vapor emerges at its saturated vapor pressure. By contrast, in variable-bypass vaporizers, the total gas flow is split between a variable bypass and the vaporizer chamber containing the anesthetic agent. The ratio of these two flows is called the splitting ratio. The splitting ratio depends on the anesthetic agent, temperature, the chosen vapor concentration set to be delivered to the patient, and the saturated vapor pressure of the anesthetic *(Ehrenwerth: Anesthesia Equipment: Principles and Applications, p 63).*

24. (D) The contribution of the fresh gas flow from the anesthesia machine to the patient's VT should be considered when setting the VT of a mechanical ventilator. Because the ventilator pressure-relief valve is closed during inspiration, both the gas from the ventilator bellows and the fresh gas flow will be delivered to the patient breathing circuit. In this question, the fresh gas flow is 6 L/min or 100 mL/sec (6000 mL/60). Each breath lasts 6 sec (60 sec/10 breaths) with inspiration lasting 2 sec (I:E ratio = 1:2). Under these conditions, the VT delivered to the patient by the mechanical ventilator will be augmented by approximately 200 mL. In some ventilators, such as the Ohmeda 7900, VT is controlled for the fresh gas flow rate such that the delivered VT is always the same as the dial setting *(Morgan: Clinical Anesthesia ed 4, pp 82-84).*

25. (C) Also see explanation to question 24. The ventilator rate is decreased from 10 to 6 breaths/min. Thus, each breath will last 10 seconds (60 sec/6 breaths) with inspiration lasting approximately 3.3 sec (I:E ratio = 1:2), i.e., 3.3 seconds times 100 mL/second. Under these conditions, the actual VT delivered to the patient by the mechanical ventilator will be 830 mL (500 mL + 330 mL) *(Morgan: Clinical Anesthesia, ed 4, pp 82-84).*

26. (D) The saturated vapor pressures of halothane and isoflurane are very similar (approximately 240 mm Hg at room temperature) and therefore could be used interchangeably in agent-specific vaporizers (see explanation and table in explanation for question 16) *(Ehrenwerth: Anesthesia Equipment: Principles and Applications, pp 60-63; Stoelting: Basics of Anesthesia, ed 5, p 79).*

27. (D) Clinically significant concentrations of carbon monoxide can result from the interaction of desiccated absorbent, both soda lime and Baralyme. The resulting carboxyhemoglobin level can be as high as 30%. Many of the reported occurrences of carbon monoxide poisoning have been observed on Monday mornings. This is thought to be the case because the absorbent granules are the driest after disuse for two days, particularly if the oxygen flow has not been turned off completely. There are several factors that appear to predispose to the production of carbon monoxide: (1) degree of absorbent dryness (completely desiccated granules produce more carbon monoxide than hydrated granules); (2) use of Baralyme versus soda lime (provided that the water content is the same in both); (3) high concentrations of volatile anesthetic (more carbon monoxide is generated at higher volatile concentrations); (4) high temperatures (more carbon monoxide is generated at higher temperatures); and (5) type of volatile used:

$$\text{desflurane} \geq \text{enflurane} > \text{isoflurane} \gg \text{halothane} = \text{sevoflurane}^*$$

(*Given that MAC level used is the same for all volatiles. If the anesthesia machine has been left on all weekend, the absorbent should be changed before the machine is used again to avoid carbon monoxide production.) *(Miller: Anesthesia, ed 6, pp 296-298).*

28. (A) NIOSH mandates that the highest trace concentration of volatile anesthetic contamination of the OR atmosphere when administered in conjunction with N_2O is 0.5 ppm *(Miller: Anesthesia, 6 ed, pp 303-304).*

29. (B) The O_2 analyzer is the last line of defense against inadvertent delivery of hypoxic gas mixtures. It should be located in the inspiratory (not expiratory) limb of the patient breathing circuit to provide maximum safety. Because the O_2 concentration in the fresh-gas supply line may be different from that of the patient breathing circuit, the O_2 analyzer should not be located in the fresh-gas supply line *(Ehrenwerth: Anesthesia Equipment: Principles and Applications, pp 216-220).*

30. (A) The ventilator pressure-relief valve (also called the spill valve) is pressure controlled via pilot tubing that communicates with the ventilator bellows chamber. As pressure within the bellows chamber increases during the inspiratory phase of the ventilator cycle, the pressure is transmitted via the pilot tubing to close the pressure-relief valve, thus making the patient breathing circuit "gastight." This valve should open during the expiratory phase of the ventilator cycle to allow the release of excess gas from the patient breathing circuit into the waste-gas scavenging circuit after the bellows has fully expanded. If the ventilator pressure-relief valve were to stick in the closed position, there would be a rapid buildup of pressure within the circle system that would be readily transmitted to the patient. Barotrauma to the patient's lungs would result if this situation were to continue unrecognized *(Eisenkraft: Potential for barotrauma or hypoventilation with the Drager AV-E ventilator. J Clin Anesth, 1:452-456, 1989; Morgan: Clinical Anesthesia, ed 4, pp 81-82).*

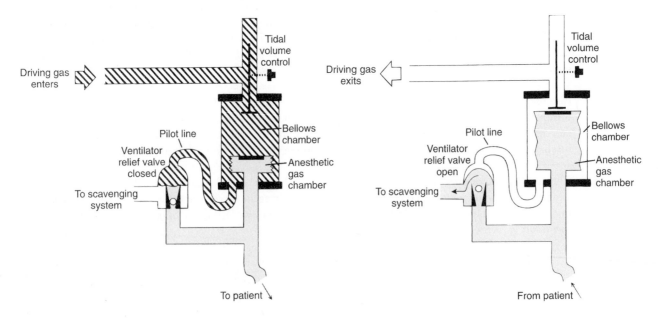

31. **(D)** Vaporizer output can be affected by the composition of the carrier gas used to vaporize the volatile agent in the vaporizing chamber, especially when nitrous oxide is either initiated or discontinued. This observation can be explained by the solubility of nitrous oxide in the volatile agent. When nitrous oxide and oxygen enter the vaporizing chamber, a portion of the nitrous oxide dissolves in the liquid agent. Thus, the vaporizer output transiently decreases. Conversely, when nitrous oxide is withdrawn as part of the carrier gas, the nitrous oxide dissolved in the volatile agent comes out of solution, thereby transiently increases the vaporizer output *(Miller: Anesthesia, ed 6, pp 286-288).*

32. **(E)** The capnogram can provide a variety of information, such as verification of the presence of exhaled CO_2 after tracheal intubation, estimation of the difference in Pa_{CO_2} and Pet_{CO_2}, abnormalities of ventilation, and the presence of hypercapnia or hypocapnia. The four phases of the capnogram are inspiratory baseline, expiratory upstroke, expiratory plateau, and inspiratory downstroke. The shape of the capnogram can be used to recognize and diagnose a variety of potentially adverse circumstances. Under normal conditions, the inspiratory baseline should be 0, indicating that there is no rebreathing of CO_2 with a normal functioning circle breathing system. If the inspiratory baseline is elevated above 0, there is rebreathing of CO_2. If this occurs, the differential diagnosis should include an incompetent expiratory valve, exhausted CO_2 absorbent, or gas channeling through the CO_2 absorbent. However, the inspiratory baseline may be elevated when the inspiratory valve is incompetent (e.g., there may be a slanted inspiratory downstroke). The expiratory upstroke occurs when the fresh gas from the anatomic dead space is quickly replaced by CO_2-rich alveolar gas. Under normal conditions the upstroke should be steep; however, it may become slanted during partial airway obstruction, if a sidestream analyzer is sampling gas too slowly, or if the response time of the capnograph is too slow for the patient's respiratory rate. Partial obstruction may be the result of an obstruction in the breathing system (e.g., by a kinked endotracheal tube) or in the patient's airway (e.g., the presence of chronic obstructive pulmonary disease or acute bronchospasm). The expiratory plateau is normally characterized by a slow but shallow progressive increase in CO_2 concentration. This occurs because of imperfect matching of ventilation and perfusion in all lung units. Partial obstruction of gas flow either in the breathing system or in the patient's airways may cause a prolonged increase in the slope of the expiratory plateau, which may continue rising until the next inspiratory downstroke begins. The inspiratory downstroke is caused by the rapid influx of fresh gas, which washes the CO_2 away from the CO_2 sensing or sampling site. Under normal conditions the inspiratory downstroke is very steep. Causes of a slanted or blunted inspiratory downstroke include an incompetent inspiratory valve, slow mechanical inspiration, slow gas sampling, and partial CO_2 rebreathing *(Ehrenwerth: Anesthesia Equipment: Principles and Applications, p 240).*

33. **(B)** Complications of tracheal intubation can be divided into those associated with direct laryngoscopy and intubation of the trachea, tracheal tube placement, and extubation of the trachea. The most frequent complication associated with direct laryngoscopy and tracheal intubation is dental trauma. If a tooth is dislodged and not found, radiographs of the chest and abdomen should be taken to determine whether the tooth has passed through the glottic opening into the lungs. Should dental trauma occur, immediate consultation with a dentist is indicated. Other complications of direct laryngoscopy and tracheal intubation include hypertension, tachycardia, cardiac dysrhythmias, and aspiration of gastric contents. The most common complication that occurs while the ETT is in place is inadvertent endobronchial intubation. Flexion, not extension, of the neck or change from the supine to the head-down position can shift the carina upward, which may convert a mid-tracheal tube placement into a bronchial intubation. Extension of the neck can cause cephalad displacement of the tube into the pharynx. Lateral rotation of the head can displace the distal end of the ETT approximately 0.7 cm away from the carina. Complications associated with extubation of the trachea can be immediate or delayed. The two most serious immediate complications associated with extubation of the trachea are laryngospasm and aspiration of gastric contents. Laryngospasm is most likely to occur in patients who are lightly anesthetized at the time of extubation. If laryngospasm occurs, positive-pressure mask-bag ventilation with 100% O_2 and forward displacement of the mandible may be sufficient treatment. However, if laryngospasm persists, succinylcholine should be administered intravenously or intramuscularly. Pharyngitis is another frequent complication after extubation of the trachea. This complication occurs most commonly in females, presumably because of the thinner mucosal covering over the posterior vocal cords compared with males. This complication usually does not require treatment and spontaneously resolves in 48 to 72 hours. Delayed complications associated with extubation of the trachea include laryngeal ulcerations, tracheitis, tracheal stenosis, vocal cord paralysis, and arytenoid cartilage dislocation *(Stoelting: Basics of Anesthesia, ed 5, pp 231-232).*

34. (B) Gas leaving a compressed-gas cylinder is directed through a pressure-reducing valve, which lowers the pressure within the metal tubing of the anesthesia machine to 45 to 55 psi *(Miller: Anesthesia, ed 6, p 276).*

35. (C) There is considerable controversy regarding the role of bacterial contamination of anesthesia machines and equipment in cross-infection between patients. The incidence of postoperative pulmonary infection is not reduced by the use of sterile disposable anesthetic breathing circuits (as compared with the use of reusable circuits that are cleaned with basic hygienic techniques). Furthermore, inclusion of a bacterial filter in the anesthesia breathing circuit has no effect on the incidence of cross-infection. Clinically relevant concentrations of volatile anesthetics have no bacteriocidal or bacteriostatic effects. Low concentrations of volatile anesthetics, however, may inhibit viral replication. Shifts in humidity and temperature in the anesthesia breathing and scavenging circuits are the most important factors responsible for killing bacteria. In addition, high O_2 concentration and metallic ions present in the anesthesia machine and other equipment have a significant lethal effect on bacteria. Acid-fast bacilli are the most resistant bacterial form to destruction. Nevertheless, there has been no case documenting transmission of tuberculosis via a contaminated anesthetic machine from one patient to another. When managing patients who can potentially cause cross-infection of other patients (e.g., patients with tuberculosis, pneumonia, or known viral infections, such as acquired immune deficiency syndrome [AIDS]) a disposable anesthetic breathing circuit should be used and nondisposable equipment should be disinfected with glutaraldehyde (Cidex). Sodium hypochlorite (bleach), which destroys the human immunodeficiency virus, should be used to disinfect nondisposable equipment, including laryngoscope blades, if patients with AIDS require anesthesia *(Ehrenwerth: Anesthesia Equipment: Principles and Applications, p 100).*

36. (B) The diameter-index safety system prevents incorrect connections of medical gas lines. This system consists of two concentric and specific bores in the body of one connection, which correspond to two concentric and specific shoulders on the nipple of the other connection *(Ehrenwerth: Anesthesia Equipment: Principles and Applications, pp 21, 30, 37).*

37. (C) The amount of anesthetic vapor (mL) in effluent gas from a vaporizing chamber can be calculated using the following equation:

$$VO = \frac{CG \times SVP_{anes}}{P_b - SVP_{anes}}$$

where VO is the vapor output (mL) of effluent gas from the vaporizer, CG is the carrier gas flow (mL/min) into the vaporizing chamber, SVP_{anes} is the saturated vapor pressure (mm Hg) of the anesthetic gas at room temperature, and P_b is the barometric pressure (mm Hg). In this question, fresh gas flow is 100 mL/min. 100 mL/min × 0.9 = 90 mL/min *(Ehrenwerth: Anesthesia Equipment: Principles and Applications, p 61).*

$$VO = \frac{100 \times 360}{760 - 360}$$

$$VO = \frac{36,000}{400}$$

$$VO = 90 \text{ mL}$$

38. (A) The output of the vaporizer will be lower at flow rates less than 250 mL/min because there is insufficient pressure to advance the molecules of the volatile agent upward. At extremely high carrier gas flow rates (>15 L/ min) there is insufficient mixing in the vaporizing chamber *(Miller: Anesthesia, ed 6, p 286).*

39. (C) Pulse oximeters estimate arterial hemoglobin saturation (Sao_2) by measuring the amount of light transmitted through a pulsatile vascular tissue bed. Pulse oximeters measure the alternating current (AC) component of light absorbance at each of two wavelengths (660 and 940 nm) and then divide this measurement by the corresponding direct current component. Then the ratio (R) of the two absorbance measurements is determined by the following equation:

$$R = \frac{AC_{660}/DC_{660}}{AC_{940}/DC_{940}}$$

Using an empirical calibration curve that relates arterial hemoglobin saturation to R, the actual arterial hemoglobin saturation is calculated. Based on the physical principles outlined above, the sources of error in SpO_2 readings can be easily predicted. Pulse oximeters can function accurately when only two hemoglobin species, oxyhemoglobin and reduced hemoglobin, are present. If any light-absorbing species other than oxyhemoglobin and reduced hemoglobin are present, the pulse oximeter measurements will be inaccurate. Fetal hemoglobin has minimal effect on the accuracy of pulse oximetry, because the extinction coefficients for fetal hemoglobin at the two wavelengths used by pulse oximetry are very similar to the corresponding values for adult hemoglobin. In addition to abnormal hemoglobins, any substance present in the blood that absorbs light at either 660 or 940 nm, such as intravenous dyes used for diagnostic purposes, will affect the value of R, making accurate measurements of the pulse oximeter impossible. These dyes include methylene blue and indigo carmine. Methylene blue has the greatest effect on SaO_2 measurements because the extinction coefficient is so similar to that of oxyhemoglobin *(Ehrenwerth: Anesthesia Equipment: Principles and Applications, pp 254-255).*

40. (B)   The mass spectrometer functions by separating the components of a stream of charged particles into a spectrum based on their mass-to-charge ratio. The amount of each ion at specific mass-to-charge ratios is then determined and expressed as the fractional composition of the original gas mixture. The charged particles are created and manipulated in a high vacuum to avoid interference by outside air and minimize random collisions among the ions and residual gases. An erroneous reading will be displayed by the mass spectrometer when a gas that is not detected by the collector plate system is present in the gas mixture to be analyzed. Helium, which has a mass charge ratio of 4, is not detected by standard mass spectrometers. Consequently, the standard gases (i.e., halothane, enflurane, isoflurane, oxygen, nitrous oxide, nitrogen, and carbon dioxide) will be summed to 100% as if helium were not present. All readings would be approximately twice their real values in the original gas mixture in the presence of 50% helium *(Ehrenwerth: Anesthesia Equipment: Principles and Applications, pp 203-205).*

41. (E)   Because halothane and isoflurane have similar saturated vapor pressures, the vaporizers for these volatile anesthetics could be used interchangeably with accurate delivery of the anesthetic concentration set by the vaporizer dial. If a sevoflurane vaporizer were filled with a volatile anesthetic that has a greater saturated vapor pressure than sevoflurane (e.g., halothane or isoflurane), a higher-than-expected concentration would be delivered from the vaporizer. If a halothane or isoflurane vaporizer were filled with a volatile anesthetic that had a lower saturated vapor pressure than halothane or isoflurane (e.g., sevoflurane, enflurane, or methoxyflurane), a lower-than-expected concentration would be delivered from the vaporizer *(Ehrenwerth: Anesthesia Equipment: Principles and Applications, pp 66-67).*

VAPOR PRESSURE AND MINIMUM ALVEOLAR CONCENTRATION

	Halothane	Enflurane	Sevoflurane	Isoflurane	Desflurane	Methoxyflurane
Vapor pressure 20° C mm Hg	243	172	160	240	669	23
MAC 30-55 yr	0.75	1.63	1.8	1.17	6.6	0.16

MAC, minimal alveolar concentration.

42. (E)   Gas density decreases with increasing altitude (i.e., the density of a gas is directly proportional to atmospheric pressure). Atmospheric pressure will influence the function of rotameters because the accurate function of rotameters is influenced by the physical properties of the gas, such as density and viscosity. The magnitude of this influence, however, depends on the rate of gas flow. At low gas flows, the pattern of gas flow is laminar. Atmospheric pressure will have little effect on the accurate function of rotameters at low gas flows because laminar gas flow is influenced by gas viscosity (which is minimally affected by atmospheric pressure) and not gas density. However, at high gas flows, the gas flow pattern is turbulent and is influenced by gas density (see explanation to question 2). At high altitudes (i.e., low atmospheric pressure), the gas flow through the rotameter will be greater than expected at high flows but accurate at low flows *(Ehrenwerth: Anesthesia Equipment: Principles and Applications, pp 38-43, 224-225).*

43. (B) Pacemakers have a three to five letter code that describes the pacemaker type and function. Since the purpose of the pacemaker is to send electrical current to the heart, the first letter identifies the chamber(s) paced; A for atrial, V for ventricle and D for dual chamber (A+V). The second letter identifies the chamber where endogenous current is sensed; A,V, D, and O for none sensed. The third letter describes the response to sensing; O for none, I for inhibited, T for triggered and D for dual (I+T). The fourth letter describes programmability or rate modulation; O for none and R for rate modulation (i.e., faster heart rate with exercise). The fifth letter describes multisite pacing (more important in dilated heart chambers); A, V or D (A+V) or O. A VDD pacemaker is used for patients with AV node dysfunction but intact sinus node activity. (*Miller: Anesthesia, ed 6, pp 1416-1418*).

44. (A) Although controversial, it is thought that chronic exposure to low concentrations of volatile anesthetics may constitute a health hazard to OR personnel. Therefore, removal of trace concentrations of volatile anesthetic gases from the OR atmosphere with a scavenging system and steps to reduce and control gas leakage into the environment are required. High-pressure system leakage of volatile anesthetic gases into the OR atmosphere occurs when gas escapes from compressed-gas cylinders attached to the anesthetic machine (e.g., faulty yokes) or from tubing delivering these gases to the anesthesia machine from a central supply source. The most common cause of low-pressure leakage of anesthetic gases into the OR atmosphere is the escape of gases from sites located between the flowmeters of the anesthesia machine and the patient, such as a poor mask seal. The use of high gas flows in a circle system will not reduce trace gas contamination of the OR atmosphere. In fact, this could contribute to the contamination if there is a leak in the circle system (*Miller: Anesthesia, ed 6, pp 3151-3153*).

45. (A) Although all of the choices in this question can contribute as sources of contamination, leakage around the anesthesia face mask poses the greatest threat (*Ehrenwerth: Anesthesia Equipment: Principles and Applications, pp 128-129; Miller: Anesthesia, ed 6, pp 3151-3153*).

46. (C) The amount of volatile anesthetic taken up by the patient in the first minute is equal to that amount taken up between the squares of any two consecutive minutes. Accordingly, 50 mL would be taken up between the 16th (4 × 4) and 25th (5 × 5) minute, and another 50 mL would be taken up between the 25th and 36th (6 × 6) minute (*Miller: Anesthesia, ed 5, p 87*).

47. (E) In evaluating SSEPs, one looks at both the amplitude or voltage of the recorded response wave as well as the latency (time measured from the stimulus to the onset or peak of the response wave). A decrease in amplitude (>50%) and/or an increase in latency (>10%) is usually clinically significant. These changes may reflect hypoperfusion, neural ischemia, temperature changes, or drug effects. All of the volatile anesthetics as well as barbiturates cause a decrease in amplitude as well as an increase in latency. Etomidate causes an increase in latency and an increase in amplitude. Midazolam decreases the amplitude but has little effect on latency. Opioids cause small and not clinically significant increases in latency and decrease in amplitude of the SSEPs. Muscle relaxants have no effect of the SSEP (*Miller: Anesthesia, ed 6, pp 1525-1537; Stoelting: Basics of Anesthesia, ed 5, pp 312-314*).

48. (E) Also see explanation to question 35. There is no evidence that the incidence of postoperative pulmonary infection is altered by the use of sterile disposable anesthesia breathing systems (compared with the use of reusable systems that are cleaned with basic hygienic techniques) or by the inclusion of a bacterial filter in the anesthesia breathing system (*Ehrenwerth: Anesthesia Equipment: Principles and Applications, p 100*).

49. (D) Vaporization of a liquid requires the transfer of heat from the objects in contact with the liquid (e.g., the metal cylinder and surrounding atmosphere). For this reason, at high gas flows, atmospheric water will condense as frost on the outside of compressed-gas cylinders (*Stoelting: Basics of Anesthesia, ed 5, p 188*).

50. (B) Pulmonary artery, esophageal, axillary, nasopharyngeal, and tympanic membrane temperature measurements correlate with central temperature in patients undergoing noncardiac surgery. Skin temperature does not reflect central temperature and does not warn adequately of malignant hyperthermia or excessive hypothermia (*Miller: Anesthesia, ed 6, p 1591*).

51. (D) Rotameters consist of a vertically positioned tapered tube that is smallest in diameter at the bottom (Thorpe tube). Gas enters at the bottom of the Thorpe tube and elevates a bobbin or float, which comes to rest when gravity on the float is balanced by the fall in pressure across the float. The rate of gas flow through the tube depends on the pressure drop along the length of the tube, the resistance to gas flow through the tube, and the physical properties (density and viscosity) of the gas. Because few gases have the same density and viscosity, rotameters cannot be used interchangeably *(Ehrenwerth: Anesthesia Equipment: Principles and Applications, pp 38-43).*

52. (A) The critical velocity for helium is greater than that for nitrogen. For this reason, there is less work of breathing when helium is substituted for nitrogen *(Ehrenwerth: Anesthesia Equipment: Principles and Applications, pp 224-225; Miller: Anesthesia, ed 6, pp 690-691).*

53. (E) The FIO_2 delivered to patients from low-flow systems (e.g., nasal prongs) is determined by the size of the O_2 reservoir, the O_2 flow, and the patient's breathing pattern. As a rule of thumb, assuming a normal breathing pattern, the FIO_2 delivered by nasal prongs increases by approximately 0.04 for each L/min increase in O_2 flow up to a maximal FIO_2 of approximately 0.45 (at an O_2 flow of 6 L/min). In general, the larger the patient's VT or faster the respiratory rate, the lower the FIO_2 for a given O_2 flow *(Miller: Anesthesia, ed 6, pp 2812-2813).*

54. (A)

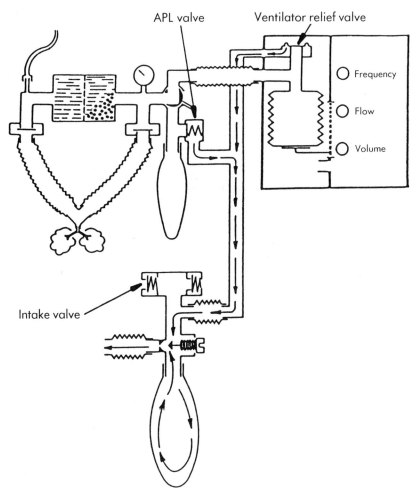

In a closed scavenging system interface, the reservoir bag should expand during expiration and contract during inspiration. During the inspiratory phase of mechanical ventilation the ventilator pressure-relief valve closes, thereby directing the gas inside the ventilator bellows into the patient breathing circuit. If the ventilator pressure-relief valve is incompetent, there will be a direct communication between the patient breathing circuit and scavenging circuit. This would result in delivery of part of the mechanical ventilator Vt directly to the scavenging circuit, causing the reservoir bag to inflate during the inspiratory phase of the ventilator cycle *(Ehrenwerth: Anesthesia Equipment: Principles and Applications, p 128).*

55. (C) The accurate function of dual-wavelength pulse oximeters is altered by nail polish. Because blue nail polish has a peak absorbance similar to that of adult deoxygenated hemoglobin (near 660 nm), blue nail polish has the greatest effect on the SpO_2 reading. Nail polish causes an artifactual and fixed decrease in the SpO_2 reading by these devices. Turning the finger probe 90 degrees and having the light shining sidewise through the finger is useful when there is nail polish on the patient's fingernails *(Miller: Anesthesia, ed 6, pp 1448-1452)*.

56. (C) The minimum macroshock current required to elicit ventricular fibrillation is 50 to 100 mA *(Brunner: Electricity, Safety, and the Patient, ed 1, pp 22-23; Miller: Anesthesia, ed 6, pp 3145-3146)*.

57. (D) The line isolation monitor alarms when grounding occurs in the OR or when the maximum current that a short circuit could cause exceeds 2 to 5 mA. The line isolation monitor is purely a monitor and does interrupt electrical current. Therefore, the line isolation monitor will not prevent microshock or macroshock *(Brunner: Electricity, Safety, and the Patient, ed 1, p 304; Miller: Anesthesia, ed 6, pp 3140-3141)*.

58. (A) A scavenging system with a closed interface is one in which there is communication with the atmosphere through positive- and negative-pressure relief valves. The positive-pressure relief valve will prevent transmission of excessive pressure buildup to the patient breathing circuit, even if there is an obstruction distal to the interface or if the system is not connected to wall suction. However, obstruction of the transfer tubing from the patient breathing circuit to the scavenging circuit is proximal to the interface. This will isolate the patient breathing circuit from the positive-pressure relief valve of the scavenging system interface. Should this occur, barotrauma to the patient's lungs can result *(Ehrenwerth: Anesthesia Equipment: Principles and Applications, pp 127-128)*.

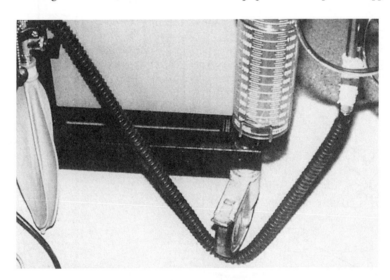

59. (B) MAC for isoflurane is 1.15% of 1 atmosphere or 8.7 mm Hg. An isoflurane vaporizer set for 1.15% will use a splitting ratio of 1:39. For purposes of illustration, imagine 100 mL of oxygen passes through the vaporizing chamber and 3900 mL through bypass chamber.

100 mL × 240/(760 - 240) = 46.1 mL of isoflurane vapor (plus 100 mL oxygen)

46.1/(3900 + 100) = 46.1/4000 = 1.15%

1.15% × 760 mm Hg = 8.7 mm Hg (1 MAC)

Consider now the same splitting ratio applied in Denver, Colo.:

100 mL × 240/(630 - 240) = 61.5 mL of isoflurane vapor (plus 100 mL oxygen)

61.5/(3900 + 100) = 61.5/4000 = 1.53%

1.53% × 630 mm Hg = 9.7 mm Hg (roughly 1.1 MAC)

MAC Equivalent (Barometric Pressure)

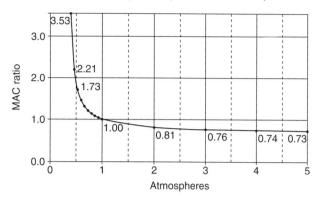

Older vaporizers are not compensated for changes in barometric pressure. As a general rule, the higher the altitude (lower the barometric pressure), the greater the vaporizer output. Conversely, the higher the barometric pressure (i.e., hyperbaric chamber), the lower the output. The graph above depicts the relationship between "dialed" MAC versus delivered MAC as a function of barometric pressure expressed in atmospheres *(Ehrenwerth: Anesthesia Equipment: Principles and Applications, p 70).*

60. (A) Automated noninvasive blood pressure (ANIBP) devices provide consistent and reliable arterial BP measurements. Variations in the cuff pressure resulting from arterial pulsations during cuff deflation are sensed by the device and are used to calculate mean arterial pressure. Then, values for systolic and diastolic pressures are derived from formulas that use the rate of change of the arterial pressure pulsations and the mean arterial pressure (oscillometric principle). This methodology provides accurate measurements of arterial BP in neonates, infants, children, and adults. The main advantage of ANIBP devices is that they free the anesthesia provider to perform other duties required for optimal anesthesia care. Additionally, these devices provide alarm systems to draw attention to extreme BP values and have the capacity to transfer data to automated trending devices or recorders. Improper use of these devices can lead to erroneous measurements and complications. The width of the BP cuff should be approximately 40% of the circumference of the patient's arm. If the width of the BP cuff is too narrow or if the BP cuff is wrapped too loosely around the arm, the BP measurement by the device will be falsely elevated. Frequent BP measurements can result in edema of the extremity distal to the cuff. For this reason, cycling of these devices should not be more frequent than every 1 to 3 minutes. Other complications associated with improper use of ANIBP devices include ulnar nerve paresthesia, superficial thrombophlebitis, and compartment syndrome. Fortunately, these complications are rare occurrences *(Miller: Anesthesia, ed 6, pp 1269-1271; Stoelting: Basics of Anesthesia, ed 5, p 307).*

61. (D) If the ventilator pressure-relief valve were to become incompetent, there would be a direct communication between the patient breathing circuit and the scavenging system circuit. This would result in delivery of part of the V_T during the inspiratory phase of the ventilator cycle directly to the scavenging system reservoir bag. Therefore, adequate positive-pressure ventilation may not be achieved and hypoventilation of the patient's lungs may result. Also see explanation to question 54 and accompanying figure *(Ehrenwerth: Anesthesia Equipment: Principles and Applications, p 120).*

62. (C) A size "E" compressed-gas cylinder completely filled with air contains 625 L and would show a pressure gauge reading of 2000 psi. Therefore, a cylinder with a pressure gauge reading of 1000 psi would be half-full, containing approximately 325 L of air. A half-full size "E" compressed-gas cylinder containing air could be used for approximately 30 minutes at a flow rate of 10 L/min (see definition of Boyle's law in explanation to question 9 and explanation and table from question 10) *(Stoelting: Basics of Anesthesia, ed 5, p 188).*

63. (E) Failure to oxygenate patients adequately is the leading cause of anesthesia-related morbidity and mortality. All of the choices listed in this question are potential causes of inadequate delivery of O_2 to the patient; however, the most frequent cause is inadvertent disconnection of the O_2 supply system from the patient (e.g., disconnection of the patient breathing circuit from the endotracheal tube) *(Miller: Anesthesia, ed 6, p 300).*

64. (A)   The esophageal detector device (EDD) is essentially a bulb that is first compressed then attached to the ETT after the tube is inserted into the patient. The pressure generated is about negative 40 cm of water. If the ETT is placed in the esophagus, then the negative pressure will collapse the esophagus and the bulb will not inflate. If the ETT is in the trachea, then the air from the lung will enable the bulb to inflate (usually in a few seconds but at times may take more than 30 seconds). A syringe that has a negative pressure applied to it has also been used. Although initial studies were very positive about its use, more recent studies show that up to 30% of correctly placed ETTs in adults may be removed because the EDD suggested esophageal placement. Misleading results have been noted in patients with morbid obesity, late pregnancy, status asthmatics and when there is copious endotracheal secretion, where the trachea tends to collapse. Its use in children younger than 1 year of age showed poor sensitivity as well as poor specificity. Although a cardiac output is needed to get CO_2 to the lungs for a CO_2 gas analyzer to function, a cardiac output is not needed for an EDD *(American Heart Association—Guidelines for CPR and ECC. Circulation Volume 112, Issue 24, pp IV-54, IV-150, IV-169, 2005; Miller: Anesthesia, ed 6, p 1648).*

65. (D)   The capnometer measures the CO_2 concentration of respiratory gases. Today this is most commonly performed by infrared absorption using a sidestream gas sample. The sampling tube should be connected as close to the patient's airway as possible. The difference between the end-tidal CO_2 ($Etco_2$) and the arterial CO_2 ($Paco_2$) is typically 5-10 mm Hg and is due to alveolar dead space ventilation. Because non-perfused alveoli do not contribute to gas exchange, any condition that increases alveolar dead space ventilation (i.e., reduces pulmonary blood flow such as a pulmonary embolism or cardiac arrest) will increase dead space ventilation and the $Etco_2$ to $Paco_2$ difference. Conditions that increase pulmonary shunt result in minimal changes in the $Paco_2$-$Etco_2$ gradient. CO_2 diffuses rapidly across the capillary-alveolar membrane *(Barash: Clinical Anesthesia, ed 5, pp 670-671; Miller: Anesthesia, ed 6, pp 1455-1462).*

66. (E)   The last gas added to a gas mixture should always be O_2. This arrangement is the safest because it assures that leaks proximal to the O_2 inflow cannot result in delivery of a hypoxic gas mixture to the patient. With this arrangement (O_2 added last), leaks distal to the O_2 inflow will result in a decreased volume of gas, but the Fio_2 of Anesthesia will not be reduced *(Stoelting: Basics of Anesthesia, ed 5, pp 188-189).*

67. (D)   Most modern Datex-Ohmeda Tec or North American Dräger Vapor vaporizers (except desflurane) are variable-bypass, flow-over vaporizers. This means that the gas that flows through the vaporizers is split into two parts depending upon the concentration selected. The gas either goes through the bypass chamber on the top of the vaporizer or the vaporizing chamber on the bottom of the vaporizer. If the vaporizer is "tipped" which might happen when a filled vaporizer is "switched out" or moved from one machine to another machine, part of the anesthetic liquid in the vaporizing chamber may get into the bypass chamber. This could result in a much higher concentration of gas than dialed. With the Datex-Ohmeda Tec 4 or the North American Drager Vapor 19.1 series it is recommended to flush the vaporizer at high flows with the vaporizer set at a low concentration until the output shows no excessive agent (this usually takes 20-30 minutes). The Drager Vapor 2000 series has a transport (T) dial setting. This setting isolates the bypass from the vaporizer chamber. The Aladin cassette vaporizer does not have a bypass flow chamber and has no "tipping" hazard *(Miller: Anesthesia ed 6, pp 285-288).*

68. (A)   Accurate delivery of volatile anesthetic concentration is dependant upon filling the agent specific vaporizer with the appropriate (volatile) agent. Differences in anesthetic potencies further necessitate this requirement. Each agent-specific vaporizer utilizes a splitting ratio that determines the portion of the fresh gas that is directed through the vaporizing chamber versus that which travels through the bypass chamber.

VAPOR PRESSURE, ANESTHETIC VAPOR PRESSURE, AND SPLITTING RATIO

	Halothane	Sevoflurane	Isoflurane	Enflurane
Vapor pressure at 20° C	243 mm Hg	160 mm Hg	240 mm Hg	172 mm Hg
VP/(BP-VP)	0.47	0.27	0.47	0.29
Splitting ratio for 1% vapor°$_{anesanes}$	1:47	1:27	1:47	1:29

V_{panes}, anesthetic vapor pressure; BP, barometric pressure.

The table above shows the calculation (fraction) that when multiplied by the quantity of fresh gas traversing the vaporizing chamber (affluent fresh gas in mL/min) will yield the output (mL/min) of anesthetic vapor in the effluent gas. When this fraction is multiplied by 100 it equals the splitting ratio for 1% for the given volatile. For example, when the isoflurane vaporizer is set to deliver 1% isoflurane, one part of fresh gas passed through the vaporizing chamber while 47 parts travel through the bypass chamber. One can determine on inspection that when a less soluble volatile like sevoflurane (or enflurane for the sake of example) is placed into an isoflurane (or halothane) vaporizer, the output in volume percent will be less than expected. How much less can be determined by simply comparing their splitting ratios 27/47 or 0.6. Halothane and enflurane are no longer used in the United States, but old halothane and enflurane vaporizers can be (and are) used elsewhere in the world to accurately deliver isoflurane and sevoflurane respectively *(Ehrenwerth: Anesthesia Equipment: Principles and Applications, p 67).*

69. (C) Two percent of 4 L/min would be 80 mL of isoflurane per minute.

VAPOR PRESSURE PER ML OF LIQUID

	Halothane	Enflurane	Isoflurane	Sevoflurane	Desflurane
mL vapor per ml liquid at 20° C	226	196	195	182	207

(Ehrenwerth: Anesthesia Equipment: Principles and Applications, p 60)

Since 1 mL of vapor produces 195 mL of gas or making the simplistic calculation of 195 × 150 mL = 29,250. It follows that 29,250/80 = 365 minutes or about 6 hours.

Note that each mL of most volatiles will yield 200 mL vapor at 20° C. Thus 150 min × 200 mL/min = 30,000 min. It follows that 30,000 min/80 mL/min = 375 minutes or ≈ 6 hours. *(Ehrenwerth: Anesthesia Equipment: Principles and Applications, p 60).*

70. (C) The human ear can perceive sound in the range of 20 Hz to 20 kHz. Frequencies above 20 kHz, inaudible to humans, are ultrasonic frequencies (ultra = Latin for "beyond" or "on the far side of"). In regional anesthesia, ultrasound is used for imaging in the frequency range of 2.5 to 10 MHz. Wavelength is inversely proportional to frequency, i.e., λ = C/f (λ = wavelength, C = velocity of sound through tissue or 1540 m/sec, f = frequency). Wavelength in millimeters can be calculated by dividing 1.54 by the Doppler frequency in megahertz. Penetration into tissue is 200 to 400 times wavelength and resolution is twice the wavelength. Therefore, a frequency of 3 MHz (wavelength .51 mm) would have a resolution of 1 mm and a penetration of up to 100 - 200 mm (10-20 cm) whereas 10 MHz (wavelength 0.15 mm) corresponds to a resolution of 0.3 mm, but penetration depth of no more than 60-120 mm (6-12 cm) *(Miller: Anesthesia, ed 6, p 1364).*

71. (A) Microshock refers to electric shock in or near the heart. A current as low as 50 μA passing through the heart can produce ventricular fibrillation. Use of pacemaker electrodes, central venous catheters, pulmonary artery catheters and other devices in the heart make are necessary prerequisites for microshock. Because the line isolation monitor has a 2 milliamps (2000 μA) threshold for alarming, it will not protect against microshock *(Miller Anesthesia, ed 6, page 3145).*

72. (E) Intraoperative awareness or recall during general anesthesia is rare (overall incidence is 0.2%, for obstetrics 0.4%, for cardiac 1-1.5%) except for major trauma which has a reported incidence up to 43%. With the EEG, trends can be identified with changes in the depth of anesthesia, however the sensitivity and specificity of the available trends are such that none serve as a sole indicator of anesthesia depth. Although using the BIS monitor may reduce the risk of recall, it, like the other listed signs as well as patient movement, does not totally eliminate recall *(Miller: Anesthesia, ed 6, pp 1230-1259).*

73. (D) The minute ventilation is five liters (0.5 L per breath at 10 breaths per minute) and 2 liters per minute to drive the ventilator for a total O_2 consumption of 7 liters per minute. A full oxygen "E" cylinder contains 625 liters. Ninety percent of the volume of the cylinder (≈ 560 L) can be delivered before the ventilator can no longer be driven. At a rate of 7 L/min, this supply would last about 80 minutes *(Stoelting: Basics of Anesthesia, ed 5, page 188).*

74. (C) After eliminating reversible causes of high peak airway pressures such as occlusion of the endotracheal tube, mainstem intubation, bronchospasm, etc., adjusting the ventilator can reduce the peak airway pressure. Increasing the inspiratory flow rate would cause the airway pressures to go up faster and would produce higher peak airway pressures. Taking the PEEP off would have no significant effect. Changing the I:E ratio from 1:3 to 1:2 will permit 8% (25% inspiratory time to 33% inspiratory time) more time for the V_T to be administered and would result in lower airway pressures. Decreasing the V_T to 300 and increasing the rate to 28 would give the same minute ventilation, but not the same alveolar ventilation. Recall that alveolar ventilation equals (frequency) times (V_T minus dead space); and since dead space is the same (about 2 mL/kg ideal weight) alveolar ventilation would be reduced, in this case to a dangerously low level. Another option is to change from volume cycled to pressure cycled ventilation, which produces a more constant pressure over time instead of the peaked pressures seen with fixed V_T ventilation. *(Barash: Clinical Anesthesia, ed 5, pp 1484-1485; Miller: Anesthesia, ed 6, pp 2820-2822).*

75. (D) The central hospital oxygen supply to the operating rooms is designed to give enough pressure and oxygen flow to run the three oxygen components of the anesthesia machine (patient fresh gas flow, the anesthesia ventilator and the oxygen flush valve). The oxygen flowmeter on the anesthesia machine is designed to run at an oxygen pressure of 50 psi and for emergency purposes the oxygen flush valve delivers 35 to 75 L/min of oxygen *(Stoelting: Basics of Anesthesia, ed 5, pp 187-189).*

76. (B) Within the respiratory system both laminar and turbulent flows exist. At low flow rates, the respiratory flow tends to be laminar, like a series of concentric tubes that slide over one another with the center tubes flowing faster than the more peripheral tubes. Laminar flow is usually inaudible and is dependent on gas viscosity. Turbulent flow tends to be faster flow, is audible and is dependent upon gas density. Gas density can be decreased by using a mixture of helium with oxygen. *(Barash: Clinical Anesthesia, ed 5, pp 794-795, Miller: Anesthesia, ed 6, p 2539).*

77. (B) Anesthesia machines have a high, intermediate and low pressure circuits. The high pressure circuit is from the oxygen cylinder to the oxygen pressure regulator (first stage regulator) which takes the oxygen pressure from a high of 2200 psi to 45 psi. The intermediate pressure circuit consists of the pipeline pressure of about 50 to 55 psi and goes to the second stage regulator, which then lowers the pressure to 14 to 26 psi (depending upon the machine). The low pressure circuit then consists of the flow tubes, vaporizer manifold, vaporizers and vaporizer check valve to the common gas outlet. The oxygen flush valve is in the intermediate pressure circuit and bypasses the low pressure circuit *(Stoelting: Basics of Anesthesia, ed 5, p 187; Miller: Anesthesia, ed 6, pp 274-276).*

78. (C) Two major problems should be noted in this case. The first obvious problem is the inspired oxygen concentration of 4%, a concentration that is not possible if the gases going to the machine are appropriate unless the oxygen analyzer is faulty. In this case, where both the oxygen analyzer and the mass spectrometer read 4%, the pipeline gas line supplying "oxygen" most likely contains something other than oxygen. Second, the oxygen line pressure is 65 psi. The pipeline pressures are normally around 50 to 55 psi, whereas the pressure from the oxygen cylinder, if the cylinder is turned on, is reduced to 45 psi. For the oxygen tank to deliver oxygen to the patient, the pipeline pressure needs to be less than 45 psi, which in this case would occur only when the pipeline is disconnected. Although we rarely think of problems with hospital gas lines, a survey of more than 200 hospitals showed about 33% had problems with the pipelines. Most common pipeline problems were low pressure, followed by high pressure and, very rarely, crossed gas lines. *(Barash: Clinical Anesthesia, ed 5, pp 563-564, Miller: Anesthesia, ed 6, pp 274-276).*

79. (D) There are many ways to monitor the electrical activity of the heart. The five-electrode system using one lead for each limb and the fifth lead for the precordium is commonly used in the operating suite. The precordial lead placed in the V5 position (anterior axillary line in the fifth intercostal space) gives the V5 tracing, which combined with the standard lead II are most common tracings used to look for myocardial ischemia *(Barash: Clinical Anesthesia, ed 5, pp 889, 1539; Miller: Anesthesia, ed 6, pp 1392-1393).*

80. (A) The DISS provides threaded, non-interchangeable connections for medical gas pipelines through the hospital as well as to the anesthesia machine. The Pin Index Safety System (PISS) has two metal pins located in different arrangements around the yoke on the back of anesthesia machines, with each arrangement for a specific gas cylinder. Vaporizers often have keyed fillers that attach to the bottle of anesthetic and the vaporizer. Vaporizers not equipped with keyed fillers occasionally have been misfilled with the wrong anesthetic liquid *(Barash: Clinical Anesthesia, ed 5, p 563; Miller: Anesthesia, ed 6, pp 276 and 288).*

81. **(C)**   Calcium hydroxide lime does not contain the monovalent hydroxide bases that are present in soda lime (namely NaOH and KOH). Sevoflurane in the presence of NaOH or KOH is degraded to trace amounts of Compound A, which is nephrotoxic to rats at high concentrations. Soda lime normally contains about 13% to 15% water, but if the soda lime is desiccated (water content < 5% — which has occurred if the machine is not used for a while and the fresh gas flow is left on) and exposed to current volatile anesthetics (isoflurane, sevoflurane and especially desflurane), carbon monoxide can be produced. Neither Compound A nor carbon monoxide are formed when calcium hydroxide lime is used. With soda lime and calcium hydroxide lime the indicator dye changes from white to purple as the granules become exhausted; however, over time, exhausted soda may revert back to white. With calcium hydroxide lime the dye once changed does not revert to normal. The two major disadvantages of calcium hydroxide lime are the expense and the fact that its absorptive capacity is about half of soda lime (10.2 L of CO_2/100 g of calcium hydroxide lime versus 26 L of CO_2/100 g of soda lime) *(Barash: Clinical Anesthesia, ed 5, pp 411-413; Miller: Anesthesia, ed 6, pp 296-298; Stoelting: Basics of Anesthesia, ed 5, pp 200-202).*

82. **(B)**   The aim of direct invasive monitoring is to give continuous arterial BPs that are similar to the intermittent noninvasive arterial BPs from a cuff, as well as to give a port for arterial blood samples. The displayed signal reflects the actual pressure as well as distortions from the measuring system (i.e., the catheter, tubing, stopcocks, amplifier). Although most of the time the signal is accurate, at times we see an underdamped or an overdamped signal. In an underdamped signal, as in this case, exaggerated readings are noted (widened pulse pressure). In an overdamped signal, readings are diminished (narrowed pulse pressure). Note however the mean BP tends to be accurate in both underdamped and overdamped signals *(Miller: Anesthesia, ed 6, pp 1272-1279).*

83. **(E)**   Rebreathing of expired gases (e.g., stuck open expiratory or inspiratory valves), faulty removal of CO_2 from the carbon dioxide absorber (e.g., exhausted CO_2 absorber, channeling through a CO_2 absorber or having the CO_2 absorber bypassed — an option in some older anesthetic machines), or adding CO_2 from a gas supply (rarely done with current anesthetic machines) can all increase inspired CO_2. Absorption of CO_2 during laparoscopic surgery when CO_2 is used as the abdominal distending gas would increase absorption of CO_2 but would not cause an increase in inspired CO_2 *(Miller: Anesthesia, ed 6, pp 1458-1461; Stoelting: Basics of Anesthesia, ed 5, pp 199-201, 314).*

84. **(B)**   **85. (A) 86. (D)**
Medical gas cylinders are color coded but may differ from one country to another. If there is a combination of two gases, the tank would have both corresponding colors, for example, a tank containing oxygen and helium would be green and brown. The only exception to the mixed gas color scheme is O_2 and N_2 in the proportion of 19.5% to 23.5% mixed with N_2, which is solid yellow (air).

GAS COLOR CODES

Gas	United States	International
Air	Yellow	White and Black
Carbon Dioxide	Gray	Gray
Helium	Brown	Brown
Nitrogen	Black	Black
Nitrous Oxide	Blue	Blue
Oxygen	Green	White

(Ehrenwerth: Anesthesia Equipment: Principles and Applications, p 7.)

87. **(A)**   **88. (D) 89. (D) 90. (E)**
There are five different types of Mapleson breathing circuits (designated A through E). These circuits vary in arrangement of the fresh-gas-flow inlet, tubing, mask, reservoir bag, and unidirectional expiratory valve. These systems are lightweight, portable, easy to clean, offer low resistance to breathing, and, because of high fresh gas inflows, prevent rebreathing of exhaled gases. In addition, with these breathing circuits, the concentration of volatile anesthetic gases and O_2 delivered to the patient can be accurately estimated. The reservoir bag enables the anesthesia provider to provide assisted or controlled ventilation of the lungs. The unidirectional expiratory valve functions to direct fresh gas into the patient and exhaled gases out of the circuit. In the Mapleson A breathing circuit, the unidirectional expiratory valve is located near the patient and the fresh-gas-flow inlet

is located proximal to the reservoir bag. This arrangement is the most efficient for elimination of CO_2 during spontaneous breathing. However, because the unidirectional expiratory valve must be tightened to permit production of positive airway pressure when the gas reservoir bag is manually compressed, this breathing circuit is less efficient in preventing rebreathing of CO_2 during assisted or controlled ventilation of the lungs. The structure of the Mapleson D breathing circuit is similar to that of the Mapleson A breathing circuit except that the positions of the fresh-gas-flow inlet and the unidirectional expiratory valve are reversed. The placement of the fresh-gas-flow inlet near the patient produces efficient elimination of CO_2, regardless of whether the patient is breathing spontaneously or the patient's ventilation is controlled. The Bain anesthesia breathing circuit is a coaxial version of the Mapleson D breathing circuit except that the fresh gas enters through a narrow tube within the corrugated expiratory limb of the circuit. The Jackson-Rees breathing circuit is a modification of the Mapleson E breathing circuit. In the Jackson-Rees breathing circuit, the adjustable unidirectional expiratory valve is incorporated into the reservoir bag and the fresh-gas-flow inlet is located close to the patient. This arrangement offers the advantage of ease of instituting assisted or controlled ventilation of the lungs, as well as monitoring ventilation by movement of the reservoir bag during spontaneous breathing *(Ehrenwerth: Anesthesia Equipment: Principles and Applications, pp 102-108; Miller: Anesthesia, ed 6, pp 293-295).*

Chapter 2

Respiratory Physiology and Critical Care Medicine

DIRECTIONS (Questions 91 through 168): Each of the questions or incomplete statements in this section is followed by answers or by completions of the statement, respectively. Select the ONE BEST answer or completion for each item.

91. A 29-year-old man is admitted to the intensive care unit (ICU) after a drug overdose. The patient is placed on a ventilator with a set tidal volume (V_T) of 750 mL at a rate of 10 breaths/min. The patient is making no inspiratory effort. The measured minute ventilation is 6 L and the peak airway pressure is 30 cm H_2O. What is the compression factor for this ventilator delivery circuit?
    A. 1 mL (cm H_2O)$^{-1}$
    B. 2 mL (cm H_2O)$^{-1}$
    C. 3 mL (cm H_2O)$^{-1}$
    D. 4 mL (cm H_2O)$^{-1}$
    E. 5 mL (cm H_2O)$^{-1}$

92. A 62-year-old male is brought to the ICU after elective repair of an abdominal aortic aneurysm. His vital signs are stable, but he requires a sodium nitroprusside infusion at a rate of 10 μg/kg/min to keep the systolic blood pressure below 110 mm Hg. The Sao_2 is 98% with controlled ventilation at 12 breaths/min and an Fio_2 of 0.60. After 3 days, his Sao_2 decreases to 85% on the pulse oximeter. Chest x-ray film and results of physical examination are unchanged. Which of the following would most likely account for this desaturation?
    A. Cyanide toxicity
    B. Thiocyanate toxicity
    C. O_2 toxicity
    D. Thiosulfate toxicity
    E. Methemoglobinemia

93. Maximizing which of the following lung parameters is the most important factor in prevention of postoperative pulmonary complications?
    A. Tidal volume (V_T)
    B. Inspiratory reserve volume
    C. Vital capacity
    D. Functional residual capacity (FRC)
    E. Inspiratory capacity

94. An 83-year-old woman is admitted to the ICU after coronary artery surgery. A pulmonary artery catheter is in place and yields the following data: central venous pressure (CVP) 5 mm Hg, cardiac output (CO) 4.0 L/min, mean arterial pressure (MAP) 90 mm Hg, mean pulmonary artery pressure (PAP) 20 mm Hg, pulmonary artery occlusion pressure (PAOP) 12 mm Hg, and heart rate 90. Calculate this patient's pulmonary vascular resistance (PVR)
    A. 40 dynes-sec-cm^{-5}
    B. 80 dynes-sec-cm^{-5}
    C. 160 dynes-sec-cm^{-5}
    D. 200 dynes-sec-cm^{-5}
    E. 240 dynes-sec-cm^{-5}

95.   A 72-year-old male patient with a history of myocardial infarction 12 months earlier is scheduled to undergo elective repair of a 6-cm abdominal aortic aneurysm under general anesthesia. When would this patient be at highest risk for another myocardial infarction?
      A. On induction of anesthesia
      B. During placement of the aortic cross-clamp
      C. Upon release of the aortic cross-clamp
      D. 24 hours postoperatively
      E. On the third postoperative day

96.   Calculate the body mass index of a male 200 cm (6 feet 6 inches) tall who weighs 100 kg (220 pounds)
      A. 20
      B. 25
      C. 30
      D. 35
      E. 40

97.   The normal FEV_1/FVC ratio is
      A. 0.95
      B. 0.80
      C. 0.60
      D. 0.50
      E. 0.40

98.   Direct current (DC) cardioversion is not useful and therefore **NOT** indicated in an unstable patient with which of the following?
      A. Supraventricular tachycardia in a patient with Wolff-Parkinson-White syndrome
      B. Atrial flutter
      C. Multifocal atrial tachycardia
      D. New-onset atrial fibrillation
      E. All of these rhythms should be DC cardioverted in an unstable patient

99.   During the first minute of apnea, the $Paco_2$ will rise
      A. 2 mm Hg/min
      B. 4 mm Hg/min
      C. 6 mm Hg/min
      D. 8 mm Hg/min
      E. 10 mm Hg/min

100. Potential complications associated with total parenteral nutrition (TPN) include all of the following **EXCEPT**
      A. Ketoacidosis
      B. Hyperglycemia
      C. Hypoglycemia
      D. Hypophosphatemia
      E. Increased work of breathing

101. O_2 requirement for a 70-kg adult is
      A. 150 mL/min
      B. 250 mL/min
      C. 350 mL/min
      D. 450 mL/min
      E. 550 mL/min

102. The FRC is composed of the
      A. Expiratory reserve volume and residual volume
      B. Inspiratory reserve volume and residual volume
      C. Inspiratory capacity and vital capacity
      D. Expiratory capacity and V_T
      E. Expiratory reserve volume and tidal volume

103. Which of the following statements correctly defines the relationship between minute ventilation ($\dot{V}_E$), dead space ventilation (V_D), and Pa_{CO_2}?
    A. If $\dot{V}_E$ is constant and V_D increases, then Pa_{CO_2} will increase
    B. If $\dot{V}_E$ is constant and V_D increases, then Pa_{CO_2} will decrease
    C. If V_D is constant and $\dot{V}_E$ increases, then Pa_{CO_2} will increase
    D. If V_D is constant and $\dot{V}_E$ decreases, then Pa_{CO_2} will decrease
    E. None of the above

104. A 22-year-old patient who sustained a closed head injury is brought to the operating room (OR) from the ICU for placement of a dural bolt. Hemoglobin has been stable at 15 g/dL. Blood gas analysis immediately before induction reveals a Pa_{O_2} of 120 mm Hg and an arterial saturation of 100%. After induction, the Pa_{O_2} rises to 150 mm Hg and the saturation remains the same. How has the oxygen content of this patient's blood changed?
    A. It has increased by 10%
    B. It has increased by 5%
    C. It has increased by less than 1%
    D. Cannot be determined without Pa_{CO_2}
    E. Cannot be determined without pH

105. Inhalation of CO_2 increases $\dot{V}_E$ by
    A. 0.5 to 1 L/min/mm Hg increase in Pa_{CO_2}
    B. 2 to 3 L/min/mm Hg increase in Pa_{CO_2}
    C. 3 to 5 L/min/mm Hg increase in Pa_{CO_2}
    D. 5 to 10 L/min/mm Hg increase in Pa_{CO_2}
    E. 10 to 20 L/min/mm Hg increase in Pa_{CO_2}

106. What is the O_2 content of whole blood if the hemoglobin concentration is 10 g/dL, the Pa_{O_2} is 60 mm Hg, and the Sa_{O_2} is 90%?
    A. 10 mL/dL
    B. 12.5 mL/dL
    C. 15 mL/dL
    D. 17.5 mL/dL
    E. 21 mL/dL

107. Each of the following will cause erroneous readings by dual-wavelength pulse oximeters **EXCEPT**
    A. Carboxyhemoglobin
    B. Methylene blue
    C. Fetal hemoglobin
    D. Methemoglobin
    E. Nail polish

108. The mechanism for the compensatory shift of the oxyhemoglobin dissociation curve toward normal in response to chronic (>24 hours) respiratory alkalosis is
    A. Increased renal excretion of HCO_3^-
    B. An influx of potassium into red blood cells
    C. Altered erythrocyte 2,3-diphosphoglycerate (2,3-DPG) metabolism
    D. Decreased sensitivity of the central nervous system to changes in Pa_{CO_2}
    E. None of the above

109. The P_{50} for normal adult hemoglobin is approximately
    A. 15 mm Hg
    B. 25 mm Hg
    C. 35 mm Hg
    D. 45 mm Hg
    E. 50 mm Hg

110. During a normal V_T (500-mL) breath, the transpulmonary pressure increases from 0 to 5 cm H_2O. The product of transpulmonary pressure and V_T is 2500 cm H_2O-mL. This expression of the pressure-volume relationship during breathing determines what parameter of respiratory mechanics?
    A. Lung compliance
    B. Airway resistance
    C. Pulmonary elastance
    D. Work of breathing
    E. Closing capacity

111. An oximetric pulmonary artery catheter is placed in a 69-year-old male patient who is undergoing surgical resection of an abdominal aortic aneurysm under general anesthesia. Before the aortic cross-clamp is placed, the mixed venous O_2 saturation decreases from 75% to 60%. Each of the following could account for the decrease in mixed venous O_2 saturation **EXCEPT**
    A. Hypovolemia
    B. Bleeding
    C. Hypoxia
    D. Sepsis
    E. Congestive heart failure

112. The normal vital capacity for a 70-kg man is
    A. 1 L
    B. 2 L
    C. 5 L
    D. 7 L
    E. 9 L

113. A 32-year-old male is found unconscious by the fire department in a room where he has inhaled 0.1% carbon monoxide for a prolonged period. His respiratory rate is 42 breaths/min, but he is not cyanotic. Carbon monoxide has increased this patient's minute ventilation by which of the following mechanisms?
    A. Shifting the O_2 hemoglobin dissociation curve to the left
    B. Increasing CO_2 production
    C. Causing lactic acidosis
    D. Decreasing Pao_2
    E. Producing methemoglobin

114. An acute increase in $Paco_2$ of 10 mm Hg will result in a decrease in pH of
    A. 0.01 pH units
    B. 0.02 pH units
    C. 0.04 pH units
    D. 0.08 pH units
    E. None of the above

115. A 20-year-old, 75-kg patient with a history of insulin-dependent diabetes mellitus arrives in the emergency room (ER) in diabetic ketoacidosis. The arterial blood gases (ABGs) while on room air are as follows: pH 6.95, $Paco_2$ 30 mm Hg, Pao_2 98 mm Hg, [HCO_3^-] 6 mEq/L. What is the total body deficit of HCO_3^- in this patient?
    A. 500 mEq
    B. 400 mEq
    C. 300 mEq
    D. 200 mEq
    E. 100 mEq

116. A 44-year-old patient is hyperventilated to a $Paco_2$ of 24 mm Hg for 48 hours. What [HCO_3^-] would you expect (normal [HCO_3^-] is 24 mEq/L)?
    A. 10 mEq/L
    B. 12 mEq/L
    C. 14 mEq/L
    D. 16 mEq/L
    E. 18 mEq/L

117. The diagram below depicts which mode of ventilation?

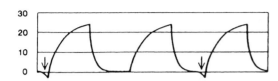

　　A. Spontaneous ventilation
　　B. Controlled ventilation
　　C. Assisted ventilation
　　D. Assisted/controlled ventilation
　　E. Synchronized intermittent mandatory ventilation

118. A 35-year-old morbidly obese patient is discharged after gastric bypass surgery. She is readmitted 4 days later after she falls and twists her ankle. She is noted in the ER to be in atrial fibrillation, she is hypotensive, but only complains of leg pain. She is admitted to the hospital and temperature on admission is 38.6° C and heart rate 105. The next step in management of her dysrhythmia should be
　　A. Ibutilide
　　B. Procainamide
　　C. Echocardiographic study
　　D. DC cardioversion
　　E. Digitalis

119. The P_{50} of sickle cell hemoglobin is
　　A. 19 mm Hg
　　B. 26 mm Hg
　　C. 31 mm Hg
　　D. 35 mm Hg
　　E. 40 mm Hg

120. The leftward shift of the oxyhemoglobin dissociation curve caused by hypocarbia is known as the
　　A. Fick principle
　　B. Bohr effect
　　C. Haldane effect
　　D. Law of Laplace
　　E. None of the above

121. Which of the following is the correct mathematical expression of Fick's law of diffusion of a gas through a lipid membrane ($\dot{V}$ = rate of diffusion, D = diffusion coefficient of the gas, A = area of the membrane, P1 – P2 = transmembrane partial pressure gradient of the gas, T = thickness of the membrane)?

　　A. $\dot{V} = D \times \dfrac{A \times T}{P_1 - P_2}$

　　B. $\dot{V} = \dfrac{A \times T}{D(P_1 - P_2)}$

　　C. $\dot{V} = D \times \dfrac{A(P_1 - P_2)}{T}$

　　D. $\dot{V} = D \times \dfrac{T(P_1 - P_2)}{A}$

　　E. $\dot{V} = \dfrac{D \times T \times A}{P_1 - P_2}$

122. Each of the following is decreased in elderly patients compared with their younger counterparts **EXCEPT**
    A. Pa_{O_2}
    B. FEV_1
    C. Ventilatory response to hypercarbia
    D. Vital capacity
    E. Closing volume

123. Calculate the V_D/V_T ratio (physiologic dead-space ventilation) based on the following data: Pa_{CO_2} 45 mm Hg, mixed expired CO_2 tension (Pe_{CO_2}) 30 mm Hg.
    A. 0.1
    B. 0.2
    C. 0.3
    D. 0.4
    E. 0.5

124. Which of the following statements concerning the distribution of O_2 and CO_2 in the upright lungs is true?
    A. Pa_{O_2} is greater at the apex than at the base
    B. Pa_{CO_2} is greater at the apex than at the base
    C. Both Pa_{O_2} and Pa_{CO_2} are greater at the apex than at the base
    D. Both Pa_{O_2} and Pa_{CO_2} are greater at the base than at the apex
    E. Pa_{CO_2} is equal throughout the lung

125. Which of the following acid-base disturbances is the least well compensated?
    A. Metabolic alkalosis
    B. Respiratory alkalosis
    C. Increased anion gap metabolic acidosis
    D. Normal anion gap metabolic acidosis
    E. Respiratory acidosis

126. What is the Pa_{O_2} of a patient on room air in Denver, Colo. (assume a barometric pressure of 630 mm Hg, respiratory quotient of 0.8, and Pa_{CO_2} of 34 mm Hg)?
    A. 40 mm Hg
    B. 50 mm Hg
    C. 60 mm Hg
    D. 70 mm Hg
    E. 80 mm Hg

127. A venous blood sample from which of the following sites would correlate most reliably with Pa_{O_2} and Pa_{CO_2}?
    A. Jugular vein
    B. Subclavian vein
    C. Antecubital vein
    D. Femoral vein
    E. Vein on posterior surface of a warmed hand

128. Which of the following pulmonary function tests is least dependent on patient effort?
    A. Forced expiratory volume in 1 second (FEV_1)
    B. Forced vital capacity (FVC)
    C. FEF 800-1200
    D. FEF 25%-75%
    E. Maximum voluntary ventilation (MVV)

129. A 33-year-old woman with 20% carboxyhemoglobin is brought to the ER for treatment of smoke inhalation. Which of the following is **LEAST** consistent with a diagnosis of carbon monoxide poisoning?
  A. Cyanosis
  B. Pao_2 105 mm Hg, oxygen saturation 80% on initial room air ABGs
  C. 98% oxygen saturation on dual-wavelength pulse oximeter
  D. Dizziness
  E. Oxyhemoglobin dissociation curve shifted far to the left

130. The $PAo_2 - Pao_2$ of a patient breathing 100% O_2 is 240 mm Hg. The estimated fraction of the cardiac output shunted past the lungs without exposure to ventilated alveoli (i.e., transpulmonary shunt) is
  A. 5%
  B. 12%
  C. 17%
  D. 20%
  E. 34%

131. Each of the following will alter the position or slope of the CO_2-ventilatory response curve **EXCEPT**
  A. Hypoxemia
  B. Fentanyl
  C. N_2O
  D. Isoflurane
  E. Ketamine

132. Which of the following statements concerning the distribution of alveolar ventilation ($\dot{V}A$) in the upright lungs is true?
  A. The distribution of $\dot{V}A$ is not affected by body posture
  B. Alveoli at the apex of the lungs (nondependent alveoli) are better ventilated than those at the base
  C. All areas of the lungs are ventilated equally
  D. Alveoli at the base of the lungs (dependent alveoli) are better ventilated than those at the apex
  E. Alveoli at the central regions of the lungs are better ventilated than those at the base or apex

133. In the resting adult, what percentage of total body O_2 consumption is due to the work of breathing?
  A. 2%
  B. 5%
  C. 10%
  D. 20%
  E. 50%

134. The anatomic dead space in a 70-kg male is
  A. 50 mL
  B. 150 mL
  C. 250 mL
  D. 500 mL
  E. 700 to 1000 mL

135. The most important buffering system in the body is
  A. Hemoglobin
  B. Plasma proteins
  C. Bone
  D. $[HCO_3^-]$
  E. Phosphate

136. A decrease in $Paco_2$ of 10 mm Hg will result in
  A. A decrease in serum potassium concentration [K+] of 0.5 mEq/L
  B. A decrease in [K+] of 1.0 mEq/L
  C. No change in [K+] under normal circumstances
  D. An increase in [K+] of 0.5 mEq/L
  E. An increase in [K+] of 1.0 mEq/L

137. An increase in $[HCO_3^-]$ of 10 mEq/L will result in an increase in pH of
    A. 0.10 pH units
    B. 0.15 pH units
    C. 0.20 pH units
    D. 0.25 pH units
    E. None of the above

138. A 28-year-old, 70-kg woman with ulcerative colitis is receiving a general anesthetic for a colon resection and ileostomy. The patient's lungs are mechanically ventilated with the following parameters: $\dot{V}_E$ 5000 mL and respiratory rate 10 breaths/min. Assuming no change in $\dot{V}_E$ how would $\dot{V}_A$ change if the respiratory rate were increased from 10 to 20 breaths/min?
    A. Increase by 500 mL
    B. Increase by 1000 mL
    C. No change
    D. Decrease by 750 mL
    E. Decrease by 1500 mL

139. Each of the following will shift the oxyhemoglobin dissociation curve to the right **EXCEPT**
    A. Volatile anesthetics
    B. Decreased Pao_2
    C. Decreased pH
    D. Increased temperature
    E. Increased red blood cell 2,3-DPG content

140. The half-life of carboxyhemoglobin in a patient breathing 100% O_2 is
    A. 5 minutes
    B. 1 hour
    C. 2 hours
    D. 4 hours
    E. 12 hours

141. Disadvantage of using propofol for prolonged sedation (days) of intubated patients in the ICU is potential
    A. Acidosis
    B. Tachyphylaxis
    C. Hyperglycemia
    D. Bradycardia
    E. Prolonged neurocognitive deficiency

142. A 17-year-old type I diabetic with history of renal failure is in the preoperative holding area awaiting an operation for acute appendicitis. Arterial blood gases are obtained with the following results: Pao_2 88 mm Hg, $Paco_2$ 32 mm Hg, pH 7.2, $[HCO_3^-]$ 12, $[Cl^-]$ 115 mEq/L, $[Na+]$ 138 mEq/L, and glucose 251 mg/dL. The most likely cause of this patient's acidosis is
    A. Renal tubular acidosis
    B. Lactic acidosis
    C. Diabetic ketoacidosis
    D. Aspirin overdose
    E. Nasogastric suction

143. Methods to decrease the incidence of central venous catheter infections include all of the following **EXCEPT**
    A. Using chlorhexidine over povidone-iodine for skin decontamination
    B. Using minocycline/rifampin impregnated catheters over chlorhexidine/silver sulfadiazine impregnated catheters for suspected long term use
    C. Using the subclavian over the internal jugular route for access
    D. Using a single lumen over a multi-lumen catheter
    E. Changing the central catheter every 3 to 4 days over a guidewire.

144. Signs of Sarin nerve gas poisoning include all of the following **EXCEPT**
   A. Diarrhea
   B. Urination
   C. Mydriasis
   D. Bronchoconstriction
   E. Lacrimation

145. Which of the following conditions would be associated with the **LEAST** risk of venous air embolism during removal of a central line?
   A. Spontaneous breathing, head up
   B. Spontaneous breathing, flat
   C. Spontaneous breathing, Trendelenburg
   D. Mechanical ventilation, head up
   E. Mechanical ventilation, Trendelenburg

146. Which of the following adverse effects is **NOT** attributable to respiratory or metabolic acidosis?
   A. Increased incidence of cardiac dysrhythmias
   B. Vasoconstriction
   C. Increased pulmonary vascular resistance
   D. Increased serum potassium concentration
   E. Increased intracranial pressure

147. Which of the following maneuvers is **LEAST** likely to raise arterial saturation in a patient in whom the endotracheal tube (ETT) is seated in the right mainstem bronchus? The patient has normal lung function.
   A. Inflating the pulmonary artery catheter balloon (in the left pulmonary artery)
   B. Raising hemoglobin from 8 mg/dL to 12 mg/dL
   C. Raising F_{IO_2} from 0.8 to 1.0
   D. Increasing cardiac output from 2 to 5 L/min
   E. Withdrawing the tube into the trachea

148. A 100-kg male patient is 24 hours status post four-vessel coronary artery bypass graft. Which of the following pulmonary parameters would be compatible with successful extubation in this patient?
   A. Vital capacity 2.5 L
   B. $Paco_2$ 44 mm Hg
   C. Maximum inspiratory pressure 38 cm H_2O
   D. Pao_2 155 mm Hg on F_{IO_2} 0.40
   E. All of the above

149. Which of the following can cause a rightward shift of the oxyhemoglobin dissociation curve?
   A. Methemoglobinemia
   B. Carboxyhemoglobinemia
   C. Hypothermia
   D. Pregnancy
   E. Alkalosis

150. A 24-year-old patient is brought to the operating room one hour after motor vehicle accident. He has C7 spinal cord transection and ruptured spleen. Regarding his neurologic injury, anesthetic concerns include
   A. Risk of hyperkalemia with succinylcholine administration
   B. Risk of autonomic hyperreflexia with urinary catheter insertion
   C. Need for fiberoptic intubation
   D. Increased risk of hypothermia
   E. All of the above

151.   After sustaining traumatic brain injury, a 37-year-old patient in the ICU develops polyuria and a plasma sodium concentration of 159 mEq/L. What pathologic condition is associated with these clinical findings?
A. Syndrome of inappropriate antidiuretic hormone (SIADH)
B. Diabetes mellitus
C. Diabetes insipidus
D. Cerebral salt wasting syndrome
E. Spinal shock

152.   Which of the following drugs is best choice for treating hypotension in the setting of severe acidemia?
A. Norepinephrine
B. Epinephrine
C. Phenylephrine
D. Vasopressin
E. Dopamine

153.   The end tidal CO_2 measured by a mass spectrometer is 35 mm Hg. An arterial blood gas sample drawn at exactly the same moment is 45 mm Hg. Which of the following is the **LEAST** plausible explanation for this?
A. Cystic fibrosis
B. Pulmonary embolism
C. Intrapulmonary shunt
D. Chronic obstructive pulmonary disease (COPD)
E. Morbid obesity

154.   A transfusion related lung injury (TRALI) reaction is suspected in 48 year old man in the ICU after a 10 hour operation for scoliosis during which multiple units of blood and factors were administered. Which of the following items is inconsistent with the diagnosis of a TRALI reaction?
A. Fever
B. Arterial to alveolar oxygen gradient of 25 mm Hg
C. Acute rise in neutrophil count after onset of symptoms
D. Bilateral pulmonary infiltrates
E. High pulmonary pressures with hyperdynamic left ventricular function

155.   If a central line located in the superior vena cava (SVC) is withdrawn such that the tip of the catheter is just proximal to the SVC, it would be located in which vessel?
A. Subclavian vein
B. Brachiocephalic vein
C. Cephalic vein
D. Internal jugular vein
E. External jugular vein

156.   The time course of anticoagulation therapy is variable after different percutaneous coronary interventions (PCI). Arrange the interventions in order starting with the one requiring the shortest course of aspirin and clopidogrel (Plavix) therapy to the one requiring the longest course.
A. Bare metal stent, percutaneous transluminal coronary angioplasty (PTCA), drug eluting stent
B. Drug eluting stent, bare metal stent, PTCA
C. PTCA, drug eluting stent, bare metal stent
D. PTCA, bare metal stent, drug eluting stent
E. Bare metal stent, drug eluting stent, PTCA

157.   Basic Life Support Working Group's single rescuer cardiac compression-ventilation ratio for infant, child and adult victims (excluding newborns) is
A. 10: 1
B. 15: 2
C. 30: 2
D. 60: 2
E. None of the above

158. Which of the features below is suggestive of weaponized anthrax exposure as opposed to a common flu-like viral illness?
  A. Widened mediastinum
  B. Fever, chills
  C. Cough
  D. Pharyngitis
  E. Myalgia

159. Which of the following factors could not explain a Pa_{O_2} of 48 mm Hg in a patient breathing a mixture of nitrous oxide and oxygen?
  A. Hypoxic gas mixture
  B. Eisenmenger syndrome
  C. Profound anemia
  D. Hypercarbia
  E. Lab error

160. During a left hepatectomy under general isoflurane anesthesia, arterial blood gases are: O_2 138, CO_2 39, pH 7.38, saturation 99%. At the same time, CO_2 on mass spectrometer is 26 mm Hg. The most plausible explanation for the difference between CO_2 measured with mass spectrometer versus arterial blood gas gradient is
  A. Mainstem intubation
  B. Atelectasis
  C. Shunting through thebesian veins
  D. Hypovolemia
  E. Ablation of hypoxic pulmonary vasoconstriction by isoflurane

161. Under which set of circumstance would energy expenditure per day be the greatest?
  A. Sepsis with fever
  B. 60% burn
  C. Multiple fractures
  D. 1 hour status post after liver transplantation
  E. After 20 days of starvation

162. Select the **FALSE** statement regarding amiodarone (Cordarone)
  A. It is shown to decrease mortality after myocardial infarction
  B. It is indicated for ventricular tachycardia and fibrillation refractory to electrical defibrillation
  C. Adverse effects include pulmonary fibrosis and thyroid dysfunction
  D. It has an elimination half-time of 29 days
  E. It is useful in treatment of torsades de pointes

163. A 58-year-old woman is awaiting orthotopic liver transplantation for primary biliary cirrhosis in the ICU. An oximetric pulmonary artery catheter is placed and an Sv_{O_2} of 90% is measured. Which of the following blood pressure interventions is the **LEAST** appropriate for treatment of hypotension in this patient?
  A. Milrinone
  B. Norepinephrine
  C. Vasopressin
  D. Phenylephrine
  E. Epinephrine

164. Recombinant human activated protein C (Xigris) is indicated in the treatment of
  A. Factor V Leiden deficiency
  B. Heparin induced thrombocytopenia
  C. Septic shock
  D. Acute respiratory distress syndrome
  E. Disseminated intravascular coagulation (DIC)

165. A 55-year-old main with polycystic liver disease undergoes an eight-hour right hepatectomy. The patient receives 5 units of packed red cell, 1000 mL Hextend and 6 L normal saline. The patient is extubated and taken to a postanesthesia care unit (PACU) where ABGs are: Pao_2 135, $Paco_2$ 44, pH 7.17, base deficit −11, Hco_3^-, 12, 97% saturation, [Cl] 119, [Na^+] 145, and [K^+] 5.6. The most likely cause for this acidosis is
      A. Lactic acid
      B. Use of normal saline
      C. Diabetic ketoacidosis
      D. Narcotics
      E. Ethylene glycol from bowel prep

166. Which of the following is the **LEAST** appropriate use of non-invasive positive pressure ventilation (NIPPV)?
      A. Acute respiratory distress syndrome (ARDS)
      B. Chronic obstructive pulmonary disease (COPD) exacerbation
      C. Obstructive sleep apnea
      D. Multiple sclerosis exacerbation
      E. Human immunodeficiency virus (HIV) patient with acute hypoxic respiratory failure

167. A 68-year-old asthmatic, drunk driver comes into the ER after being in a motor vehicle accident. After a difficult intubation you fail to observe end-tidal CO_2 on the monitor. Reasons for this include all of the following **EXCEPT**
      A. You intubated the esophagus by mistake
      B. You forgot to ventilate the patient
      C. The connection between the circuit and monitor has become disconnected
      D. The patient also has a pneumothorax and high airway pressures are needed to adequately ventilate the patient
      E. The patient has also sustained a cardiac arrest

168. A 30-year-old woman has undergone a 2 hour abdominal surgical procedure and is sent to the ICU intubated for postoperative monitoring due to suspected sepsis. Three hours later, the ventilator malfunctions and the resident disconnects the patient from the ventilator and hand ventilates the patient with 100% oxygen. The patient has good bilateral breath sounds, the chest rises nicely and moisture is seen in the endotracheal tube. Shortly thereafter, the patient's heart rate slows. The heart rate is 30 and the blood pressure is 50 systolic. The next thing that should be done in addition to chest compressions is
      A. Atropine
      B. Epinephrine
      C. Isoproterenol infusion
      D. External pacing
      E. Recheck the endotracheal tube position

Respiratory Physiology and Critical Care

Answers, References, and Explanations

91. (E) A volume-cycled ventilator set to deliver a volume of 750 mL at a rate of 10/min would deliver a minute ventilation of 7.5 L. The measured minute ventilation, however, is only 6 L; therefore, 1.5 L must be absorbed by the breathing circuit. This volume is known as the compression volume. If one divides the volume by 10 (number of breaths/min), then one determines the compression volume/breath. This number (mL) can be further divided by the peak inflation pressure (cm H_2O) to determine the actual compression factor, which in this case is 5 mL (cm $H_2O)^{-1}$ (*Stoelting: Basics of Anesthesia, ed 5, p 195*).

$$\text{Compression Volume} = \frac{(\dot{V}_{delivered} - \dot{V}_{measured}) / \text{Respiratory Rate}}{\text{Peak Airway Pressure (cm } H_2O)} = 5 \text{ mL (cm } H_2O)^{-1}$$

92. (E) The metabolism of nitroprusside in the body requires the conversion of oxyhemoglobin (Fe^{++}) to methemoglobin (Fe^{+++}). The presence of sufficient quantities of methemoglobin in the blood will cause the pulse oximeter to read 85% saturation regardless of the true arterial saturation. Cyanide toxicity is also a possibility in any patient who is receiving nitroprusside. Cyanide toxicity should be suspected when the patient develops metabolic acidosis or becomes resistant to the hypotensive effects of this drug despite a sufficient infusion rate. This can be confirmed by measuring the mixed venous Pao_2, which would be elevated in the presence of cyanide toxicity. Thiocyanate toxicity is also a potential hazard of nitroprusside administration in patients with renal failure. Patients suffering from thiocyanate toxicity display nausea, mental confusion, and skeletal-muscle weakness (*Miller: Anesthesia, ed 6, pp 1450, 2187; Stoelting: Pharmacology and Physiology, ed 4, pp 357-358*).

93. (D) FRC is composed of expiratory reserve volume plus residual volume. It is essential to maximize FRC in the postoperative period to ensure that it will be greater than closing volume. Closing volume is that lung volume at which small-airway closure begins to occur. Maximizing FRC, therefore, reduces atelectasis and lessens the incidence of arterial hypoxemia and pneumonia. Maneuvers aimed at increasing FRC include early ambulation, incentive spirometry, deep breathing, and intermittent positive pressure breathing (*Barash: Clinical Anesthesia, ed 5, pp 804-805*).

94. (C)

$$PVR = \frac{(PAP_{mean} - PAOP)}{CO} \times 80$$

where PVR is the pulmonary vascular resistance, PAP_{mean} is the mean pulmonary artery pressure, PAOP is the mean pulmonary capillary occlusion pressure, and CO is the cardiac output.

$$PVR = \frac{(20-12)}{4} \times 80 = 160 \text{ dynes-sec-cm}^{-5}$$

The normal range for PVR is 50 to 150 dynes-sec-cm^{-5} (*Miller: Anesthesia, ed 6, pp 1333-1334*).

95. (E) For reasons that are not fully understood, patients who have sustained a myocardial infarction and subsequently undergo surgery are most likely to have another infarction on the third postoperative day (*Stoelting: Basics of Anesthesia, ed 5, p 367*).

96. (B) Calculation of body mass index (BMI) is a convenient way to define obesity and morbid obesity (>31 kg/m^2). Obesity, defined as a weight 25% greater than ideal body weight, would correspond to a BMI of 27 for women and 28 for men.

$$BMI = \frac{mass \ (kg)}{(Height)^2 \ (meters)}$$

$$BMI = \frac{100}{(2)^2} = 25$$

All major organ systems are affected as a consequence of obesity. The greatest concerns for the anesthesiologist are, however, related to the heart and lungs. Cardiac output must increase about 0.1 L/min for each extra kilogram of adipose tissue. As a consequence, obese patients frequently are hypertensive, and many ultimately develop cardiomegaly and left-sided heart failure. FRC is reduced in obese patients and management of the airway often can be difficult (*Miller: Anesthesia, ed 6, pp 1028-1029*).

97.   (B)   The forced expiratory volume in 1 second (FEV_1) is the total volume of air that can be exhaled in the first second. Normal healthy adults can exhale approximately 75% to 85% of their forced vital capacity (FVC) in the first second, 94% in 2 seconds and 97% in 3 seconds. Therefore, the normal FEV_1/FVC ratio is 0.75 or higher. In the presence of obstructive airway disease, the FEV_1/FVC ratio less than 70% reflects mild obstruction, less than 60% moderate obstruction and less than 50% severe obstruction. This ratio can be used to determine the severity of obstructive airway disease and to monitor the efficacy of bronchodilator therapy (*Barash: Clinical Anesthesia, ed 5, p 805; Miller: Anesthesia, ed 6, pp 1000-1001*).

98.   (C)   Multifocal atrial tachycardia (MAT) is a non-reentrant, ectopic atrial rhythm often seen in patients with chronic obstructive pulmonary disease (COPD). It is frequently confused with atrial fibrillation but, in contrast to atrial fibrillation, atrial flutter, and paroxysmal supraventricular tachycardia, DC cardioversion is ineffective in converting it to normal sinus rhythm. Ectopic atrial tachydysrhythmias are not amenable to cardioversion because they lack the reentrant mechanism, which is necessary for successful termination with electrical counter shock (*Miller: Anesthesia, ed 6, pp 2930-2933*).

99.   (C)   During apnea, the Pa_{CO_2} will increase approximately 6 mm Hg during the first minute and then 3 to 4 mm Hg each minute thereafter (*Miller: Anesthesia, ed 6, p 1901*).

100.   (A)   Total parenteral nutrition (TPN) therapy is associated with numerous potential complications. Blood sugars need to be carefully monitored since hyperglycemia may develop due to the high glucose load and require treatment with insulin, and hypoglycemia may develop if TPN is abruptly stopped (i.e., infusion turned off or mechanical obstruction in the IV tubing). Other complications include electrolyte disturbances (e.g., hypokalemia, hypophosphatemia, hypomagnesemia, hypocalcemia), volume overload, catheter-related sepsis, renal and hepatic dysfunction, thrombosis of the central veins, and nonketotic hyperosmolar coma. Increased work of breathing is related to increased production of CO_2 most frequently due to overfeeding. Acidosis in these patients is hyperchloremic metabolic acidosis resulting from formation of HCl during metabolism of amino acids. Ketoacidosis is not associated with TPN therapy (*Hines: Stoelting's Anesthesia and Co-Existing Disease, ed 5, p 312*).

101.   (B)   The O_2 requirement for an adult is 3 to 4 mL/kg/min. The O_2 requirement for a newborn is 7 to 9 mL/kg/min. Alveolar ventilation (V_A) in neonates is double that of adults to help meet their increased O_2 requirements. This increase in V_A is achieved primarily by an increase in respiratory rate as V_T is similar to that of adults (i.e., 7 mL/kg). Although CO_2 production also is increased in neonates, the elevated V_A maintains the Pa_{CO_2} near 38 to 40 mm Hg (*Barash: Clinical Anesthesia, ed 5, pp 1186-1187*).

102.   (A)   A comprehensive understanding of respiratory physiology is important for understanding the effects of both regional and general anesthesia on respiratory mechanics and pulmonary gas exchange. The volume of gas remaining in the lungs after a normal expiration is called the functional residual capacity. The volume of gas remaining in the lungs after a maximal expiration is called the residual volume. The difference between these two volumes is called the expiratory reserve volume. Therefore, the FRC is composed of the expiratory reserve volume and residual volume (*Barash: Clinical Anesthesia, ed 5, pp 804-805; Stoelting: Pharmacology and Physiology in Anesthetic Practice, ed 4, pp 776-777*).

LUNG VOLUMES AND CAPACITIES

Measurement	Abbreviation	Normal Adult Value
Tidal volume	V_T	500 mL (6-8 mL/kg)
Inspiratory reserve volume	IRV	3000 mL
Expiratory reserve volume	ERV	1200 mL
Residual volume	RV	1200 mL
Inspiratory capacity	IC	3500 mL
Functional residual capacity	FRC	2400 mL
Vital capacity	VC	4500 mL (60-70 mL/kg)
Forced exhaled volume in 1 second	FEV_1	80%
Total lung capacity	TLC	5900 mL

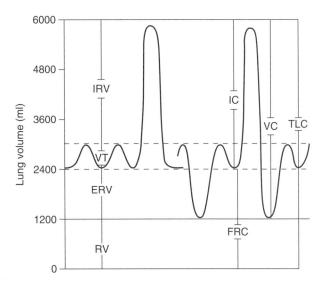

103. (A) The volume of gas in the conducting airways of the lungs (and not available for gas exchange) is called the anatomic dead space. The volume of gas in ventilated alveoli that are unperfused (and not available for gas exchange) is called the functional dead space. The anatomic dead space together with the functional dead space is called the physiologic dead space. Physiologic dead-space ventilation (V_D) can be calculated by the Bohr dead-space equation, which is mathematically expressed as follows:

$$V_D/V_T = \frac{(Pa_{CO_2} - Pe_{CO_2})}{Pa_{CO_2}}$$

where V_D/V_T is the ratio of V_D to V_T, and the subscripts a and E represent arterial and mixed expired, respectively. Of the choices given, only the first is correct. A large increase in V_D will result in an increase in Pa_{CO_2} (*Barash: Clinical Anesthesia, ed 5, pp 801-803; Miller: Anesthesia, ed 6, pp 697-698; West: Respiratory Physiology, ed 6, pp 16-18*).

104. (C) The oxygen content of blood can be calculated with the following formula:

O_2 content = (1.39 × hemoglobin × arterial saturation) + (0.003 × Pa_{O_2})

First oxygen content = (1.39 × 15 × 1.0) + 0.003 × 120 = 21.21 mL/dL

Second oxygen content = (1.39 × 15 × 1.0) + 0.003 × 150 = 21.30 mL/dL

The difference in the oxygen content is 0.09 mL/dL. This represents a change of 0.42% (*Stoelting: Basics of Anesthesia, ed 5, p 327*).

105.   **(B)**   The degree of ventilatory depression caused by volatile anesthetics can be assessed by measuring resting Pa_{CO_2}, the ventilatory response to hypercarbia, and the ventilatory response to hypoxemia. Of these techniques, the resting Pa_{CO_2} is the most frequently used index. However, measuring the effects of increased Pa_{CO_2} on ventilation is the most sensitive method of quantifying the effects of drugs on ventilation. In awake unanesthetized humans, inhalation of CO_2 increases minute ventilation $\dot{V}_E$ by approximately 2 to 3 L/min/mm Hg increase in Pa_{CO_2}. Using this technique, halothane, isoflurane, enflurane, and N_2O cause a dose-dependent depression of the ventilation (*Miller: Anesthesia, ed 6, pp 178-179; Stoelting: Basics of Anesthesia, ed 5, pp 92-93; Stoelting: Pharmacology and Physiology in Anesthetic Practice, ed 4, pp 60-61, 780*).

106.   **(B)**   The amount of O_2 in blood (O_2 content) is the sum of the amount of O_2 dissolved in plasma and the amount of O_2 combined with hemoglobin. The amount of O_2 dissolved in plasma is directly proportional to the product of the blood/gas solubility coefficient of O_2 (0.003) and Pa_{O_2}. The amount of O_2 bound to hemoglobin is directly related to the fraction of hemoglobin that is saturated. One gram of hemoglobin can bind 1.39 mL of O_2. The mathematical expression of O_2 content is as follows:

$$O_2 \text{ content} = 1.39 \times [\text{Hgb}] \times Sa_{O_2} + (0.003 \times Pa_{O_2})$$

where [Hgb] is the hemoglobin concentration (g/dL), Sa_{O_2} is the fraction of hemoglobin saturated with O_2, and $(0.003 \times Pa_{O_2})$ is the amount of O_2 dissolved in plasma. In this case $(1.39 \times 10 \times 0.9) + (0.003 \times 60) = 12.51 + 0.18 = 12.69$ or approximately 13 mL/dL (*Miller: Anesthesia, ed 6, p 2812; Stoelting: Basics of Anesthesia, ed 5, p 327*).

107.   **(C)**   The presence of hemoglobin species other than oxyhemoglobin can cause erroneous readings by dual-wavelength pulse oximeters. Hemoglobin species such as carboxyhemoglobin and methemoglobin, dyes such as methylene blue and indocyanine green, and some colors of nail polish will cause erroneous readings. Because the absorption spectrum of fetal hemoglobin is similar to that of adult oxyhemoglobin, fetal hemoglobin does not significantly affect the accuracy of these types of pulse oximeters. High levels of bilirubin have no significant effect on the accuracy of dual-wavelength pulse oximeters, but may cause falsely low readings by nonpulsatile oximeters (*Miller: Anesthesia, ed 6, pp 1450-1452*).

108.   **(C)**   The compensatory shift of the oxyhemoglobin dissociation curve toward normal in response to chronic acid-base abnormalities is a result of altered erythrocyte-2,3-DPG metabolism (*Miller: Anesthesia, ed 6, p 701*).

109.   **(B)** P_{50} is the Pa_{O_2} required to produce 50% saturation of hemoglobin. The P_{50} for adult hemoglobin at a pH of 7.4 and body temperature of 37° C is 26 mm Hg (*Stoelting: Pharmacology and Physiology in Anesthetic Practice, ed 4, pp 788-789*).

110.   **(D)**   The work of breathing is defined as the product of transpulmonary pressure and V_T. The work of breathing is related to two factors: the work required to overcome the elastic forces of the lungs and the work required to overcome airflow or frictional resistances of the airways (*Barash: Clinical Anesthesia, ed 5, pp 793-794; Miller: Anesthesia, ed 6, pp 692-693*).

111.   **(D)**   The normal mixed venous O_2 saturation is 75%. Physiologic factors that affect mixed venous O_2 saturation include hemoglobin concentration, arterial Pa_{O_2}, cardiac output, and O_2 consumption. Anemia, hypoxia, decreased cardiac output, and increased O_2 consumption decrease mixed venous O_2 saturation. During sepsis with adequate volume resuscitation, the cardiac output is increased and maldistribution of perfusion (distributive shock) results in an elevated mixed-venous O_2 saturation. Mixed venous O_2 saturation ($S\bar{v}_{O_2}$) is related to a number of factors, as shown in this equation:

$$S\bar{v}_{O_2} = Sa_{O_2} - \left(\frac{\dot{V}_{O_2}}{13.9 \times \dot{Q} \times \text{Hgb}} \right)$$

where Hgb is hemoglobin concentration, 13.9 is a constant (O_2 combining power of Hgb [mL/10 g]), $\dot{Q}$ is cardiac output, and $\dot{V}_{O_2}$ is the oxygen consumption (*Barash: Clinical Anesthesia, ed 5, p 679; Miller: Anesthesia, ed 6, pp 1331-1332*).

112. (C) The volume of gas exhaled during a maximum expiration is the vital capacity. In a normal healthy adult, the vital capacity is 60 to 70 mL/kg. In a 70-kg patient, the vital capacity is approximately 5 L (*Stoelting: Pharmacology and Physiology in Anesthetic Practice, ed 4, p 776; Barash: Clinical Anesthesia, ed 5, p 804*).

113. (C) Carbon monoxide inhalation is the most common immediate cause of death from fire. Carbon monoxide binds to hemoglobin with an affinity 200 times greater than that of oxygen. For this reason very small concentrations of carbon monoxide can greatly reduce the oxygen-carrying capacity of blood. In spite of this, the arterial Pao_2 often is normal. Because the carotid bodies respond to arterial Pao_2, there would not be an increase in minute ventilation until tissue hypoxia were sufficient to produce lactic acidosis (*Hines: Stoelting's Anesthesia and Co-Existing Disease, ed 5, pp 552-553; Miller: Anesthesia, ed 6, pp 2671-2672; West: Respiratory Physiology, ed 6, pp 66-69*).

114. (D) Respiratory acidosis is present when the $Paco_2$ exceeds 44 mm Hg. Respiratory acidosis is caused by decreased elimination of CO_2 by the lungs (i.e., hypoventilation) or increased metabolic production of CO_2. An acute increase in $Paco_2$ of 10 mm Hg will result in a decrease in pH of approximately 0.08 pH units. The acidosis of arterial blood will stimulate ventilation via the carotid bodies and the acidosis of cerebrospinal fluid will stimulate ventilation via the medullary chemoreceptors located in the fourth cerebral ventricle. Volatile anesthetics greatly attenuate the carotid body-mediated and aortic body-mediated ventilatory responses to arterial acidosis, but they have little effect on the medullary chemoreceptor-mediated ventilatory response to cerebrospinal fluid acidosis (*Stoelting: Basics of Anesthesia, ed 5, p 321; West: Respiratory Physiology, ed 6, pp 72-74*).

115. (B) Metabolic acidosis occurs when the pH is less than 7.36 and $[HCO_3^-]$ is less than 24 mEq/L. A decrease in $[HCO_3^-]$ is caused by decreased elimination of [H+] by the renal tubules (e.g., renal tubular acidosis) or increased metabolic production of [H+] relative to $[HCO_3^-]$ (e.g., lactic acidosis, ketoacidosis, or uremia). Total body deficit in $[HCO_3^-]$ can be estimated using the following formula:
Total body deficit (mEq) = Total body weight (kg) × Deviation of $[HCO_3^-]$ from 24 mEq/L × Extracellular fluid volume as a fraction of body mass (0.3)
The total body deficit in $[HCO_3^-]$ in this patient is 75 × (24 − 6) × 0.3 = 405 mEq. When administering sodium bicarbonate, half the calculated dose is administered and repeat measurements are made to determine the need for further treatment (*Barash: Clinical Anesthesia, ed 5, pp 177-178; Stoelting: Basics of Anesthesia, ed 5, p 323*).

116. (D) Respiratory alkalosis is present when the $Paco_2$ is less than 36 mm Hg. There are three compensatory mechanisms responsible for attenuating the increase in pH that accompanies respiratory alkalosis. First, there is an immediate shift in the equilibrium of the $[HCO_3^-]$ buffer system, which results in the production of CO_2. Second, alkalosis stimulates the activity of phosphofructokinase, which increases glycolysis and the production of pyruvate and lactic acid. Third, there is a decrease in reabsorption of $[HCO_3^-]$ by the proximal and distal renal tubules. These three compensatory mechanisms result in a maximum decrease in $[HCO3^-]$ of approximately 5 mEq/L for every 10 mm Hg decrease in $Paco_2$ less than 40 mm Hg (*Stoelting: Basics of Anesthesia, ed 5, pp 320-321*).

117. (D) Mechanical ventilation of the lungs can be accomplished by various modes. These modes are categorized as controlled, assisted, assisted/controlled, controlled with positive end-expiratory pressure (PEEP), and assisted/controlled using intermittent mandatory ventilation (IMV). Assisted/controlled modes of mechanical ventilation are best used in patients when the muscles of respiration require rest because minimal breathing efforts are required. IMV exercises inspiratory muscles and decreases mean thoracic pressure and thus is used most frequently when weaning patients from mechanical ventilation. With the assisted/controlled mode of ventilation, positive-pressure ventilation is triggered by small breathing efforts produced by the patient. The airway pressure tracing shown is typical of that of a patient requiring assisted/controlled ventilation (*Hines: Stoelting's Anesthesia and Co-Existing Disease, ed 5, pp 187-188*).

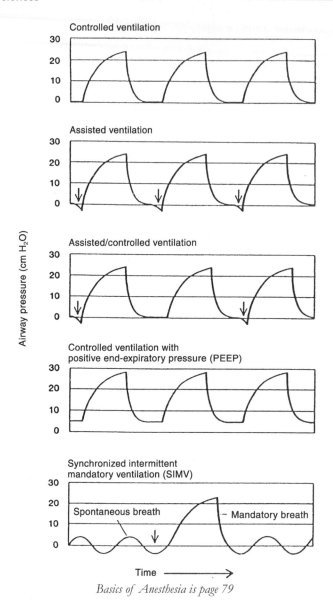

Basics of Anesthesia is page 79

118.   **(C)**   The first step in evaluating any patient with a tachycardia is to determine if the patient is hemodynamically stable or unstable (serious signs or symptoms are chest pain or congestive heart failure due to the tachycardia). In the unstable patient, DC cardioversion should be performed for rapid heart rate control regardless of the duration of atrial fibrillation. In this case, where the patient is reasonably stable, the three major goals in the management of atrial fibrillation should be considered. These goals are control of ventricular rate, assessment of anticoagulation needs, and conversion to sinus rhythm. In addition, the underlying cause of atrial fibrillation should be sought and treated. Because this patient is febrile and may be dehydrated, an intravenous (IV) line for fluid resuscitation should be initiated. Because we do not know when atrial fibrillation developed (after 48 hours embolic events may occur with conversion to sinus rhythm), it would be best not to convert the atrial fibrillation to sinus rhythm using either ibutilide or procainamide until the patient is adequately anticoagulated. Adequate anticoagulation should usually be therapeutic for at least 3 weeks. In marginal cases where the duration of atrial fibrillation is uncertain, cardiac consultation and transesophageal echocardiography to exclude atrial thrombus should be performed before cardioversion. This patient should undergo cardiac echocardiographic study to look for intra-atrial thrombus and to determine the ejection fraction (EF) of the ventricle. After adequate hydration, rate control could be improved with calcium channel blockers or beta-blockers in patients with preserved left ventricular function (EF > 40%) or with digoxin, diltiazem, or amiodarone if EF is less than 40% (*2005 AHA Guidelines for CPR and Emergency Cardiovascular Care: Circulation 112 (Suppl. I): IV 67 - IV 77, 2005*).

119.   **(C)**   A P_{50} less than 26 mm Hg defines a leftward shift of the oxyhemoglobin dissociation curve. This means that at any given Pao_2, hemoglobin has a higher affinity for O_2. A P_{50} greater than 26 mm Hg describes a rightward

shift of the oxyhemoglobin dissociation curve. This means that at any given Pa_{O_2}, hemoglobin has a lower affinity for O_2. Conditions that cause a rightward shift of the oxyhemoglobin dissociation curve are metabolic and respiratory acidosis, hyperthermia, increased erythrocyte 2,3-DPG content, pregnancy, and abnormal hemoglobins, such as sickle cell hemoglobin or thalassemia. Alkalosis, hypothermia, fetal hemoglobin, abnormal hemoglobin species, such as carboxyhemoglobin, methemoglobin, and sulfhemoglobin, and decreased erythrocyte 2,3-DPG content will cause a leftward shift of the oxyhemoglobin dissociation curve. Also see explanation to question 109 (*Miller: Anesthesia, ed 6, pp 699-701; Stoelting: Pharmacology and Physiology in Anesthetic Practice, ed 4, pp 788-789*).

120. (B) The effects of Pa_{CO_2} and pH on the position of the oxyhemoglobin dissociation curve is known as the Bohr effect. Hypercarbia and acidosis shift the curve to the right, and hypocarbia and alkalosis shift the curve to the left. The Bohr effect is attributed primarily to the action of CO_2 and pH on erythrocyte 2,3-DPG metabolism (*Miller: Anesthesia, ed 6, p 703*).

121. (C) The rate at which a gas diffuses through a lipid membrane is directly proportional to the area of the membrane, the transmembrane partial pressure gradient of the gas, and the diffusion coefficient of the gas, and it is inversely proportional to the thickness of the membrane. The diffusion coefficient of the gas is directly proportional to the square root of gas solubility and is inversely proportional to the square root of the molecular weight of the gas. This is known as Fick's law of diffusion (*Barash: Clinical Anesthesia, ed 5, p 1154*).

122. (E) Aging is associated with reduced ventilatory volumes and capacities, and decreased efficiency of pulmonary gas exchange. These changes are caused by progressive stiffening of cartilage and replacement of elastic tissue in the intercostal and intervertebral areas, which decreases compliance of the thoracic cage. In addition, progressive kyphosis or scoliosis produces upward and anterior rotation of the ribs and sternum, which further restricts chest wall expansion during inspiration. With aging, the FRC, residual volume, and closing volume are increased, whereas the vital capacity, total lung capacity, maximum breathing capacity, FEV_1, and ventilatory response to hypercarbia and hypoxemia are reduced. In addition, age-related changes in lung parenchyma, alveolar surface area, and diminished pulmonary capillary bed density cause ventilation/perfusion mismatch, which decreases resting Pa_{O_2} (*Hines: Stoelting's Anesthesia and Co-Existing Disease, ed 4, p 641; Stoelting: Basics of Anesthesia, ed 5, pp 519-520*).

123. (C) Physiologic dead-space ventilation can be estimated using the Bohr equation (described in the explanation to question 103):

$$V_D/V_T = \frac{45 \text{ mm Hg} - 30 \text{ mm Hg}}{45 \text{ mm Hg}} = \frac{15 \text{ mm Hg}}{45 \text{ mm Hg}} = 0.33$$

(*Barash: Clinical Anesthesia, ed 5, pp 801-803; Miller: Anesthesia, ed 6, pp 697-698.*)

124. (A) The ventilation/perfusion ratio is greater at the apex of the lungs than at the base of the lungs. Thus, dependent regions of the lungs are hypoxic and hypercarbic compared to the nondependent regions. Also see explanation to question 132 (*Miller: Anesthesia, ed 6, pp 679-683; West: Respiratory Physiology, ed 6, pp 18, 19, 37, 38*).

125. (A) The degree to which a person can hypoventilate to compensate for metabolic alkalosis is limited; hence, this is the least well-compensated acid-based disturbance. Respiratory compensation for metabolic alkalosis is rarely more than 75% complete. Hypoventilation to a Pa_{CO_2} greater than 55 mm Hg is the maximum respiratory compensation for metabolic alkalosis. A Pa_{CO_2} greater than 55 mm Hg most likely reflects concomitant respiratory acidosis (*Stoelting: Basics of Anesthesia, ed 5, p 323*).

126. (E) Pa_{O_2} can be estimated using the alveolar gas equation, which is given as follows:

$$Pa_{O_2} = (P_B - 47)F_{IO_2} - \frac{Pa_{CO_2}}{R}$$

where P_B is the barometric pressure (mm Hg), F_{IO_2} is the fraction of inspired O_2, Pa_{CO_2} is the arterial CO_2 tension (mm Hg), and R is the respiratory quotient (*Barash: Clinical Anesthesia, ed 5, p 803; West: Respiratory Physiology, ed 6, p 47*).

127. (E) When arterial sampling is not possible, "arterialized" venous blood can be used to estimate ABG tensions. Because blood in the veins on the back of the hands has very little O_2 extracted, the O_2 content in this blood best approximates the O_2 content in a sample of blood obtained from an artery (*Stoelting: Basics of Anesthesia, ed 5, p 324*).

128. (D) Pulmonary function tests can be divided into those that assess ventilatory capacity and those that assess pulmonary gas exchange. The simplest test to assess ventilatory capacity is the FEV1/FVC ratio. Other tests to assess ventilatory capacity include the maximum mid-expiratory flow (FEF 25%-75%), MVV, and flow-volume curves. The most significant disadvantage of these tests is that they are dependent on patient effort. However, because the FEF 25%-75% is obtained from the mid-expiratory portion of the flow-volume loop, it is least dependent on patient effort. Also see explanation to question 97 (*Barash: Clinical Anesthesia, ed 5, p 805; Miller: Anesthesia, ed 6, pp 1000-1001*).

129. (A) Carbon monoxide binds to hemoglobin with an affinity greater than 200 times that of oxygen. This stabilizes the oxygen-hemoglobin complex and hinders release of oxygen to the tissues, leading to a leftward shift of the oxyhemoglobin dissociation curve. The diagnosis is suggested when there is a low oxygen hemoglobin saturation in the face of a normal Pa_{O_2}. The two-wave pulse oximeter cannot distinguish oxyhemoglobin from carboxyhemoglobin so that a normal oxyhemoglobin saturation would be observed in the presence of high concentrations of carboxyhemoglobin. Carbon monoxide poisoning is not associated with cyanosis. See also explanations for questions 113 and 140. (*Hines: Stoelting's Anesthesia and Co-Existing Disease, ed 5, pp 552-553; Miller: Anesthesia, ed 6, pp 1447-1448, 2671-2672*).

130. (B) The fraction of total cardiac output that traverses the pulmonary circulation without participating in gas exchange is called the transpulmonary shunt. It can be calculated exactly by the equation:

$$\dot{Q}_s/\dot{Q}_T = \frac{Cc'_{O_2} - Ca_{O_2}}{Cc'_{O_2} - C\bar{v}_{O_2}}$$

where Cc', Ca, and $C\bar{v}_{O_2}$ stand for the content of oxygen in the alveolar capillary, artery, and mixed venous samples respectively. This information is not provided in the question; however, the alveolar to arterial partial pressure of oxygen difference is using high inspired oxygen concentrations. The alveolar to arterial oxygen difference can be used to estimate venous admixture, most commonly transpulmonary shunt. For every increase in alveolar-arterial O_2 of 20 mm Hg, there is an increase in shunt fraction of 1% of the cardiac output. In the example, 240/20 = 12 and the transpulmonary shunt can be estimated at 12% (*Miller: Anesthesia, ed 6, pp 701-703*).

131. (E) Measuring the ventilatory response to increased Pa_{CO_2} is a sensitive method for quantifying the effects of drugs on ventilation. In general, all volatile anesthetics (including N_2O), narcotics, benzodiazepines, and barbiturates depress the ventilatory response to increased Pa_{CO_2} in a dose-dependent manner. The magnitude of ventilatory depression by volatile anesthetics is greater in patients with COPD than in healthy patients. Arterial blood gases (ABGs) may need to be monitored during recovery from general anesthesia in patients with COPD. Ketamine causes minimal respiratory depression. Typically, respiratory rate is decreased only 2 to 3 breaths/min and the ventilatory response to changes in Pa_{CO_2} is maintained during ketamine anesthesia. Also see explanation to question 105 (*Miller: Anesthesia, ed 6, pp 178-179; Stoelting: Basics of Anesthesia, ed 5, pp 92-93; Stoelting: Pharmacology and Physiology in Anesthetic Practice, ed 4, pp 60-61, 173, 780*).

132. (D) The orientation of the lungs relative to gravity has a profound effect on efficiency of pulmonary gas exchange. Because alveoli in dependent regions of the lungs expand more per unit change in transpulmonary pressure (i.e., are more compliant) than alveoli in nondependent regions of the lungs, $\dot{V}_A$ increases from the top to the bottom of the lungs. Because pulmonary blood flow increases more from the top to the bottom of the lungs than does $\dot{V}_A$, the ventilation/perfusion ratio is high in nondependent regions of the lungs and is low in dependent regions of the lungs. Therefore, in the upright lungs, the Pa_{O_2} and pH are greater at the apex, whereas the Pa_{CO_2} is greater at the base (*Barash: Clinical Anesthesia, ed 5, p 801; Miller: Anesthesia, ed 6, pp 679-683; West: Respiratory Physiology, ed 6, pp 18, 19, 37, 38*).

133. (A) The work required to overcome the elastic recoil of the lungs and thorax, along with airflow or frictional resistances of the airways, contributes to the work of breathing. When the respiratory rate or airway resistance is high or pulmonary or chest wall compliance is reduced, a large amount of energy is spent overcoming the work of breathing. In the healthy resting adult, only 1% to 3% of total O_2 consumption is used for the work

of breathing at rest, but up to 50% may be needed in patients with pulmonary disease. Also see explanation to question 110. (*Miller: Anesthesia, ed 6, pp 692-693*).

134. (B)   The conducting airways (trachea, right and left mainstem bronchi, and lobar and segmental bronchi) do not contain alveoli and therefore do not take part in pulmonary gas exchange. These structures constitute the anatomic dead space. In the adult, the anatomic dead space is approximately 2 mL/kg. The anatomic dead space increases during inspiration because of the traction exerted on the conducting airways by the surrounding lung parenchyma. In addition, the anatomic dead space depends on the size and posture of the subject. Also see explanation to question 103 (*Barash: Clinical Anesthesia, ed 5, pp 801-803; Miller: Anesthesia, ed 6, pp 697; Stoelting: Pharmacology and Physiology in Anesthetic Practice, ed 4, p 778*).

135. (D)   There are three main mechanisms that the body has to prevent changes in pH. The buffer systems (immediate), the ventilatory response (takes minutes) and the renal response (takes hours to days). The buffer systems represent the first line of defense against adverse changes in pH. The $[HCO_3^-]$ buffer system is the most important system and represents greater than 50% of the total buffering capacity of the body. Other important buffer systems include hemoglobin, which is responsible for approximately 35% of the buffering capacity of blood, phosphates, plasma proteins, and bone (*Stoelting: Basics of Anesthesia, ed 5, pp 318-319; Stoelting: Pharmacology and Physiology in Anesthetic Practice, ed 4, pp 794-799*).

136. (A)   Cardiac dysrhythmias are a common complication associated with acid-base abnormalities. The etiology of these dysrhythmias is related partly to the effects of pH on myocardial potassium homeostasis. As a general rule, there is an inverse relationship between [K+] and pH. For every 0.08 unit change in pH there is a reciprocal change in [K+] of approximately 0.5 mEq/L (*Miller: Anesthesia, ed 6, pp 1105-1106*).

137. (B)   There are several guidelines that can be used in the initial interpretation of ABGs that will permit rapid recognition of the type of acid-base disturbance. These guidelines are as follows: 1) a 1 mm Hg change in $Paco_2$ above or below 40 mm Hg results in a 0.008 unit change in the pH in the opposite direction; 2) the $Paco_2$ will decrease by about 1 mm Hg for every 1 mEq/L reduction in $[HCO_3^-]$ below 24 mEq/L; 3) a change in $[HCO_3^-]$ of 10 mEq/L from 24 mEq/L will result in a change in pH of approximately 0.15 pH units in the same direction (*Stoelting: Basics of Anesthesia, ed 5, p 321*).

138. (E)   A patient with a VD of 150 mL and a VA of 350 mL (assuming a normal VT of 500 mL) will have a VD minute ventilation (V̇D) of 1500 mL and a VA minute ventilation (V̇A) of 3500 mL (V̇E of 5000 mL) at a respiratory rate of 10 breaths/min. If the respiratory rate is doubled but V̇E remains unchanged, then the V̇D would double to 3000 mL and there would be an increase in V̇D of 1500 mL and decrease in V̇A of 1500 mL. Also see explanation to questions 103 and 134 (*Barash: Clinical Anesthesia, ed 5, pp 801-803; Miller: Anesthesia, ed 6, pp 697-698; West: Respiratory Physiology, ed 6, pp 14-15*).

139. (B)   In addition to the items listed in this question, other factors that shift the oxyhemoglobin dissociation curve to the right include pregnancy and all abnormal hemoglobins such as hemoglobin S (sickle cell hemoglobin). For reasons unknown, volatile anesthetics increase the P_{50} of adult hemoglobin by 2 to 3.5 mm Hg. A rightward shift of the oxyhemoglobin dissociation curve will decrease the transfer of O_2 from alveoli to hemoglobin and improve release of O_2 from hemoglobin to peripheral tissues. Also see explanation to questions 108 and 109 (*Miller: Anesthesia, ed 6, pp 700-701; Stoelting: Pharmacology and Physiology in Anesthetic Practice, ed 4, pp 788-789; West: Respiratory Physiology, ed 6, pp 64-67*).

140. (B)   The most frequent immediate cause of death from fires is carbon monoxide toxicity. Carbon monoxide is a colorless, odorless gas that exerts its adverse effects by decreasing O_2 delivery to peripheral tissues. This is accomplished by two mechanisms. First, because the affinity of carbon monoxide for the O_2 binding sites on hemoglobin is more than 200 times that of O_2, O_2 is readily displaced from hemoglobin. Thus, O_2 content is reduced. Second, carbon monoxide causes a leftward shift of the oxyhemoglobin dissociation curve, which increases the affinity of hemoglobin for O_2 at peripheral tissues. Treatment of carbon monoxide toxicity is administration of 100% O_2. Supplemental oxygen decreases the half-time of carboxyhemoglobin from 4 to 6 hours with room air to about 1 hour with 100% oxygen. Breathing 100% oxygen at 3 Atm in a hyperbaric chamber reduces the half-time even more to 15-30 minutes. See also explanations for questions 113 and 129 (*Barash: Clinical Anesthesia, ed 5, p 1280; Hines: Stoelting's Anesthesia and Co-Existing Disease, ed 5, pp 552-553; Miller: Anesthesia, ed 6, pp 2671-2672*).

141. (A) Propofol infusion syndrome is a rare condition associated with prolonged (greater than 48 hour) administration of propofol at a dose of 5 mg/kg/hr (83 μg/kg/min) or higher. This syndrome was first described in children, but later observed in critically ill adults as well. It is manifested by cardiomyopathy with acute cardiac failure, metabolic acidosis, skeletal muscle myopathy, hepatomegaly, hyperkalemia and lipidemia. It is thought to be related a failure of free fatty acid transport into the mitochondria and failure of the mitochondrial respiratory chain. Bradycardia can be a late sign with this syndrome and heralds a bad prognosis (*Miller: Anesthesia, ed 6, p 326*).

142. (A) Calculating the anion gap (i.e., the unmeasured anions in the plasma) is helpful in determining the cause of a metabolic acidosis. Anion gap = [Na+] - ([Cl-] + [HCO$_3$-]) and is normally 10 to 12 nmol/L. In this case the anion gap = 138 - (115 + 12) = 11, a normal anion gap. Causes of a high anion gap metabolic acidosis include: lactic acidosis, ketoacidosis, acute and chronic renal failure, as well as toxins (e.g., salicylates, ethylene glycol, methanol). Nonanion gap metabolic acidosis include: renal tubular acidosis, expansion acidosis (e.g., rapid saline infusion), GI bicarbonate loss (e.g., diarrhea, small bowel drainage), drug-induced hyperkalemia and acid loads (e.g., ammonium chloride, hyperalimentation). Vomiting and nasogastric drainage are some of the many causes of metabolic alkalosis (*Kasper: Harrison's Principles of Internal Medicine, ed 16, pp 263-268*).

143. (E) Bloodstream infectious complications with central venous catheters are the most common late complication seen with central catheters (>5%). Current Centers for Disease Control and Prevention (CDC) guidelines do not recommend replacing central venous catheters. All the other statements are true. In addition, evidence is suggesting that the use of ultrasound may decrease the time needed to place catheters and the number of skin punctures needed for central vein access and may also decrease infections *Miller: Anesthesia, ed 6, pp 1289-1296, 2797; O'Grady NP, Alexander M, Dellinger EP, et al: Guidelines for the prevention of intravascular catheter-related infections. Centers for Disease Control and Prevention. MMWR Recomm Rep, 51(RR10):1-29, 2002.*

144. (C) Sarin (also called GB), like GA (Tabun), GD (Soman), GF, VR and VX are all clear liquid organophosphates that vaporize at room temperatures. These chemical nerve gases mainly bind with acetylcholinesterase and produce clinical signs of excessive parasympathetic activity. The term DUMBELS – *D*iarrhea, *U*rination, *M*iosis, *B*ronchorrhea and bronchoconstriction, *E*mesis, *L*acrimation and *S*alivation) can help you remember several of the signs. Note the eye signs are pupillary constriction (miosis) and not pupillary dilation (mydriasis). Other signs relate to the cardiovascular system and include bradycardia, prolonged QT interval as well as ventricular dysrhythmias. These chemicals also affect the GABA and NMDA receptors and may also cause central nervous system (CNS) excitation (i.e., convulsions) (*Barash: Clinical Anesthesia, ed 5, pp 1533-1534; Miller: Anesthesia, ed 6, pp 2504-2509*).

145. (E) Venous air embolism occurs when air enters the venous system through an incised or cannulated vein. When cannulating or decannulating central veins, it is important to keep a positive venous-to-atmospheric pressure gradient. This is usually accomplished by placing the site below the level of the heart (i.e., Trendelenburg position). In addition, under mechanical ventilation or when the spontaneously breathing patient exhales or valsalvas, the venous-to-atmospheric pressure is greater than if a spontaneously breathing patient inhales, a time when the venous pressure may be less than atmospheric pressure (*Lobato: Complications in Anesthesiology, pp 198-200*).

146. (B) Adverse physiologic effects of respiratory or metabolic acidosis include CNS depression and increased intracranial pressure (ICP), cardiovascular system depression (partially offset by increased secretion of catecholamines and elevated [Ca^{++}]), cardiac dysrhythmias, vasodilation, hypovolemia (which is a result of decreased precapillary and increased postcapillary sphincter tone), pulmonary hypertension, and hyperkalemia (*Miller: Anesthesia, ed 6, p 1603; Stoelting: Basics of Anesthesia, ed 5, p 322*).

147. (C) Withdrawing the tube into the trachea obviously would improve arterial saturation and is the treatment of choice for inadvertent mainstem intubation. Short of pulling the ETT back, all other successful options address ways of improving arterial oxygenation during one-lung ventilation. In essence, any maneuver that improves the saturation of the venous blood will also improve the saturation of arterial blood (in this question). Normal pulmonary circulation is in series with the systemic circulation. Blood exiting the lungs is nearly 100% oxygenated regardless of the saturation of the venous blood when it exits the right ventricle and enters the lungs via the pulmonary artery. In one-lung ventilation, deliberate or accidental, blood exiting the ventilated side of the lungs (the right side in this question) is also essentially fully saturated, but it mixes with non-oxygenated blood. The non-oxygenated blood has effectively bypassed the lungs by passing through an area that is perfused but not ventilated, that is, a shunt. When the blood from the ventilated lung (nearly 100% oxygenated) mixes with the shunted blood, a mixture will be formed that has saturation less than 100%, but higher than the mixed venous O_2 saturation.

$$Svo_2 = Sao_2 - \dot{V}O_2/\dot{Q} \times 1.39 \times Hgb$$

where Svo_2 = mixed venous hemoglobin saturation and Sao_2 = arterial oxygen saturation

$$O_2 \text{ content} = 1.39 \times [Hgb] \times Sao_2 + (0.003 \times Pao_2)$$

The exact saturation of the arterial blood in this question depends on the ratio of blood exiting the right lung versus that exiting the left lung. Fortunately, during one-lung ventilation, the non-ventilated lung collapses and in so doing raises its resistance to blood flow. This results in preferentially directing blood to the right ventilated lung. A second factor to consider is how well saturated the shunted blood is. "Red" blood from the right lung mixes with "blue" blood from the left lung to give a mixture of partially saturated blood. The saturation of the shunted "blue" blood depends on the hemoglobin concentration and cardiac output. From equation 1 above you can see that raising either of these would improve the mixed venous oxygen saturation and ultimately the arterial saturation during one-lung ventilation. Inflating the PA catheter balloon located in the non-ventilated (left) lung would also improve arterial saturation by limiting blood flow to the left lung. Raising the F_{IO_2} from 80% to 100% percent will do little if anything to improve arterial saturation since the blood exiting the "working" lung is already fully saturated. The small rise in Pao_2 which would result from an increase in F_{IO_2}, once multiplied by .003 (see equation 2 above) would be a very small and insignificant number. In other words, raising F_{IO_2} does not improve arterial saturation in the presence of a shunt (*Miller: Anesthesia, ed 6, pp 1331-1332, 1440; Stoelting: Basics of Anesthesia, ed 5, pp 422, 569*).

148. (E) The decision to stop mechanical support of the lungs is based on a variety of factors that can be measured. Guidelines suggesting that cessation of mechanical inflation of the lungs is likely to be successful include a vital capacity greater than 15 mL/kg, arterial Pao_2 greater than 60 mm Hg ($F_{IO_2} < 0.5$), A – a gradient less than 350 mm Hg ($F_{IO_2} = 1.0$), arterial pH greater than 7.3, $Paco_2$ less than 50 mm Hg, dead space/tidal volume ratio less than 0.6, and maximum inspiratory pressure of at least –20 cm H_2O. In addition to these guidelines, the patient should be hemodynamically stable, conscious, and oriented, and be in good nutritional status (*Morgan: Clinical Anesthesiology, ed 4, pp 1029, 1036; Stoelting: Basics of Anesthesia, ed 5, pp 596-597*).

149. (D) A shift to the left in the oxyhemoglobin dissociation curve occurs with fetal hemoglobin, alkalosis, hypothermia, carboxyhemoglobin, methemoglobin, decreased levels of 2,3 diphosphoglycerate (2,3-DPG). Storage of blood lowers 2,3-DPG levels in acid-citrate-dextrose stored blood, but minimal changes are seen in 2,3-DPG with citrate-dextrose-stored blood. A shift to the right occurs with acidosis, hyperthermia, increased levels of 2,3 diphosphoglycerate (2,3-DPG), inhaled anesthetics and pregnancy (*Hines: Stoelting's Anesthesia and Co-Existing Disease, ed 5, p 415; Miller: Anesthesia, ed 6, pp 700-701*).

150. (D) With acute spinal cord injuries the major anesthetic concerns are airway management and management of hemodynamic perturbations associated with interruption of the sympathetic nervous system below the level of the transection. Hyperkalemia in response to succinylcholine does not occur until at least 24 hours after the injury. Autonomic hyperreflexia is not a concern in the acute management of patients with spinal cord injuries. There is no evidence that awake intubation (fiberoptic) is superior to direct laryngoscopy as long as in-line traction is held in both cases. These patients are more susceptible to hypothermia compared with patients without spinal cord injuries because they lack thermoregulation below the level of the cord injury (*Hines: Stoelting's Anesthesia and Co-Existing Disease, ed 5, pp 240-241; Stoelting: Basics of Anesthesia, ed 5, pp 461-462*).

151. (C) Polyuria of neurogenic (rather than nephrogenic) diabetes insipidus is caused by diminished or absent antidiuretic hormone (ADH) synthesis or release following injury to the hypothalamus, pituitary stalk or posterior pituitary gland. Hemoconcentration resulting in hypernatremia often results. In contrast, SIADH is associated with excessive amounts of ADH which in turn causes hyponatremia. Cerebral salt wasting syndrome results from release of brain natriuretic peptide in subarachnoid hemorrhage patients. The resulting natriuresis-mediated electrolyte perturbation is hyponatremia. Diabetes mellitus and spinal shock do not cause hypernatremia (*Kasper: Harrison's Principles of Internal Medicine, ed 16, pp 254-258; Lobato: Complications in Anesthesiology, pp 461-466*).

152. (D) Vasopressin, also known as antidiuretic hormone, is a naturally occurring peptide synthesized in the hypothalamus and stored in the posterior pituitary. It is used clinically to treat diabetes insipidus, and in the ICU it is used to treat hypotension. Patients with severe sepsis and septic shock have a relative deficiency of vasopressin and these patients may be sensitive to vasopressin. Vasopressin interacts with a different receptor and, unlike the catecholamines, it is effective even in the presence of acidemia (*Stoelting: Basics of Anesthesia, ed 5, p 605*).

153. (C) Confusion may exist between the concepts of shunt versus dead space. Both of these are forms of $\dot{V}/\dot{Q}$ mismatch. With shunts, there is a gradient between arterial oxygen saturation and Pao_2 (PA is calculated from the alveolar gas equation). The $Paco_2$ with shunt is compensated and is usually normal even in the presence of a significant $\dot{V}/\dot{Q}$ mismatch. Dead space refers to the portion of a breath that does not reach perfused alveoli. In pathological conditions, such as COPD, morbid obesity and pulmonary embolism, dead space is increased because air passes into alveoli, which are ventilated, but not perfused. This air does not participate in gas exchange and simply exits these unperfused alveoli and "dilutes" the carbon dioxide exiting the lungs from the perfused alveoli. Under these circumstances the mixed expired CO_2 measured with capnometry will be less than the actual arterial CO_2 (*Miller: Anesthesia, ed 6, pp 697-698; Stoelting: Basics of Anesthesia, ed 5, p 59*).

154. (C) Transfusion related lung injury (TRALI) reactions are a serious complication of transfusing any product containing plasma, that is, FFP, whole blood, packed RBC's, platelets or factor concretes derived from human blood. The clinical diagnosis is made 1 to 2 hours after transfusion (but may occur up to 6 hours later in the ICU). The key features include wide A-a gradient, non-cardiogenic pulmonary edema and leukopenia (not leukocytosis) secondary to sequestration in the lungs. Transfusion relate lung injury (TRALI) reactions are one of the leading causes of transfusion-related mortality (*Stoelting: Basics of Anesthesia, ed. 5, p 569*).

155. (B) The right internal jugular vein and the right subclavian vein form the right brachiocephalic vein, similarly the left internal jugular vein and the left subclavian vein form the left brachiocephalic vein. These two brachiocephalic veins form the superior vena cava (*Netter: Atlas of Human Anatomy, plates 68, 195, 201*).

156. (D) Patients who have undergone a PCI are placed on a course of a thienopyridine (ticlopidine or clopidogrel) and aspirin. The thienopyridine is used for at least two weeks after PTCA, one month after a bare-metal stent is placed and one year after a drug eluting stent is placed. Aspirin is continued for a longer period of time. This is to decrease the chance of thrombosis of the treated coronary artery (*ACC/AHA 2007 Guidelines on Perioperative Cardiovascular Evaluation and Care for Noncardiac Surgery: Executive Summary. Anesth and Analg, 106:685-712, 2008*).

157. (C) The universal compression-ventilation ratio for infant, child and adult victims (excluding newborns) is 30 chest compressions to two breath cycles (5 cycles in 2 minutes). Once an advanced airway is in place two rescuers no longer deliver "cycles", but compressions at a rate of 100/minute and ventilation is 8 to 10/min. For newborns the ratio is 3:1 (90 compressions and 30 breaths/min. (*2005 American Heart Association guidelines for cardiopulmonary resuscitation and emergency cardiovascular care. Circulation, 2005;112, p IV-12-13, 192*).

158. (A) After an incubation period commonly within 2 weeks, inhalational anthrax symptoms initially look like viral flu (fever, chills, myalgia, and a non-productive cough). Although leucocytosis is common with anthrax and rare with viral flu, WBC counts initially may be normal at the time the patient presents. After a short while the patient suddenly appears critically ill and without treatment, death can occur within a few days. Substernal chest pain, hypoxemia, cyanosis, dyspnea, abdominal pain and sepsis syndrome are common with inhaled anthrax but rare with viral flu. After the anthrax spores are inhaled, macrophages phagocytize the spores and transport them to mediastinal lymph nodes where the spores germinate, producing enlarged nodes and a widened mediastinum on the chest x-ray film. A widened mediastinum is not seen with viral flu. Pharyngitis is common with viral flu and occasionally is seen with anthrax (*Kasper: Harrison's Principles of Internal Medicine ed 16, pp 1280-1281; Stoelting: Basics of Anesthesia, ed 5, pp 622-623*).

159. (C) To answer this question it is helpful to review the alveolar gas equation:

$$Pao_2 = Fio_2\,(Pb - PH_2O) - Pao_2/R$$

Pao_2 = partial pressure of oxygen in the alveolar gas; Fio_2 = fraction of inhaled oxygen; Pb = barometric pressure; R = respiratory quotient.

Any factor that lowers Pao_2 (below 100 mm Hg or so) will also lower Pao_2. Hypoxic gas mixture lowers Fio_2, hence Pao_2. Hypercarbia makes the term $Paco_2/R$ larger and therefore reduces Pao_2. Eisenmenger syndrome results in a larger shunt fraction and lower Pao_2 on that basis (see explanation to question 147). In normally functioning lungs, anemia has a minimal impact on Pao_2 because physiologic shunt is normally only 2% to 5% of cardiac output (*Barash: Clinical Anesthesia, ed 5, pp 803-804*).

160. (D)   The difference between the $Paco_2$ and the CO_2 value measured by the mass spectrometer is a function of the patient's physiologic dead space. Physiologic dead space is equal to anatomic dead space plus alveolar dead space. Anatomic dead space is roughly 1 mL/pound of body weight. Since anatomic dead space is relatively "fixed," changes in physiologic dead space are mainly attributable to changes in alveolar dead space. Alveoli that are ventilated, but not perfused, add to alveolar dead space. In essence, air goes into these alveoli, but does not participate in gas exchanges and merely exits the alveoli upon exhalation. Ventilation of dead space serves no useful purpose, but does result in "dilution" of the exhaled CO_2, thus explaining why the CO_2 seen on the mass spectrometer can be substantially lower than that obtained from arterial blood gas analysis. Several factors increase dead space such as lung diseases like COPD, cystic fibrosis, and pulmonary emboli. In addition, decreased alveolar perfusion from low cardiac output or hypovolemia may also contribute to increased dead space. Mainstem intubation, atelectasis, shunting through the besian veins and ablation of hypoxic pulmonary vasoconstriction by isoflurane are various causes of shunting. Shunting is also a mismatch between ventilation and perfusion, but, in contrast to $\dot{V}/\dot{Q}$ mismatch from dead space ventilation, shunting results in a normal or nearly normal $Paco_2$, but a larger than expected A-a O_2 gradient. The only choice in this question that would explain an increase in dead space ventilation is hypovolemia (*Barash: Clinical Anesthesia, ed 5, pp 802-803; Stoelting: Basics of Anesthesia, ed 5, p 322*).

161. (B)   The normal man's resting energy expenditure as well as the postoperative state is about 1800 kcal/24 hr. With starvation (20 days), energy expenditure decreases to about 1080 kcal/day (60% of normal). Patients who have sustained multiple fractures (2160 kcal/day or 120% of normal), major sepsis (2520 kcal/day or 140% normal) and burns have increased energy expenditures. The energy expenditure in a patient with a major burn also depends on the temperature of the room. The highest energy expenditure is at a room temperature of 25° C (3819 kcal/day or 212% normal) and is lower at 33° C (342 kcal/day or 185% normal) and at 21° C (3600 kcal/day or 200% normal) (*Miller: Anesthesia, ed 6, p 2906*).

162. (E)   Amiodarone is useful in the treatment of a variety of supraventricular and ventricular cardiac arrhythmias. For the treatment of ventricular tachycardia or fibrillation that is refractory to electrical defibrillation, the recommended dose is 300 mg IV. Similar to β blockers, amiodarone decreases mortality after myocardial infarctions. About 5% to 15% of treated patients develop pulmonary toxicity (especially when doses are > 400 mg/day, or underlying lung disease is present) and 2% to 4% develop thyroid dysfunction (amiodarone is a structural analogue of thyroid hormone). It has a prolonged elimination half-time of 29 hours and a large volume of distribution. Because it prolongs the QTc interval, it may lead to the production of ventricular tachydysrhythmias and thus is not useful in treating torsades de pointes (*Hardman: Goodman and Gilman's The Pharmacological Basis of Therapeutics, ed 10, pp 953-957; Stoelting: Pharmacology and Physiology, ed 4, pp 381-383*).

163. (A)   Patients with cirrhosis have hyperdynamic circulations as noted here with the elevated Svo_2 of 90%. The cardiac output is usually increased, peripheral vascular resistance is low, intravascular volume is increased and arteriovenous shunts are present. Hypotension is common. Milrinone is a positive inotrope with vasodilating properties, something this patient does not need. If a treatment for hypotension is needed, drugs with α-agonist properties may be helpful. In addition, vasopressin is also a good choice since it increases SVR, but does not increase the already high cardiac output (*Morgan: Clinical Anesthesiology, ed 4, p 794; Stoelting: Basics of Anesthesia, ed 5, p 432; Stoelting: Pharmacology and Physiology in Anesthetic Practice, ed 4, pp 317-318*).

164. (C)   Recombinant human activated protein C is a naturally occurring serum protein with anticoagulant properties indicated for the treatment of septic shock. APC is indicated for patients with APACHE scores greater than or equal to 25. Its mechanism is inhibition of factors Va and VIIIa. Inhibition of these proteins directly or indirectly reduces inflammation and microthrombi. APC also blocks production of tissue necrosis factor and it can bind selectins that promote inflammation on endothelial surfaces by activation of neutrophils. The major side effect of this drug is hemorrhage (*Hines: Stoelting's Anesthesia and Co-Existing Disease, ed 5, p 480; Miller: Anesthesia, ed 6, p 2796*).

165. **(B)** This patient has a metabolic acidosis. Recall that anion gap = $[Na+] - ([Cl^-] + [HCO_3^-])$ and is normally 10 to 12 nmol/L. In this case the anion gap = $145 - (119+12) = 14$, which is slightly above the normal anion gap range. In looking at this case, the acidosis is quite profound and would most likely be related to the rapid infusion of normal saline. Lactic acid, ketoacidosis and ethylene glycol produce a high anion gap metabolic acidosis. Narcotics may produce respiratory but not metabolic acidosis. See also question 142 (*Kasper: Harrison's Principles of Internal Medicine, ed 16, pp 263-268*).

166. **(A)** Noninvasive positive pressure ventilation (NIPPV) refers to delivering positive pressure ventilation to patients by way of a nasal mask, or full face mask, without the placement of an endotracheal or tracheostomy tube. This mode of therapy requires conscious and cooperative patients and does not protect the airway. NIPPV has been very useful in COPD patients and in immunosuppressed patients in acute respiratory failure. It most likely will fail (i.e., intubation would be needed) in patients with pneumonia and ARDS. (*Miller: Anesthesia, ed 6, pp 2825-2828*).

167. **(D)** Capnography has been a valuable monitor for the cardiac and pulmonary systems as well as checking the anesthetic equipment. Forgetting to ventilate the patient, intubating the esophagus as well as having the sensing tube become disconnected from the monitor quickly will show no CO_2 detected. Any significant reduction in lung perfusion (i.e., air embolism, decreased cardiac output or decreased blood pressure) increases alveolar dead space and leads to a lowering of the detected CO_2. A cardiac arrest where there is no blood flow to the lungs and hence no carbon dioxide going to the lungs would also give you no detectable CO_2. As CPR is started, detectable CO_2 would be a sign of lung perfusion and ventilation. A patient with a pneumothorax and high airway pressures would still give you CO_2 readings (*Morgan: Clinical Anesthesiology, ed 4, pp 141-143*).

168. **(E)** Always confirm an adequate *A*irway and *B*reathing before treating a *C*ardiac rhythm (A,B before C). Having the endotracheal tube in proper position for several hours does not ensure that it remains in proper position. In this case, the endotracheal tube slipped out of the trachea and went into the esophagus. The only way you know the endotracheal tube is in the trachea is to see the tube passing between the vocal cords directly with a conventional laryngoscope or by putting a fiberoptic bronchoscope through the tube and seeing carina. Other forms of confirmation such as bilateral breath sounds, adequate chest rise, and moisture in the tube are helpful, but could also be seen with an esophageal intubation. Getting a consistent and adequate end tidal CO_2 on a monitor confirms some gas exchange, but in cases where blood does not get to the lungs, as in a cardiac arrest, CO_2 cannot be removed from the lungs. The first part in the treatment of bradycardia is adequate ventilation with oxygen. After that the other choices may be indicated (*Miller: Anesthesia, ed 6, p 1648*).

Chapter 3

Pharmacology and Pharmacokinetics of Intravenous Drugs

169. Which of the following muscle relaxants is eliminated the most by renal excretion?
   A. Pancuronium
   B. Vecuronium
   C. d-Tubocurare
   D. Rocuronium
   E. Atracurium

170. Special considerations for patients with porphyria cutanea tarda would include which of the following?
   A. Avoidance of regional techniques because of neurotoxicity
   B. Avoidance of sodium pentothal
   C. Need for higher doses of nondepolarizing neuromuscular blocking drugs
   D. Special attention to skin pressure
   E. Need for reduced doses of renally metabolized drugs

171. Which of the following β-adrenergic antagonists is a nonselective β_1 and β_2 blocker?
   A. Atenolol
   B. Betaxolol
   C. Esmolol
   D. Metoprolol
   E. Nadolol

172. A 78-year-old patient with Parkinson's disease undergoes a cataract operation under general anesthesia. In the recovery room, the patient has two episodes of emesis and complains of severe nausea. Which of the following antiemetics would be the best choice for treatment of nausea in this patient?
   A. Droperidol
   B. Promethazine
   C. Ondansetron
   D. Thiethylperazine
   E. Metoclopramide

173. Which of the following diseases is associated with increased resistance to neuromuscular blockade with succinylcholine?
   A. Myasthenia gravis
   B. Myasthenic syndrome
   C. Huntington's chorea
   D. Polymyositis
   E. Duchenne's muscular dystrophy (pseudohypertrophic muscular dystrophy)

174. At what intravenous dose does dopamine increase renal blood flow?
   A. 0.5 to 3 μg/kg/min
   B. 3 to 10 μg/kg/min
   C. 10 to 20 μg/kg/min
   D. 20 to 50 μg/kg/min
   E. Greater than 50 μg/kg/min

175. Which of the following intravenous anesthetics is converted from a water-soluble to a lipid-soluble drug after exposure to the bloodstream?
   A. Propofol
   B. Thiopental
   C. Etomidate
   D. Ketamine
   E. Midazolam

176. A 33-year-old, 70-kg patient is brought to the operating room for resection of an anterior pituitary prolactin-secreting tumor. Anesthesia is induced with sevoflurane, nitrous oxide, and oxygen. The patient is intubated and nitrous oxide is discontinued. Anesthesia is maintained with 1.2 minimum alveolar concentration (MAC) sevoflurane in oxygen. The surgeon plans to inject epinephrine into the nasal mucosa to minimize bleeding. What is the maximum volume of a 1:100,000 epinephrine solution that can be administered safely to this patient without producing ventricular arrhythmias?
   A. 55 mL
   B. 45 mL
   C. 35 mL
   D. 25 mL
   E. 15 mL

177. Patients receiving antihypertensive therapy with propranolol are at increased risk for each of the following **EXCEPT**
   A. Blunted response to hypoglycemia
   B. Bronchoconstriction
   C. Rebound tachycardia after discontinuation
   D. Orthostatic hypotension
   E. Atrioventricular heart block

178. Atropine causes each of the following **EXCEPT**
   A. Decreased gastric acid secretion
   B. Inhibition of salivary secretion
   C. Tachycardia
   D. Mydriasis
   E. Increased lower esophageal sphincter tone

179. Which of the following drugs is capable of crossing the blood-brain barrier?
   A. Neostigmine
   B. Pyridostigmine
   C. Edrophonium
   D. Physostigmine
   E. None of the above

180. Which drug exerts its main central nervous system (CNS) action by inhibiting the *N*-methyl-D-aspartate (NMDA) receptors?
   A. Thiopental
   B. Midazolam
   C. Etomidate
   D. Ketamine
   E. Propofol

181. Which of the following opioid-receptor agonists has anticholinergic properties?
   A. Morphine
   B. Fentanyl
   C. Sufentanil
   D. Meperidine
   E. Oxymorphone

182. Which of the following statements about ketamine is **FALSE?**
   A. In the United States, it is a racemic mixture of two isomers
   B. It is a potent cerebral vasodilator and can increase intracranial pressure (ICP)
   C. Respiratory depression rarely occurs with induction doses
   D. It can be given intravenously, intramuscularly, orally, nasally and rectally
   E. Its metabolite norketamine is more potent than the parent compound

183. Which of the following vasopressor agents increases systemic blood pressure indirectly by stimulating the release of norepinephrine from sympathetic nerve fibers and directly by binding to adrenergic receptors?
   A. Dobutamine
   B. Ephedrine
   C. Epinephrine
   D. Phenylephrine
   E. Methoxamine

184. Which of the following narcotics causes the greatest decrease in myocardial contractility when administered in large doses alone?
   A. Morphine
   B. Meperidine
   C. Sufentanil
   D. Alfentanil
   E. Fentanyl

185. Select the **FALSE** statement about ketamine.
   A. Purposeful skeletal muscle movements may occur
   B. Visceral pain is better controlled than somatic pain
   C. Blood pressure and cardiac output may increase
   D. It can be given intramuscularly, orally and intravenously
   E. It is metabolized by the liver

186. Which of the following anesthetics is most likely to cause myocardial depression?
   A. Propofol
   B. Thiopental
   C. Etomidate
   D. Ketamine
   E. Midazolam

187. Which of the following drugs should be administered with caution to patients receiving echothiophate for the treatment of glaucoma?
   A. Atropine
   B. Succinylcholine
   C. Ketamine
   D. Pancuronium
   E. Neostigmine

188. When one of four thumb twitches in the train-of-four (TOF) stimulation of the ulnar nerve can be elicited, how much suppression would there be if you were measuring a single twitch?
    A. 5 to 10
    B. 20 to 25
    C. 45 to 55
    D. 75 to 80
    E. 90 to 95

189. Which of the following muscle relaxants causes slight histamine release at 2 to 3 times the ED95 dose?
    A. Doxacurium
    B. Rocuronium
    C. Pancuronium
    D. Atracurium
    E. Cisatracurium

190. Termination of action of the neurotransmitter norepinephrine is achieved predominately by which mechanism?
    A. Reuptake into postganglionic sympathetic nerve endings (uptake 1)
    B. Uptake by the innervated organ (uptake 2)
    C. Metabolism by catechol-*O*-methyltransferase (COMT)
    D. Metabolism by monoamine oxidase (MAO)
    E. Dilution by diffusion away from receptors

191. The incidence of unpleasant dreams associated with emergence from ketamine anesthesia can be reduced by the administration of
    A. Atropine
    B. Droperidol
    C. Physostigmine
    D. Midazolam
    E. Glycopyrrolate

192. Which of the following premedications is associated with extrapyramidal side effects?
    A. Metoclopramide
    B. Cimetidine
    C. Scopolamine
    D. Glycopyrrolate
    E. Diazepam

193. Succinylcholine, when administered to patients with renal failure, will increase serum [K+] by approximately
    A. No increase in [K+]
    B. 0.5 mEq/L
    C. 1.5 mEq/L
    D. 2.5 mEq/L
    E. Greater than 2.5 mEq/L

194. Each of the following drugs can enhance the neuromuscular blockade produced by nondepolarizing muscle relaxants **EXCEPT**
    A. Calcium
    B. Aminoglycoside antibiotics
    C. Magnesium
    D. Dantrolene
    E. Intravenous lidocaine

195. Discontinuation of which of the following medications is strongly recommended before elective surgery?
    A. Clonidine
    B. Propranolol
    C. Monoamine oxidase inhibitors (MAOIs)
    D. Tricyclic antidepressants
    E. None of the above

196. Laudanosine is a metabolite of
   A. Atracurium
   B. d-Tubocurarine
   C. Vecuronium
   D. Pancuronium
   E. Rocuronium

197. Pretreatment with a nondepolarizing muscle relaxant is **LEAST** effective in attenuating which of the following side effects of succinylcholine?
   A. Increased intragastric pressure
   B. Increased ICP
   C. Hyperkalemia
   D. Myalgias
   E. Bradycardia

198. Which of the following antibiotics does **NOT** augment neuromuscular blockade?
   A. Clindamycin
   B. Neomycin
   C. Streptomycin
   D. Erythromycin
   E. Gentamicin

199. Time of onset from most rapid to least rapid
   A. Edrophonium, pyridostigmine, neostigmine
   B. Edrophonium, neostigmine, pyridostigmine
   C. Neostigmine, edrophonium, pyridostigmine
   D. Neostigmine, pyridostigmine, edrophonium
   E. Pyridostigmine, neostigmine, edrophonium

200. The pH of commercially available thiopental is
   A. 4.5
   B. 5.5
   C. 7.4
   D. 8.5
   E. 10.5

201. In which of the following situations is succinylcholine most likely to cause severe hyperkalemia?
   A. 24 hours after a right hemisphere stroke
   B. 14 days after a severe burn injury
   C. 24 hours after a mid-thoracic spinal cord transection
   D. 2 days with a severe abdominal infection
   E. Chronic renal failure

202. The most common minor side effect reported after flumazenil administration in anesthesia is
   A. Nausea and/or vomiting
   B. Dizziness
   C. Tremors
   D. Hypertension
   E. Pain on injection

203. The most appropriate combination of drugs, in terms of a stable heart rate, during reversal of nondepolarizing neuro-muscular blockade is
   A. Edrophonium and glycopyrrolate
   B. Edrophonium and atropine
   C. Neostigmine and atropine
   D. Pyridostigmine and atropine
   E. None of the above

204. A 37-year-old patient with a history of acute intermittent porphyria is scheduled for knee arthroscopy under general anesthesia. Which of the following drugs is contraindicated in this patient?
   A. Pyridostigmine
   B. Isoflurane
   C. Propofol
   D. Thiopental
   E. Succinylcholine

205. The combination of dantrolene and verapamil administered intravenously places the patient at increased risk for
   A. Hyperkalemia
   B. Constipation
   C. Hepatotoxicity
   D. Profound muscular weakness
   E. Increased prothrombin time (PT) and partial thromboplastin time (PTT)

206. If etomidate were accidentally injected into a left-sided radial arterial line, the most appropriate step to take would be
   A. Left stellate ganglion block
   B. Administer intra-arterial clonidine
   C. Administer intra-arterial guanethidine
   D. Slowly inject dilute (0.1 mEq/L) $[HCO_3^-]$
   E. Observe

207. The most important reason for the more rapid onset and shorter duration of action of fentanyl compared with morphine is the difference in
   A. Volume of distribution
   B. Hepatic clearance
   C. Renal clearance
   D. Lipid solubility
   E. Protein binding

208. The term azeotrope refers to
   A. A mixture of two volatile anesthetics
   B. A mixture of a volatile anesthetic plus N_2O
   C. A mixture of volatile anesthetic plus N_2
   D. Radioactively labeled N_2O
   E. Radioactively labeled N_2

209. All the following agents inhibit cerebrospinal fluid (CSF) production **EXCEPT**
   A. Furosemide
   B. Halothane
   C. Acetazolamide
   D. Hypothermia
   E. Enflurane

210. The unique advantage of rocuronium over other muscle relaxants is its
   A. Short duration of action
   B. Metabolism by pseudocholinesterase
   C. Onset of action
   D. Lack of need for reversal
   E. Lack of potentiation with aminoglycoside antibiotics

211. Which of the following statements concerning the effect of an acute decrease in serum potassium levels regarding neuromuscular blockade is correct?
   A. No effect with depolarizing or nondepolarizing muscle relaxants
   B. Resistance to effects of both depolarizing or nondepolarizing muscle relaxants
   C. Increased sensitivity to effects of both depolarizing or nondepolarizing muscle relaxants
   D. Resistance to depolarizing muscle relaxants and increased sensitivity to nondepolarizing muscle relaxants
   E. Resistance to nondepolarizing muscle relaxants and increased sensitivity to depolarizing muscle relaxants

212. Which of the following neuromuscular blocking drugs causes the greatest release of histamine when administered intravenously?
    A. Succinylcholine
    B. d-Tubocurarine
    C. Doxacurium
    D. Atracurium
    E. Cisatracurium

213. A 58-year-old patient is brought to the emergency room with the following symptoms: miosis, abdominal cramping, salivation, loss of bowel and bladder control, bradycardia, ataxia, and skeletal muscle weakness. The most likely diagnosis is
    A. Central anticholinergic syndrome
    B. Malignant neuroleptic syndrome
    C. Anticholinesterase poisoning
    D. Digitalis overdose
    E. Thorazine overdose

214. Flumazenil
    A. Is contraindicated in narcotic addicts
    B. Partially antagonizes thiopental
    C. Can produce seizures in chronic benzodiazepine users
    D. Has a longer elimination half-life compared to midazolam
    E. Can be given orally as well as intravenously

215. What percentage of neuromuscular receptors could be blocked and still allow patients to carry out a 5-second head lift?
    A. 5%
    B. 15%
    C. 25%
    D. 50%
    E. 75%

216. Methohexital has a shorter elimination half-time than thiopental because methohexital
    A. Is more lipid soluble
    B. Is more ionized in blood
    C. Has greater protein binding
    D. Has greater hepatic extraction
    E. None of the above

217. Which of the following drugs can prevent tachyarrhythmias in patients with Wolff-Parkinson-White (WPW) syndrome?
    A. Droperidol
    B. Pancuronium
    C. Ketamine
    D. Verapamil
    E. Meperidine

218. The half-life of pseudocholinesterase is
    A. 3 minutes
    B. 1 hour
    C. 12 hours
    D. 1 week
    E. 2 weeks

219. A 29-year-old patient undergoes a herniorrhaphy under general anesthesia. Ketorolac 30 mg is administered intramuscularly after the patient is induced and intubated. Intravenous morphine 4 mg also is administered. The operation is carried out uneventfully. The patient is extubated and taken to the recovery room. One hour later she is resting quietly and complains of no pain. The effects of ketorolac on transmission of painful stimuli are exerted at which part in the afferent sensory pathway?
    A. At the level of peripheral sensory receptors
    B. At the dorsal route ganglia
    C. At the spinal thalamic tract
    D. At the thalamus
    E. At the sensory cortex

220. Which of the following equals the anti-inflammatory activity of 50 mg of prednisone (Deltasone)?
    A. 100 mg cortisol (Solu-Cortef)
    B. 80 mg methylprednisolone (Solu-Medrol)
    C. 7.5 mg dexamethasone (Decadron)
    D. 4 mg betamethasone (Celestone)
    E. 20 mg prednisolone (Delta-Cortef)

221. The recovery index (RI) of which of the following nondepolarizing muscle relaxants is not altered by aging?
    A. Atracurium
    B. Vecuronium
    C. d-Tubocurarine
    D. Pancuronium
    E. Rocuronium

222. Side effects associated with cyclosporine therapy include each of the following **EXCEPT**
    A. Nephrotoxicity
    B. Pulmonary toxicity
    C. Hypertension
    D. Limb paresthesias
    E. Seizures

223. What is the predominant mechanism for succinylcholine-induced tachycardia in adults?
    A. Histamine release from mast cells
    B. Stimulation of nicotinic receptors at autonomic ganglia
    C. Blockade of nicotinic receptors at autonomic ganglia
    D. Direct vagolytic effect at postjunctional muscarinic receptors
    E. Direct sympathomimetic effect at postjunctional muscarinic receptors

224. Bradycardia observed after administration of succinylcholine to children is attributable to which mechanism?
    A. Nicotinic stimulation at the autonomic ganglia
    B. Nicotinic blockade at the autonomic ganglia
    C. Muscarinic stimulation at the sinus node
    D. Muscarinic blockade at the sinus node
    E. Stimulation of the vagus nerve centrally

225. A 72-year-old retired farmer with essential hypertension takes 100 mg of guanethidine daily. Which of the following most accurately describes this patient's blood pressure response to direct- and indirect-acting sympathomimetic agents?
    A. Normal response to indirect-acting agents; exaggerated response to direct-acting agents
    B. Reduced response to indirect-acting agents; exaggerated response to direct-acting agents
    C. Exaggerated response to both direct- and indirect-acting agents
    D. Reduced response to both direct- and indirect-acting agents
    E. Normal response to both direct- and indirect-acting agents

226. Succinylcholine is contraindicated for routine tracheal intubation in children because of an increased incidence of which of the following side effects?
    A. Hyperkalemia
    B. Malignant hyperthermia
    C. Masseter spasm
    D. Sinus bradycardia
    E. Severe myalgias

227. From **MOST** to **LEAST** rapid, select the correct temporal sequence of neuromuscular blockade in the adductor of the thumb, the orbicularis oculi, and the diaphragm after administration of an intubating dose of vecuronium to an otherwise healthy patient.
    A. Diaphragm, orbicularis oculi, thumb
    B. Orbicularis oculi, diaphragm, thumb
    C. Orbicularis oculi, thumb, diaphragm
    D. Thumb, orbicularis oculi, diaphragm
    E. Orbicularis oculi same as diaphragm, thumb

228. Select the true statement regarding interaction of nondepolarizing neuromuscular blocking drugs when durations of action are dissimilar.
    A. If a long-acting drug is administered after an intermediate-acting drug, the duration of the long-acting drug will be longer than normal
    B. If a long-acting drug is administered after an intermediate-acting drug, the duration of the long-acting drug will be about the same as expected
    C. If an intermediate-acting drug is administered after a long-acting drug, the duration of the intermediate-acting drug will be about the same as expected
    D. If an intermediate-acting drug is administered after a long-acting drug, the duration of action of the intermediate-acting drug will be shorter than expected
    E. If an intermediate-acting drug is administered after a long-acting drug, the duration of action of the intermediate-acting drug will be longer than expected

229. Select the correct statement regarding the effects of volatile anesthetics on nondepolarizing neuromuscular blocking drugs and the reversal agents.
    A. Volatile anesthetics potentiate neuromuscular blockade but retard reversal agents
    B. Volatile anesthetics potentiate both neuromuscular blocking drugs and reversal agents
    C. Volatile anesthetics retard both neuromuscular blocking drugs and reversal agents
    D. Volatile anesthetics retard neuromuscular blocking drugs but potentiate reversal agents
    E. Volatile anesthetics have no effect on both neuromuscular blocking drugs and reversal agents

230. Meperidine is contraindicated in patients taking which of the following drugs for Parkinson's disease?
    A. Bromocriptine
    B. Levodopa
    C. Selegiline (Eldepryl)
    D. Amantadine (Symmetrel)
    E. Trihexyphenidyl (Artane)

231. Which of the following benzylisoquinolinium nondepolarizing neuromuscular blocking drugs is unique among this class of drugs in that it does not cause release of histamine?
    A. d-Tubocurarine
    B. Cisatracurium
    C. Rocuronium
    D. Atracurium
    E. Pipecuronium

232. The most common reason for patients to rate anesthesia with etomidate as unsatisfactory is
    A. Postoperative nausea and vomiting
    B. Pain on injection
    C. Recall of intubation
    D. Myoclonus
    E. Postoperative hiccups

233. Which of the following muscle relaxants inhibits the reuptake of norepinephrine by the adrenergic nerves?
    A. Pancuronium
    B. Pipecuronium
    C. Rocuronium
    D. Doxacurium
    E. Vecuronium

234. The most common side effect of oral dantrolene used to prevent malignant hyperthermia is
    A. Nausea and vomiting
    B. Muscle weakness
    C. Blurred vision
    D. Hepatitis
    E. Diarrhea

235. If not discontinued 24 hours before surgery, there is a risk of developing intraoperative lactic acidosis with which of the following oral hypoglycemic drugs?
    A. Metformin (Glucophage)
    B. Glyburide (DiaBeta, Micronase)
    C. Glipizide (Glucotrol)
    D. Tolbutamide (Orinase)
    E. Chlorpropamide (Diabinese)

236. A 37-year-old man is brought to the operating room for repair of a broken mandible sustained in a motor vehicle accident. No other injuries are significant. The patient has been in treatment for alcohol abuse and takes disulfiram and naltrexone. Which of the following would be the best technique for management of this patient's postoperative pain?
    A. Continue naltrexone with round-the-clock low-dose methadone
    B. Continue naltrexone with small doses of morphine every 4 hours as needed
    C. Continue naltrexone with small doses of nalbuphine every 4 hours as needed
    D. Discontinue naltrexone and treat pain with morphine as needed
    E. Discontinue naltrexone and treat pain with acetaminophen as needed

237. Which of the following muscle relaxants is most suitable for rapid intubation in a patient in whom succinylcholine is contraindicated?
    A. d-Tubocurare
    B. Rocuronium
    C. Doxacurium
    D. Pipecuronium
    E. Vecuronium

238. The neuromuscular effects of an intubation dose of vecuronium are terminated by
    A. Pseudocholinesterase
    B. Nonspecific plasma cholinesterases
    C. The kidneys
    D. The liver
    E. Diffusion from the neuromuscular junction back into the plasma

239. Respiratory depression produced by which of the following analgesics is not readily reversed by administration of naloxone?
    A. Propoxyphene
    B. Methadone
    C. Hydromorphone
    D. Buprenorphine
    E. Opium

240. Which of the following intravenous anesthetic agents is associated with the highest incidence of nausea and vomiting?
    A. Thiopental
    B. Etomidate
    C. Ketamine
    D. Propofol
    E. Midazolam

241. If naloxone were administered to a patient who is receiving ketorolac for postoperative pain, the most likely result would be
    A. Bradycardia
    B. Hypotension
    C. Pain
    D. Somnolence
    E. None of the above

242. Which drug produces strong pulmonary arterial dilation with the least amount of systemic artery dilation?
    A. Nitroprusside
    B. Prostaglandin E_1
    C. Phentolamine
    D. Nitric oxide
    E. Nitroglycerin IV

243. The action of succinylcholine at the neuromuscular junction is terminated by which mechanism?
    A. Hydrolysis by pseudocholinesterase
    B. Hydrolysis by acetylcholinesterase
    C. Reuptake into nerve tissue
    D. Reuptake into muscle tissue
    E. Diffusion into extracellular fluid

244. The **LEAST** likely side effect of dexmedetomidine in a healthy patient is
    A. Hypertension
    B. Bradycardia
    C. Sinus arrest
    D. Hypotension
    E. Respiratory arrest

245. The advantage of fospropofol (Lusedra) over propofol is the absence of
    A. Pain on injection
    B. Risk of hypertriglyceridemia
    C. Risk of pulmonary embolism
    D. Risk of infection, sepsis, or both
    E. All of the above

246. Which of the following features of chronic morphine therapy is **NOT** subject to tolerance?
    A. Analgesia
    B. Respiratory depression
    C. Constipation
    D. Nausea
    E. Euphoria

247. Intravenous cimetidine (Tagamet) 300 mg is administered to an obese 78-year-old woman with a history of reactive airways disease. It is administered 30 minutes before induction of anesthesia for an exploratory laparotomy. Possible side effects associated with this drug include all of the following **EXCEPT**
    A. Bradycardia
    B. Elevation of aminotransaminase enzymes
    C. Confusion
    D. Increased metabolism of diazepam
    E. Delayed awakening

248. Intraoperative allergic reactions are **LEAST** common after patient exposure to
    A. Ketamine
    B. Latex
    C. Muscle relaxants
    D. Hydroxyethyl starch
    E. Radiocontrast media

249. Which of the following medications would be useful in the definitive treatment of Sarin nerve gas poisoning?
    A. Sodium nitroprusside
    B. Methylene blue
    C. Nitroglycerin
    D. Atropine
    E. Any of the above could be used to treat this toxicity

250. Alfentanil
    A. Has a more rapid onset of action compared to fentanyl
    B. Has a longer duration of action compared with fentanyl
    C. Is more potent than fentanyl
    D. Is excreted unchanged in the urine
    E. Undergoes little hepatic metabolism

251. Which of the following medications is **NOT** useful in the immediate management of status asthmaticus?
    A. Terbutaline
    B. Subcutaneous (SQ) epinephrine
    C. Magnesium sulfate
    D. Cromolyn
    E. Isoflurane

252. Clonidine
    A. Is an α_2 blocker
    B. Increases CNS sympathetic response to painful stimuli
    C. Can be given orally as well as IV, but not epidurally or intrathecally
    D. Decreases postanesthetic shivering
    E. Should be discontinued 24 hours or more prior to elective surgery

253. The plasma half-times of which of the following drugs is prolonged in patients with end-stage cirrhotic liver disease?
    A. Diazepam
    B. Pancuronium
    C. Alfentanil
    D. Procaine
    E. All are prolonged

254. A 24-year-old, 100-kg patient is brought to the ER by the fire department after suffering smoke inhalation and third degree burns on abdomen, chest and thighs 30 minutes earlier. The best muscle relaxant choice for the most rapid intubation would be
   A. 2 mg vecuronium followed by succinylcholine
   B. 1 mg of vecuronium, then 2 to 4 minutes later 9 mg vecuronium
   C. Rocuronium
   D. d-Tubocurarine
   E. Succinylcholine

255. Clonidine is useful in each of the following applications **EXCEPT**
   A. Reducing blood pressure with pheochromocytoma
   B. Treatment of postoperative shivering
   C. Use as sole analgesic in a spinal
   D. Agent for prolonging bupivacaine spinal
   E. Protection against perioperative myocardial ischemia

256. A 79-year-old male patient is brought to the operating room for elective repair of bilateral inguinal hernias. The patient has a history of awareness during general anesthesia and refuses regional anesthesia. The patient is preoxygenated before induction of general anesthesia; 5 mg of midazolam and 500 mg of fentanyl are administered. One minute later the patient loses consciousness and chest wall stiffness develops to the extent that positive-pressure ventilation is very difficult. The most appropriate therapy for reversal of chest wall stiffness at this point could include
   A. Flumazenil
   B. Naloxone
   C. Thiopental
   D. Albuterol
   E. Succinylcholine

257. Respiratory depression is **LEAST** after the induction dose of which of the following drugs?
   A. Etomidate
   B. Ketamine
   C. Methohexital
   D. Propofol
   E. Thiopental

258. A 64-year-old man with colon cancer is anesthetized for hepatic resection of liver metastasizes. Medical history is significant for ileal conduit surgery for bladder cancer, diabetes treated with glyburide, 50 pack per year smoking history, and family history of malignant hyperthermia. Anesthesia is provided with morphine, midazolam, oxygen and a propofol infusion. After 3 unit packed red blood cell (RBC) transfusion and 8 hours of surgery, the following blood gas values are recorded: pH 7.2, CO_2 34, [HCO_3^-] 14, base deficit -13, [Na^+] 135, [K^+] 5, Cl 95, glucose 240 mg/dL. The most likely cause of this patient's acidosis is
   A. Ureteroenteric fistula (ileal conduit)
   B. Renal tubular acidosis
   C. Propofol infusion syndrome
   D. Diabetic ketoacidosis
   E. Excessive infusion of normal saline

259. Treatment of neuroleptic malignant syndrome may be carried out with administration of the following drugs **EXCEPT**
   A. Amantadine
   B. Dantrolene
   C. Bromocriptine
   D. Physostigmine
   E. Stopping haloperidol administration

260. A patient with a normal quantity of pseudocholinesterase (plasma cholinesterase) has a dibucaine number of 57. A 1 mg/kg dose of intravenous succinylcholine would likely result in
    A. Hyperkalemic cardiac arrest
    B. Paralysis lasting 5 to 10 minutes
    C. Paralysis lasting 20 to 30 minutes
    D. Paralysis lasting more than 1 to 3 hours
    E. No effect

261. Cyanide toxicity may be treated with all of the following drugs **EXCEPT**
    A. Sodium nitrite
    B. Hydroxycobalamine
    C. Sodium thiosulfate
    D. Methylene blue
    E. Amyl nitrite

262. A prolonged neuromuscular block with succinylcholine can be seen in all of the following patients **EXCEPT**
    A. Chronically exposed to malathion
    B. Treated with echothiophate for glaucoma
    C. Treated with cyclophosphamide for metastatic cancer
    D. Genetically homozygous for atypical pseudocholinesterase
    E. Having a C_5 isoenzyme variant

263. Which of the following statements concerning midazolam is **FALSE**?
    A. Midazolam has greater amnestic properties than sedative properties
    B. It produces anterograde amnesia
    C. It produces retrograde amnesia
    D. It facilitates the inhibitory neurotransmitter GABA's actions in the CNS
    E. Its breakdown is inhibited by cimetidine

264. After a 2 hour vertical gastric banding procedure under desflurane, oxygen and remifentanil anesthesia, the trocar is removed and the wound is closed. Upon emergence, the most likely scenario is
    A. Adequate analgesia for 2 hours
    B. Delayed emergence from narcotic
    C. Pain
    D. Respiratory depression in postanesthesia care unit (PACU)
    E. Chest wall stiffness

265. An oral surgeon is about to perform a full mouth extraction on a 70-kg, 63-year-old man under conscious sedation. He inquires as to the maximum dose of lidocaine with epinephrine that he can safely infiltrate.
    A. 200 mg
    B. 300 mg
    C. 400 mg
    D. 500 mg
    E. 600 mg

266. Postanesthetic shivering can be treated with all of the following **EXCEPT**
    A. Meperidine
    B. Physostigmine
    C. Magnesium sulfate
    D. Dexmedetomidine
    E. Naloxone

267. The main disadvantage of Sugammadex (ORG 25969) compared with neostigmine is
    A. Recurarization
    B. Profound bradycardia
    C. Not effective with benzylisoquinoline relaxants
    D. High incidence of allergic reactions
    E. Contraindicated with renal failure

268. Treatment for accidental intra-arterial injection of thiopental could include
    A. Stellate ganglion block
    B. Heparin administration
    C. Intra-arterial injection of lidocaine
    D. Intra-arterial injection of papaverine
    E. All are useful

269. Above which infusion rate does cyanide toxicity become a concern in a healthy adult receiving sodium nitroprusside?
    A. 0.5 µg/kg/min
    B. 2 µg/kg/min
    C. 10 µg/kg/min
    D. 20 µg/kg/min
    E. Never

270. Important interactions involving chlorpromazine include all of the following **EXCEPT**
    A. Potentiation of the depressant effects of narcotics
    B. Lowering of the seizure threshold
    C. Interference with the antihypertensive effects of guanethidine
    D. Potentiation of neuromuscular blockade
    E. Prolongation of the QT interval

271. Amrinone
    A. Is a positive inotropic drug
    B. Is antagonized by esmolol
    C. Is a vasoconstrictor
    D. Has weak antidysrhythmic properties
    E. Is a catecholamine

272. Which statements concerning tricyclic antidepressants in patients receiving general anesthesia is **TRUE**
    A. They should be discontinued two weeks before elective operations
    B. They may decrease the requirement for volatile anesthetics (decrease MAC)
    C. Meperidine may produce hyperpyrexia in patients taking tricyclic antidepressants
    D. They may exaggerate the response to ephedrine
    E. They produce cholinergic side effects

273. Which of the following types of insulin preparations has the fastest onset of action if administered subcutaneously (SQ)?
    A. Glargine (Lantus)
    B. Lispro (Humalog)
    C. Regular (Humulin-R)
    D. NPH (Humulin-N)
    E. Ultralente

274. Which of the following intravenous adrenergic blockers would be the most suitable drug for the treatment of hypertension and tachycardia in a 68-year-old patient with a reactive airway disease?
    A. Propranolol
    B. Nadolol
    C. Atenolol
    D. Pindolol
    E. Timolol

275. The duration of action of remifentanil is attributable to which mode of metabolism?
    A. Spontaneous degradation in blood (Hoffman elimination)
    B. Hydrolysis by nonspecific plasma esterases
    C. Hydrolysis by pseudocholinesterase
    D. Rapid metabolism in the large intestine
    E. Urinary excretion

276. Pain at the intravenous site is **LEAST** with which IV drug
   A. Diazepam
   B. Etomidate
   C. Methohexital
   D. Propofol
   E. Thiopental

277. A 35-year-old patient with history of grand mal seizures is anesthetized for thyroid biopsy under general anesthesia consisting of 4 mg midazolam with infusion of propofol (150 μg/kg/min) and remifentanil (1 μg/kg/min). The patient takes phenytoin for control of seizures. After 30 minutes, the infusion is stopped and the patient is transported intubated to the recovery room where he is arousable, but not breathing. The most reasonable course of action would be
   A. Administer naloxone
   B. Administer flumazenil
   C. Administer naloxone and flumazenil
   D. Place on flumazenil infusion
   E. Ventilate by hand

278. Which of the following α-antagonists produces an irreversible blockade?
   A. Phentolamine
   B. Prazosin
   C. Yohimbine
   D. Phenoxybenzamine
   E. Tolazoline

279. Which of the following drugs should not be used in the treatment of severe bradycardia induced by an excess of β-adrenergic receptor blockade?
   A. Atropine
   B. Dobutamine
   C. Dopamine
   D. Glucagon
   E. Isoproterenol

280. A dose of 150 mg of IV dantrolene is administered to a 24-year-old male (75-kg) patient in whom incipient malignant hyperthermia is suspected. An expected consequence of this therapy would be
   A. Muscle spasticity in the postoperative period
   B. Hypothermia
   C. Cardiac dysrhythmias
   D. Diuresis
   E. Emergence delirium

281. Atracurium differs from cis-atracurium in which way?
   A. Molecular weight
   B. Formation of laudanosine
   C. Histamine release
   D. No renal metabolism
   E. No hepatic metabolism

282. Signs and symptoms of opioid withdrawal include all of the following **EXCEPT**
   A. Increased blood pressure (BP) and heart rate
   B. Seizures
   C. Abdominal cramps
   D. Jerking of the legs
   E. Hyperthermia

DIRECTIONS (Questions 283 through 320): Each group of questions consists of several numbered statements followed by lettered headings. For each numbered statement, select the **ONE** lettered heading that is most closely associated with it. Each lettered heading may be selected once, more than once, or not at all.

Group 283-287

283. Adrenal suppression

284. Thrombosis, phlebitis, specific antagonist available

285. Pain on injection, severe hypotension in elderly

286. Increases ICP

287. Lactic acidosis may develop with prolonged use
   A. Thiopental
   B. Diazepam
   C. Etomidate
   D. Propofol
   E. Ketamine

Group 288-292

288. Reduces MAC

289. Is associated with pericardial effusion and cardiac tamponade

290. With high doses may cause a systemic lupus erythematosus-like syndrome

291. Produces α-adrenergic receptor and β-adrenergic receptor blockade

292. May result in severe rebound hypertension when abruptly discontinued
   A. Captopril
   B. Hydralazine
   C. Minoxidil
   D. Labetalol
   E. Clonidine

Group 293-297

293. Increases systemic vascular resistance at low and high doses. Cardiac output is usually unchanged or decreased. Heart rate and blood flow to the kidneys are decreased

294. At low doses lowers systemic vascular resistance, at high doses increases systemic vascular resistance. Cardiac output increases at all doses. Decreases renal blood flow, and has a significant effect on metabolism.

295. Lowers systemic vascular resistance and mean arterial pressure, with marked tachycardia.

296. Little change in systemic vascular resistance with mild increases in heart rate and mean arterial pressure.

297. Little change in systemic vascular resistance, at low or intermediate doses increases renal blood flow, but at high doses decreases renal blood flow.
   A. Dopamine (5 μg/kg/min)
   B. Norepinephrine (10 μg/min)
   C. Epinephrine (10 μg/min)
   D. Isoproterenol (10 μg/min)
   E. Dobutamine (10 μg/kg/min)

Group 298-301

298.   Analgesia (supraspinal and spinal)

299.   Supraspinal analgesia and prolactin release

300.   Depressed ventilation and marked constipation

301.   Little respiratory depression but dysphoria and diuresis
    A. μ (mu), $\varkappa$ (kappa), and δ (delta) opioid receptors
    B. μ_1 (mu$_1$) opioid receptors
    C. μ_2 (mu$_2$) opioid receptors
    D. δ (delta) opioid receptors
    E. $\varkappa$ (kappa) opioid receptors

Group 302-305

302.   Block is antagonized with anticholinesterase drugs

303.   Block is enhanced with anticholinesterase drugs

304.   Post-tetanic facilitation occurs

305.   Sustained response to tetanic stimulus is seen
    A. True of nondepolarizing blockade only
    B. True of phase I depolarizing blockade only
    C. True of phase II depolarizing blockade only
    D. True of nondepolarizing and phase II depolarizing blockade
    E. True of phase I and phase II depolarizing blockade

Group 306-315

306.   Amphetamines

307. α_2 Agonists (clonidine, dexmedetomidine)

308.   Hyperthyroidism

309.   Ethanol

310.   Lidocaine

311.   Lithium

312.   Opioids

313.   Duration of anesthesia

314.   Pregnancy

315.   Pao$_2$ 35 mm Hg
    A. No change in MAC
    B. Increases MAC
    C. Decreases MAC
    D. Acute administration increases MAC; chronic administration decreases MAC
    E. Acute administration decreases MAC; chronic administration increases MAC

Group 316-320

316. Least effective antisialagogue

317. Produces best sedation

318. Increases gastric fluid pH at usual clinical doses

319. Does not produce central anticholinergic syndrome

320. May produce mydriasis and cycloplegia when placed topically in the eye
   A. Atropine
   B. Glycopyrrolate
   C. Scopolamine
   D. Atropine and scopolamine
   E. None of the above

Pharmacology and Pharmacokinetics of Intravenous Drugs

Answers, References, and Explanations

169. (A) The duration of action of neuromuscular blocking drugs is related to the dose administered, as well as how the drug is metabolized or handled in the body. Succinylcholine normally is rapidly metabolized by plasma cholinesterase and has an ultrashort duration of action. The intermediate-duration neuromuscular blockers atracurium and cisatracurium undergo chemical breakdown in the plasma (Hofmann elimination), as well as ester hydrolysis. Vecuronium and rocuronium also have intermediate duration of actions and undergo primarily hepatic metabolism and biliary excretion with limited renal excretion (10% to 25%). Only the long-duration neuromuscular blockers d-tubocurarine, pancuronium, doxacurium, and pipecuronium are primarily excreted in the urine (>70%). In patients with renal failure, the duration of action of neuromuscular blockers is not prolonged with atracurium or cisatracurium; is slightly prolonged with vecuronium and rocuronium; and is markedly prolonged with d-tubocurarine, pancuronium, doxacurium, and pipecuronium. Of the long-duration drugs, 80% of pancuronium, 70% of doxacurium, 70% of pipecuronium are renally excreted unchanged in the urine. D-tubocurarine has a little more liver excretion and a little less renal elimination compared with pancuronium (*Miller: Anesthesia, ed 6, pp 505-511; Stoelting: Pharmacology and Physiology in Anesthetic Practice, ed 4, pp 209-245*).

COMPARATIVE PHARMACOLOGY OF NONDEPOLARIZING NEUROMUSCULAR-BLOCKING DRUGS (%)

Duration	Drug	Renal Excretion	Biliary Excretion	Hepatic Degradation	Plasma Hydrolysis	Chemodegradation (Hofmann Elimination)
Intermediate	Atracurium	10	NS	?	Yes	Yes
	Cisatracurium	NS	NS	0	No	Yes
	Vecuronium	15-25	40-75	20-30	No	No
	Rocuronium	10-25	50-70	10-20	No	No
Long	Pancuronium	80	5-10	10	No	No
	Pipercuronium	70	20	10	No	No
	Doxacurium	70	30	?	No	No

NS, not significant.
(*Stoelting: Pharmacology and Physiology in Anesthetic Practice, ed 4, p 212.*)

170. (D) Porphyrias are caused by a defect in heme synthesis (usually autosomal dominant inheritance pattern) and are commonly classified into inducible and noninducible forms. Only the inducible forms (e.g., acute intermittent porphyria, variegate porphyria, hereditary coproporphyria) show acute symptoms (e.g., neurologic, gastrointestinal) from drug exposure (e.g., barbiturates). Propofol, neuromuscular relaxants, inhalation agents, and opioids are safe in all forms of porphyrias. Although local anesthetics are believed to be safe, some avoid regional anesthesia in inducible porphyrias to avoid confusion if a neurologic complication develops in the postoperative period. Porphyria cutanea tarda is a noninducible form (not affected by drugs) and most often appears as photosensitivity in males older than 35 years. Because the skin often is very friable in these patients, special attention is required to avoid excessive pressure or irritation of the skin (e.g., during mask ventilation or with taping of the endotracheal tube, IV catheters, or eyes) (*Barash: Clinical Anesthesia, ed 5, pp 549-550; Hines: Stoelting's Anesthesia and Co-Existing Disease, ed 5, pp 312-319*).

171. (E) β-Adrenergic receptor antagonists are of two main classes: nonselective blockers (β_1 and β_2 receptors) and cardioselective blockers (β_1 receptors). The selectivity is dose dependent and with large doses the selectivity can be lost. Propranolol, nadolol, pindolol and timolol are nonselective antagonists. Atenolol, acebutolol, betaxolol, bisoprolol, esmolol and metoprolol are cardioselective β₁ antagonists (*Stoelting: Pharmacology and Physiology in Anesthetic Practice, ed 4, pp 323-330*).

172. **(C)** Parkinson's disease (paralysis agitans or shaking palsy) is a degenerative CNS disease. It is caused by greater than 80% destruction of dopaminergic neurons in the substantia nigra of the basal ganglia. Dopamine acts as a neurotransmitter to inhibit the rate of firing of neurons that control the extrapyramidal motor system. The imbalance of neurotransmitters that results leads to the extrapyramidal symptoms of this disease. Symptoms include bradykinesia (slowness of movement), muscular rigidity, resting tremor (that lessens with voluntary movement), and impaired balance. Drugs that can produce extrapyramidal effects, such as the dopamine antagonists droperidol, promethazine, and thiethylperazine, as well as the dopamine and serotonin antagonist metoclopramide, are contraindicated. Ondansetron, a 5-HT₃ receptor antagonist, is the preferred drug to treat nausea and vomiting for this patient (*Barash: Clinical Anesthesia, ed 5, pp 513-514; Hardman: Goodman & Gilman's The Pharmacological Basis of Therapeutics, ed 10, pp 552-560, 1029-1031; Hines: Stoelting's Anesthesia and Co-Existing Disease, ed 5, pp 227-228, 644*).

173. **(A)** In order for depolarizing muscle relaxants such as succinylcholine to work, the drug must interact with the receptor at the myoneural junction. Patients with myasthenia gravis have fewer acetylcholine receptors on the muscle and are more resistant to succinylcholine but are much more sensitive to nondepolarizing muscle relaxants. Patients with myasthenic syndrome (Eaton-Lambert syndrome) have a decreased release of acetylcholine at the myoneural junction; however, the number of receptors is normal. Patients with myasthenic syndrome are more sensitive to both depolarizing and nondepolarizing muscle relaxants. Huntington's chorea is a degenerative CNS disease that is associated with decreased plasma cholinesterase activity, and prolonged responses to succinylcholine use have been seen. The response to depolarizing and nondepolarizing muscle relaxants appears to be unchanged in patients with polymyositis. Succinylcholine is contraindicated in patients with Duchenne's muscular dystrophy because of the risks of rhabdomyolysis, hyperkalemia, and cardiac arrest. Nondepolarizing muscle relaxants have a normal response in patients with Duchenne's muscular dystrophy, although some patients have prominent coexisting skeletal muscle weakness (*Hines: Stoelting's Anesthesia and Co-Existing Disease, ed 5, pp 229, 445-455*).

174. **(A)** Dopamine can directly stimulate dopamine, and β- and α-adrenergic receptors. Because of its rapid metabolism and marked potency, it is only administered intravenously. The pharmacologic effects of dopamine are dose related. Dopamine receptors stimulated at the low dose of 0.5 to 3 μg/kg/min produce renal vasodilation and an increase in renal blood flow. When the dose is increased to 3 to 10 μg/kg/min, β-adrenergic stimulation occurs as well. At doses between 10 and 20 μg/kg/min, both β- and α-adrenergic stimulation are seen (i.e., increased cardiac output and systemic vascular resistance). When the dose is greater than 20 μg/kg/min, α-adrenergic effects predominate (*Miller: Anesthesia, ed 6, pp 798-799; Stoelting: Pharmacology and Physiology in Anesthetic Practice, ed 4, p 300*).

175. **(E)** Diazepam is a benzodiazepine drug that is not water soluble and must be mixed with propylene glycol to become soluble. This intravenous mixture is quite painful. Midazolam (pH 3.5) is a water-soluble drug that is converted to a lipid-soluble drug when exposed to the blood's pH and has very quickly replaced diazepam in clinical practice because of the lack of pain on injection and the shorter half-life. The lipid-soluble form of midazolam can readily cross the blood-brain barrier and exert its pharmacologic effects. None of the other drugs changes form when exposed to blood (*Miller: Anesthesia, ed 6, p 335; Stoelting: Pharmacology and Physiology in Anesthetic Practice, ed 4, pp 142-147*).

176. **(C)** The amount of submucosally injected epinephrine required to produce ventricular cardiac dysrhythmias (i.e., three or more premature ventricular contractions during or after injection) varies with the volatile anesthetic administered. Patients under halothane anesthesia are particularly sensitive to ventricular arrhythmias, whereas patients with isoflurane, desflurane and sevoflurane are less sensitive to epinephrine. Fifty percent of patients have ventricular arrhythmias when a dose of 2.1 μg/kg of epinephrine is administered submucosally into patients under halothane anesthesia. Ventricular arrhythmias do not seem to occur when a dose of up to 5 μg/kg of epinephrine is injected submucosally into patients under 1.2 MAC of sevoflurane or isoflurane in oxygen anesthesia. However, when the dose of epinephrine is increased to between 5 and 15 μg/kg, then about one third of patients will exhibit ventricular ectopy under sevoflurane or isoflurane anesthesia. Thus, using the 5 μg/kg maximum dose, a 70-kg patient could receive up to 350 μg of epinephrine (70 kg × 5 μg/kg) or 35 mL of this 1:100,000 solution (10 μg/mL) without ventricular arrhythmias (*Johnston: A comparative interaction of* *epinephrine with enflurane, isoflurane and halothane in man. Anesth Analg, 55:709-712, 1976; Navarro: Humans anesthetized with sevoflurane or isoflurane have similar arrhythmic response to epinephrine. Anesthesiology, 80:545-549, 1994; Stoelting: Pharmacology and Physiology in Anesthetic Practice, ed 4, pp 54-56).*

177. **(D)** β-Adrenergic receptor antagonists are effective in the treatment of essential hypertension and angina pectoris. They can be used to decrease mortality in patients suffering myocardial infarctions; to treat hyperthyroidism, or hypertrophic obstructive cardiomyopathy; and to prevent migraine headaches. Although they are useful drugs, their use is limited by many side effects, which include bronchoconstriction, suppression of insulin secretion, blunting of the catecholamine response to hypoglycemia, excessive myocardial depression, atrioventricular heart block, accentuated increases in plasma concentrations of potassium with intravenous infusion of potassium chloride, fatigue, and rebound tachycardia associated with abrupt drug discontinuation. An important advantage of β-adrenergic receptor antagonists used in treating hypertension is the lack of orthostatic hypotension (*Miller: Anesthesia, ed 6, pp 654-657; Stoelting: Basics of Anesthesia, ed 5, pp 74-75*).

178. **(E)** Anticholinergics are rarely given with premedication today unless a specific effect is needed (e.g., drying of the mouth before fiberoptic intubation, prevention of bradycardias, and rarely as a mild sedative). Side effects are many and include relaxation or a decrease of the lower esophageal sphincter tone that may make patients more likely to regurgitate gastric contents. Although these drugs can decrease gastric acid secretion and increase gastric pH, the pH effects are small and the dose needed to accomplish this is much higher than clinically used. The following table compares the effects of various anticholinergics (*Miller: Anesthesia, ed 6, pp 660-662; Stoelting: Basics of Anesthesia, ed 5, pp 171-173; Stoelting: Pharmacology and Physiology in Anesthetic Practice, ed 4, pp 268-273*).

COMPARATIVE EFFECTS OF ANTICHOLINERGICS ADMINISTERED INTRAMUSCULARLY AS PHARMACOLOGIC PREMEDICATION

	Atropine	Scopolamine	Glycopyrrolate
Antisialagogue effect	+	+++	++
Sedative and amnesic effects	+	+++	0
Increase in heart rate	+++	+	++
Decreased gastric hydrogen ion secretion	+	+	+
Prevent motion-induced nausea	+	+++	0
Central nervous system toxicity	+	++	0
Relaxation of lower esophageal sphincter tone	++	++	++
Mydriasis, cycloplegia	+	+++	0

0, none; +, mild; ++, moderate; +++, marked.
(*Stoelting: Basics of Anesthesia, ed 5, p172; Stoelting: Pharmacology and Physiology in Anesthetic Practice, ed 4, p 268.*)

179. **(D)** Neostigmine, pyridostigmine, edrophonium, and physostigmine are anticholinesterase drugs. Neostigmine, pyridostigmine, and edrophonium are quaternary ammonium compounds and do not pass the blood-brain barrier. However, physostigmine is a tertiary amine and does cross the blood-brain barrier. This property makes physostigmine useful in the treatment for central anticholinergic syndrome (also called postoperative delirium or atropine toxicity) (*Barash: Clinical Anesthesia, ed 5, pp 300-302; Miller: Anesthesia, ed 6, p 662*).

180. **(D)** Whereas propofol, barbiturates, etomidate, and benzodiazepines exert much, if not all of their pharmacologic effects via the GABA receptors, ketamine has only weak activity on the GABA receptors. Ketamine's mechanism of action is complex with most of the effects due to interaction with NMDA receptors. Ketamine also interacts with monoaminergic, muscarinic and opioid receptors as well as voltage-sensitive calcium ion channels (*Barash: Clinical Anesthesia, ed 5, pp 344-345; Miller: Anesthesia, ed 6, pp 346-347; Stoelting: Basics of Anesthesia, ed 5, pp 98-109; Stoelting: Pharmacology and Physiology in Anesthetic Practice, ed 4, pp 167-168*).

181. **(D)** All of the drugs listed are opioids. Meperidine is structurally similar to atropine and possesses mild anticholinergic properties. In contrast to other opioid-receptor agonists, meperidine rarely causes bradycardia but can increase heart rate. Normeperidine, a metabolite of meperidine with some CNS-stimulating properties, may cause delirium and seizures if the level is high enough. This is more likely in patients who have renal impairment and are receiving meperidine over several days (*Stoelting: Pharmacology and Physiology in Anesthetic Practice, ed 4, pp 102-104*).

182. **(E)** In the United States, ketamine is prepared as a mixtures of the two isomers S(+) and R(-). In some countries the S(+) isomer, which is more potent and has fewer side effects, is available. All of the statements are true except for E. Norketamine (ketamine's primary active metabolite) is one fifth to one third as potent as ketamine and can contribute to prolonged effects (*Miller: Anesthesia, ed 6, pp 345-350; Stoelting: Basics of Anesthesia, ed 5, pp 106-108*).

183. **(B)** Direct-acting sympathomimetic drugs work directly on the receptors. Indirect-acting sympathomimetic drugs have their effects primarily by entering the neurons then displacing norepinephrine and causing the release of norepinephrine from the postganglionic sympathetic nerve fibers. Ephedrine, mephentermine, and metaraminol are primarily indirect-acting sympathomimetic agents that may have some direct-acting properties as well. The following table summarizes the sympathomimetic agents and their effects on the adrenergic receptors (*Stoelting: Basics of Anesthesia, ed 5, pp 66-71; Stoelting: Pharmacology and Physiology in Anesthetic Practice, ed 4, pp 292-309*).

CLASSIFICATION AND COMPARATIVE PHARMACOLOGY OF SYMPATHOMIMETICS

Sympathomimetic	α	β_1	β_2	Mechanism of Action
Amphetamine	++	+	+	Indirect
Dobutamine	0	+++	0	Direct
Dopamine	++	++	+	Direct
Ephedrine	++	+	+	Indirect and some direct
Epinephrine	+	++	++	Direct
Isoproterenol	0	+++	+++	Direct
Mephentermine	++	+	+	Indirect
Metaraminol	++	+	+	Indirect and some direct
Methoxamine	+++	0	0	Direct
Norepinephrine	+++	++	0	Direct
Phenylephrine	+++	0	0	Direct

0, no change; +, mild stimulation; ++, moderate stimulation; +++, marked stimulation.
(*Stoelting: Pharmacology and Physiology in Anesthetic Practice, ed 4, p 293.*)

184. **(B)** Opioids in general produce less direct negative effects on myocardial contractility than the IV induction agents propofol and thiopental, or the volatile inhalation agents. The physiologic effects of meperidine on the cardiovascular system are different from those of most other opioid-receptor agonists. These effects are related to its atropine-like effects and its local anesthetic properties. Meperidine rarely causes bradycardia, even in high doses, but it can cause an increase in heart rate. A decrease in contractility can be seen with large doses of meperidine. This decrease in contractility appears to be unique among the opioids and may be related to meperidine's local anesthetic properties (*Morgan: Clinical Anesthesia, ed 4, p 195; Stoelting: Pharmacology and Physiology in Anesthetic Practice, ed 4, pp 93-112*).

185. **(B)** Ketamine is a nonbarbiturate anesthetic/analgesia drug that is a derivative of phencyclidine. Patients who have received ketamine have a strong feeling of dissociation from their environment and hence the term dissociative anesthesia is commonly used. With adequate induction dose (i.e., not responsive), patients may appear awake (i.e., breathing but still and eyes may remain open). Ketamine may produce varying degrees of hypertonus, purposeful skeletal muscle movements, increased salivation, marked amnesia, and intense analgesia. Although the analgesia produced by ketamine is intense, there is evidence that analgesia is greater for somatic than for visceral pain. Ketamine can stimulate the sympathetic nervous system; can produce increases in systemic and pulmonary artery blood pressures, heart rate, cardiac output, cardiac work, and myocardial oxygen requirement; and can produce bronchodilation. Ketamine is metabolized almost exclusively in the liver by cytochrome P-450 enzymes to norketamine, which is one-fifth to one-third as potent as ketamine. It can be administered by a variety of routes, including intravenous, intramuscular, rectal, nasal, and oral. Because many patients have unpleasant hallucinations, especially if the drug is used alone, it is not widely administered (*Hardman: Goodman & Gilman's The Pharmacological Basis of Therapeutics, ed 10, pp 346-347; Miller: Anesthesia, ed 6, pp 345-350; Stoelting: Pharmacology and Physiology in Anesthetic Practice, ed 4, pp 167-174*).

186. **(B)** Myocardial depression can occur with a variety of anesthetic drugs, with volatile anesthetics being more depressant than intravenous anesthetics. Of the intravenous drugs listed in this question, thiopental is most likely to cause a dose dependent negative inotropic effect which results from a decrease in calcium influx into the myocardial cells (*Miller: Anesthesia, ed 6, pp 323-340*).

187. (B)   Echothiophate is an organophosphate that irreversibly inhibits acetylcholinesterase, which is responsible for the metabolism of succinylcholine and ester-type local anesthetics. It does this by forming a phosphorylated complex with acetylcholinesterase. The topical solution is instilled in the eye for treatment of refractory open angle glaucoma. The amount of drug absorbed may be sufficient to inhibit acetylcholinesterase and cause prolongation in the duration of action of succinylcholine or mivacurium. Because of this, it is "recommended" to wait at least 3 weeks after the stoppage of echothiophate before the administration of these two muscle relaxants. One must wonder about these "recommendations" because clinical cases have shown that when cholinesterase activity is decreased (from echothiophate) to no activity, the increase in duration of neuromuscular block from succinylcholine was less than 25 minutes (*Stoelting: Basics of Anesthesia, ed 5, p 464; Miller: Anesthesia, ed 6, pp 1125-1126, 2536-2537*).

188. (E)   Monitoring neuromuscular blockade for nondepolarizing muscle relaxants can be done a variety of ways. The simplest way is to measure the reduction or suppression of a single twitch height. This is commonly performed by observing the twitch response of the thumb's adductor pollicis muscle, after ulnar nerve stimulation. At 90% to 95% reduction of twitch height (i.e., ED_{90} to ED_{95}) there is good muscle relaxation for intubation and intra-abdominal surgery. However, measuring the reduction of twitch height is not practical. Because there is good correlation between reduction of twitch height and the number of thumb twitches that can be elicited by TOF stimulation, TOF stimulation is more commonly used where 4 twitches are administered over 2 seconds. If only one twitch of a TOF is demonstrated, single twitch height is depressed at least 85%; with two to four thumb twitches 70% to 85% depression is seen. Note that the presence of four twitches does not mean that neuromuscular function has completely recovered; in fact, a significant number of receptors may still be occupied by the muscle relaxant (*Barash: Clinical Anesthesia, ed 5, pp 440-441*).

189. (D)   There are two major chemical classes of nondepolarizing muscle relaxants, the aminosteroids (-onium drugs) and the benzylisoquinolinium (-urium) drugs. In general, the aminosteroids cause no significant histamine release (at the clinical doses of 2 to $3 \times ED_{95}$), whereas some of the benzylisoquinolinium drugs can. The histamine release primarily occurs with rapid administration of atracurium but does not occur with cisatracurium or doxacurium. The amount of histamine released is rarely of clinical significance. The cardiovascular effects of neuromuscular blocking drugs occur by three main mechanisms: (1) drug-induced histamine release; (2) effects at cardiac muscarinic receptors; or (3) effects on nicotinic receptors at autonomic ganglia. The following table summarizes the mechanisms for the cardiovascular effects of muscle relaxants (*Miller: Anesthesia, ed 6, p 512; Stoelting: Basics of Anesthesia, ed 5, pp 142-145; Stoelting: Pharmacology and Physiology in Anesthetic Practice, ed 4, p 223*).

MECHANISMS OF NEUROMUSCULAR-BLOCKING DRUG-INDUCED CARDIOVASCULAR EFFECTS

Drug*	Histamine Release Receptors	Cardiac Muscarinic Receptors	Nicotinic Receptors at Autonomic Ganglia
Succinylcholine	Slight	Modest stimulation	Modest stimulation
Vecuronium	None	None	None
Atracurium	Slight†	None	None
Cisatracurium	None	None	None
Rocuronium	None	None	None
d-Tubocurarine	Moderate	None	Blocks
Pancuronium	None	Modest blockade	None
Pipecuronium	None	None	None
Doxacurium	None	None	None

*ED_{90} or ED_{95} doses.
†Occurs only with doses of 2 to $3 \times ED_{90}$ or ED_{95}.
(*Stoelting: Pharmacology and Physiology in Anesthetic Practice, ed 4, p 223; Miller: Anesthesia, ed 6, p 512.*)

190. (A)   Postganglionic sympathetic nerve fibers release norepinephrine from the synaptic vesicles in the nerve terminals. Eighty percent of the released norepinephrine rapidly undergoes reuptake into the sympathetic nerve terminals (uptake 1) and reenters storage vesicles for future release. Only a small amount of the norepinephrine that is reabsorbed is metabolized in the cytoplasm by MAO. Twenty percent of the norepinephrine is diluted by diffusion away from the receptors and can gain access to the circulation. COMT, which is located primarily in the liver, metabolizes this norepinephrine (*Miller: Anesthesia, ed 6, p 633; Stoelting: Pharmacology and Physiology in Anesthetic Practice, ed 4, pp 700-701*).

191. (D) Administration of ketamine may be associated with visual, auditory, and proprioceptive hallucinations. These unpleasant side effects of ketamine occur on emergence and may progress to delirium. The incidence of emergence delirium from ketamine is dose dependent and occurs in approximately 5% to 30% of patients. Emergence delirium is less frequent after repeated administrations of ketamine. The most effective prevention for emergence delirium is administration of a benzodiazepine (midazolam being more effective than diazepam) about 5 minutes before induction of anesthesia with ketamine. Atropine and droperidol given perioperatively may increase the incidence of emergence delirium (*Miller: Anesthesia, ed 6, pp 347-349; Stoelting: Pharmacology and Physiology in Anesthetic Practice, ed 4, pp 173-174*).

192. (A) Extrapyramidal side effects are seen most often with antipsychotic drugs (e.g., phenothiazines, thioxanthenes, and butyrophenones), but they also can be seen with administration of metoclopramide. Metoclopramide, a dopamine antagonist, increases lower esophageal sphincter tone and stimulates gastric and upper intestinal tract motility. Side effects associated with metoclopramide use include mild sedation, dysphoria, agitation, dry mouth, and, in rare instances, dystonic extrapyramidal reactions (oculogyric crises, trismus, torticollis). Akathisia, or the feeling of unease and motor restlessness, has occurred following IV metoclopramide, which may result in cancellation of elective surgery (*Stoelting: Pharmacology and Physiology in Anesthetic Practice, ed 4, pp 499-502*).

193. (B) Succinylcholine is a depolarizing muscle relaxant that chemically resembles acetylcholine and attaches to the postjunctional membrane ion channel receptors. Sustained opening of ion channels produced by succinylcholine (as opposed to a transient opening with acetylcholine) is associated with leakage of potassium from the interior of cells sufficient to increase plasma concentrations of potassium by about 0.5 mEq/L in normal patients. This slight increase of potassium levels in patients with renal failure is similar to patients with normal renal function (*Miller: Anesthesia, ed 6, p 489; Stoelting: Basics of Anesthesia, ed 5, pp 141-142; Stoelting: Pharmacology and Physiology in Anesthetic Practice, ed 4, p 220*).

194. (A) Many drugs can enhance the neuromuscular block produced by nondepolarizing muscle relaxants. These include volatile anesthetics, aminoglycoside antibiotics, magnesium, intravenous local anesthetics, furosemide, dantrolene, calcium channel blockers, and lithium. Calcium does not enhance neuromuscular blockade and, in fact, actually antagonizes the effects of magnesium. In patients with hyperparathyroidism and hypercalcemia there is a decreased sensitivity to nondepolarizing muscle relaxants and shorter durations of action (*Miller: Anesthesia, ed 6, pp 514-518; Stoelting: Pharmacology and Physiology in Anesthetic Practice, ed 4, pp 224-226, 395*).

195. (E) None of these drugs should be abruptly stopped. Clonidine is a centrally active alpha-adrenergic agonist that is used in the treatment of hypertension. Severe rebound hypertension can be seen between 8 and 36 hours after the last dose, especially in patients receiving more than 1.2 mg/day. Rebound hypertension, as well as cardiac ischemia, can be seen after discontinuation of β-blocker therapy (e.g., propranolol). In the past, it was recommended to stop MAOIs 2 to 3 weeks before elective surgery because of the possibility of developing hypertensive crisis during surgery. More recently it has become acceptable to use these drugs up to the time of surgery, because their discontinuance could place the patient at risk for suicide. Certain drug interactions may occur with MAOI use, including skeletal muscle rigidity or hyperpyrexia with meperidine, as well as an exaggerated hypertensive response with the indirect-acting vasopressor ephedrine. Abrupt withdrawal of chronic high-dose tricyclic antidepressant therapy can be associated with withdrawal (i.e., malaise, chills, coryza, skeletal muscle aching) and is not recommended (*Stoelting: Basics of Anesthesia, ed 5, pp 72-75; Stoelting: Pharmacology and Physiology in Anesthetic Practice, ed 4, pp 401-407*).

196. (A) Cisatracurium and atracurium are metabolized in blood primarily by the processes of Hofmann elimination and ester hydrolysis. Hofmann elimination is a chemical (pH and temperature dependent) and not a biologic process. Ester hydrolysis of atracurium occurs via plasma cholinesterases different from pseudocholinesterase, the enzymes that metabolize succinylcholine. Therefore, in contrast to succinylcholine, patients with atypical pseudocholinesterase will not experience prolonged paralysis after administration of atracurium. The principal metabolite of atracurium is laudanosine, a tertiary amine that can pass the blood-brain barrier and cause CNS stimulation at very high, usually nonclinical levels. Because laudanosine is dependent on the kidney and liver for excretion, levels may become high in patients who received atracurium for several hours in the intensive care area who also have significant renal or hepatic clearances. Because cisatracurium is 4 to 5 times more potent than atracurium, significantly lower levels of laudanosine are produced at equivalent muscle relaxant doses (*Miller: Anesthesia, ed 6, pp 501, 509-510; Stoelting: Pharmacology and Physiology in Anesthetic Practice, ed 4, pp 232-233*).

197. (C) Succinylcholine is associated with numerous potential adverse side effects, including cardiac arrhythmias (sinus bradycardia, junctional rhythm, and, rarely, sinus arrest), increased gastric pressure, increased intraocular pressure, increased ICP, hyperkalemia, myalgias, and myoglobinuria (mainly in children). Other side effects that are genetically related include prolonged muscle paralysis (abnormal pseudocholinesterase) and malignant hyperthermia. These side effects may be serious and may limit or contraindicate succinylcholine use in certain patients. Pretreatment with a nondepolarizing muscle relaxant (e.g., about 1 mL for a 70-kg patient with d-tubocurarine, pancuronium, or atracurium) 3 to 5 minutes before administration of succinylcholine attenuates but does not eliminate cardiac dysrhythmias, elevations in intragastric pressure or ICP, or myalgia. However, the potassium increase seen with succinylcholine use, as well as prolonged muscle paralysis or malignant hyperthermia, are not attenuated by pretreatment (*Barash: Clinical Anesthesia, ed 5, pp 428-429; Miller: Anesthesia, ed 6, pp 489-491; Stoelting: Pharmacology and Physiology in Anesthetic Practice, ed 4, pp 220-221*).

198. (D) Several antibiotics potentiate neuromuscular blockade. The aminoglycosides (neomycin, streptomycin, gentamicin, and tobramycin) and the lincosamines (clindamycin and lincomycin) can augment neuromuscular blockade. The only drug in this question that does not affect neuromuscular blockade is erythromycin (of the macrolide antibiotic group). In addition, tetracyclines, penicillins and cephalosporins do not affect neuromuscular blockade (*Barash: Clinical Anesthesia, ed 5, p 438; Miller: Anesthesia, ed 6, p 516*).

199. (B) Edrophonium, neostigmine, and pyridostigmine are anticholinesterase drugs used to antagonize the neuromuscular blockade induced by nondepolarizing neuromuscular blocking drugs. These drugs do not cross the blood-brain barrier. They produce an increase in acetylcholine not only at the myoneural junction but also at the cholinergic neurons of the autonomic nervous system (preganglionic sympathetic, preganglionic and postganglionic parasympathetic). Prevention of the cholinergic side effects is the reason why these drugs are routinely administered with atropine or glycopyrrolate. Edrophonium has a rapid (1 to 2 minutes) onset of action, neostigmine an intermediate onset (7 to 11 minutes), and pyridostigmine a delayed (16 minutes) onset. The difference in onset of action may be related to the mechanism of action of these drugs. Edrophonium primarily has a presynaptic (acetylcholine release) action, whereas neostigmine and pyridostigmine appear to work primarily postsynaptically (acetylcholinesterase inhibition). Because edrophonium has a rapid onset of action, it is used with atropine (atropine has a faster onset of action than glycopyrrolate). Neostigmine and pyridostigmine can be used with either atropine or glycopyrrolate, although from the onset of action standpoint glycopyrrolate is more appropriate if a stable heart rate is desired with these two anticholinesterase drugs (*Miller: Anesthesia, ed 6, p 521; Stoelting: Pharmacology and Physiology in Anesthetic Practice, ed 4, pp 258-259*).

200. (E) Thiopental is a short-acting thiobarbiturate most commonly used intraoperatively to induce general anesthesia. Thiopental is prepared commercially for clinical use in a 2.5% sodium salt solution. Concentrations greater than 2.5% are not used because of the possibility of significant tissue damage if the drug is inadvertently injected subcutaneously or intra-arterially. The high alkaline pH of thiopental solutions (pH 10.5) makes this drug incompatible for mixture with acidic-type drugs (e.g., opioids, catecholamines, and neuromuscular blocking drugs). The high alkaline pH of thiopental solutions is responsible for its bacteriostatic properties (i.e., sterile for at least 6 days at 22° C) (*Hardman: Goodman & Gilman's The Pharmacological Basis of Therapeutics, ed 10, pp 342-343; Stoelting: Pharmacology and Physiology in Anesthetic Practice, ed 4, p 127*).

201. (B) In normal patients, potassium levels increase about 0.5 mEq/L after the administration of succinylcholine. However, in some acquired conditions the potassium level may increase 5 to 7 mEq/L above the baseline potassium level after administration of succinylcholine. This marked elevation of potassium may lead to cardiac arrest. These acquired conditions include the following: (1) denervation injury as caused by spinal cord injury leading to skeletal muscle atrophy; (2) skeletal muscle injury resulting from third-degree burns (until scarring occurs); (3) acute upper motor neuron injury such as stroke; (4) severe skeletal muscle trauma; and (5) severe abdominal infections. In these acquired conditions the potential to increase potassium levels after succinylcholine usually takes a few days to develop, peaks 10 to 50 days after the initial injury, and may persist for 6 months or more. All factors considered, it might be prudent to avoid administration of succinylcholine to any patient more than 24 hours after the conditions listed here. This vulnerability to hyperkalemia may reflect a proliferation of extrajunctional cholinergic receptors, which provide more sites for potassium to leak outward across the cell membrane during depolarization. Some have suggested that the number of receptors is unchanged but that the receptors themselves have altered affinity to acetylcholine or drugs. Similar marked elevations of potassium may develop in cases of undiagnosed myopathy (*Hines: Stoelting's Anesthesia and Co-Existing Disease, ed 5, pp 240-242; Miller: Anesthesia, ed 6, pp 489-490; Stoelting: Pharmacology and Physiology in Anesthetic Practice, ed 4, pp 220-221*).

202. (A) Although flumazenil (a specific benzodiazepine antagonist) inhibits the activity at the GABA receptor, it works only at the benzodiazepine recognition site and has no effect in reversing other drugs that work on the GABA site (e.g., barbiturates, etomidate, propofol). It has a fast onset (within minutes), with peak brain levels occurring within 6 to 10 minutes, and a relatively short duration of action. Flumazenil can reverse all benzodiazepine CNS effects, including sedative, amnestic, muscle relaxant, and anticonvulsant effects. Side effects are rare, the most common being nausea, vomiting, or both (about 10%). Nausea occurs more commonly when flumazenil is given to patients after general anesthesia than after conscious sedation. Patients receiving flumazenil should be monitored for possible resedation and respiratory depression due to its short clinical duration of action (*Miller: Anesthesia, ed 6, pp 343-345; Physicians Desk Reference, ed 63, 2009, pp 2646-2649*).

203. (B) The onset of action of edrophonium is fast (1 to 2 minutes), neostigmine is intermediate (7 to 11 minutes), and pyridostigmine is slow (about 16 minutes). If these drugs are given without an anticholinergic drug, marked cholinergic activity (e.g., bradycardia, increased salivation) is seen, along with the reversal of neuromuscular blockade. The onset of action of atropine (7 μg/kg) is very rapid and is similar to that of edrophonium (0.5 mg/kg). Little change in heart rate is usually noted with this combination. Since glycopyrrolate has a slow onset of action compared to atropine, it is better suited for use with the slower onset neostigmine or pyridostigmine. If glycopyrrolate is used with edrophonium, a marked bradycardia will initially develop (*Miller: Anesthesia, ed 6, p 523; Stoelting: Pharmacology and Physiology in Anesthetic Practice, ed 4, pp 254-259*).

204. (D) Acute intermittent porphyria is the most serious form of porphyria. This disease affects both the central and peripheral nervous systems. An acute intermittent porphyria attack can be triggered by a variety of conditions, including starvation, dehydration, stress, sepsis, and some drugs (especially barbiturates such as thiopental). Drugs that are safe or probably safe include local anesthetics, inhaled anesthetics, neuromuscular blocking drugs, some intravenous anesthetics (propofol and ketamine), some analgesics (acetaminophen, aspirin, morphine, fentanyl, sufentanil), antiemetics (droperidol, H_2 blockers, metoclopramide, ondansetron), and some benzodiazepines (midazolam, lorazepam). Drugs that are contraindicated include some intravenous anesthetics (barbiturates and perhaps etomidate), some analgesics (ketorolac, pentazocine), some benzodiazepines (diazepam), and hydantoin anticonvulsants. Etomidate is potentially porphyrinogenic in animal studies, despite its safe use in humans. Also see explanation to question 170 (*Barash: Clinical Anesthesia, ed 5, pp 549-550; Hines: Stoelting's Anesthesia and Co-Existing Disease, ed 5, pp 312-318*).

205. (A) Both verapamil and dantrolene have the ability to inhibit intracellular calcium flux and excitation-contraction coupling. This combination suggests that it might be useful in the treatment of malignant hyperthermia. Clinically however, calcium antagonists do not increase survival. Calcium has been useful in treating severe hyperkalemia during episodes of malignant hyperthermia. In laboratory animals and in case reports, administration of dantrolene in the presence of verapamil has resulted in hyperkalemia and, at times, cardiovascular collapse. Dantrolene can produce hepatitis in less than 1% of patients treated chronically for more than 60 days (*Miller: Anesthesia, ed 6, p 1184, Stoelting: Pharmacology and Physiology in Anesthetic Practice, ed 4, pp 396, 596-597*).

206. (E) Although etomidate causes pain on intravenous injection in up to 80% of patients, the unintentional administration of etomidate into an artery does not result in detrimental effects to the artery (*Miller: Anesthesia, ed 6, p 354*).

207. (D) Fentanyl is more lipid soluble than morphine, so it passes through the blood-brain barrier more easily and has a faster onset of action. Fentanyl also has a larger volume of distribution, slower plasma clearance, and longer elimination half-life than morphine. However, the duration of action of fentanyl (when given in small doses) is much shorter than that of morphine because fentanyl is rapidly redistributed from the brain to inactive tissue sites (e.g., lipid sites). In larger doses, these tissue sites can become saturated, and the pharmacologic action of fentanyl becomes considerably prolonged (*Miller: Anesthesia, ed 6, p 401; Stoelting: Pharmacology and Physiology in Anesthetic Practice, ed 4, pp 104-105*).

208. **(A)** An azeotrope is a mixture of two vapors that evaporates to provide a gas mixture from the agents present in the same ratio that occurs in a solution. This type of anesthesia was briefly popular after the introduction of halothane. The idea was to mix it with diethyl ether and to reap the advantages of two agents having counteracting side effects. However, presently the subject of azeotropes commonly arises when the wrong anesthetic is used to fill a half-empty vaporizer (*Miller: Anesthesia, ed 2, pp 83-84*).

209. **(E)** Cerebrospinal fluid (CSF) secretion or production can be reduced with certain drugs such as furosemide, acetazolamide, halothane, etomidate, and hypothermia. The clinical effect of reducing CSF secretion by these methods is transient; therefore, their use in long-term management of intracranial hypertension has not been substantiated. In animal studies, volatile anesthetics have various effects on CSF secretion and absorption. Halothane decreases CSF secretion and absorption; isoflurane has no effect on CSF secretion but increases CSF absorption; and enflurane increases the rate of CSF secretion but decreases the rate of CSF absorption. Although the time course of enflurane's effect on CSF dynamics is slow, this observation suggests that enflurane may not be appropriate during prolonged closed cranium procedures in patients with reduced intracranial compliance. Similarly, desflurane may not be appropriate in similar circumstances because desflurane also appears to increase secretion of CSF (but this may occur only with hypocapnia) and does not seem to affect CSF absorption (*Barash: Clinical Anesthesia, ed 5, pp 400, 749-750; Miller: Anesthesia, ed 6, p 832*).

210. **(C)** The first two letters of the name rocuronium stands for rapid onset. Of the nondepolarizing muscle relaxants currently available, it has the most rapid onset of action at clinically useful dosages. Rocuronium is a nondepolarizing neuromuscular relaxant with an intermediate duration of action similar to vecuronium, atracurium, and cisatracurium. At an ED_{95} dose (0.3 mg/kg), the onset time is 1.5 to 3 minutes, whereas with the other intermediate nondepolarizing muscle relaxants, the onset time is 3 to 7 minutes. At larger doses (i.e., $2 \times ED_{95}$ or 0.6 mg/kg), onset time can be reduced to 1 to 1.5 minutes (*Barash: Clinical Anesthesia, ed 5, pp 427, 435-436*).

211. **(D)** An acute decrease in serum potassium causes hyperpolarization of cell membranes. This causes resistance to depolarizing neuromuscular blockers and an increased sensitivity to non-depolarizing neuromuscular blockers. (*Stoelting: Pharmacology and Physiology in Anesthetic Practice, ed 4, pp 226-227*).

212. **(B)** Succinylcholine and the benzylisoquinolinium neuromuscular blocker drug atracurium (but not cisatracurium or doxacurium) can release histamine when given as a rapid intravenous bolus. The amount of histamine released is rarely of clinical significance. However, the benzylisoquinolinium drug d-tubocurarine can produce significant decreases in arterial blood pressure when given rapidly. This is principally the result of histamine release and is why large bolus doses of d-tubocurarine are not given. Also see explanation to question 189 (*Miller: Anesthesia, ed 6, p 512; Stoelting: Basics of Anesthesia, ed 5, pp 142-145; Stoelting: Pharmacology and Physiology in Anesthetic Practice, ed 4, p 223*).

213. **(C)** The symptoms described in this patient are consistent with cholinergic stimulation or increased levels of acetylcholine that occur with anticholinesterase poisoning. Stimulation of the parasympathetic nervous system activation produces miosis, abdominal cramping, excess salivation, loss of bowel and bladder control, bradycardia, and bronchoconstriction. These symptoms are treated with atropine. The acetylcholinesterase reactivator pralidoxime sometimes is added to treat the nicotinic effects of elevation of acetylcholine at the neuromuscular junction of skeletal muscle (i.e., skeletal muscle weakness, apnea). CNS effects of elevated acetylcholine levels can include confusion, ataxia, and coma. In addition, supportive therapy (the ABCs of resuscitation [Airway, Breathing, Circulation, etc.]) is provided as needed (*Stoelting: Pharmacology and Physiology in Anesthetic Practice, ed 4, pp 262-263*).

214. **(C)** Flumazenil is a benzodiazepine antagonist used to antagonize the benzodiazepine effects on the CNS. It does not reverse the effects of barbiturates, opiates, or alcohol. Seizures can be precipitated in patients who have been on benzodiazepines for long term sedation or patients showing signs of serious cyclic antidepressant overdosage (e.g., twitching, rigidity, widened QRS complex, hypotension). Flumazenil has a shorter elimination half-life (0.7 to 1.3 hours) compared with midazolam (2 to 2.5 hours). Flumazenil is poorly absorbed orally (*Miller: Anesthesia, ed 6, pp 343-345; Physicians Desk Reference ed 63, 2009, pp 2646-2649*).

215. (D) Adequate recovery from neuromuscular blockade is believed to occur when 50% or less of receptors are occupied with muscle relaxants. This can be measured with sustained tetanus at 100 Hz, but this test is very painful. Another method requires patient cooperation and consists of a sustained head lift for 5 seconds in the supine position. The "head lift" test is the standard test to determine adequate muscular function (*Miller: Anesthesia, ed 6, pp 484-487*).

216. (D) The onsets of action (<30 seconds) of thiopental and methohexital are similar. The clearance time for methohexital (11 mL/kg/min) is approximately three times faster than the time for thiopental (3.4 mL/kg/min). The shorter elimination half-time of methohexital compared with that of thiopental reflects the greater hepatic metabolism of methohexital (*Miller: Anesthesia, ed 6, p 329; Stoelting: Basics of Anesthesia, ed 5, pp 99-104*).

217. (A) Patients with WPW syndrome are predisposed to develop supraventricular arrhythmias. Sympathetic stimulation (e.g., anxiety, hypovolemia), as well as many drugs (e.g., pancuronium, meperidine, ketamine, ephedrine, digoxin, verapamil), can induce tachyarrhythmias, often by enhancing conduction through accessory atrial pathways. Although verapamil is used to treat supraventricular tachyarrhythmias because of its depressant effects on alveolar nodal conduction, it actually may increase the heart rate in patients with WPW syndrome because it can increase conduction of the accessory pathways. Droperidol, in addition to its antidopaminergic properties, has antidysrhythmic properties that protect against epinephrine-induced dysrhythmias. Proposed mechanisms include alpha-adrenergic receptor blockade and mild local anesthetic effects. Large doses of droperidol (0.2 to 0.6 mg/kg) can reduce impulse transmission via the accessory pathways responsible for the tachyarrhythmias that occur in patients with WPW syndrome (*Barash: Clinical Anesthesia, ed 5, p 1545; Hines: Stoelting's Anesthesia and Co-Existing Disease, ed 5, p 72; Morgan: Clinical Anesthesiology, ed 4, pp 435-440; Stoelting: Pharmacology and Physiology in Anesthetic Practice, ed 4, pp 413-415, 766*).

218. (C) Pseudocholinesterase (also called plasma cholinesterase) is an enzyme found in plasma and most other tissues (except erythrocytes). Pseudocholinesterase metabolizes the acetylcholine released at the neuromuscular junction, as well as certain drugs such as succinylcholine, mivacurium, and ester-type local anesthetics. It is produced in the liver and has a half-life of approximately 8 to 16 hours. Pseudocholinesterase levels may be reduced in patients with advanced liver disease. The decrease must be greater than 75% before significant prolongation of neuromuscular blockade occurs with succinylcholine (*Barash: Clinical Anesthesia, ed 5, pp 546-549; Miller: Anesthesia, ed 6, pp 487-488*).

219. (A) Ketorolac is a nonsteroidal anti-inflammatory drug (NSAID) that inhibits the enzyme cyclooxygenase, which is necessary for prostaglandin synthesis. Prostaglandins are mediators of pain and inflammation and act at the site of injury; therefore, inhibition of cyclooxygenase is a peripheral effect (*Stoelting: Basics of Anesthesia, ed 5, pp 582-583*).

220. (C) The adrenal cortex secretes two classes of steroids, the corticosteroids (glucocorticoids and mineralocorticoids) and the androgens. The main glucocorticoid is hydrocortisone, also called cortisol. The glucocorticoids are used primarily for their anti-inflammatory and immunosuppressive effects, but they also have mineralocorticoid activity (i.e., sodium-retaining effects). These drugs differ in potency, amount of mineralocorticoid effect, and duration of action. The normal amount of cortisol produced daily is about 10 mg, but under stress, the level can increase tenfold. The main mineralocorticoid is aldosterone. The normal amount of aldosterone produced daily is about 0.125 mg. Because fludrocortisone has such significant mineralocorticoid activity it is used only for its mineralocorticoid activity. The following table compares several corticosteroids. In this case, 50 mg of prednisone is equivalent in glucocorticoid activity to 7.5 mg of dexamethasone and 200 mg of hydrocortisone (*Hardman: Goodman & Gilman's The Pharmacological Basis of Therapeutics, ed 10, pp 1655-1666; Stoelting: Pharmacology and Physiology in Anesthetic Practice, ed 4, pp 461-464*).

COMPARATIVE PHARMACOLOGY OF CORTICOSTEROIDS

Agent	Anti-inflammatory Potency	Equivalent Glucocorticoid Dose (mg)	Sodium-Retaining Potency	Duration of Action (Hr)
Hydrocortisone or Cortisol (Cortef)	1	20	1	8-12
Cortisone (Cortone)	0.8	25	0.8	8-36
Prednisolone (Hydeltrasol)	4	5	0.8	12-36

(Continued)

COMPARATIVE PHARMACOLOGY OF CORTICOSTEROIDS—cont'd

Agent	Anti-inflammatory Potency	Equivalent Glucocorticoid Dose (mg)	Sodium-Retaining Potency	Duration of Action (Hr)
Prednisone (Deltasone)	4	5	0.8	18-36
Methylprednisolone (Solu-Medrol)	5	4	0.5	12-36
Triamcinolone (Kenalog)	5	4	0	12-36
Betamethasone (Celestone)	25	0.75	0	36-54
Dexamethasone (Decadron)	25	0.75	0	36-54
Fludrocortisone (Florinef)	10	2	250	24
Aldosterone	0	NA	3000	

(Stoelting: Pharmacology and Physiology in Anesthetic Practice, ed 4, p 462.)

221. (A) The RI of neuromuscular blocking drugs is the time needed for spontaneous recovery of a twitch height from 25% to 75% of the baseline height. The elderly, who tend to have reduced renal and hepatic function, have a prolonged RI for nondepolarizing muscle relaxants that are dependent upon renal or hepatic elimination (e.g., vecuronium, d-tubocurarine, pancuronium, rocuronium). The RI for atracurium and cisatracurium which are broken down in the plasma, are not prolonged in the elderly (*Barash: Clinical Anesthesia, ed 5, pp 432-436; Miller: Anesthesia, ed 6, pp 526-527*).

222. (B) Cyclosporine is a drug that selectively inhibits helper T-lymphocyte–mediated but not B-lymphocyte–mediated immune responses. It is mainly used alone or in combination with corticosteroids to prevent or treat organ rejection. Other uses include the treatment of Crohn's disease, uveitis, psoriasis, and rheumatoid arthritis. Side effects that may accompany the administration of cyclosporine include nephrotoxicity (25% to 38%), hypertension, limb paresthesias (50%), headaches, confusion, somnolence, seizures, elevation of liver enzymes, allergic reactions, gum hyperplasia, hirsutism, and hyperglycemia. There appears to be no pulmonary toxicity associated with cyclosporine therapy (*Miller: Anesthesia, ed 6, pp 2271-2273; Stoelting: Pharmacology and Physiology in Anesthetic Practice, ed 4, pp 469-470*).

223. (B) Succinylcholine is basically two acetylcholine molecules hooked together. Succinylcholine may exert cardiovascular effects by: (1) inducing histamine release from mast cells; (2) stimulating autonomic ganglia, which increases neurotransmission at both the sympathetic and parasympathetic nervous systems; and (3) directly stimulating postjunctional cardiac muscarinic receptors. The effect of succinylcholine on heart rate is variable, with both bradycardias and tachycardias being possible. The final heart rate depends upon many factors, including the amount of nicotinic stimulation of the sympathetic and parasympathetic ganglia, which is greater for the nondominant autonomic nervous system. For example, when sympathetic nervous system tone is high (as in children), bradycardia is more likely to develop when succinylcholine is administered. When parasympathetic nervous system tone is high (as in many adults), tachycardia, although not common, is more likely to occur when succinylcholine is administered. Cardiac bradycardias are more likely to occur when a second intravenous dose of succinylcholine is administered 4 to 5 minutes after the first dose, especially when difficult laryngoscopy (e.g., intense vagal stimulation) is being performed (*Miller: Anesthesia, ed 6, p 489; Stoelting: Pharmacology and Physiology in Anesthetic Practice, ed 4, p 220*).

224. (C) Succinylcholine is chemically two acetylcholine molecules hooked together and has many effects similar to acetylcholine. In addition to causing neuromuscular blockade, succinylcholine stimulates all cholinergic autonomic receptors, including the nicotinic receptors of the sympathetic and parasympathetic ganglia, as well as the muscarinic receptors in the sinus node of the heart. It is this muscarinic effect that causes the bradycardia that can be seen after the administration of succinylcholine in children. Also see explanation to question 223 (*Miller: Anesthesia, ed 6, p 489*).

225. (B) Guanethidine is a peripheral postganglionic adrenergic blocker. It can be used orally or intravenously in the treatment of moderate-to-severe hypertension, including hypertensive crisis, and as an intravenous sympathetic blocker for the treatment of complex regional pain syndrome. Guanethidine produces its antihypertensive effect by entering the sympathetic neurons and replacing norepinephrine in the storage vesicles. When the neuron is stimulated it is released instead of norepinephrine and acts as an inactive neurotransmitter. Intravenously it may initially release some norepinephrine and cause some initial hypertension (contraindicated in patients with pheochromocytoma) before its antihypertensive activity. With chronic oral administration of guanethidine, a denervation hypersensitivity phenomenon occurs, which may result in a hypertensive crisis if direct-acting sympathomimetic agents are administered. Conversely, the vasopressor response to indirect-acting sympatho-mimetic agents, such as ephedrine, is attenuated because norepinephrine stores within sympathetic nerve fibers are depleted (*Hardman: Goodman & Gilman's The Pharmacological Basis of Therapeutics, ed 10, p 143; Miller: Anesthesia, ed 6, p 658*).

226. (A) Hyperkalemia, malignant hyperthermia, masseter spasm, sinus bradycardia, nodal rhythms, and myalgias are side effects that can be seen after the administration of succinylcholine. In recent years, there have been several case reports of intractable cardiac arrest in apparently healthy children after the administration of succinylcholine. In these cases, hyperkalemia, rhabdomyolysis, and acidosis were documented. Later, muscle biopsy samples demonstrated many of these cases were subclinical cases of Duchenne muscular dystrophy. It is for this reason of occasional severe hyperkalemia that succinylcholine is contraindicated for routine tracheal intubation in children (*Miller: Anesthesia, ed 6, p 525*).

227. (E) To make intubation easier, it is important to know when the muscles of the airway are maximally relaxed after administration of a neuromuscular relaxant. This often is done with neuromuscular monitoring. However, which muscles you monitor is important because neuromuscular blockade develops faster, lasts a shorter time, and recovers more quickly in the central muscles of the airway (i.e., the larynx, jaw, and diaphragm) than in the more peripheral abductor muscles of the thumb (e.g., ulnar nerve monitoring). Also important is the observation that the pattern of blockade in the orbicularis oculi (e.g., facial nerve monitoring) is similar to that of the laryngeal muscles and the diaphragm. Therefore, when the orbicular oculi muscles are maximally relaxed, intubation would be optimal. When the adductor of the thumb's function returns to normal, the diaphragm and laryngeal muscles will have recovered (*Miller: Anesthesia, ed 6, pp 484-485*).

228. (E) Rarely it is necessary to change from one nondepolarizing drug to another. A general rule to determine the duration of action of a drug given after another drug of different duration is a matter of simple kinetics. Three half-lives will be required for a clinical changeover so that 95% of the first drug will have cleared for the block duration to begin to take on the characteristics of the second drug. For example, if an intermediate-acting muscle relaxant such as vecuronium is given after a long-acting agent such as pancuronium, the duration of action of vecuronium is prolonged after the first two maintenance doses of vecuronium. After the third maintenance dose the duration of vecuronium is not prolonged (*Miller: Anesthesia, ed 6, pp 514-515*).

229. (A) Volatile anesthetics enhance neuromuscular blockade in a dose-dependent fashion. Recent studies have suggested that antagonism of neuromuscular block is slowed by volatile anesthetics; thus, volatile anesthetic vapor concentrations should be reduced as much as possible at the end of the case to help ensure that reversal will take place as promptly as possible (*Miller: Anesthesia, ed 6, pp 515-516, 522*).

230. (C) Selegiline is an MAOI that is sometimes used in the treatment of Parkinson's disease. Meperidine is contraindicated in patients taking MAOIs because of the possibility of excitation (e.g., agitation, skeletal muscle rigidity, hyperpyrexia) or depression (e.g., hypotension, depressed ventilation, coma) that may result (*Stoelting: Pharmacology and Physiology in Anesthetic Practice, ed 4, pp 405-407*).

231. (B) Rocuronium and pipecuronium (as well as the other amino-steroidal neuromuscular blocking drugs) do not release histamine. Of the listed benzylisoquinolinium drugs, d-tubocurarine, cisatracurium and atracurium, only cisatracurium does not cause histamine release. Also see explanation to question 189 (*Miller: Anesthesia, ed 6, p 512*).

232. (A) Etomidate, an imidazole derivative, is used most often for induction of general anesthesia, but it also can be used for maintenance of general anesthesia. Etomidate has a relatively short duration of action and provides very stable hemodynamics, even in patients with limited cardiovascular reserve. However, it is associated with several adverse effects. These adverse effects include a high incidence of nausea and vomiting (greater than after thiopental), pain on injection, thrombophlebitis, myoclonic movements, and, sometimes, hiccups. Nausea and vomiting constitute the most common reason patients rate anesthesia with etomidate as unsatisfactory. The addition of fentanyl to etomidate to decrease the pain of injection also increases the incidence of nausea and vomiting (*Miller: Anesthesia, ed 6, p 354*).

233.   **(A)**   Pancuronium tends to increase the heart rate, mean arterial blood pressure, and cardiac output. This may be related to several mechanisms, including a moderate vagolytic effect, norepinephrine release, and decreased reuptake of norepinephrine by adrenergic nerves. The other listed drugs rarely cause direct adrenergic stimulation and do not inhibit the uptake of norepinephrine by adrenergic nerves (*Miller: Anesthesia, ed 6, p 512; Stoelting: Pharmacology and Physiology in Anesthetic Practice, ed 4, pp 228-230*).

234.   **(B)**   Dantrolene is a muscle relaxant used orally to help control skeletal muscle spasticity in patients with upper motor neuron lesions, and it can be used acutely in the prevention of malignant hyperthermia in patients undergoing anesthesia. It is given intravenously in the treatment of malignant hyperthermia. Dantrolene has little or no effect on smooth or cardiac muscle at clinical doses. Dantrolene works directly on skeletal muscle by decreasing the amount of calcium released from the sarcoplasmic reticulum. This decreases the excitation-contraction coupling needed for the muscle to contract. The most common side effect of dantrolene administration is skeletal muscle weakness. Other acute side effects include nausea, diarrhea, and blurred vision. When the drug is given intravenously, a brisk diuresis occurs and is related to the mannitol added to make the intravenous solution isotonic. With chronic oral use, patients may rarely develop hepatitis and pleural effusions (*Stoelting: Pharmacology and Physiology in Anesthetic Practice, ed 4, pp 596-597*).

235.   **(A)**   Diabetes mellitus is a disease characterized by altered metabolism of carbohydrates (usually manifested by hyperglycemia), lipids, and proteins. Ninety percent of diabetic patients in the United States have non–insulin-dependent diabetes mellitus (NIDDM) or type II diabetes and a relative deficiency in circulating insulin. Diabetics also can have a decreased tissue response to circulating insulin (insulin resistance). Oral hypoglycemic agents, most commonly of the sulfonylurea chemical class, can be used in patients with NIDDM. These sulfonylurea drugs have many metabolic effects, including the initial stimulation of the pancreas to release insulin (chronically, insulin secretion is not increased but the hypoglycemic effects are maintained). Tolbutamide (Orinase) and chlorpropamide (Diabinese) are first-generation analogues. The half-life of tolbutamide is 4 to 7 hours, whereas the half-life of chlorpropamide is 24 to 48 hours. Second-generation sulfonylureas are about 100 times more potent and include glyburide (DiaBeta, Micronase) and glipizide (Glucotrol). The half-life of the second-generation drugs is about 1.5 to 5 hours, but their hypoglycemic effects are longer, about 12 to 24 hours. Because of the hypoglycemic effects, you need to watch for hypoglycemia in the perioperative period, especially with drugs having long half-lives. The biguanides metformin (Glucophage) and phenformin work by increasing the action of circulating insulin on peripheral tissues and are called antihyperglycemic, not hypoglycemic, agents. Phenformin was withdrawn from the market because of an association with lactic acidosis. This is less common but possible with metformin, especially if metformin is administered within 48 hours of surgery (*Hardman: Goodman & Gilman's The Pharmacological Basis of Therapeutics, ed 10, pp 1701-1706; Hines: Stoelting's Anesthesia and Co-Existing Disease, ed 5, pp 368-369; Miller: Anesthesia, ed 6, p 1779; Stoelting: Basics of Anesthesia, ed 5, p 439*).

236.   **(D)**   Disulfiram and naltrexone occasionally are administered orally in alcoholic rehabilitation programs. Disulfiram alters the metabolism of alcohol by irreversibly inactivating the enzyme aldehyde dehydrogenase. If the patient drinks alcohol there is a buildup of acetaldehyde in the blood. This produces the unpleasant effects of flushing, headache, nausea, vomiting, chest pain, tachycardia, hypotension, and confusion. The alcohol sensitivity with disulfiram use may last up to 2 weeks after the drug is stopped. Naltrexone is used with disulfiram in the treatment of alcohol addiction. It appears to block some of the reinforcing properties of alcohol. Patients taking naltrexone with disulfiram have a lower rate of relapse for alcohol. Naltrexone is a pure opioid antagonist. Patients taking naltrexone at the time of surgery will have markedly elevated opioid requirements if opioids are chosen for pain relief. The duration of action of naltrexone is 24 hours, and the drug should be stopped during the hospitalization to allow better pain control with narcotics, as would be desirable in this major surgical procedure (*Hardman: Goodman & Gilman's The Pharmacological Basis of Therapeutics, ed 10, pp 602-604; Hines: Stoelting's Anesthesia and Co-Existing Disease, ed 5, p 542; Miller: Anesthesia, ed 6, pp 421, 440-441*).

237.   **(B)**   Rapid-sequence inductions are performed in cases where rapid control of the airway is needed. Usually this is performed to secure the airway in a patient who should be easily intubated and has a "full stomach." In these cases, after adequate preoxygenation and suctioning of the airway can be readily performed, an intravenous induction of general anesthesia is performed with cricoid pressure and a muscle relaxant with a short onset time is administered. Succinylcholine has the fastest onset time of all neuromuscular relaxants and is the drug of choice. However, in some cases, succinylcholine is contraindicated and another neuromuscular blocker is chosen. Of the drugs listed, rocuronium is the best choice because of its rapid onset. Although the onset time of other nondepolarizing neuromuscular relaxants can be sped up with priming (a technique where 10% of the intubating dose is followed 2 to 4 minutes later with an intravenous induction of general anesthesia and the remaining 90% of the relaxant), rocuronium is fast enough without priming and much simpler to use. In patients who may be difficult to intubate, even with adequate muscle relaxation, an awake intubation should be strongly considered. D-tubocurare should never have an intubating dose bolused because it causes significant histamine release, and it should be given incrementally over several minutes if used to intubate (*Miller: Anesthesia, ed 6, pp 502-505*).

238. (E) The effects of nondepolarizing neuromuscular drugs are based on the drug being at the receptor. After intravenous injection of a muscle relaxant, plasma drug concentration immediately starts to decrease. To produce paralysis, the drug must diffuse from the plasma to the neuromuscular junction after injection and bind to the receptors. The drug effect is later terminated by diffusion of drug back into the plasma. Recovery of neuromuscular function occurs when the muscle relaxant diffuses from the neuromuscular junction back into the plasma to be metabolized and/or eliminated from the body (*Miller: Anesthesia, ed 6, pp 498-500*).

239. (D) Buprenorphine (Buprenex) is a mixed agonist-antagonist opioid with a very strong affinity for μ receptors. Because of its strong affinity (50 times greater than morphine) and slow dissociation from the receptors, it has a prolonged duration of effect (>8 hours) and shows resistance to reversal from naloxone. In rare cases of respiratory depression, reversal may not be achieved with high doses of naloxone (*Hardman: Goodman & Gilman's The Pharmacological Basis of Therapeutics, ed 10, pp 601-602; Miller: Anesthesia, ed 6, pp 418-419; Stoelting: Pharmacology and Physiology in Anesthetic Practice, ed 4, p 119*).

240. (B) Nausea and vomiting can be associated with all of the drugs listed. However of the listed drugs in this question, etomidate has the highest incidence of nausea and vomiting with some reporting an incidence as high as 40% (*Barash: Clinical Anesthesia, ed 5, p 1398; Miller: Anesthesia, ed 6, p 354; Stoelting: Pharmacology and Physiology in Anesthetic Practice, ed 4, pp 158, 165*).

241. (E) Naloxone is a pure opioid antagonist (affinity but no intrinsic activity) at all opioid receptors. It is used mainly to reverse narcotic induced toxicity. In large doses, naloxone may reverse the effects of endogenous opioids that are elevated in conditions of stress (e.g., shock or stroke). Naloxone has no effect on NSAIDs (e.g., ketorolac) (*Hardman: Goodman & Gilman's The Pharmacological Basis of Therapeutics, ed 10, pp 574, 602-604, 709; Miller: Anesthesia, ed 6, pp 420-421, 2719-2720*).

242. (D) Nitric oxide, nitroglycerin, nitroprusside, phentolamine, amrinone, milrinone, and prostaglandin E all have a vasodilatory effect on the pulmonary arterial tree. However, only nitric oxide has basically no effect on the systemic circulation. The following table compares the relative efficacy of various intravenous vasodilators (*Miller: Anesthesia, ed 5, p 1794; Stoelting: Pharmacology and Physiology in Anesthetic Practice, ed 4, pp 321, 352-365*).

RELATIVE EFFICACY OF INTRAVENOUS VASODILATORS ON HEMODYNAMIC VARIABLES

	Dilation			
	Venous	Pulmonary Arterial	Systemic Arterial	Cardiac Output
Nitric oxide	0	+++	0	±
Nitroglycerin IV	+++	+	+	I, D*
Nitroprusside	+++	+++	+++	I, D*
Phentolamine	+	+	+++	I
Hydralazine	0	?	+++	I
Nicardipine	0	?	+++	I
Amrinone†	+	+	+	I
Milrinone†	+	+	+	I
Prostaglandin E1‡	+	+++	+++	I, D*

*Effect on cardiac output depends on net balance of effects on preload, afterload, and myocardial oxygenation.
†Amrinone and milrinone are inodilators (have inotropic plus vasodilating effects).
‡Prostaglandin E_1 almost always requires left atrial infusion of norepinephrine to sustain adequate systemic blood pressure.
0, none; ±, small and variable; +, mild; +++, strongest effect of that particular drug; I, increase; D, decrease.
(*Miller: Anesthesia, ed 5, p 1794.*)

243. **(E)** Succinylcholine is rapidly metabolized in the blood by pseudocholinesterase (plasma cholinesterase). This accounts for the large dose required to facilitate intubation. Since pseudocholinesterase is not present at the neuromuscular junction, succinylcholine's action is terminated after it diffuses into the extracellular fluid (*Stoelting: Basics of Anesthesia, ed 5, p 140*).

244. **(E)** Dexmedetomidine is a highly selective α_2 adrenergic agonist that is mainly used for sedation. It has a rapid onset of action (<5 minutes) and a peak effect in about 15 minutes. In normovolemic healthy patients, the cardiovascular effects include a decrease in heart rate and cardiac output. The heart-rate changes can be profound and occasionally sinus arrest may develop. After an IV injection, the blood pressure initially increases (due to peripheral α stimulation), then within 15 minutes returns to normal and is followed by approximately a 15% decrease in blood pressure by an hour. This is related to its CNS α adrenergic stimulation overriding the peripheral effects. Respiratory changes are minimal providing excessive sedation does not produce obstructive apnea. At clinical doses of 1 to 2 μg/kg/min only a mild decrease in tidal volume (V_T) is seen, with no change in respiratory rate. With high doses, the $Paco_2$ may increase about 20% and is due to a decrease in V_T as the respiratory rate increases (*Barash: Clinical Anesthesiology ed 5, p 315-316; Miller: Anesthesia, ed 6, pp 355-357*).

245. **(E)** Fospropofol (Lusedra), approved in December 2008 for monitored anesthesia care is a prodrug of propofol that after IV infusion is rapidly converted into propofol. Because it is water soluble, the problems associated with a lipid vehicle (pain on injection, risk of hypertriglyceridemia, risk of pulmonary embolism, risk of sepsis) are gone. (*Eisai Corporation product information; Stoelting: Pharmacology and Physiology in Anesthetic Practice, ed 4, p 155*).

246. **(C)** In addition to analgesia, respiratory depression, nausea and euphoria, tolerance to sedation with chronic analgesic therapy with morphine will develop after 2 to 3 weeks of treatment. Miosis and constipation occur with narcotic administration regardless of length of therapy. The concept of tolerance is not applicable to these two side effects. (*Stoelting: Pharmacology and Physiology in Anesthetic Practice, ed 4, p 101*).

247. **(D)** H_2-receptor antagonists (e.g., cimetidine, ranitidine, famotidine, nizatidine) can be used preoperatively to increase gastric fluid pH before induction of anesthesia. Elevation of gastric fluid pH (above 2.5) is desirable to decrease the incidence and severity of lung damage if aspiration of gastric contents occurs. H_2-receptor antagonists are not uncommonly used as a premedication for parturients, patients with symptomatic gastroesophageal reflux, and obese patients (who tend to have very acidic gastric fluid compared to nonobese patients). H_2-receptor antagonists, in contrast to metoclopramide, have no effect on lower esophageal sphincter tone, intestinal motility, or gastric emptying. Although the incidence of side effects is low, side effects occasionally may develop in patients, especially when the drug is administered intravenously and when the drugs are administered to the elderly or to patients with hepatic or renal dysfunction. Bradycardia may develop and may be related to the effects on cardiac H_2 receptors. Reversible elevation of plasma aminotransaminase enzymes may occur. H_2-receptor antagonists cross the blood-brain barrier and may lead to mental confusion or delayed awakening. Cimetidine impairs the metabolism of drugs such as lidocaine, propranolol, and diazepam. This impairment may be related to the binding of cimetidine to the cytochrome P-450 enzymes (*Stoelting: Pharmacology and Physiology in Anesthetic Practice, ed 4, pp 435-441*).

248. **(A)** Drug sensitivity has been reported to occur in about 3% to 4% of anesthetic related deaths. Allergic drug reactions have been reported to occur to most drugs administered during anesthesia, with the exception of ketamine and the benzodiazepines. Although most drug-induced allergic reaction occur within 5 to 10 minutes of exposure, latex reactions may take longer than 30 minutes to develop (*Hines: Stoelting's Anesthesia and Co-Existing Disease, ed 5, pp 526-530*).

249. **(D)** Atropine is administered in doses of 2 to 6 mg and is repeated every 5 to 10 minutes until secretions begin to decrease. In most cases, 2 mg every 8 hours is needed. However, doses of 15 to 20 mg are not uncommon and occasionally doses over 1000 mg have been needed. Pralidoxime 600 mg removes the organophosphate compounds from acetylcholinesterase and is often used in conjunction with atropine. Benzodiazepines are often administered to counter the affects of the nerve gases on the GABA system (*Barash: Clinical Anesthesiology, ed 5, pp 1533-1534; Miller: Anesthesia, ed 6, pp 2504-2509*).

250. **(A)** Alfentanil (a fentanyl analogue) is less potent (1/5 to 1/10), has a more rapid onset (within 1.5 minutes) and a shorter duration of action than fentanyl. The brief duration of action of alfentanil is a result of redistribution to inactive tissue sites and its rapid hepatic metabolism (96% cleared within 1 hour). Renal failure does not alter the clearance of alfentanil (*Stoelting: Pharmacology and Physiology in Anesthetic Practice, ed 4, pp 110-112*).

251. (D) Asthma is an inflammatory illness associated with bronchial hyperreactivity and bronchospasm. Medications effective in the management of acute exacerbations of bronchial asthma include the rapid onset inhaled β_2-adrenergic receptor agonists (e.g., albuterol, pirbuterol, terbutaline), anticholinergic drugs (e.g., inhaled ipratropium), and IV corticosteroids. In an acute attack, ipratropium (slower in onset than β_2-adrenergic receptor agonists) can be effective when used in combination with the rapid onset β_2 agonists. When unresolving bronchospasm occurs and is considered life threatening, the diagnoses of status asthmaticus is made. Although treatment often starts with β_2 agonists (2-4 puffs every 15 to 20 minutes), when alveolar ventilation is reduced, inhaled agents may not be successful. In this case subcutaneous (SQ) epinephrine (adult dose of 0.2 to 1 mg or 0.2 to 1 mL of 1:1000 solution) can be given. Corticosteroids enhance and prolong the response to β_2 agonists and in status asthmaticus, IV corticosteroids such as cortisol (Solu-Cortef) 2 mg/kg IV bolus followed by 0.5 mg/kg/hr, or methylprednisolone (Solu-Medrol) 60 to 125 mg every 6 hours, are administered early in the treatment (but may take several hours to work). Supplemental oxygen is given to keep the oxygen saturation greater than 90%. Since Heliox (70% helium and 30% oxygen) is one-third the density of oxygen, it can be tried. IV terbutaline starting at a rate of 0.1 μg/kg/min and increased until improvement is seen or significant tachycardia develops may be useful. Magnesium sulfate at a dose of 25 to 40 mg/kg (maximum of 2 grams) administered over 20 minutes has been used. Broad spectrum antibiotics are also started. In severe cases where fatigue sets in and the $Paco_2$ is rising (e.g., >70-80 mm Hg), general anesthesia with mechanical ventilation may be needed. The volatile anesthetics such as isoflurane, halothane or sevoflurane can be used not only to sedate but also to relax the smooth muscle in the constricted airways. Cromolyn, however, does not relieve bronchospasm. Cromolyn is used prophylactically because it inhibits antigen-induced release of histamine and other autocoids, such as leukotrienes, from mast cells. Aminophylline once was widely used to treat acute asthma but is rarely used today because it adds little to β_2-agonist activity and has significant side effects (*Hardman: Goodman & Gilman's The Pharmacological Basis of Therapeutics, ed 10, pp 733-749; Hines: Stoelting's Anesthesia and Co-Existing Disease, ed 5, pp 163-166; Miller: Anesthesia, ed 6, pp 2852-2853*).

252. (D) Clonidine is an α_2-adrenergic agonist. Unlike many peripherally acting antihypertensive drugs (e.g., guanethidine, propranolol, captopril), clonidine primarily stimulates central adrenergic receptors and decreases the sympathetic response. As with other drugs that affect the central release of catecholamines, clonidine not only reduces anesthetic requirements (as represented by a decrease in MAC) but also decreases extremes in arterial blood pressure during anesthesia. Clonidine has analgesic properties and reduces the requirements for opioids. Clonidine has been given orally, intravenously, epidurally, intrathecally and in peripheral nerve blocks and potentiates the analgesic effect of local anesthetics. α_2-Adrenergic agonists can reduce the muscle rigidity seen with the administration of narcotics and can be used to decrease postanesthetic shivering. Patients chronically taking clonidine should not have it discontinued prior to surgery and should keep taking clonidine to prevent clonidine withdrawal and hypertensive crisis (*Miller: Anesthesia, ed 6, pp 650-651, 1582-1583*).

253. (E) Chronic liver disease may interfere with the metabolism of drugs because of the decreased number of enzyme-containing hepatocytes, decreased hepatic blood flow, or both. Prolonged elimination half-times for morphine, alfentanil, diazepam, lidocaine, pancuronium, and, to a lesser extent, vecuronium have been demonstrated in patients with cirrhosis of the liver. In addition, severe liver disease may decrease the production of cholinesterase (pseudocholinesterase) enzyme, which is necessary for the hydrolysis of ester linkages in drugs such as succinylcholine, and the ester local anesthetics such as procaine (*Hines: Stoelting's Anesthesia and Co-Existing Disease, ed 5, p 271; Stoelting: Basics of Anesthesia, ed 5, pp 431-434*).

254. (E) Succinylcholine is the drug of choice (unless contraindicated) when rapid sequence tracheal intubation in needed. Although hyperkalemic cardiac arrest is a complication of succinylcholine administrations to patients who have sustained burns (as well as crush injuries, spinal cord trauma or other denervation injuries, chronic illness polyneuropathy and chronic illness myopathy), the susceptibility for hyperkalemia after a burn injury peaks at 7 to 10 days, but may begin as early as 2 days after sustaining a thermal injury. The first 24 hours after the injury is considered safe. Adding a defasciculating dose of a non-depolarizing neuromuscular blocking drug prior to succinylcholine use to the regimen would slow down achievement of paralysis. Although the "priming" technique of giving 10% of the intubating dose followed by 2 to 4 minutes with the rest of the intubating dose has been used to speed conditions for intubation, it is still slower than succinylcholine and this technique is rarely done because rocuronium (which provides the most rapid intubating conditions among the non-depolarizing neuromuscular blocking drugs, and is a close second behind succinylcholine) is available. An intubating dose of d-tubocurarine should never be given as a bolus because of its moderate histamine release (*Miller: Anesthesia, ed 6, pp 491, 501-505, 530; Stoelting: Basics of Anesthesia, ed 5, p 141*).

255. **(A)**   Clonidine, a centrally acting α agonist, decreases sympathetic nervous system outflow and decreases plasma catecholamine concentrations in normal patients, but has no effect in patients with pheochromocytomas. It is used as an antihypertensive agent for treating essential hypertension, an analgesic when injected epidurally or into the subarachnoid space alone, a drug that prolongs the effect of regional local anesthetics, a drug that can be used to stop shivering (75 μg IV), a drug that can help protect against perioperative myocardial ischemia (when given preop and typically for four days after surgery), and a drug that can help decrease the symptoms of narcotic and alcohol withdrawal (*Stoelting: Pharmacology and Physiology in Anesthetic Practice, ed 4, pp 340-344*).

256. **(E)**   Skeletal muscle spasm, particularly of the thoracoabdominal muscles ("stiff chest" syndrome), may occur when large doses of opioids are given rapidly. This may be significant enough to prevent adequate ventilation. Although the administration of a muscle relaxant or an opioid antagonist such as naloxone will terminate the skeletal muscle rigidity, reversing the narcotic effect may not be desirable if surgery is needed (*Stoelting: Basics of Anesthesia, ed 5, p 116*).

257. **(B)**   One of the advantages of ketamine is the minimal effect on respirations. After the intravenous induction dose of 2 mg/kg, general anesthesia is induced within 30 to 60 seconds with, at most, a transient decrease in respirations ($Paco_2$ rarely increases more than 3 mm Hg). With unusually high doses or if opioids are also administered, apnea can occur (*Miller: Anesthesia, ed 6 pp 347-348; Stoelting: Pharmacology and Physiology in Anesthetic Practice, ed 4, pp 170-173*).

258. **(C)**   This patient has a partially compensated metabolic acidosis. Metabolic acidosis is commonly divided into those with a normal ion gap, also called hyperchloremic metabolic acidosis (bicarbonate loss is counterbalanced by an increase in chloride levels), and those with a high anion gap. The anion gap can be calculated by determining the difference between the sodium concentration and the sum of the chloride and bicarbonate concentrations (i.e., $[Na^+] - [Cl^-] + [HCO_3^-]$) and is normally 8 to 14 mEq/L. In this case the anion gap is $135 - [95 + 14] = 26$. This patient, therefore, has a high anion gap acidosis. This question has two forms of acidosis that have a high anion gap: diabetic ketoacidosis (DKA) and propofol infusion syndrome which causes a lactic acidosis. Since this patient is a type II (non-insulin dependant diabetic) DKA is less likely and the cause more likely would be propofol infusion syndrome (*Hines: Stoelting's Anesthesia and Co-Existing Disease, ed 5, pp 361-362, 372-373; Stoelting: Pharmacology and Physiology in Anesthetic Practice, ed 4, p 162*).

259. **(D)**   Neuroleptic malignant syndrome (NMS) can be seen in up to 1% of patients treated with antipsychotic drugs. The syndrome has many features that resemble the condition malignant hyperthermia, including increased metabolism, tachycardia, muscle rigidity, rhabdomyolysis, fever, and acidosis. The mortality rate may be 20% to 30%. There are many differences between NMS and malignant hyperthermia. NMS is not inherited and usually takes 24 to 72 hours to develop after the use of neuroleptic drugs (e.g., phenothiazines, haloperidol), whereas malignant hyperthermia presents more acutely. Stopping the antipsychotic medication is obviously needed. Because dopamine depletion appears to play a role in causing NMS, the dopamine agonists bromocriptine and amantadine appear useful in the treatment. Abrupt withdrawal of levodopa may also cause this syndrome. Succinylcholine and volatile anesthetics, which are known triggers for malignant hyperthermia, are not triggers for NMS. Dantrolene has been used to treat this condition (*Barash: Clinical Anesthesia, ed 5, p 533; Stoelting: Pharmacology and Physiology in Anesthetic Practice, ed 4, pp 412-413*).

260. **(C)**   Normal pseudocholinesterase is inhibited 80% by dibucaine (dibucaine number of 80), whereas patients with atypical cholinesterase show only 20% inhibition (dibucaine number of 20). Patients who are heterozygous for atypical pseudocholinesterase (as in this case) have intermediate dibucaine numbers ranging from 50 to 60%. Succinylcholine paralysis after an intubating dose of 1 mg/kg lasts up to 10 minutes with normal pseudocholinesterase, up to 30 minutes in patients with the atypical heterozygous pseudocholinesterase, and in patients who have atypical cholinesterase paralysis may persist for 3 hours or longer (*Stoelting: Pharmacology and Physiology in Anesthetic Practice, ed 4, pp 218-220*).

261. **(D)**   Cyanide (hydrocyanic acid [HCN], prussic acid) is a rapidly acting poison. Cyanide is commercially used as a pesticide, but it can be released as a gas from burning nitrogen-containing plastics. Sodium nitroprusside (SNP)

is metabolized to cyanide and nitric oxide. The cyanide produced from SNP usually is rapidly metabolized to relatively nontoxic thiocyanate (SCN⁻), which is excreted into the urine. Although rare, cyanide and/or thiocyanate toxicity can develop in patients receiving prolonged high-dose infusions of nitroprusside. Cyanide binds to iron in the ferric state and inhibits cellular respiration. This produces severe lactic acidosis and cytotoxic hypoxia. Because oxygen is not used well, the venous blood is well oxygenated (elevated central venous oxygen levels and patients are not cyanotic). Treatment (adult doses in parenthesis) can include sodium nitrite (NaNO$_2$ — 300 mg IV over 3 minutes), amyl nitrite (inhalation), sodium thiosulfate (12.5 g IV over 10 minutes), and hydroxocobalamin (5 g IV over 15 minutes). Nitrite converts hemoglobin to methemoglobin which competes with cytochrome oxidase for the cyanide ion forming cyanmethemoglobin. Nitrite can be administered IV as sodium nitrite or by inhalation with amyl nitrite. Sodium thiosulfate (Na$_2$S$_2$O$_3$), the preferred drug, is a sulfur donor that converts cyanide to thiocyanate.

$$Na_2S_2O_3 + CN^- \leftrightarrow SCN^- + Na_2S_2O_3$$

Hydroxocobalamin combines with cyanide to form cyanocobalamin or vitamin B$_{12}$. Methylene blue is not an antidote for cyanide toxicity and can complicate therapy by converting methemoglobin back to hemoglobin and releasing free cyanide. Although oxygen alone (even under hyperbaric conditions) has little benefit, it should be used since it dramatically potentiates the activity of thiosulfate and nitrites (*Hardman: Goodman & Gilman's The Pharmacological Basis of Therapeutics, ed 10, pp 1892-1893; Miller: Anesthesiology, ed 6, pp 2513-2514*).

262. (E) The duration of neuromuscular block by succinylcholine can be markedly prolonged when the total amount of plasma cholinesterase is very low, the amount is normal but of an abnormal type (i.e., atypical plasma cholinesterase), or an anticholinesterase drug (e.g., neostigmine, echothiophate, or the organophosphate insecticide malathion) is administered. To evaluate a prolonged response to succinylcholine you need to evaluate both the total amount of cholinesterase (i.e., quantitative test) and the type of cholinesterase (i.e., qualitative test). Atypical plasma cholinesterase is an inherited disorder that occurs in approximately 1 of every 480 patients with heterozygous genome and in approximately 1 of 3200 patients with homozygous genome. The local anesthetic dibucaine can inhibit normal plasma cholinesterase enzyme better than an abnormal enzyme. In patients with normal plasma cholinesterase, the dibucaine inhibition test reports a number around 80 or produces 80% inhibition. Heterozygotes have a dibucaine number of around 50, and patients who are homozygous for the atypical plasma cholinesterase have a number around 20. Total plasma cholinesterase levels can be reduced with decreased production, as occurs with severe chronic liver disease or with the use of some chemotherapeutic drugs (e.g., cyclophosphamide). The dibucaine number is normal when the total plasma cholinesterase levels are reduced, as well as after the use of anticholinesterase drugs. Patients with a C$_5$ isoenzyme variant have increased plasma cholinesterase activity, a more rapid breakdown of succinylcholine and a shorter duration of action (*Stoelting: Basics of Anesthesia, ed 5, p 140; Stoelting: Pharmacology and Physiology in Anesthetic Practice, ed 4, pp 216-220*).

263. (C) Benzodiazepines are drugs that have the chemical structure of a benzene ring attached to a seven-member diazepine ring. Midazolam, lorazepam, oxazepam, and diazepam are benzodiazepine agonists and flumazenil is an antagonist. Benzodiazepine agonists all are sedatives and possess a number of favorable pharmacologic characteristics, including production of sedation, anxiolysis, anterograde amnesia (acquisition of new information), and anticonvulsant activity. The amnestic properties are greater than the sedative properties, which is why patients sometimes forget what you tell them after the benzodiazepine is given, despite their having what appears to be a lucid discussion with you. They do not produce retrograde amnesia (stored information). They rarely cause significant respiratory or cardiovascular depression and rarely are associated with the development of significant tolerance or physical dependence. The agonist actions of benzodiazepines most likely reflect the ability of these drugs to facilitate the inhibitory neurotransmitter GABA actions in the CNS. Midazolam and diazepam undergo oxidative metabolism and their metabolites are conjugated with glucuronide before renal excretion. Cimetidine inhibits oxidative metabolism and may prolong the duration of these drugs. Lorazepam and oxazepam primarily undergo conjugation with glucuronic acid, which is not influenced by cimetidine usage or alterations in hepatic function (*Stoelting: Pharmacology and Physiology in Anesthetic Practice, ed 4, pp 140-153*).

264. (C) Remifentanil is an ultrashort-acting opioid that is most commonly administered by an IV infusion. Its short duration of action is due to its ester linkage which allows for rapid breakdown by nonspecific plasma and tissue esterases. The clinical elimination half-time is less than 6 minutes. For monitored anesthesia care sedation after 2 mg of midazolam, an infusion rate of 0.05-0.1 μg/kg/min is used in healthy adults. For analgesia during general anesthesia with controlled respirations, a rate of 0.05 to 2 μg/kg/min is commonly used. A loading dose of 1 μg/kg of remifentanil (or 0.5 μg/kg, if a benzodiazepine was also given) can be given IV over 60 to 90 seconds prior to starting the infusion. Although it effectively suppresses autonomic and hemodynamic responses to painful stimuli and decreases respirations well, its rapid dissipation of opioid effect produces rapid onset of postoperative pain (in painful surgical operations), unless other analgesics are administered for postoperative pain before stopping the infusion (*Miller: Anesthesia, ed 6, pp 403, 411-412; Stoelting: Pharmacology and Physiology in Anesthetic Practice, ed 4, pp 112-115*).

265. **(D)**   The maximum recommended single dose of lidocaine given by infiltration is 300 mg of lidocaine without epinephrine and 500 mg of lidocaine with epinephrine. Careful injection in the mouth is recommended due to the vascular nature of that area (*Stoelting: Pharmacology and Physiology in Anesthetic Practice, ed 4, p 195*).

266. **(E)**   Postoperative shivering can be caused by many factors, including hypothermia, transfusion reactions, and pain, as well as anesthetics. It is uncomfortable for patients and can make monitoring more difficult, but it also can lead to significant increases in oxygen consumption (up to 200%). The exact etiology in many cases is unclear but after routine skin surface warming, pharmacologic treatment may be needed. Clonidine, dexmedetomidine, propofol, ketanserin, tramadol, physostigmine, magnesium sulfate and narcotics (especially meperidine) have been used. Naloxone use may increase pain and does not help decrease shivering (*Barash: Clinical Anesthesia, ed 5, p 1400; Miller: Anesthesiology, ed 6, pp 1582-1583; Stoelting: Pharmacology and Physiology in Anesthetic Practice, ed 4, p 103*).

267. **(C)**   Sugammadex is a cyclodextrin (cyclic oligosaccharide) compound that encapsulates nondepolarizing steroidal muscle relaxants (rocuronium > vecuronium >> pancuronium) and produces rapid reversal of profound block (e.g., reversal of 0.6 mg/kg rocuronium in three minutes). Because it has no effect on acetylcholinesterase, there is no need to combine it with the anticholinergics atropine or glycopyrrolate. It works only with steroidal muscle relaxants and has no effect on reversing the benzylisoquinolinium relaxants (e.g., atracurium, cisatracurium, doxacurium, d-tubocurarine). There appears to be no cardiovascular effects with Sugammadex. It is being used in clinical trials at present (*Miller: Anesthesia, ed 6, pp 524-525; Stoelting: Basics of Anesthesia, ed 5, p 153*).

268. **(E)**   Intra-arterial injection of thiopental may result in excruciating pain and intense vasoconstriction that may lead to gangrene (especially if the concentration is >2.5%). Treatment of this complication should include immediate dilution with saline or administration of a drug that will produce vasodilation (e.g., lidocaine, papaverine, or phenoxybenzamine). This should be done through the needle in the artery. If the needle has been removed from the artery, consider a more proximal injection of the artery affected. Other treatments to consider include intra-arterial heparin or urokinase injection or an upper extremity sympathectomy if the artery is in the upper extremity (i.e., stellate ganglion block or brachial plexus block) (*Stoelting: Pharmacology and Physiology in Anesthetic Practice, ed 4, p 137*).

269. **(B)**   Sodium nitroprusside (SNP) is a rapid-acting, direct-acting peripheral vasodilator that is composed of 5 cyanide moieties for every NO (nitric oxide) moiety. Sodium nitroprusside undergoes rapid metabolism to release NO as the active ingredient. Healthy adults can easily eliminate the cyanide produced during SNP rates of less than 2 μg/kg/min. Above 2 μg/kg/min and especially if the infusion rate is greater than 10 μg/kg/min for 10 minutes, you should be concerned about cyanide toxicity. An early sign of cyanide toxicity is resistance to the hypotensive effects of SNP infusion, especially when the rate is less than 2 μg/kg/min. Other signs include metabolic acidosis and an elevation of mixed venous PO_2 values (*Stoelting: Pharmacology and Physiology in Anesthetic Practice, ed 4, pp 355-358*).

270. **(D)**   Phenothiazines, such as chlorpromazine (Thorazine), are effective antipsychotic (neuroleptic) drugs that block D_2 dopaminergic receptors in the brain. Extrapyramidal effects are not uncommon with these drugs. They also possess antiemetic effects. Phenothiazines with low potency, such as chlorpromazine, have prominent sedative effects, which gradually decreases with treatment. The effects of CNS depressants (e.g., narcotics and barbiturates) are enhanced by concomitant administration of phenothiazines. Lowering the seizure threshold is more common with aliphatic phenothiazines with low potency (e.g., chlorpromazine) compared with piperazine phenothiazines. These drugs are associated with cholestatic jaundice, impotence, dystonia, and photosensitivity. Electrocardiographic abnormalities, such as prolongation of the QT or PR intervals, blunting of T waves, depression of the ST segment, and, on rare occasions, premature ventricular contractions and torsades de pointes, are seen. The antihypertensive effects of guanethidine and guanadrel are blocked by phenothiazines. These drugs have no effect on neuromuscular blockade (*Hardman: Goodman & Gilman's The Pharmacological Basis of Therapeutics, ed 10, pp 492, 497; Miller: Anesthesia, ed 6, p 1123*).

271. (A) Amrinone is a noncatecholamine, nonglycoside cardiac inotropic drug that works as a selective phosphodiesterase III (PDE III) inhibitor. Amrinone increases cyclic adenosine monophosphate (cAMP) levels by decreasing cAMP breakdown in the myocardium and vascular smooth muscle. Because the actions of PDE III inhibitors work by a different mechanism than catecholamines (cAMP levels are increased by β-adrenergic receptor stimulation), amrinone can work in the presence of β-blockade, and in cases where patients become refractory to catecholamine use. The catecholamine actions can be enhanced with PDE III inhibitors. Amrinone produces both positive inotropic and vasodilatory effects but has no antidysrhythmic effects (*Stoelting: Pharmacology and Physiology in Anesthetic Practice, ed 4, p 317*).

272. (D) Tricyclic antidepressants often are administered as the initial treatment of mental depression; however, the more recently developed selective serotonin uptake inhibitors (SSRIs) are more frequently used because of fewer side effects. Tricyclic antidepressants work by inhibiting the reuptake of released norepinephrine (and serotonin) into the nerve endings. Although at one time it was recommended to stop tricyclic antidepressants before elective surgery, this has not been shown to be necessary. However, alterations in patient responses to some drugs should be anticipated. The increased availability of neurotransmitters in the CNS can result in increased anesthetic requirement (i.e., increased MAC). In addition, the increased availability of norepinephrine at postsynaptic receptors in the peripheral sympathetic nervous system can be responsible for an exaggerated blood pressure response after administration of an indirect-acting vasopressor such as ephedrine. If a vasopressor is required, a direct-acting drug such as phenylephrine may be preferred. If hypertension occurs and requires treatment, deepening the anesthetic or adding a peripheral vasodilator such as nitroprusside may be needed. The potential for an exaggerated blood pressure response (i.e., hypertensive crisis) is greatest during the acute treatment phase (the first 14 to 21 days). Chronic treatment is associated with down-regulation receptors and a decreased likelihood of an exaggerated blood pressure responses after administration of a sympathomimetic. Tricyclics have significant anticholinergic side effects (e.g., dry mouth, blurred vision, increased heart rate, urinary retention,) and caution is especially important in elderly patients who may develop anticholinergic delirium despite the therapeutic doses administered. Caution is advised with the use of meperidine in patients taking MAOIs (not tricyclic antidepressants) because of the possibility of inducing seizure, hyperpyrexia, or coma (*Hardman: Goodman & Gilman's The Pharmacological Basis of Therapeutics, ed 10, pp 451-459, 466; Hines: Stoelting's Anesthesia and Co-Existing Disease, ed 5, pp 533-536; Stoelting: Pharmacology and Physiology in Anesthetic Practice, ed 4, pp 401-405*).

273. (B) For normal nondiabetic patients, about 40 units of insulin are secreted every day. There are many subcutaneous insulin preparations available. After subcutaneous administration the onset of action is very rapid with Lispro and Aspart (15 minutes); rapid with Regular (30 minutes); intermediate with NPH or Lente (1-2 hours); and slow with Glargine (1.5 hours) and Ultralente (4-6 hours) (*Hines: Stoelting's Anesthesia and Co-Existing Disease, ed 5, pp 370-372; Miller: Anesthesia, ed 6, p 1777; Physicians Desk Reference, ed 63, 2009, pp 1829-1833, 1846-1850, 2359-2364, 2749-2756; Stoelting: Pharmacology and Physiology in Anesthetic Practice, ed 4, pp 479-480*).

INSULIN PREPARATIONS

Insulin Preparation		Hours after Subcutaneous (SQ) Administration		
		Onset	Peak	Duration
Very Rapid Acting				
	Lispro (Humalog)	0.25	1-2	3-6
	Aspart (NovoLog)	0.25	1-2	3-6
Rapid Acting				
	Regular (Humulin-R, Novolin-R)	0.5	2-4	5-8
Intermediate Acting				
	NPH (Humulin-N)	1-2	6-10	10-20
	Lente	1-2	6-10	10-20
Long Acting				
	Glargine (Lantus)	1-2	peakless	about 24
	Ultralente	4-6	8-20	24-48

(Hines: Stoelting's Anesthesia and Co-Existing Disease, ed 5, p 371.)

274. (C) Adrenergic-receptor antagonists often are used to treat hypertension and tachycardia. Variations exist among adrenergic blocking agents with regard to β_1-, β_2-, and α-adrenergic blocking activity. Alpha-blockade alone (e.g., phentolamine) tends to decrease peripheral vascular resistance but leads to a reflex increase in the heart rate. β_1-Agonist activity includes stimulatory effects on the heart, whereas β_2-agonist activity includes relaxation of the bronchial smooth muscle. β-Blockers can be nonselective (both β_1- and β_2-blocking activity) or β_1 selective (primarily but not totally β_1-blocking activity). The nonselective β-blockers (e.g., propranolol, nadolol, timolol, pindolol) would decrease heart rate and blood pressure but may lead to bronchospasm, especially in patients with reactive airway disease. The selective β_1-blockers (e.g., atenolol, acebutolol, betaxolol, bisoprolol, esmolol, metoprolol) may decrease heart rate and blood pressure without causing bronchospasm. Selective β_1 blockade is not always complete, and some β_2 blockade may occur (bronchoconstriction may still be possible), especially if high doses are used. Also see explanation to question 177 (*Stoelting: Pharmacology and Physiology in Anesthetic Practice, ed 4, pp 321-337*).

275. (B) Remifentanil is rapidly hydrolyzed by nonspecific plasma and tissue esterases, making it ideal for an infusion where precise control is sought. The onset and offset of remifentanil is rapid (clinical half-time of <6 minutes). Because the activity of these nonspecific esterases is not usually affected by liver and renal failure, remifentanil is well suited for such patients (*Stoelting: Pharmacology and Physiology in Anesthetic Practice, ed 4, p 114*).

276. (E) Pain with the intravenous injection is common with diazepam, etomidate, methohexital and propofol. It is very rare after thiopental and ketamine (*Miller: Anesthesia, ed 6, p 326; Stoelting: Pharmacology and Physiology in Anesthetic Practice, ed 4, pp 147, 163-164, 170*).

277. (E) Patients anesthetized with total intravenous anesthesia (TIVA), in this case consisting of midazolam, remifentanil and propofol, sometimes require a few minutes to resume breathing after the infusions are stopped. Although it may seem appropriate to reverse this patient and avoid the need for hand ventilation, reversing benzodiazepines (midazolam) with flumazenil may precipitate seizures in epileptic patients and because remifentanil has such a short elimination half-life (<6 minutes), reversal with naloxone is not necessary. The patient needs a brief period to allow the propofol to wear off during which hand or mechanical ventilation will be necessary (until the patient breathes spontaneously). Also muscle weakness must be ruled out if a muscle relaxant had been used, and normocapnia should be assured since hyperventilation may reduce the arterial CO_2 below the apneic threshold (*Stoelting: Pharmacology and Physiology in Anesthetic Practice, ed 4, pp 114, 152, 161*).

278. (D) Phentolamine, prazosin, yohimbine, tolazoline and terazosin are competitive and reversible α-adrenergic antagonists. Phenoxybenzamine produces an irreversible α-adrenergic blockade. Once phenoxybenzamine's α-blockade develops, even massive doses of sympathomimetics are ineffective until phenoxybenzamine's action is terminated by metabolism. Phentolamine and phenoxybenzamine are nonselective α_1 and α_2 antagonists, prazosin is a selective α_1 antagonist and yohimbine is a selective α_2 antagonist (*Stoelting: Pharmacology and Physiology in Anesthetic Practice, ed 4, pp 321-323*).

279. (C) Symptomatic bradycardia as a result of excessive β-adrenergic receptor blockade can be treated with a variety of drugs, as well as with a pacemaker. Treatment depends upon severity of symptoms. Atropine can block any parasympathetic nervous system contribution to the bradycardia. If atropine is not effective, then a pure β-adrenergic receptor agonist can be tried. For excessive cardioselective β_1 blockade, dobutamine can be used; for a noncardiac selective β_1 and β_2 blockade, isoproterenol can be chosen. Dopamine is not recommended because the high doses needed to overcome β-adrenergic receptor blockade will cause significant α-adrenergic receptor-induced vasoconstriction. Glucagon at an initial dose of 1 to 10 mg intravenously followed by an infusion of 5 mg/hr often is believed to be the drug of choice for β-adrenergic blockade overdosage. Glucagon increases myocardial contractility and heart rate, primarily by increasing cAMP formation (not via β-adrenergic receptor stimulation) and to a lesser extent, by stimulating the release of catecholamines. Other drugs that have been used include aminophylline and calcium chloride. Aminophylline inhibits phosphodiesterase, resulting in an increase in cyclic AMP. Thus, like glucagon, aminophylline increases cardiac output and heart rate via a non–β-adrenergic receptor-mediated mechanism. Calcium chloride may prove useful to counteract any decrease in myocardial contractility induced by the β-blockade; however, this effect may be transient (*Stoelting: Pharmacology and Physiology in Anesthetic Practice, ed 4, pp 331-332*).

280. (D) Dantrolene is a skeletal muscle relaxant that is effective in the treatment of malignant hyperthermia (MH). Dantrolene is formulated with mannitol (300 mg mannitol/20 mg dantrolene) so that diuresis is promoted during dantrolene therapy. Myoglobinuria from MH-associated muscle breakdown accumulates in the renal tubules and can cause kidney failure if urine output is not maintained. Dantrolene works within the muscle cell to reduce intracellular levels of calcium. In the usual clinical doses, dantrolene has little effect on cardiac muscle contractility. In fulminant MH, cardiac dysrhythmias may occur, but this is related to perturbations in pH and electrolytes. (Verapamil should not be used, because it interacts with dantrolene and may produce hyperkalemia and myocardial depression. Lidocaine appears safe.) Some side effects of short-term administration include muscle weakness (which may persist for 24 hours after dantrolene therapy is discontinued), nausea and vomiting, diarrhea, blurred vision and phlebitis. Hypothermia may also occur with MH treatment, but is related to ice packing, not to dantrolene administration per se. When decreasing the fever, cooling should be stopped when core temperature reaches 38° C to avoid hypothermia. Hepatotoxicity has been demonstrated only with long-term use of oral dantrolene (*Barash: Clinical Anesthesia, ed 5, pp 538-539; Stoelting: Pharmacology and Physiology in Anesthetic Practice, ed 4, p 625*).

281. (C) Cis-atracurium is a stereoisomer of atracurium and as such has the same molecular weight. Both drugs undergo Hoffman elimination and form laudanosine. Atracurium is also estimated to undergo two thirds of its metabolism via ester hydrolysis catalyzed by nonspecific plasma esterases (not pseudocholinesterase). Neither drug requires renal or hepatic input for its degradation, hence both can be used with renal or hepatic failure. Atracurium causes histamine release whereas cis-atracurium does not (*Stoelting: Basics of Anesthesia, ed 5, pp 147-148*).

282. (B) Withdrawal from opioids is rarely life threatening but may complicate postoperative care. Opioid withdrawal may spontaneously start within 6 to 12 hours after the last dose of a short-acting opioid and as long as 72 to 84 hours after a long-acting opioid in addicted patients. The duration of withdrawal symptoms also depends on the opioid, for heroin withdrawal symptoms last 5 to 10 days, and for methadone, even longer. Opioid withdrawal can be precipitated within seconds if naloxone is administered intravenously to an addict (naloxone is contraindicated in opioid addicts for this reason). Signs and symptoms of withdrawal include craving for opioids, restlessness, anxiety, irritability, nausea, vomiting, abdominal cramps, muscle aches, insomnia, sympathetic stimulation (increased heart rate, increased blood pressure, mydriasis, diaphoresis) as well as tremors, jerking of the legs (origin of the term "kicking the habit") and hyperthermia. Seizures however, are very rare and if seizures occur, you should think that withdrawal from other drugs may also be occurring (i.e., from barbiturates) or an underlying seizure disorder may also exist (*Hardman: Goodman & Gilman's The Pharmacological Basis of Therapeutics, ed 10, pp 631-634; Hines: Stoelting's Anesthesia and Co-Existing Disease, ed 5, pp 544-546*).

For questions 283-287: Side effects of each of the intravenous induction agents (thiopental, diazepam, etomidate, propofol, and ketamine) occur. Some are unique for each drug.

283. (C) Etomidate is unique among the intravenous induction agents because it can cause adrenocortical suppression by inhibiting the conversion of cholesterol to cortisol. This can occur after a single induction dose and may persist for greater than 24 hours. The clinical significance of this temporary adrenocortical suppression is unclear. However, in the intensive care unit (ICU) with prolonged sedation, clinical adrenal insufficiency may develop (i.e., hypotension, hyponatremia and hyperkalemia), here corticosteroids should be administered in stress doses (e.g., cortisol 100 mg/day) (*Miller: Anesthesia, ed 6, p 1041; Stoelting: Pharmacology and Physiology in Anesthetic Practice, ed 4, pp 166-167, 283*).

284. (B) Diazepam is a benzodiazepine drug and was widely used intravenously for anesthesia until midazolam was developed. Although an effective sedative and amnestic drug, diazepam causes significant pain on injection and at times venous irritation and thrombophlebitis. This does not seem to occur with midazolam. Benzodiazepines do not suppress the adrenal gland. The most significant problem with benzodiazepines is respiratory depression. Benzodiazepines are unique among the intravenous sedatives because a specific benzodiazepine receptor antagonist is available (flumazenil). One problem with flumazenil is its relatively short duration of action (half-life about 1 hour), which is shorter than that of diazepam (21 to 37 hours) and midazolam (1 to 4 hours) (*Miller: Anesthesia, ed 6, pp 342-343; Stoelting: Pharmacology and Physiology in Anesthetic Practice, ed 4, pp 147-150, 152*).

285. (D) Pain on injection is common with diazepam, etomidate, and propofol; and rare with thiopental and ketamine. However, hemodynamic stability is common with etomidate and diazepam, whereas hypotension is common after propofol and thiopental, especially in patients who are volume depleted or elderly. Hypertension may develop with ketamine use due to its sympathetic nervous system stimulation (*Miller: Anesthesia, ed 6, pp 318-355; Stoelting: Pharmacology and Physiology in Anesthetic Practice, ed 4, pp 127-172*).

286. (E)   Intracranial pressure (ICP) tends to fall after the administration of thiopental, etomidate, and propofol and can either fall or remain unchanged with benzodiazepines. Ketamine, however, can increase ICP and should be avoided in patients with intracranial mass lesions and elevated ICP because it can further increase the ICP (*Miller: Anesthesia, ed 6, pp 347, 352, 2130; Stoelting: Basics of Anesthesia, ed 5, pp 107, 456-457*).

287. (D)   Propofol infusion syndrome (lactic acidosis) may develop when high dose infusions (i.e., >75 μg/kg/min) are infused for greater than 24 hours. Early signs include tachycardia; later on severe metabolic acidosis, bradyarrhythmias and myocardial failure may develop. The cause appears to be related to impaired fatty acid oxidation in the mitochondria (*Lobato: Complications in Anesthesiology, pp 859-860; Stoelting: Pharmacology and Physiology in Anesthetic Practice, ed 4, p 162*).

For questions 288-292: Antihypertensive agents are used primarily in the treatment of essential hypertension to reduce blood pressure toward normal. These agents include direct-acting smooth muscle relaxants or vasodilators (e.g., hydralazine, minoxidil), centrally acting α₂ sympathetic receptor agonists (e.g., clonidine), peripheral adrenergic receptor antagonists (e.g., labetalol), calcium channel blockers, diuretics, and angiotensin-converting enzyme (ACE) inhibitors (e.g., captopril, lisinopril) (Stoelting: Basics of Anesthesia, ed 5, pp 71-73; Stoelting: Pharmacology and Physiology in Anesthetic Practice, ed 4, pp 338-349).

288. (E)   Central-acting sympathomimetic agents such as clonidine produce some sedative effects and can reduce the anesthetic requirement or MAC.

289. (C)   Side effects associated with minoxidil include pulmonary hypertension (which most likely reflects fluid retention), pericardial effusion, cardiac tamponade, and hair growth.

290. (B)   About 10% to 20% of patients who are chronically taking hydralazine (i.e., >6 months) develop a systemic lupus erythematosus-like syndrome, especially if the daily dose is high (e.g., >200 mg). The systemic lupus erythematosus-like syndrome will resolve once hydralazine therapy is discontinued.

291. (D)   Labetalol is an α₁-adrenergic receptor and nonselective β-adrenergic receptor antagonist.

292. (E)   Abrupt discontinuation of chronically administered clonidine (especially if the dose is >1.2 mg/day) may result in severe rebound hypertension within 8 to 36 hours after the last dose.

For questions 293-297: There are five catecholamines commonly used that have sympathomimetic effects. All are positive inotropes. The physiologic effects are many and affect many organ systems. Norepinephrine, epinephrine, and dopamine are endogenous catecholamines, and isoproterenol and dobutamine are exogenous catecholamines. The clinical response observed depends upon the characteristics of each drug, the physiologic state of the patient, and the dose of the drug administered. With respect to the cardiovascular system, the physiologic response seen (e.g., cardiac output) depends upon the following four factors: (1) preload; (2) afterload; (3) contractility; and (4) heart rate and rhythm. Afterload (the stress on the left ventricle) is related to the systemic vascular resistance if the aortic valve is normal (Hardman: Goodman & Gilman's The Pharmacological Basis of Therapeutics, ed 10, pp 215-229; Stoelting: Basics of Anesthesia, ed 5, pp 66-69).

293. (B)   Norepinephrine has α- and β₁-agonist activity (with little β₂ activity). However, the α effects of norepinephrine are significantly stronger than the β₁ effects. Both low and high doses increase systemic vascular resistance. The net result is marked increase in afterload demonstrated by a marked increase in blood pressure and a baroreceptor-mediated decrease in heart rate. Cardiac output is usually unchanged or decreased. In addition, renal blood flow tends to be markedly reduced.

294. (C)   Epinephrine has potent α- and β-agonist activity. Its actions are complex and mimic the stress response. At low doses the β receptors in the muscle causes vasodilation and overall lowers the systemic vascular resistance, but at high doses the α receptors are activated, causing muscle vasoconstriction and an increase in systemic vascular resistance. Cardiac output, mean arterial pressure, preload, afterload, contractility, and heart rate tend to increase and cardiac dysrhythmias become more frequent, whereas renal blood flow tends to decrease. Of the five catecholamines, epinephrine has the most significant effect on metabolism. For example, hyperglycemia usually is seen after administration of epinephrine or with the stress of surgery.

295. (D)   Isoproterenol is a nonselective β-adrenergic receptor agonist with almost no α-adrenergic activity. Increases in contractility and heart rate, as well as a marked decrease in afterload, resulting in an increase in cardiac output. Mean arterial blood pressure and renal blood flow usually are mildly decreased.

296. (E)   Dobutamine's actions are complex, but primarily activate $β_1$-receptors (with some effect on the alpha receptors). Dobutamine has more prominent inotropic than chronotropic effects compared to isoproterenol. It increases cardiac output with little change in systemic vascular resistance. Mild increases in heart rate and mean arterial pressure are seen.

297. (A)   At low doses, dopamine produces increases in contractility, heart rate, cardiac output, and renal blood flow, with little change in systemic vascular resistance. Mean arterial pressure is mildly elevated. At moderate doses, dopamine takes on the characteristics of epinephrine and at high doses, takes on the characteristics of norepinephrine, with a decrease in renal blood flow.

For questions 298-301: The clinical pharmacology of opioid-receptor agonists and antagonists is mediated by their interaction with the three classical types of opioid receptors in the CNS (μ - MOP, δ – DOP and ϰ - KOP). These classical types have subtypes (e.g., $μ_1$, $μ_2$, $δ_1$ and $δ_2$) and several other receptor types have been described, such as nociceptin/orphanin FQ (N/OFQ), epsilon, iota, lambda, zeta (Hardman: Goodman & Gilman's The Pharmacological Basis of Therapeutics, ed 10, pp 569-589; Stoelting: Pharmacology and Physiology in Anesthetic Practice, ed 4, pp 88-89).

298. (A)   Both supraspinal and spinal analgesia can be produced at the μ, ϰ and δ receptors.

299. (B)   Supraspinal analgesia occurs with agonists at the $μ_1$, $δ_1$, $δ_2$, and ϰ receptors. Only the $μ_1$-receptor agonists increase prolactin release. This may partially explain the menstrual cycle disruption that occurs in women who use heroin.

300. (C)   Respiratory depression (due to a reduced responsiveness to carbon dioxide blood levels) is a characteristic of both μ and δ receptors, but constipation is marked mainly with $μ_2$ stimulation and minimal with δ stimulation.

301. (E)   Respiratory depression which is characteristic at the μ and δ receptors is less so at the ϰ receptors. Both dysphoria and diuresis (inhibition of ADH) occurs with stimulation of ϰ agonists. $μ_2$ receptor stimulation tends to produce ADH effects.

For questions 302-305: Depolarizing neuromuscular blockade usually is described as having two phases. Phase I blockade occurs with depolarization of the postjunctional membrane. Phase II blockade occurs when the postjunctional membranes have become repolarized but do not respond normally to acetylcholine (i.e., often called desensitized but other factors are involved). This can occur when the dose of succinylcholine is greater than 2 to 4 mg/kg. The response of a muscle to electrical nerve stimulation for a phase II block is similar to that for a nondepolarizing block. Nondepolarizing neuromuscular blockade is only of one type (Miller: Anesthesia, ed 6, pp 484-486, 1552-1563; Stoelting: Pharmacology and Physiology in Anesthetic Practice, ed 4, pp 217-218, 222).

302. (D)   Although the mechanisms of a nondepolarizing and a phase II depolarizing block likely are different, they both can be antagonized with anticholinesterase drugs.

303. (B)   Only a phase I depolarizing block is enhanced with the use of anticholinesterase drugs.

304. (D)   Post-tetanic facilitation occurs when a single twitch that is induced a short period of time after tetanic stimulation is larger than the amplitude of the tetanus. This occurs with a phase II depolarizing blockade as well as with a nondepolarizing blockade.

305. (B)   The amplitude of the muscle response to sustained tetanic stimulation remains the same with phase I depolarizing blockade, but it shows a marked fade with a phase II depolarizing blockade or a nondepolarizing blockade.

SUMMARY OF MUSCULAR RESPONSES TO NERVE STIMULATION WITH DIFFERENT TYPES OF BLOCKADE

Stimulation	Phase I Depolarizing	Phase II Depolarizing	Nondepolarizing
Single twitch	Decreased	Decreased	Decreased
Tetanic stimulation	Decreased height but no fade	Fade	Fade
Post-tetanic facilitation	None	Yes	Yes
Train of four	All twitches same, decrease in height	Marked fade	Marked fade
Train-of-four ratio	>0.7	<0.4	<0.7
Anticholinesterase	Enhances	Antagonizes	Antagonizes

For questions 306-315: A simple way to measure the potency of inhaled drugs is to measure their MAC values. MAC is the minimum alveolar concentration of an inhaled drug at 1 atmosphere (1 atm = 760 mm Hg) where 50% of patients do not move in response to a painful stimulus. It is commonly measured as the end-expired drug concentration. Various physiologic or pharmacologic factors can increase or decrease MAC. In general, factors that increase metabolic function of the brain (e.g., hyperthermia) or in patients with an elevation of brain catecholamines (e.g., MAOIs, tricyclic antidepressants, cocaine, acute amphetamine use) increase MAC and factors that depress function (e.g., intravenous anesthetics, acute ethanol use, narcotics, hypothermia) decrease MAC. Recently, it has been suggested that there might be a genetic component to MAC, since redheaded females have about a 20% increase in MAC compared with dark-haired females (Barash: Clinical Anesthesia, ed 5, pp 397-398; Stoelting: Basics of Anesthesia, ed 5, pp 83, 116, 479).

306. **(D)**   Acute amphetamine use increases MAC, whereas chronic amphetamine use decreases MAC.

307. **(C)** α_2-Agonists decrease MAC.

308. **(A)**   Changes in thyroid function (e.g., hyperthyroidism, hypothyroidism) do not seem to affect MAC. However, the cardiovascular response to volatile drugs is altered with thyroid function.

309. **(E)**   With acute administration, ethanol is a CNS depressant and decreases MAC. Chronic ethanol administration increases MAC.

310. **(C)**   Lidocaine use decreases MAC.

311. **(C)**   Patients on lithium therapy have lower MAC values. This may be related to the lower catecholamine levels in the brain.

312. **(C)**   Opioids produce a dose dependent decrease in MAC (up to about 50%).

313. **(A)**   The duration of anesthesia, as well as the gender of the patient, does not affect MAC.

314. **(C)**   Pregnancy lowers MAC. This may be related to the sedative effects of progesterone. Pregnant patients also are very sensitive to local anesthetics.

315. **(C)**   Severe hypoxia (Pao_2 of 38 mm Hg), as well as severe anemia (<4.3 mL/oxygen/dL of blood), decreases MAC.

For questions 316-320: The goals of pharmacologic premedication must be individualized to meet each patient's requirements. Some of these goals include amnesia, relief of anxiety, sedation, analgesia, reduction of gastric fluid volume, elevation of gastric fluid pH, prophylaxis against allergic reactions, and reduction of oral and respiratory secretions. The drugs most commonly used to achieve these goals include benzodiazepines, barbiturates, opioids, H_2-receptor antagonists, nonparticulate antacids, antihistamines, and anticholinergic agents. The anticholinergics atropine, scopolamine, and glycopyrrolate are rarely given with premedication today unless a specific effect is needed (e.g., drying of the mouth before fiberoptic intubation, prevention of bradycardias, and, rarely, as a mild sedative). Atropine and scopolamine are tertiary compounds that can readily cross lipid membranes such as the blood-brain *barrier. These tertiary amines can produce sedation, amnesia, CNS toxicity (central anticholinergic syndrome manifested as delirium or prolonged somnolence after anesthesia), mydriasis, and cycloplegia (whereas glycopyrrolate, a quaternary compound, does not cross lipid membranes well). All three anticholinergics can cause drying of airway secretions by inhibiting salivation, can cause tachycardia (although bradycardia can be seen in some patients), can decrease the lower esophageal sphincter tone, and can increase body temperature by inhibiting sweating. The main differences are listed in the table following the explanation to question 178 (Physicians Desk Reference ed 63, 2009, pp 2206-2208; Stoelting: Basics of Anesthesia, ed 5, pp 171-173; Stoelting: Pharmacology and Physiology in Anesthetic Practice, ed 4, pp 268-273).*

316. (A)   All three anticholinergics can cause drying of airway secretions by inhibiting salivation, but atropine is the least effective of these drugs.

317. (C)   To produce sedation, the drug must pass the blood-brain barrier. This is much more prominent with scopolamine and much less so with atropine. Glycopyrrolate does not cause any sedation.

318. (E)   Although these drugs can decrease gastric acid secretion and increase gastric pH, the pH effects are small and the dose needed to do this is much higher than clinically used.

319. (B)   Glycopyrrolate does not cross the blood-brain barrier and cannot cause any CNS effects, including the toxic state known as central anticholinergic syndrome.

320. (D)   Both atropine and scopolamine can cause ocular effects (scopolamine more so than atropine), including mydriasis and cycloplegia when applied topically to the eye. Caution is suggested when scopolamine is given IM to patients with glaucoma. IV administration of atropine to prevent or treat bradycardia appears to have little effect on the eye. If a scopolamine patch is placed to help prevent postoperative nausea and vomiting, you need to carefully wash your hands after application, since rubbing one of your eyes with any scopolamine on your fingers may lead to unilateral mydriasis.

Chapter 4

Pharmacology and Pharmacokinetics of Volatile Anesthetics

DIRECTIONS (Questions 321 through 377): Each of the questions or incomplete statements in this section is followed by answers or by completions of the statement, respectively. Select the ONE BEST answer or completion for each item.

321. The minimum alveolar concentration (MAC) is highest in neonates (0 to 30 days old) versus other age groups with which of the following?
    A. Isoflurane
    B. Sevoflurane
    C. Desflurane
    D. Halothane
    E. None of the above

322. The rate of increase in the alveolar concentration of a volatile anesthetic relative to the inspired concentration (FA/FI) plotted against time is steep during the first moments of inhalation with all volatile anesthetics. The reason for this observation is that
    A. Volatile anesthetics decrease blood flow to the liver
    B. There is minimal anesthetic uptake from the alveoli into pulmonary venous blood
    C. Volatile anesthetics increased cardiac output initially
    D. The volume of the anesthetic breathing circuit is small
    E. Volatile anesthetics reduce alveolar ventilation (VA)

323. During spontaneous breathing, volatile anesthetics
    A. Increase tidal volume (VT) and decrease respiratory rate
    B. Increase VT and increase respiratory rate
    C. Decrease VT and decrease respiratory rate
    D. Decrease VT and increase respiratory rate
    E. None of the above

324. Each of the following volatile anesthetics is an ether derivative **EXCEPT**
    A. Halothane
    B. Enflurane
    C. Isoflurane
    D. Desflurane
    E. Sevoflurane

325. The reason desflurane is not used for inhalation induction in clinical practice is because of
    A. Its low blood/gas partition coefficient
    B. Its propensity to produce hypertension in high concentrations
    C. Its propensity to produce airway irritability
    D. Its propensity to produce tachyarrhythmias
    E. Its propensity to produce nodal rhythms

326. A medical group planning a trip to South American has a large supply of old enflurane vaporizers (vapor pressure [VP] = 170 mm Hg). Which volatile could be delivered through an enflurane vaporizer such that the dialed setting equaled the vaporizer's output?
   A. Halothane
   B. Sevoflurane
   C. Isoflurane
   D. Desflurane
   E. Both halothane and isoflurane

327. Select the true statement regarding blood pressure when 1.5 MAC N_2O-isoflurane is substituted for 1.5 MAC isoflurane-oxygen.
   A. Blood pressure is less than awake value, but greater than that seen with isoflurane-O_2
   B. Blood pressure is equal to awake value
   C. Blood pressure is greater than awake value
   D. Blood pressure is less than isoflurane-O_2 pressure
   E. Blood pressure is unchanged

328. Which of the following groups of volatile anesthetics decrease systemic vascular resistance?
   A. Desflurane, sevoflurane, and isoflurane
   B. Halothane and isoflurane
   C. Desflurane and halothane
   D. Halothane and isoflurane
   E. Halothane only

329. With which of the following inhalational agents is cardiac output moderately increased?
   A. Halothane
   B. Sevoflurane
   C. Desflurane
   D. Isoflurane
   E. Nitrous oxide

330. Select the **FALSE** statement about isoflurane ($\leq$ 1 MAC).
   A. May attenuate bronchospasm
   B. Produces a 2- to 3-fold increase in skeletal muscle blood flow
   C. Decreases mean arterial pressure
   D. Decreases cardiac output
   E. Increases right atrial pressure

331. Abrupt and large increases in the delivered concentration of which of the following inhalational anesthetics may produce transient increases in systemic blood pressure and heart rate?
   A. Desflurane
   B. Isoflurane
   C. Sevoflurane
   D. Halothane
   E. Nitrous oxide

332. Discontinuation of 1 MAC of which volatile anesthetic followed by immediate introduction of 1 MAC of which second volatile anesthetic would temporarily result in the greatest combined anesthetic potency?
   A. Halothane followed by desflurane
   B. Sevoflurane followed by desflurane
   C. Halothane followed by isoflurane
   D. Isoflurane followed by desflurane
   E. Isoflurane followed by halothane

333. Cardiogenic shock has the greatest impact on the rate of increase in Fᴀ/Fɪ for which of the following volatile anesthetics?
      A. Isoflurane
      B. Desflurane
      C. Sevoflurane
      D. N_2O
      E. The impact will be about the same for all agents

334. The vessel-rich group receives what percent of the cardiac output?
      A. 45%
      B. 60%
      C. 75%
      D. 90%
      E. 95%

335. Which of the following volatile anesthetics undergoes the greatest degree of metabolism?
      A. Enflurane
      B. Isoflurane
      C. Halothane
      D. Desflurane
      E. Sevoflurane

336. With a properly functioning circle system, each of the following is a potential disadvantage to low flow anesthesia **EXCEPT**
      A. Hypercarbia
      B. Hypoxia
      C. Increased compound A exposure
      D. Increased carbon monoxide exposure
      E. Higher serum fluoride levels

337. How would a right mainstem intubation affect the rate of increase in arterial partial pressure of volatile anesthetics?
      A. It would be reduced to the same degree for all volatile anesthetics
      B. It would be accelerated to the same degree for all volatile anesthetics
      C. There would be no change if Pao_2 is 60 mm Hg or greater
      D. It would be reduced the most for poorly soluble agents
      E. It would be reduced the most for highly soluble agents

338. Halothane, unlike desflurane and isoflurane, does not cause tachycardia. The most reasonable explanation for this observation is that halothane
      A. Lacks intrinsic sympathomimetic properties
      B. Lacks vagolytic properties
      C. Causes direct cardiac depression
      D. Has intrinsic parasympathomimetic properties
      E. Inhibits baroreceptor reflexes

339. Isoflurane, when administered to healthy patients in concentrations less than 1.0 MAC, will decrease all the following **EXCEPT**
      A. Cardiac output
      B. Myocardial contractility
      C. Stroke volume
      D. Systemic vascular resistance
      E. Ventilatory response to changes in $Paco_2$

340. Increased Vᴀ will accelerate the rate of rise of the Fᴀ/Fɪ ratio the most for
      A. Desflurane
      B. Sevoflurane
      C. Isoflurane
      D. Halothane
      E. It was accelerate Fᴀ/Fɪ for all of these equally

341. Select the correct order from greatest to least for anesthetic requirement.
   A. Adults > infants >neonates
   B. Adults > neonates > infants
   C. Neonates >infants > adults
   D. Neonates > adults > infants
   E. Infants > neonates >adults

342. Which of the following inhalational agents is **MOST** likely to produce a decrease in systemic blood pressure by causing a junctional rhythm?
   A. Desflurane
   B. Halothane
   C. Isoflurane
   D. Sevoflurane
   E. Nitrous oxide

343. A 31-year-old moderately obese female is receiving a general anesthetic for cervical spinal fusion. After induction and intubation, the patient is mechanically ventilated with isoflurane at a vaporizer setting of 2.4%. The nitrous oxide flow is set at 500 mL/min and the oxygen flowmeter is set at 250 mL/min. The mass spectrometer displays an inspired isoflurane concentration of 1.7% and an expired isoflurane concentration of 0.6%. Approximately how many MAC of anesthesia would be represented by the alveolar concentration of anesthetic gases?
   A. 0.5 MAC
   B. 0.85 MAC
   C. 1.1 MAC
   D. 1.8 MAC
   E. 2.1 MAC

344. The graph in the figure depicts

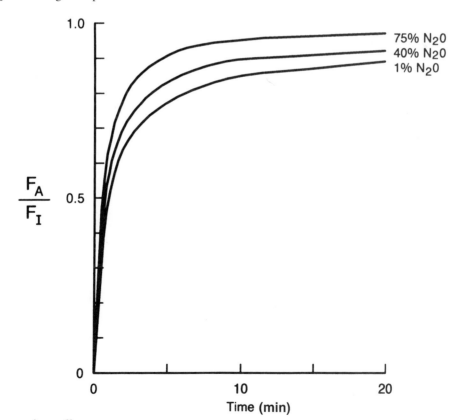

   A. The second gas effect
   B. The concentration effect
   C. The concentrating effect
   D. The effect of solubility on the rate of rise of F_A/F_I
   E. Diffusion hypoxia

345. The rate of induction of anesthesia with isoflurane would be slower than expected in patients
   A. With anemia
   B. With chronic renal failure
   C. In shock
   D. With cirrhotic liver disease
   E. With a right-to-left intracardiac shunt

346. A right-to-left intracardiac shunt would have the greatest impact on the rate of inhalation induction with which of the following inhalation anesthetics?
   A. Halothane
   B. Desflurane
   C. Isoflurane
   D. It would speed up induction for all agents equally
   E. It would slow down induction for all agents equally

347. A left-to-right tissue shunt, such as arteriovenous fistula, physiologically most resembles which of the following?
   A. A left-to-right intracardiac shunt
   B. A right-to-left intracardiac shunt
   C. Ventilation of unperfused alveoli
   D. A pulmonary embolism
   E. None of the above

348. A fresh-gas flow rate of 2 L/min or greater is recommended for administration of sevoflurane because
   A. The vaporizer cannot accurately deliver the volatile at lesser flow rates
   B. It prevents the formation of fluoride ions
   C. It prevents formation of compound A
   D. It diminishes rebreathing
   E. None of the above

349. Metabolism plays an important role on the rate of rise of F_A/F_I during induction of anesthesia for which of the following anesthetics?
   A. Isoflurane
   B. N_2O
   C. Halothane
   D. Desflurane
   E. None of the above

350. Smokers are most likely to show a mild, but transient increase in airway resistance following intubation and general anesthesia with which of the following?
   A. Isoflurane
   B. Sevoflurane
   C. Halothane
   D. Desflurane
   E. None of the above

351. Which of the following reasons best explains the more rapid alveolar washout of halothane compared with isoflurane?
   A. Differences in blood solubility
   B. Differences in the blood/brain partition coefficient
   C. Differences in the oil/gas partition coefficient
   D. The fact that halothane is not an ether
   E. Increased metabolism of halothane

352.

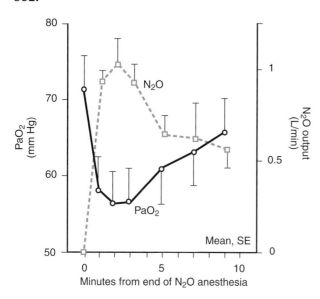

The graph above depicts which of the following?
A. Diffusion hypoxia
B. Second gas effect
C. Context sensitive half time of desflurane
D. Concentration effect
E. Uptake of N_2O

353. Which of the following organs is **NOT** considered a member of the vessel rich group?
A. Lungs
B. Brain
C. Heart
D. Liver
E. Kidney

354. In isovolumic normal human subjects, 1 MAC of isoflurane anesthesia depresses mean arterial pressure by approximately 25%. The single **BEST** explanation for this is
A. Reduction in heart rate
B. Venous pooling
C. Myocardial depression
D. Decreased systemic vascular resistance
E. Poor ventricular filling secondary to tachycardia

355. If cardiac output and alveolar ventilation are doubled, the effect on the rate of rise of F_A/F_I for isoflurane compared with that which existed immediately before these interventions would be
A. Doubled
B. Somewhat increased
C. Unchanged
D. Somewhat decreased
E. Halved

356. Which of the following characteristics of inhaled anesthetics most closely correlates with recovery from inhaled anesthesia?
A. Blood/gas partition coefficient
B. Brain/blood partition coefficient
C. Fat/blood partition coefficient
D. MAC
E. Vapor pressure

357. Which of the following inhalational anesthetics is most likely to produce a coronary steal syndrome by preferentially dilating small coronary arterial resistance vessels?
   A. Halothane
   B. Isoflurane
   C. Desflurane
   D. Sevoflurane
   E. Nitrous oxide

358. An unconscious, spontaneously breathing patient is brought to the operating room from the intensive care unit (ICU) for wound debridement. Which of the following maneuvers would serve to slow induction of inhalational anesthesia through the tracheostomy?
   A. Using sevoflurane instead of isoflurane (using MAC-equivalent inspired concentrations)
   B. Increasing fresh gas flow from 2 to 6 L/min
   C. Esmolol 30 mg IV
   D. Increasing minute ventilation
   E. None of the above

359. Which of the settings below would give the highest arterial oxygen concentration during inhalation induction of general anesthesia with sevoflurane?

		Oxygen	Air	N_2O
A.	L/min	1	2	0
B.	L/min	2	0	2
C.	L/min	2	2	2
D.	L/min	4	10	1
E.	L/min	2	3.5	0

360. Inhalational anesthetics, which produce decreases in arterial pressure primarily by reduction in left ventricular afterload, include each of the following **EXCEPT**
   A. Sevoflurane
   B. Desflurane
   C. Isoflurane
   D. Halothane
   E. Sevoflurane and desflurane

361. An anesthesia circuit is primed in preparation for an inhalation induction (with open adjustable pressure-limiting [APL] valve). The anesthesia hose is occluded with a flow of 6 L/min. The anesthesia circuit (canisters, hoses, mask, anesthesia bag) contains 6 L. A machine malfunction allows administration of 100% N_2O. Approximately how much N_2O would there be in the circuit when the malfunction is discovered at the one minute mark?
   A. 32%
   B. 48%
   C. 63%
   D. 86%
   E. 95%

362. Which of the following factors lowers MAC for volatile anesthetics?
   A. Serum sodium 151 mEq/L
   B. Red hair
   C. Body temperature 38° C
   D. Acute ethanol ingestion
   E. Acute amphetamine ingestion

363. Each of the following factors can influence the partial pressure gradient necessary for the achievement of anesthesia **EXCEPT**
    A. Inspired anesthetic concentration
    B. Cardiac output
    C. Alveolar ventilation (VA)
    D. The volume of the anesthetic breathing circuit
    E. Ventilation of nonperfused alveoli (dead space)

364. Which of the following volatile anesthetics is unique in containing preservative?
    A. Sevoflurane
    B. Desflurane
    C Isoflurane
    D. Halothane
    E. N_2O

365. If the alveolar to venous partial pressure difference of a volatile anesthetic (PA-Pv) is positive (i.e., PA > Pv) and the arterial to venous partial pressure difference (Pa-Pv) is negative (i.e., Pv > Pa) which of the following scenarios is most likely to be true?
    A. The vaporizer has been shut off at the end of the case
    B. Induction has just started
    C. Steady state has been achieved
    D. The volatile anesthetic has been turned down from steady state, but not off
    E. The vaporizer was shut off during emergence, then suddenly turned up because the patient moved before closure of the incision

366. Anesthetic loss to the plastic and rubber components of the anesthetic circuit hindering achievement of an adequate inspired concentration is a factor with which of the following anesthetics?
    A. Desflurane
    B. Nitrous oxide
    C. Sevoflurane
    D. Isoflurane
    E. All of the above

367. Factors predisposing to formation and/or rebreathing of compound A include each of the following **EXCEPT**
    A. Low fresh gas flow
    B. Use of a soda lime rather than Baralyme
    C. High absorbent temperatures
    D. Fresh absorbent
    E. Higher concentrations of sevoflurane

368. The effects of a left to right shunt such as an arteriovenous fistula on inhalation induction of anesthesia is to
    A. Speed up induction
    B. Slow down induction
    C. Slow down inhalation induction only if an intracardiac (right to left) shunt also exists
    D. Speed up inhalation induction only if an intracardiac (right to left) shunt also exists
    E. Have no effect on induction time

369. The following volatiles are correctly matched with their degree of metabolism (determined by metabolite recovery)
    A. Halothane 20%
    B. Sevoflurane 2%
    C. Isoflurane 0.2%
    D. Desflurane 0.02%
    E. All are correctly matched

370. Which of the components below is **NOT** considered in the process of "washin" of the anesthesia circuit at the onset of administration?
   A. Inspiratory limb
   B. Expiratory limb
   C. Anesthesia bag
   D. CO_2 absorber
   E. Mass spectrometer tubing and reservoir

371. Which of the following maneuvers would **NOT** increase the rate of an inhalation induction?
   A. Increasing alveolar ventilation
   B. Substitution of desflurane for isoflurane
   C. Overpressurizing
   D. Carrying out the induction in San Diego instead of Denver
   E. Placement of patient on an inotropic infusion

372. Which of the following anesthetics would undergo 90% elimination the most rapidly after a 6 hour Whipple procedure under one MAC for the duration of the operation?
   A. Isoflurane
   B. Sevoflurane
   C. Halothane
   D. Desflurane
   E. Sevoflurane and desflurane are tied

373. After induction and intubation of a healthy patient and placement on a ventilator, the sevoflurane vaporizer is set at 2% and fresh gas flow is 1 L/minute (50% N_2O and 50% O_2). The inspired concentration on the mass spectrometer one minute later is 1.4%. The **MAIN** reason for the difference between the dial setting and the concentration shown on the mass spectrometer is
   A. Rapid uptake of sevoflurane
   B. Insufficient fresh gas flow for correct vaporizer function
   C. Second gas effect
   D. Dilution
   E. Improper vaporizer calibration

374. After cessation of general anesthesia which consisted of air, oxygen and volatile only, the patient is placed on 100% oxygen. Each of the following serves as a reservoir for volatile anesthesia and may delay emergence **EXCEPT**
   A. Rebreathed exhaled gases
   B. The absorbent
   C. The patient
   D. The plastic components of the anesthesia circuit
   E. Gases emerging from the common gas outlet

375. Which of the following characteristics of volatile anesthetics is necessary for calculation of the time constant?
   A. Blood/gas partition coefficient
   B. Brain/blood partition coefficient
   C. Oil/gas partition coefficient
   D. Minimum alveolar concentration (MAC)
   E. Saturated vapor pressure

376. The concept of "context sensitive half time" emphasizes the importance of the relationship between half time and
   A. Alveolar ventilation
   B. Blood solubility
   C. Concentration
   D. Duration
   E. Anesthetic metabolism

377. Select the **FALSE** statement regarding time constants for volatile anesthetics. After 3 time constants
    A. 6 to 12 minutes have elapsed for "modern anesthetics"
    B. The A-V$_D$ for the brain is very small
    C. The expired volatile concentration will rise much less slowly than the preceding 12 minutes
    D. The venous blood will contain 95% of volatile content of arterial blood.
    E. The A-V$_D$ for the rectus abdominal muscle is large

DIRECTIONS (Questions 378 through 381): Match the volatile agents with the characteristics to which they most closely correspond. Each lettered heading (A through E) may be selected once, more than once, or not at all.

---

378. Halothane (1 MAC)

379. Isoflurane (1 MAC)

380. Desflurane (1 MAC)

381. Sevoflurane (1 MAC)

	Heart rate	Systemic vascular resistance	Cardiac index
A.	No change	No change	Decreased
B.	Decreased	Decreased	Decreased
C.	No change	Decreased	Decreased
D.	Increased	Decreased	Decreased
E.	Increased	Decreased	No change or slight increase

Pharmacology and Pharmacokinetics of Volatile Anesthetics

Answers, References, and Explanations

321. (B) The MAC for inhalation agents varies with age. For most volatile anesthetics, the highest MAC values are for infants 1 to 6 months old. In infants younger than 1 month or older than 6 months, the MAC is lower for isoflurane, halothane, and desflurane. Sevoflurane is different. For sevoflurane the MAC for neonates 0 to 30 days old is 3.3%, for infants 1 to 6 months old is 3.2%, and for infants 6 to 12 months old is 2.5% (*Coté: A Practice of Anesthesia for Infants and Children, ed 3, pp 133-141*).

322. (B) Alveolar partial pressure of a volatile anesthetic, which ultimately determines the depth of general anesthesia, is determined by the relative rates of input to removal of the anesthetic gases to and from the alveoli. Removal of anesthetic gases from the alveoli is accomplished by uptake into the pulmonary venous blood, which is most dependent upon an alveolar partial pressure difference. During the initial moments of inhalation of an anesthetic gas, there is no volatile anesthetic in the alveoli to create this partial pressure gradient. Therefore, uptake for all volatile anesthetic gases will be minimal until the resultant rapid increase in alveolar partial pressure establishes a sufficient alveolar-to-venous partial pressure gradient to promote uptake of the anesthetic gas into the pulmonary venous blood. This will occur in spite of other factors, which are discussed in the explanation to question 333 (*Miller: Anesthesia, ed 6, pp 133-135*).

323. (D) At concentrations of 1 MAC or less, volatile anesthetics, as well as the inhaled anesthetic N_2O, will produce dose-dependent increases in the respiratory rate in spontaneously breathing patients. This trend continues at concentrations greater than 1 MAC for all of the inhaled anesthetics except isoflurane. With the exception of N_2O, the evidence suggests this effect is caused by direct activation of the respiratory center in the central nervous system rather than by stimulating pulmonary stretch receptors. Additionally, volatile anesthetics decrease V_T and significantly alter the breathing pattern from the normal awake pattern of intermittent deep breaths separated by varying time intervals to one of rapid, shallow, regular, and rhythmic breathing (*Miller: Anesthesia, ed 6, pp 170-171; Stoelting Pharmacology and Physiology in Anesthetic Practice, ed 4, p 60*).

324. (A) Halothane is derived from the hydrocarbon ethane by substitution with the halogens fluorine, bromine, and chlorine. The structure of this halogenated hydrocarbon makes halothane nonflammable and provides for low blood solubility, molecular stability, and anesthetic potency (*Miller: Anesthesia, ed 6, p 160; Stoelting: Pharmacology and Physiology in Anesthetic Practice, ed 3, p 38*).

325. (C) Although desflurane has a low blood/gas partition coefficient (0.42) and should produce rapid induction of anesthesia, its marked pungency and airway irritation make inhalation inductions very difficult. Not only do patients dislike the scent, but the airway irritation often leads to coughing, increased salivation, breath holding, and sometimes laryngospasm (especially if the concentration is rapidly increased). In addition, with abrupt increases in concentration, patients often develop tachycardia and hypertension, thought to be due to increased sympathetic discharge (*Barash: Clinical Anesthesia, ed 5, pp 395-396; Stoelting: Basics of Anesthesia, ed 5, pp 93, 408*).

326. (B) A vaporizer's specificity is based on the vapor pressure of the anesthetic agent for which it is made. Filling a vaporizer with an agent with a higher vapor pressure results in a higher concentration in the vaporizer's output. Similarly, a volatile agent with a lower vapor pressure produces an output with a lower concentration than seen on the dial. Enflurane vapor pressure of 172 mm Hg (20° C) most closely approximates the vapor pressure of sevoflurane, which is 160 mm Hg (*Miller: Anesthesia, ed 6, p 284; Stoelting: Basics of Anesthesia, ed 5, p 79*).

327. (A)   When N_2O is substituted for an equal MAC value of isoflurane, the resulting blood pressure is greater than that seen with the same MAC value achieved with isoflurane as the sole anesthetic agent. When administered alone, N_2O does not alter arterial blood pressure, stroke volume, systemic vascular resistance, or baroreceptor reflexes. Administration of N_2O increases heart rate slightly, which may result in a mild increase in cardiac output. In vitro, N_2O has a dose-dependent direct depressant effect on myocardial contractility, which is probably overcome in vivo by sympathetic activation (*Miller: Anesthesia, ed 6, pp 212-215; Stoelting: Basics of Anesthesia, ed 5, p 88*).

328. (A)   All of the present-day volatile anesthetics reduce blood pressure in a dose dependent fashion. Desflurane, sevoflurane and isoflurane do this primarily through reductions in systemic vascular resistance. Halothane and the obsolete agent, enflurane, produce hypotension via direct myocardial depression (*Miller: Anesthesia, ed 6, pp 201-202; Stoelting: Pharmacology and Physiology in Anesthetic Practice, ed 4, p 51*).

329. (E)   Halothane tends to decrease the cardiac output, whereas sevoflurane, desflurane, and isoflurane tend to maintain cardiac output. Nitrous oxide tends to increase cardiac output primarily because of the mild increase in sympathetic tone (*Stoelting: Pharmacology and Physiology in Anesthetic Practice, ed 4, p 53*).

330. (D)   At concentrations of 1 MAC, isoflurane may attenuate antigen-induced bronchospasm, presumably by decreasing vagal tone. At similar concentrations, isoflurane will not reduce cardiac output in patients with normal left ventricular function. Additionally, isoflurane will decrease stroke volume, mean arterial pressure, and systemic vascular resistance in a dose-dependent manner. Cardiac output remains unchanged because decreases in systemic vascular resistance result in a reflex increase in heart rate that is sufficient to offset the decrease in stroke volume. However, dose-dependent decreases in both stroke volume and cardiac index can be seen when isoflurane is administered in concentrations greater than 1 MAC (*Miller: Anesthesia, ed 6, pp 159-160; Stoelting: Pharmacology and Physiology in Anesthetic Practice, ed 4, pp 51-54, 60*).

331. (A)   Desflurane can (but does not always) produce an increase in blood pressure and heart rate when the concentrations are rapidly increased. This may be related to airway irritation and a sympathetic response. This has also occurred with isoflurane, but to a much less frequent and usually lower extent. The other agents listed do not cause this sympathetic response with a rapid increase in concentration. If desflurane is increased slowly or a prior dose of narcotic is given, this increase in blood pressure and heart rate may not occur (*Stoelting: Basics of Anesthesia, ed 5, pp 89-90*).

332. (A)   Of all the options listed, desflurane has the lowest solubility constant, which results in a very rapid rise in F_A/F_I. The rate of rise is very similar to that seen with nitrous oxide and results in the most rapid attainment of 1 MAC concentration once the new volatile anesthetic has been initiated. Halothane has the highest blood/gas solubility coefficient of all the options, reflecting the largest quantity of gas stored in the blood. This reservoir will result in the slowest decline in the alveolar concentration of this volatile upon discontinuation. The combination of these different solubilities ultimately will result in the highest combined MAC when 1 MAC of halothane is discontinued and 1 MAC of desflurane is introduced (*Miller: Anesthesia, ed 6, pp 237-239; Stoelting: Pharmacology and Physiology in Anesthetic Practice, ed 4, p 43*).

333. (A)   The alveolar partial pressure of an anesthetic is determined by the rate of input relative to removal of the anesthetic from the alveoli as explained in question 322. During induction, the anesthetic gas is removed from the alveoli by uptake into the pulmonary venous blood. The rate of uptake is influenced by cardiac output, the blood/gas solubility coefficient, and the alveolar-to-venous partial pressure difference of the anesthetic. At a lower cardiac output, a slower rate of uptake of volatile anesthetic from the alveoli into the pulmonary venous blood results in a faster rate of increase in the alveolar concentration. This will result in an increased alveolar inspired gas concentration (F_A/F_I). Uptake of poorly soluble anesthetic gases from the alveoli is minimal and the rate of rise of F_A/F_I is rapid and virtually independent of cardiac output. Uptake of the more soluble anesthetics, such as isoflurane, from the alveoli into the pulmonary venous blood can be considerable and will be reflected by a slower rate of rise of the F_A/F_I ratio. Cardiogenic shock will have the smallest impact on the most insoluble agents, such as desflurane, sevoflurane, and N_2O, whereas the impact on the rate of rise of F_A/F_I of the relatively soluble anesthetic gases, such as isoflurane, will be more profound.

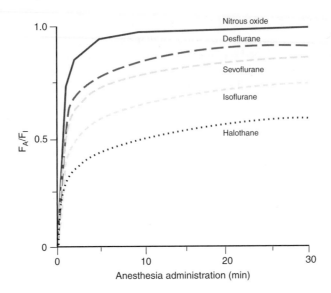

Changes in cardiac output have a profound effect on the FA/FI ratio for soluble anesthetics, but very little impact on the FA/FI ratio for the insoluble ones (*Miller: Anesthesia, ed 6, pp 132-134, 137*).

334. (C) The vessel-rich group that receives approximately 75% of the cardiac output is composed of the brain, heart, spleen, liver, splenic bed, kidneys, and endocrine glands. It constitutes, however, only 10% of the total body weight. Because of this large blood flow relative to tissue mass, these organs take up a large volume of volatile anesthetic and equilibrate with the partial pressure of the volatile anesthetic in the blood and alveoli during the earliest moments of induction (*Miller: Anesthesia, ed 6, pp 133-134; Stoelting: Pharmacology and Physiology in Anesthetic Practice, ed 4, pp 10, 725*).

335. (C) Of the choices listed, halothane undergoes oxidative metabolism to the greatest extent (approximately 20%), followed by sevoflurane (approximately 3%), isoflurane (approximately 0.2%), enflurane (approximately 3%), and desflurane (approximately 0.02%). Enflurane and sevoflurane may produce fluoride ions, which can be of concern during longer cases because of their potential for nephrotoxicity. Fluoride ion-induced nephrotoxicity is characterized by the inability of the kidneys to concentrate urine, presumably by direct inhibition of adenylate cyclase activity, which is necessary for the normal function of antidiuretic hormone (ADH) at the distal convoluted tubules. This results in ADH-resistant diabetes insipidus, that is, nephrogenic diabetes insipidus characterized by polyuria, dehydration, hypernatremia, and increased serum osmolarity (*Miller: Anesthesia, ed 6, pp 237-239; Stoelting: Pharmacology and Physiology in Anesthetic Practice, ed 4, pp 66-72*).

336. (A) Hypoxia is always a concern with low flow or closed circuit anesthesia especially if N_2O is used. Carbon monoxide can be formed when volatiles (desflurane, enflurane, isoflurane worst offenders) are exposed to desiccated CO_2 absorbents containing KOH and NaOH (Baralyme and soda lime). Similarly, halothane and sevoflurane are unstable in hydrated CO_2 absorbents and form compound A (with sevoflurane and a similar compound with halothane). Fluoride ions are formed in the metabolism of the obsolete volatile, enflurane as well as with isoflurane, sevoflurane and halothane (with reductive metabolism). These unwanted byproducts are ordinarily found in low concentrations with high flow anesthetic techniques because the large volumes of fresh gas wash them away. With low flow or closed circuit anesthetic techniques, such molecules can accumulate. Since low flow or closed circuit anesthetics require, by definition, a circle system that always includes a CO_2 absorber, hypercarbia is no more a concern than with high flow anesthetics. Regardless of technique chosen, hypercarbia can exist if the absorbents are exhausted or if the one-way valves fail (*Miller: Anesthesia, ed 6, p 143; Stoelting: Pharmacology and Physiology in Anesthetic Practice, ed 4, pp 69-72*).

337. (D) The situation described in this question is that of a transpulmonary shunt. In patients with transpulmonary shunting, blood emerging from unventilated alveoli contains no anesthetic gas. This anesthetic-deficient blood mixes with blood from adequately ventilated, anesthetic-containing alveoli producing an arterial anesthetic partial pressure considerably less than expected. Because uptake of anesthetic gas from the alveoli into pulmonary venous blood will be less than normal, transpulmonary shunting accelerates the rate of rise in the FA/FI ratio but reduces the rate of increase in the arterial partial pressure of all volatile anesthetics. The degree to which these changes occur depends on the solubility of the given volatile anesthetic. For poorly soluble anesthetics, such as N_2O, transpulmonary shunting only slightly accelerates the rate of rise in FA/FI ratio, but significantly reduces the rate of increase in arterial anesthetic partial pressure. The opposite occurs with highly soluble volatile anesthetics, such as halothane and isoflurane (*Miller: Anesthesia, ed 6, pp 132-133, 139; Stoelting: Pharmacology and Physiology in Anesthetic Practice, ed 4, pp 27, 30-31*).

338. (E) In unanesthetized subjects, a reduction in arterial blood pressure will elicit an increase in heart rate via the carotid and aortic baroreceptor reflexes. In contrast to isoflurane, desflurane and sevoflurane halothane profoundly inhibits these baroreceptor reflex responses. Therefore, despite reductions in arterial blood pressures by halothane, heart rate usually remains unchanged (*Miller: Anesthesia, ed 6, p 201; Stoelting: Pharmacology and Physiology in Anesthetic Practice, ed 4, pp 51-52, 727*).

339. (A) (*Miller: Anesthesia, ed 6, pp 178-179, 191-202; Stoelting: Pharmacology and Physiology in Anesthetic Practice, ed 4, pp 51-54, 60-61*).

340. (D) The rate of input of volatile anesthetics from the anesthesia machine to the alveoli is influenced by three factors: VA; the inspired anesthetic partial pressure; and the characteristics of the anesthetic breathing system. Increased VA will accelerate the rate of increase in FA/FI for all volatile anesthetics. However, the magnitude of this effect is dependent on the solubility of the volatile anesthetic. The rate of increase in FA/FI depends very little on VA for poorly soluble anesthetics because the uptake of these is minimal. In contrast, the rate of increase in FA/FI for highly soluble volatile anesthetics depends significantly on VA. Halothane is the most soluble volatile anesthetic listed in this question (blood/gas solubility coefficient 2.54). Therefore, an increase in VA will accelerate the rate of increase in FA/FI the most for halothane. Blood/gas solubility coefficients for the other volatile anesthetics are as follows: enflurane 1.90, isoflurane 1.46, sevoflurane 0.69, desflurane 0.42, and N_2O 0.46 (*Miller: Anesthesia, ed 6, pp 132-134, 151; Stoelting: Pharmacology and Physiology in Anesthetic Practice, ed 4, pp 25-28*).

341. (E) Anesthetic requirement increases from birth until approximately age 3 to 6 months. Then, with the exception of a slight increase at puberty, anesthetic requirement progressively declines with aging. For example, the MAC for halothane in neonates is approximately 0.87%, in infants it is approximately 1.2%, and in young adults approximately 0.75%. A notable exception to this pattern is seen with sevoflurane. Here MAC is the highest with neonates. If the question only pertained to sevoflurane, the correct response would have been C. Please review the answer to question 321 (*Miller: Anesthesia, ed 6, p 108; Stoelting: Pharmacology and Physiology in Anesthetic Practice, ed 4, pp 33-34*).

342. (B) Although a junctional rhythm can develop after any of the drugs listed, it is most common with halothane (*Stoelting: Basics of Anesthesia, ed 5, p 91*).

343. (C) Two principles of MAC must be considered in this situation. First, MAC is additive, so the fraction of MAC of each individual gas must be added to arrive at total MAC. The second is that alveolar concentrations of soluble agents are reflected more accurately by end-expiratory concentrations rather than either inspiratory concentrations or gradients between inspiratory and expiratory concentrations. Because nitrous oxide is very insoluble, it is reasonable to assume equilibrium will be established early. The inspiratory concentration of nitrous oxide, approximately 0.6 MAC, should approximate the alveolar concentration. However, the expiratory concentrations of the more soluble volatile anesthetics should be used to estimate the alveolar concentration. The end-expiratory isoflurane concentration of 0.6 reflects approximately 0.5 MAC, which in addition to 0.6 MAC of nitrous oxide would be closest to answer C, 1.1 MAC (*Miller: Anesthesia, ed 6, pp 107-109, 116; Stoelting: Pharmacology and Physiology in Anesthetic Practice, ed 4, pp 33-34*).

344. (B) The figure shown in this question depicts the concentration effect. Note that the inspired anesthetic concentration not only influences the maximum alveolar concentration that can be attained but also the rate at which the maximum alveolar concentration can be attained. The greater the inhaled anesthetic concentration, the faster the increase in FA/FI (*Miller: Anesthesia, ed 6, pp 135-136; Stoelting: Pharmacology and Physiology in Anesthetic Practice, ed 4, pp 24-25*).

345. (E) The depth of general anesthesia is directly proportional to the alveolar anesthetic partial pressure. The faster the rate of increase in FA/FI, the faster the induction of anesthesia. With the exception of a right-to-left intracardiac shunt (see explanation to question 337 on effect of shunt on the rate of increase in FA/FI and explanation to question 346 on the effect of shunt on arterial anesthetic partial pressure and rate of induction of anesthesia), all of the conditions listed in this question will accelerate the rate of increase in FA/FI and, thus, the rate of induction of anesthesia (*Stoelting: Pharmacology and Physiology in Anesthetic Practice, ed 4, p 30*).

346. (B) In general, a right-to-left intracardiac shunt or transpulmonary shunt will slow the rate of induction of anesthesia. This occurs because of a dilutional effect of shunted blood, which contains no volatile anesthetic, on the arterial anesthetic partial pressure coming from ventilated alveoli. The impact of a right-to-left shunt on the rate of increase in pulmonary arterial anesthetic partial pressure and, ultimately, the rate of induction of anesthesia is greatest for poorly soluble volatile anesthetics. This occurs because uptake of poorly soluble volatile anesthetics into pulmonary venous blood is minimal; thus, the dilutional effect of the shunt on pulmonary venous anesthetic partial pressure is essentially unopposed. In contrast, the uptake of highly soluble volatile anesthetics is sufficient to partially offset the dilutional effect. Of the anesthetics listed in the question, desflurane is the least soluble (*Stoelting: Pharmacology and Physiology in Anesthetic Practice, ed 4, pp 27, 30*).

347. (A) Both a left-to-right intracardiac shunt and a left-to-right tissue shunt, such as an arteriovenous fistula, will result in a higher partial pressure of anesthetic gas in the blood returning to the lungs, ultimately resulting in a more rapid rise in FA/FI. However, this effect is minimal and in most cases clinically insignificant (*Stoelting: Pharmacology and Physiology in Anesthetic Practice, ed 4, p 30*).

348. (D) Sevoflurane is a highly insoluble volatile anesthetic that combines with carbon dioxide absorbents to form a vinyl ether known as compound A. The blood/gas partition coefficient for sevoflurane is 0.69. The vaporizer manufactured by Ohmeda is capable of delivering concentrations ranging from 0.2% to 8% at fresh-gas flow rates of 0.2 to 15 L/min. Its vapor pressure is 160 mm Hg at 20° C, which is similar to the vapor pressure for the other volatile anesthetics with the exception of desflurane (664 mm Hg at 20° C). Gas flows greater than 2 L/min prevent rebreathing compound. A. (not formation of it), thus reducing the possibility of renal toxicity associated with it (*Miller: Anesthesia, ed 6, pp 251-254, 1490-1491; Stoelting: Pharmacology and Physiology in Anesthetic Practice, ed 4, pp 45-46, 70-72*).

349. (E) Metabolism may play an important role in emergence from anesthesia when one of the more soluble agents is used. However, this is not the case on induction. Factors that affect the rate of induction include the inspiratory concentration of anesthetic gas, alveolar ventilation, the characteristics of the anesthetic breathing system, solubility of the anesthetic gas, cardiac output, and the alveolar venous partial pressure difference (*Miller: Anesthesia, ed 6, pp 136, 147-149; Stoelting: Pharmacology and Physiology in Anesthetic Practice, ed 4, pp 23-24, 31-32*).

350. (D) Volatile anesthetics produce minimal bronchodilation unless airway resistance is increased (bronchospasm). This is explained by the fact that airway smooth muscle tone is ordinarily low and additional bronchodilation is difficult to demonstrate. The irritating effects of desflurane can be reduced by prior administration of fentanyl or morphine (*Stoelting: Basics of Anesthesia, ed 5, p 93; Stoelting: Pharmacology and Physiology in Anesthetic Practice, ed 4, pp 63-64*).

351. (E) Halothane undergoes significant metabolism compared to isoflurane (15% to 20% vs 0.2%). Metabolism increases total elimination of halothane (which occurs mainly in the liver but also occurs in the lung), resulting in a more rapid alveolar washout (*Miller: Anesthesia, ed 6, pp 147-150; Stoelting: Pharmacology and Physiology in Anesthetic Practice, ed 4, pp 75-79*).

352. **(A)** This classic graph depicts the effect of switching from 21% oxygen and 79% N_2O to 21% oxygen and 79% nitrogen, that is, air. When this occurs large volumes of N_2O are released into the lungs and dilute all gases including oxygen and CO_2. The reduction in O_2 results in hypoxia and the resulting fall in CO_2 reduces the drive to breathe. This combination occurs at a time when most patient have narcotics and other respiratory depressants on board. For this reason it is wise to administer 100% oxygen to patients for several minutes after emergence form general anesthesia (*Miller: Anesthesia, ed 6, p 150*).

353. **(A)** The vessel rich group receives 75% of the cardiac output and represents 10% of the weight of a lean adult. In a sense, the lungs receive virtually 100% of the cardiac output, but this is the right sided CO (the supply side for oxygen) and therefore doesn't "count" in the classic definition. Lung parenchyma, ironically, uses a very small quantity of oxygen compared with the brain, liver, kidney and myocardium (*Stoelting: Basics of Anesthesia, ed 5, p 86*).

354. **(D)** At 1 MAC concentrations, isoflurane depresses mean arterial pressures primarily by decreasing systemic vascular resistance. The decrease in mean arterial pressure may be greater than that seen with the administration of halothane. However, heart rate will be increased and stroke volume will decrease to a lesser extent than seen with administration of 1 MAC halothane (*Miller: Anesthesia, ed 6, pp 201-202; Stoelting: Pharmacology and Physiology in Anesthetic Practice, ed 4, pp 53-54, 58*).

355. **(B)** Changes in both cardiac output and alveolar ventilation will affect the rates of rise of F_A/F_I but in opposite directions. An increase in cardiac output will decrease the rate of F_A/F_I whereas an increase in alveolar ventilation will increase the rate of F_A/F_I. However, these two opposing options do not completely offset one another because the increased cardiac output also accelerates the equilibrium of the anesthetic between the blood and the tissues. This equilibrium results in a narrowing of the alveolar-to-venous partial pressure difference and attenuates the impact of the increased cardiac output on uptake. The net result will be a slight increase in the rate of rise of F_A/F_I.

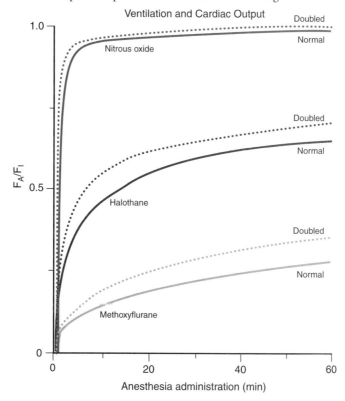

(*Miller: Anesthesia, ed 6, pp 136-138; Stoelting: Pharmacology and Physiology in Anesthetic Practice, ed 4, pp 24-25, 30*).

356. **(A)** Blood/gas partition coefficient is the option listed that most closely correlates with recovery from inhaled anesthesia. A higher blood/gas partition coefficient reflects a larger quantity of gas dissolved in the blood for a given alveolar concentration. Other factors that affect emergence from anesthesia include alveolar ventilation, cardiac output, tissue concentrations, and metabolism (*Miller: Anesthesia, ed 6, pp 132, 147-151; Stoelting: Pharmacology and Physiology in Anesthetic Practice, ed 4, pp 27, 31-33*).

357. (B) If an inhalation agent causes coronary artery vasodilation, it is theoretically possible to cause a condition called coronary steal syndrome. In this condition, when the perfusion pressure of the coronary artery is reduced, only blood vessels capable of dilation will dilate to compensate for the reduction in blood flow. Because atherosclerotic vessels cannot effectively dilate, they would be less likely to be able to compensate for a reduction in blood flow and hence become ischemic. The redistribution of blood causes the "steal." Of the listed drugs, only isoflurane produces significant coronary dilation. This was once thought to be of great clinical significance but over time has been shown to be of little significance (*Stoelting: Pharmacology and Physiology in Anesthetic Practice, ed 4, pp 56, 754-755*).

358. (E) Four main factors affect the total or rate of rise of the alveolar concentration of anesthetic (FA) and hence the inhalation induction of anesthetics. These factors are the inspired concentration of anesthetic (FI), the solubility of the anesthetic, the alveolar ventilation and the cardiac output. The rate of rise in FA/FI is faster with the less soluble anesthetics, as noted by the blood:gas partition coefficients. The blood:gas partition coefficient measured at 37° C is the least with desflurane (0.45) followed closely for nitrous oxide (0.47), then sevoflurane (0.65), isoflurane (1.4), enflurane (1.8), halothane (2.5) and highest with ether (12). Thus, replacing isoflurane with sevoflurane would speed up induction. Increasing the minute ventilation as well as increasing the fresh gas flow rate allow more of the anesthetic to get into the lungs and offsets the uptake of anesthetic by the blood, also speeding the induction of inhalational anesthesia. Decreasing the cardiac output accelerates the rise of FA/FI resulting in a faster inhalation induction (decrease amount of blood exposed to the lung and decreases the uptake of anesthesia) (*Miller: Anesthesia, ed 6, pp 131-138, Stoelting: Basics of Anesthesia, ed 5, pp 83-84*).

359. (B) The table below contains a fifth column, "FIO$_2$". It would appear that choices B and E are tied at 50%. The question asks for arterial oxygen concentration (not FIO$_2$). During induction of general anesthesia, N$_2$O is rapidly taken up into the blood, resulting in the so called second gas effect and concentrating effect. Concentration of oxygen in this manner is termed "alveolar hyperoxygenation" and results in a transient increase in Pao$_2$ of approximately 10% (*Stoelting: Basics of Anesthesia, ed 5, p 84*).

		Oxygen	Air	N$_2$O	F$_I$o$_2$
A.	L/min	1	2	0	0.47
B.	L/min	2	0	2	0.50
C.	L/min	2	2	2	0.40
D.	L/min	4	10	1	0.41
E.	L/min	2	3.5	0	0.50

360. (D) Halothane produces reductions in arterial pressure primarily by reducing cardiac output. Desflurane, sevoflurane, and isoflurane lower arterial blood pressure through reduction in system vascular resistance with relative preservation of cardiac output (*Miller: Anesthesia, ed 5, pp 104-105; Stoelting: Pharmacology and Physiology in Anesthetic Practice, ed 3, pp 46-47*).

361. (C) Calculation of the washin of N$_2$O requires use of the concept of time constant. Given a volume of 6 liters for the circle system, the time constant is 6L/(6L × min^{-1}) or one minute. The numbers to remember for time constants are 63%, 84% and 95% for 1, 2 and 3 time constant respectively. A properly functioning anesthesia machine would never allow administration of 100% N$_2$O, but this nightmare scenario is given purely for illustrative purposes (*Barash: Clinical Anesthesia, ed 5, p 389*).

362. (D) Acute ethanol ingestion is the only factor listed that will reduce MAC. Acute amphetamine ingestion raises MAC, as do hypernatremia, hyperthermia and the presence of (naturally occurring) red hair. Gender, thyroid function, and Paco$_2$ between 15 and 95 mm Hg and Pao$_2$ greater than 38 mm Hg have no effect on MAC (*Stoelting: Pharmacology and Physiology in Anesthetic Practice, ed 4, p 34*).

363. (E) This table summarizes the factors that influence the partial pressure gradients. A right to left intrapulmonary shunt affects delivery of inhaled aesthetics, but lung dead space does not, because the latter does not produce a dilutional effect on the arterial partial pressure of the anesthetic in question (*Stoelting: Basics of Anesthesia, ed 5, pp. 83-86*).

FACTORS DETERMINING PARTIAL PRESSURE GRADIENTS NECESSARY FOR ESTABLISHMENT OF ANESTHESIA

Input from Anesthesia Machine to Alveoli	Uptake from Alveoli to Pulmonary Blood	Uptake from Arterial Blood to Brain
Inspired anesthetic concentration	Blood gas partition coefficient	Brain/blood partition coefficient
Alveolar ventilation	Cardiac output	Cerebral blood flow
Characteristics of the anesthesia breathing system	Alveolar-to-venous partial pressure difference	Arterial-to-venous partial pressure difference

(*Stoelting: Basics of Anesthesia, ed 4, p 26.*)

364. **(D)** Halothane is the only modern volatile anesthetic (methoxyflurane also contained a preservative) that contains a preservative, thymol. Because halothane may undergo degradation into chloride, hydrochloric acid, bromide, hydrobromic acid, and phosgene, it is stored in amber-colored bottles and thymol is added to prevent spontaneous oxidation (*Stoelting: Pharmacology and Physiology in Anesthetic Practice, ed 4, p 4; Stoelting: Basics of Anesthesia, ed 5, pp*).

365. **(E)** The delivery of anesthetic gases to a patient is a complex series of events that starts with the anesthesia machine and culminates with achievement of an anesthetic partial pressure in the brain (PBr). The partial pressure measured in the blood for any volatile is either rising (at first rapidly, then more slowly) or falling (rapidly at first then more slowly). The vessel-rich group reaches steady state in about 12 minutes (for any dialed level of volatile). The rest of the body, however, approaches, but virtually never reaches, equilibrium (e.g. the equilibrium half time for the fat group is 30 hours for sevoflurane). Hence, a true zero gradient is never achieved in the steady state. When the anesthetic is discontinued or reduced, there is a fall in the arterial partial pressure such that it is less than the venous partial pressure. In fact, when the venous partial pressure exceeds the arterial partial pressure it means the volatile has been reduced (or shut off) because the lungs are "cleansing" the blood as the volatile filled blood passes through them. The newly "cleansed" blood then finds it way to the left ventricle with a very low Pa for the volatile in question. The present example can only be explained if the volatile had just been turned off or down (lungs cleansing) then suddenly turned back up. In this brief "window" the alveolar partial pressure gradient would exceed the venous partial pressure because there is a net transfer of anesthetic into the blood exiting the lungs (pulmonary vein). Since this just happened (turned up), the body has not had sufficient time to reverse the gradient in the left sided arterial and venous system. Moments later, the left sided arterial volatile partial pressure will exceed the venous partial pressure and the patient will become "deeper" (*Miller: Anesthesia, ed 6, pp 132-134, Stoelting: Basics of Anesthesia, ed 5, pp 82-83*).

366. **(D)** Anesthetic agents are soluble in the rubber and plastic components found in the anesthesia machine. This fact can impede the development of anesthetic concentrations of these drugs. The worst offender is the obsolete volatile methoxyflurane. However, both isoflurane and halothane are soluble in rubber and plastic, but to a lesser degree. Sevoflurane, desflurane, and nitrous oxide have little or no solubility in rubber or plastic. A different but important issue should be borne in mind regarding loss of sevoflurane. This agent can be destroyed in appreciable quantities by Baralyme and soda lime, but not calcium hydroxide lime (Amsorb). It is therefore recommended that fresh gas flow rates exceed 2 L/min when sevoflurane is administered (*Miller: Anesthesia, ed 6, p 142*).

367. **(B)** Compound A is an ether that forms when sevoflurane interacts with absorbent granules. In rats, compound A is a nephrotoxin that causes damage to the proximal renal tubule. It is believed that compound A is not nephrotoxic in humans, at least not at the concentrations that are achieved clinically (even with fresh gas flows as low as 1 L/min). The factors that lead to increased concentrations of compound A are use of fresh absorbent, use of Baralyme instead of soda lime, high absorbent temperatures, higher concentrations of sevoflurane in the anesthesia system, and closed circuit or low-flow anesthesia. Desiccated Baralyme favors the formation of compound A, whereas desiccated soda lime decreases compound A formation (*Miller: Anesthesia, ed 6, p 296*).

368. **(D)** A left to right peripheral shunt such as an arteriovenous fistula delivers volatile containing venous blood to the lungs. This action offsets the dilutional effect of a right to left intracardiac or pulmonary shunt and speeds up induction. The increase in the anesthetic partial pressure from an AV fistula is only detectable in the setting of a concomitant right to left shunt (*Stoelting: Basics of Anesthesia, ed 5, p 86*).

369. **(E)** Each of the volatiles is correctly paired with its percentage of recovered metabolites. Sevoflurane is metabolized 2% to 5% through oxidative pathways utilizing the cytochrome P-450 enzyme pathway. Likewise the other volatiles are all oxidatively metabolized in varying degrees. The obsolete anesthetic methoxyflurane underwent 50% metabolism resulting in high concentrations of fluoride ions and resultant renal failure in some patients. Halothane is unique among the volatiles agents in that it can undergo reductive metabolism in the face of low oxygen availability in the liver (*Barash: Clinical Anesthesia, ed 5, p 386; Stoelting: Pharmacology and Physiology in Anesthetic Practice, ed 4, pp 77-80*).

370. **(E)** By definition, the washin of the anesthesia circuit refers to the filling of the components of the circuit with anesthetic gases. The total washin volumes are around 7 L and break down as follows: anesthesia bag 3 L; anesthesia hoses, 2 L; and anesthesia absorbent compartment, 2 L. All of the components listed are part of the anesthesia circuit except the mass spectrometer tubing. The mass spectrometer takes away from incoming gases through aspiration, but does not dilute them (*Miller: Anesthesia, ed 6, p 142*).

371. **(E)** Increasing minute ventilation is one of two methods for manipulating ventilation to increase the rate of establishing anesthesia. Another method is increasing inspired concentration, which can be achieved by turning up the dial above desired steady state concentration (overpressurizing) to reach steady state more quickly, or increasing fresh gas flow to reduce or eliminate rebreathing (dilution). Substituting a less soluble anesthetic, such as sevoflurane for isoflurane, also establishes anesthesia more rapidly. Carrying out the induction in San Diego instead of Denver constitutes administering the anesthetic at higher atmospheric (barometric) pressure, which decreases the uptake and hence increases the rate of rise of F_A/F_I, that is, accelerates the establishment of anesthesia. Administration of an inotrope increases cardiac output, which also increases uptake and slows the rate of induction.

$$\text{uptake} = \frac{\lambda \dot{Q}(P_A - P_V)}{BP}$$

where λ is the blood/gas partition coefficient, $\dot{Q}$ is the cardiac output, ($P_A - P_V$) is the alveolar-to-pulmonary venous blood partial pressure difference, and BP is the barometric pressure (*Barash: Clinical Anesthesia, ed 5, p 391; Miller: Anesthesia, ed 6, pp 131-133*).

372. **(D)** In comparing pharmacokinetics of elimination for volatile anesthetics, desflurane is the fastest. The time for a 50% reduction (decrement) in the alveolar partial pressure of the "modern" anesthetics is roughly the same, about 5 minutes, regardless of anesthetic duration. For longer anesthetics, however, the 80% and 90% decrement times becomes markedly different. In the present example, the 90% decrement time for desflurane after a six hour anesthetic is 14 minutes. This is in stark contrast to sevoflurane (65 minutes) and isoflurane (86 minutes). Please see question and explanation 376 (*Stoelting: Basics of Anesthesia, ed 5, pp 87-88*).

373. **(D)** A properly functioning vaporizer will produce the concentration set on the dial (plus or minus a small tolerance) provided the fresh gas flow rate is greater than 250 mL/min and less than 15 L/min. The 1 L/min rate in this question is well within the limits of the vaporizer. The fact that rebreathing occurs with a circular anesthesia system causes a significant dilutional effect. It is true that uptake would enhance dilution, but it (uptake), per se, is not the main reason for this discrepancy. Uptake is considered when discussing the F_A/F_I ratio. This question addresses the characteristics of the anesthesia machine and the relationship between dial setting and delivered concentration. To achieve a desired concentration, e.g., 2%, you must either raise the fresh gas flow to convert the system to a non-rebreathing system or set the vaporizer to a higher level than is actually desired, the concept of overpressurization. In this era of cost containment, the later is more economical (*Barash: Clinical Anesthesia, ed 5, p 390, 572; Stoelting: Basics of Anesthesia, ed 5, p 195*).

374. **(E)** The anesthesia circuit can delay emergence significantly if the patient is not disconnected (functionally) from it. Anesthetic gases become dissolved in the rubber and plastic components of the breathing circuit. Likewise the soda lime can serve as a depository for anesthetics as well as the patient's own exhaled gases. To reduce these effects to nearly zero, fresh gas flow should be raised to at least 5 L/min. Fresh gases emerge via the common gas outlet and do not contain volatile agents or N_2O since these (volatiles and N_2O) are shut off during emergence. (*Miller: Anesthesia, ed 5, p 151*).

375. (B) The time constant is defined as capacity divided by flow. The time constant for a volatile anesthetic is determined by the capacity of a tissue to hold the anesthetic relative to the tissue blood flow. The capacity of a tissue to hold a volatile anesthetic depends both on the size of the tissue and on the affinity of the tissue for the anesthetic. The brain time constant of a volatile anesthetic can be estimated by doubling the brain/blood partition coefficient for the volatile anesthetic. For example, the time constant of halothane (brain/blood partition coefficient of 2.6) for the brain (mass of approximately 1500 g, blood flow of 750 mL/min) is approximately 5.2 minutes (*Eger: Anesthetic Update and Action, pp 85-87*).

376. (D) This concept highlights the fact that the difference in half time values among the volatile anesthetics is similar for all volatiles if anesthetic duration is very brief. With administration of volatile anesthetics for longer periods of time, differences in recovery time become more profound. For example, after a 1 hour anesthetic with desflurane (blood: gas tissue coefficient 0.45), a 95% reduction in the alveolar concentration can be reached in 5 minutes. With an hour-long sevoflurane anesthetic (blood: gas tissue coefficient 0.65), a 95% reduction requires 18 minutes and an hour-long isoflurane anesthetic (blood: gas tissue coefficient 1.4) requires greater than 30 minutes to reach 95% reduction in the alveolar concentration (*Miller: Anesthesia, ed 6, pp 132, 147-148*).

377. (D) After of period of time equal to 3 time constants, the venous blood exiting the vessel rich group will be at 95% level, but the blood as a whole will have a level of less than 95%. The venous blood contains a mixture of blood from the vessel rich group, the muscle group, the fat group and the vessel poor group and at the 3 time constant mark will be less than 95% (*Stoeling: Basics of Anesthesia, ed 5, p 86*).

378. (A)   379. (E)   380. (D)   381. (B)

The information for these questions is summarized in the graphs below. Halothane is unique among the volatiles listed in that it does not affect heart rate or systemic vascular resistance in the MAC ranges studied. Sevoflurane reduces heart rate until about 1 MAC, at which time it produces a dose-dependent increase in heart rate (*Stoelting: Pharmacology and Physiology in Anesthetic Practice, ed 4, pp 44-46*).

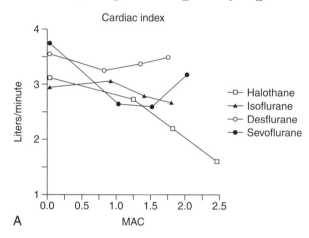

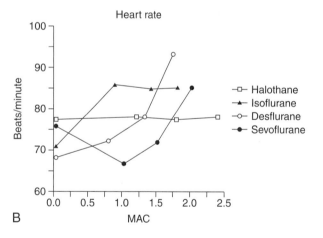

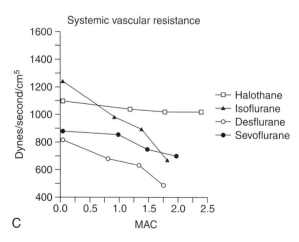

Chapter 5

Blood Products, Transfusion, and Fluid Therapy

DIRECTIONS (Questions 382 through 415) Each of the questions or incomplete statements in this section is followed by answers or by completions of the statement, respectively. Select the ONE BEST answer or completion for each item.

382. Each of the following treatments might be useful in restoring a prolonged prothrombin time (PT) to the normal range **EXCEPT**
    A. Recombinant factor VIII
    B. Vitamin K
    C. Fresh frozen plasma
    D. Stopping warfarin (Coumadin)
    E. Cryoprecipitate

383. Proper processing of platelet concentrates (to avoid future hemolytic transfusion reactions) before administration involves
    A. Type and crossmatch
    B. ABO and Rh matching
    C. Rh matching only
    D. ABO matching only
    E. Platelets can be administered without regard to any antigen system

384 The most common inherited coagulopathy is
    A. Hemophilia A
    B. Hemophilia B
    C. von Willebrand disease
    D. Factor V deficiency
    E. Factor II deficiency

385. In a 70-kg patient, 1 unit of platelet concentrate should increase the platelet count by
    A. 2000 to 5000/mm^3
    B. 5000 to 10,000/mm^3
    C. 15,000 to 20,000/mm^3
    D. 20,000 to 25,000/mm^3
    E. Greater than 25,000/mm^3

386. A 68-year-old patient receives a one unit transfusion of packed red blood cells (RBCs) in the recovery room after a laparoscopic prostatectomy. As the blood is slowly dripping into his peripheral IV, the patient complains of itching on his chest and arms, but his vital signs remain stable. The antibody most likely responsible for this is directed against
  A. Rh
  B. ABO
  C. MN, P & Lewis
  D. Kell, Duffy & Kidd
  E. None of the above

387. The likelihood of a clinically significant hemolytic transfusion reaction resulting from administration of type-specific blood is less than
  A. 1 in 10
  B. 1 in 250
  C. 1 in 500
  D. 1 in 1000
  E. 1 in 10,000

388. Frozen erythrocytes can be stored for
  A. 1 year
  B. 3 years
  C. 5 years
  D. 10 years
  E. They can be stored indefinitely

389. Which of the following clotting factors has the shortest half-life?
  A. Factor II
  B. Factor V
  C. Factor VII
  D. Factor IX
  E. Factor X

390. Which of the following clotting factors is not synthesized by the liver?
  A. Factor II
  B. Factor VII
  C. Factor VIII
  D. Factor IX
  E. Factor X

391. A 42-year-old woman is anesthetized for resection of a large (22 Kg), highly vascular sarcoma located in the abdomen. During the course of the resection, 20 units of RBC, 6 units of platelets, 10 units of cryoprecipitate, 5 units FFP and 1 liter of albumin are administered. At the conclusion of the operation, vital signs are stable and the patient is transported to the intensive care unit (ICU). Three and a half hours later, a diagnosis of sepsis is made and antibiotic therapy is started. Which of the items below would be the most likely cause of sepsis in this patient?
  A. Packed RBCs
  B. Cryoprecipitate
  C. Platelets
  D. Fresh frozen plasma
  E. Albumin

392. Blood is routinely screened (serologically) for
  A. Hepatitis A
  B. Severe acute respiratory syndrome (SARS)
  C. Malaria
  D. West Nile virus
  E. Bovine spongiform encephalitis (BSE, or mad cow disease)

393. The blood volume of a 10-kg, 1-year-old infant is
   A. 600 mL
   B. 800 mL
   C. 1000 mL
   D. 1300 mL
   E. 1500 mL

394. Which of the infections below is the most common transfusion related infection?
   A. West Nile virus
   B. Hepatitis B
   C. Hepatitis C
   D. Human immunodeficiency virus (HIV)
   E. Cytomegalovirus (CMV)

395. A 40-year-old, 78 kg patient with hemophilia A is scheduled for a right total knee arthroplasty. His laboratory test results show a hematocrit of 40, a factor VIII level of 0%, and no inhibitors to factor VIII. How much factor VIII concentrate do you need to give him to bring his factor VIII level to 100%?
   A. 1000 units
   B. 1500 units
   C. 2000 units
   D. 2500 units
   E. 3000 units

396. A 38-year-old male is undergoing a total colectomy under general anesthesia. Urine output has been 20 mL/hr for the last 2 hours. Volume replacement has been adequate. The rationale for administering 5 to 10 mg of furosemide to this patient is to
   A. Offset the effects of increased antidiuretic hormone (ADH)
   B. Improve renal blood flow
   C. Convert oliguric renal failure to nonoliguric renal failure
   D. Offset the effects of increased renin
   E. Promote renal venodilation

397. A 65-year-old male involved in a motor vehicle accident is brought to the emergency room with a blood pressure of 60 mm Hg. He is transfused with 4 units of type O, Rh-negative whole blood and 4 L of normal saline solution. After the patient is brought to the operating room his blood type is determined to be A positive. Which of the following is the most appropriate blood type for further intraoperative transfusions?
   A. Type A, Rh-positive whole blood
   B. Type A, Rh-positive RBCs
   C. Type O, Rh-positive whole blood
   D. Type O, Rh-negative whole blood
   E. Type O, Rh-negative RBCs

398. The criteria used to determine how long blood can be stored before transfusion is
   A. 90% of transfused erythrocytes must remain in circulation for 24 hours
   B. 70% of transfused erythrocytes must remain in circulation for 24 hours
   C. 70% of transfused erythrocytes must remain in circulation for 72 hours
   D. 75% of transfused erythrocytes must remain in circulation for 7 days
   E. 50% of transfused erythrocytes must remain in circulation for 7 days

399. The rational for storage of platelets at room temperature (22° C) is
   A. It maintains platelet count
   B. It optimizes platelet function
   C. It reduces the chance for infection
   D. It decreases the incidence of allergic reactions
   E. There is less splenic sequestration

400. An 18-year-old female involved in a motor vehicle accident is brought to the emergency room in shock. She is transfused with 10 units of type O, Rh-negative whole blood over 30 minutes. After infusion of the first 5 units, bleeding is controlled and her blood pressure rises to 85/51 mm Hg. During the next 15 minutes, as the remaining 5 units are infused, her blood pressure slowly falls to 60 mm Hg. The patient remains in sinus tachycardia at 120 beats/min, but the QT interval is noted to increase from 310 to 470 msec, and the central venous pressure increases from 9 to 20 mm Hg. Her breathing is rapid and shallow. The most likely cause of this scenario is
- **A.** Citrate toxicity
- **B.** Hyperkalemia
- **C.** Hemolytic transfusion reaction
- **D.** Cardiac tamponade
- **E.** Tension pneumothorax

401. A 20-kg, 5-year-old child with a hematocrit of 40% could lose how much blood and still maintain a hematocrit of 30%?
- **A.** 140 mL
- **B.** 250 mL
- **C.** 350 mL
- **D.** 450 mL
- **E.** 550 mL

402. A 100-kg male patient has a measured serum sodium concentration of 105 mEq/L. How much sodium would be needed to bring the serum sodium to 120 mEq/L?
- **A.** 600 mEq
- **B.** 900 mEq
- **C.** 1200 mEq
- **D.** 2400 mEq
- **E.** 3600 mEq

403. The likelihood of a clinically significant hemolytic transfusion reaction resulting from administration of erythrocytes to a patient with a negative antibody screen is less than
- **A.** 1 in 100
- **B.** 1 in 1000
- **C.** 1 in 10,000
- **D.** 1 in 100,000
- **E.** 1 in 1,000,000

404. A 23-year-old female who has been receiving total parenteral nutrition (15% dextrose, 5% amino acids, and intralipids) for 3 weeks is scheduled for surgery for severe Crohn's disease. Induction of anesthesia and tracheal intubation are uneventful. After establishing peripheral intravenous access, the old central line is removed and a new central line is placed at a different site. At the end of the operation, a large volume of fluid is discovered in the chest cavity on chest x-ray film. Arterial blood pressure is 105/70 mm Hg, heart rate is 150 beats/min, and Sao_2 is 96% (pulse oximeter). The most appropriate initial step in the management of this patient is to
- **A.** Place a chest tube
- **B.** Change the single-lumen to a double-lumen endotracheal tube
- **C.** Start a dopamine infusion
- **D.** Check a blood glucose level
- **E.** Administer esmolol intravenously

405. In an emergency when there is a limited supply of type O-negative RBCs, type O-positive RBCs are reasonable for transfusion for each of the following patients **EXCEPT**
- **A.** A 60-year-old woman with diabetes who was involved in a motor vehicle accident
- **B.** A 23-year-old man who sustained a gunshot wound to the upper abdomen
- **C.** An 84-year-old man with a ruptured abdominal aortic aneurysm
- **D.** A 5-year-old boy involved in a pedestrian-automobile accident
- **E.** A 21-year-old, gravida 2, para 1 woman with placenta previa who is bleeding profusely

406. Hetastarch interferes with coagulating through interacting with
   A. Antithrombin III
   B. Factor VIII
   C. Fibrinogen
   D. Protein S
   E. Prostacyclin

407. All of the following characterize packed RBCs that have been stored for 35 days at 4° C in citrate phosphate dextrose adenine-1 (i.e., CPDA-1) anticoagulant preservative **EXCEPT**
   A. Serum potassium greater than 70 mEq/L
   B. pH less than 7.0
   C. Blood glucose less than 100 mg/dL
   D. P_{50} of 28
   E. 2,3-diphosphoglycerate (2,3-DPG) less than 1 μM/L

408. What is the storage life of whole blood stored with citrate phosphate dextrose (CPD)?
   A. 14 days
   B. 21 days
   C. 35 days
   D. 42 days
   E. 49 days

409. What is the storage life of RBCs stored with Adsol?
   A. 14 days
   B. 21 days
   C. 35 days
   D. 42 days
   E. 49 days

410. Anticoagulation with low-molecular-weight heparin (LMWH) can be best monitored through which of the following laboratory tests?
   A. Activated partial thromboplastin time (aPTT)
   B. Prothrombin time (PT)
   C. Thrombin time
   D. Reptilase test
   E. Anti-Xa assay

411. Heparin resistance is likely in patients with which of the following heritable conditions?
   A Factor V Leiden mutation
   B Protein C deficiency
   C Protein S deficiency
   D Antithrombin or antithrombin III (AT3) deficiency
   E Prothrombin *G20210A* gene mutation

412. von Willebrand's disease could be treated by any of the following **EXCEPT**
   A. Cryoprecipitate
   B. Fresh frozen plasma
   C. Factor VIII concentrates
   D. Recombinant factor VIII
   E. Desmopressin (DDAVP)

413. The significance of IgA antibodies in transfusion medicine is related to
   A. Allergic reaction
   B. Immediate hemolytic reaction
   C. Febrile reaction
   D. Delayed hemolytic reaction (immune extravascular reaction)
   E. Diagnosis of transfusion-related acute lung injury (TRALI) reaction

414. The No. 1 cause of mortality associated with administration of blood is:
   A. ABO hemolytic transfusion reaction
   B. Non-ABO hemolytic transfusion reaction
   C. Microbial infection
   D. Transfusion associated circulatory overload (TACO)
   E. Transfusion related acute lung injury (TRALI)

415. Fluid resuscitation during major abdominal surgery with which of the following agents is associated with the best survival data?
   A. 5% Albumin
   B. 6% Hydroxyethyl starch
   C. Dextran 70
   D. Hypertonic saline
   E. None of the above

DIRECTIONS (questions 416 and 417) Choose the correct response below for the following questions:

416. Which of the following processes reduces the possibility of transmission of CMV to a susceptible recipient via red cell transfusion?

417. Process aimed at reducing graft versus host disease in transfusion recipients
   A. Washing erythrocytes
   B. Leukocyte reduction
   C. Irradiation
   D. Storage in ADSOL
   E. Treatment with ultraviolet light

Blood Products, Transfusion and Fluid Therapy

Answers, References, and Explanations

382. (A) The PT and the activated partial thromboplastin time (aPTT) are common tests used to evaluate coagulation factors. The PT primarily tests for factor VII in the extrinsic pathway, as well as factors I, II, V, and X of the common pathway. The aPTT primarily tests for factors VIII and IX of the intrinsic pathway, as well as factors I, II, V, and X of the common pathway. Although the PT is prolonged with deficient function of factors I, II, V, VII, or X, it is more sensitive to deficiencies of factor VII and less so with deficiencies of factor I or II. In fact, the PT is not prolonged until the level of fibrinogen (factor I) is less than 100 mg/dL and may only be prolonged 2 seconds when the level of factor II (prothrombin) is 10% of normal. Factors II, VII, IX, and X are vitamin-K-dependent factors and their formation is blocked with Coumadin therapy. Administering factor VIII will not help a prolonged PT (*Barash: Clinical Anesthesia, ed 5, pp 222-224, 228*).

383. (C) Platelet concentrates contain a fair amount of plasma and white blood cells (WBCs) but relatively few RBCs. Although ABO-compatible platelet transfusions are preferred (platelets survive better and crossmatching for subsequent RBCs is easier), in emergencies it has been noted that platelets often give adequate hemostasis without regard to ABO compatibility. Even though there are only small quantities of RBCs in platelets, the RBCs present can cause Rh immunization if Rh-positive platelet concentrates are injected into Rh-negative patients. Thus, until childbirth is no longer possible, Rh-negative females should only receive Rh-negative platelets (*Miller: Anesthesia, ed 6, pp 1822-1823; Stoelting: Pharmacology and Physiology in Anesthetic Practice, ed 4, p 625*).

384. (C) Coagulopathies can be inherited or acquired. Of the inherited coagulopathies, von Willebrand's disease is the most common, affecting 1 in 100 to 500 people. Both hemophilia A (Factor VIII) deficiency and hemophilia B (Factor IX or Christmas disease) are X-linked recessive disorders. Hemophilia A occurs in 1 to 2 per 10,000 males and hemophilia B occurs in 1 per 100,000 males. Factor V, Factor VII, Factor X, and prothrombin (Factor II) are exceedingly rare autosomal recessive disorders. (*Kasper: Harrison's Principles of Internal Medicine, ed 16, pp 680-682; Stoelting: Anesthesia and Co-Existing Disease, ed 4, pp 490-493*).

385. (B) Platelet count is increased about 5000 to 10,000/mm^3 per unit of platelet concentrate in the typical 70-kg patient. Each unit contains greater than 5.5×10^{10} platelets (*Barash: Clinical Anesthesia, ed 5, p 216; Harmening: Modern Blood Banking and Transfusion Practices, ed 5, pp 14-15; Miller: Anesthesia, ed 6, pp 1822-1823*).

386. (E) This is an example of a typical allergic reaction. All of the other choices in this question may be involved in hemolytic reactions. Allergic reactions are a form of nonhemolytic transfusion reactions, which are thought to be caused by foreign proteins in the transfused blood. The reactions occur in about 3% of all transfusions and present with urticaria, erythema, pruritus, fever and sometimes respiratory symptoms. When it occurs, the transfusion is stopped and supportive therapy including antihistamines is administered. If the symptoms resolve and there are no signs of a hemolytic reaction (no free hemoglobin in the plasma or urine) or a severe anaphylactic reaction, the transfusion can be resumed (*Lobato: Complications in Anesthesiology, p 512; Miller: Anesthesia, ed 6, p 1817; Stoelting: Basics of Anesthesia, ed 5, p 361*).

387. (D) Hemolytic transfusion reactions are often the result of clerical error. There are three main blood compatibility tests that can be performed to reduce the chance of a hemolytic reaction: ABO Rh typing, antibody screening, and crossmatching. With correct ABO and Rh typing, the possibility of an incompatible transfusion is less than 1 per 1000. If you add a type and screen, the possibility of an incompatible transfusion is less than 1 per 10,000. Optimal safety occurs when crossmatching is performed (*Barash: Clinical Anesthesia, ed 5, pp 219-220; Miller: Anesthesia, ed 6, pp 1804-1817*).

388. (D) Blood is most often stored as a liquid at about 4° C but can also be frozen for prolonged storage. Because of the added expense of frozen blood, it is used primarily for rare blood types and for autologous use. Blood that has already been collected has a cryoprotective agent (e.g., glycerol) added and is then frozen and stored at a temperature of –65° C (when 40% glycerol is used) or –120° C (when 20% glycerol is used). Currently, the U.S. Food and Drug Administration (FDA) allows frozen blood to be used up to 10 years from the time of collection (*Harmening: Modern Blood Banking and Transfusion Practices, ed 5 pp 7-11*).

389. (C) Factor VII is one of the four vitamin-K-dependent clotting factors (factors II, VII, IX, and X). It also has the shortest half-life of all the clotting factors (4 to 6 hours) and is the first factor to become deficient in patients with severe hepatic failure, Coumadin anticoagulation therapy, and vitamin K deficiency. The PT is most sensitive to decreases in factor VII (*Barash: Clinical Anesthesia, ed 5, pp 224-228; Stoelting: Pharmacology and Physiology in Anesthetic Practice, ed 4, p 861*).

390. (C) Factors IV (ionized calcium) and VIII are not synthesized by the liver. Factor VIII is synthesized by vascular endothelial cells and megakaryocytes and is involved in promoting coagulation via the intrinsic clotting (*Barash: Clinical Anesthesia, ed 5, pp 222-224; Miller: Anesthesia, ed 6, p 749*).

391. (C) Of the five blood products listed in this question, platelets are the most likely to cause bacterial sepsis. Platelet-related sepsis is estimated to occur in 1 case per 12,000. The source of bacteria can be from donor blood, or from contamination during the collection, processing and storage of the blood. If platelets are cooled, then rewarmed, the platelets tend not to function very effectively. Because platelets are stored at room temperature of 20° C to 24° C, bacteria tend to survive and multiply. All other listed blood products are cooled; whole blood and packed RBC's are cooled to 4° C (unless they are frozen which would be colder), fresh frozen plasma and cryoprecipitate are frozen to below -70° C. Albumin is heat sterilized, making it a sterile preparation that then can be safely stored at room temperatures (*Barash: Clinical Anesthesia, ed 5, p 210; Miller: Anesthesia, ed 6, pp 1815-1825*).

392. (D) Hepatitis A transmission is very rare and is screened for by history alone (not serologically) because there is no carrier state for the virus and the disease is relatively mild. A decrease in the transmission for various other infectious agents has been attributed to the recent addition of nucleic acid testing (NAT), see table. At present, there are no screening tests available for malaria, Chagas, SARS, variant Creutzfeldt-Jakob Disease (vCJD) or BSE disease (*Barash: Clinical Anesthesia, ed 5, pp 209-210; Miller: Anesthesia, ed 6, pp 1817-1820*).

TESTS USED FOR DETECTING INFECTIOUS AGENTS IN ALL UNITS OF BLOOD, 2004

Virus	RNA Minipool	Antibody To
Human immunodeficiency virus (HIV)	Nucleic acid technology	HIV-1, HIV-2
Hepatitis C virus (HCV)	Nucleic acid technology	HCV
Hepatitis B virus (HBV)		HBV
Human T-cell lymphotropic virus (HTLV)		HTLV-1, HTLV-2
West Nile virus	Nucleic acid technology	

(Miller: Anesthesia, ed 6 p 1818)

393. (B) Blood volume decreases with age. A preterm newborn has a blood volume of 100 to 120 mL/kg; a term newborn has a blood volume of about 90 mL/kg; an infant (3 to 12 months) has a blood volume of 80 mL/kg; a child older than one year has a blood volume of 70 mL/kg; and an adult has a blood volume of 65 mL/kg. This 10-kg, 1-year-old infant would have an estimated blood volume of 800 mL (*Barash: Clinic Anesthesia, ed 5, p 1214; Miller: Anesthesia, ed 6, p 2389*).

394. (E) Risk of transfusion-transmitted infection with a unit of screened blood in the United States varies from study to study but is less than 1% for CMV, 1 in 200,000 for hepatitis B, 1 in 600,000 for hepatitis C, 1 in 800,000 for HIV, 1 in 641,000 for human T-cell lymphotropic virus (HTLV), and 1 in more than 1,000,000 for West Nile virus. Thus, the most common transfusion associated infection in the United States is CMV. Antibodies to CMV are found in 40% to 90% of asymptomatic patients and show that in most patients, CMV infection is benign. However, in immunocompromised patients or premature newborns, CMV infection can be serious and at times fatal. Because the CMV's infectious form is carried in white blood cells, transfusion of CMV-negative blood or leukocyte-depleted blood can be used. Risk of seroconversion for CMV is about 0.38% per unit of seropositive donor blood. The infective agent for syphilis does not survive at 4° C, making transmission unlikely for whole blood, packed RBCs, fresh frozen plasma, or cryoprecipitate. It is possible for platelets (stored at room temperature) to transmit syphilis (*Barash: Clinical Anesthesia, ed 5, pp 209-210; Miller: Anesthesia, ed 6, pp 1817-1820; Stoelting: Basics of Anesthesia, ed 5, p 359*).

395. (E) The most common type of hemophilia is hemophilia A, an X-linked recessive disease causing a reduction in factor VIII activity. The disease occurs with a frequency of 1 in 5000 males. This disease can be severe (<1% factor VIII), moderate (1% to 4% factor VIII), or mild (5% to 30% factor VIII). Patients with mild hemophilia rarely have spontaneous bleeding. Laboratory studies show a normal platelet count and normal PT but a prolonged aPTT. The primary goal of preoperative preparation of patients with hemophilia A is to increase plasma factor VIII activity to a level that will ensure adequate hemostasis (i.e., 50% to 100%), then maintain a level (>40% factor VIII levels) for 7 to 10 days. One unit of factor VIII is equal to 1 mL of 100% activity of normal plasma. Thus, to calculate the initial dose you first calculate the patient's blood and then plasma volume. Then calculate the amount of activity needed to increase the factor VIII level. In this case, the blood volume is 78 kg × 65 mL/kg or about 5000 mL. Knowing the RBC volume is 40% (i.e., hematocrit is 40) makes the plasma volume 60%. Thus, the plasma volume is 5000 mL × 0.6 or about 3000 mL. Because the patient is starting at 0% activity and you wish to raise it to 100% activity, you will need 3000 units. (If you wished to raise the activity by 40%, then 3000 mL of plasma × 0.4 for 40% activity = 1200 units.) In addition, because the half-life of factor VIII is about 12 hours, about 1500 units will remain after 12 hours. An infusion of 1500 units in 12 hours, or 125 units per hour, will be a good starting maintenance infusion rate. Factor VIII can be administered as factor VIII concentrate or cryoprecipitate (about 10 units/mL). Patients with factor VIII inhibitors (10% to 20% of hemophiliacs) require more factor VIII. Hematology consultation should be considered for all hemophiliacs and routine checking of factor VIII levels should be performed (*Barash: Clinical Anesthesia, ed 5, p 233; Harmening: Modern Blood Banking and Transfusion Practices, ed 5, p 308; Miller: Anesthesiology, ed 6, pp 1116-1117; Stoelting: Pharmacology and Physiology in Anesthetic Practice, ed 4, p 627*).

396. (A) Serum ADH levels increase during painful stimulation associated with surgery, as well as during positive-pressure mechanical ventilation. Small doses of furosemide (i.e., 0.1 mg/kg) will counteract this effect during surgery (*Hines: Stoelting's Anesthesia and Co-Existing Disease, ed 5, pp 350-351, 404*).

397. (E) Type O, Rh-negative blood is also called universal donor blood because the transfused RBCs lacks the antigens needed to be hemolyzed. Because O-negative blood's plasma contains anti-A and anti-B antibodies, it is preferable to administer packed RBCs (with little plasma) over whole blood (lot of plasma) in an emergency. However, if two or more units of type O-negative, uncrossmatched whole blood are administered to a patient and subsequent blood typing reveals the patient's blood type to be A, B, or AB, then switching back to the patient's own blood type could lead to major intravascular hemolysis of the transfused RBCs and, therefore, is not advised. Use of type O-negative universal donor whole blood or preferably RBCs is recommended. In the male patient or the older female patient who will not have more children, type O-positive whole blood can be administered if few type O, Rh-negative units are available and massive transfusion is anticipated. Only after it is determined that the patient has low enough levels of transfused anti-A and anti-B antibodies should the correct type blood be administered (*Harmening: Modern Blood Banking and Transfusion Practices, ed 5, pp 273-274*).

398. (B) The requirement for blood storage states that at least 70% of the erythrocytes must remain in circulation for 24 hours after a transfusion for the transfusion to be successful. Erythrocytes that survive longer than 24 hours after transfusion appear to have a normal life span (*Harmening: Modern Blood Banking and Transfusion Practices, ed 5, p 7; Miller: Anesthesia, ed 6, pp 1804-1805*).

399.   **(B)**   At a pH below 6.0 or in cold temperatures such as 4° C (the temperature used for blood storage), platelets undergo irreversible shape changes. The optimal temperature for platelet storage is 22° C ± 2° C, or room temperature. There are two major problems with platelet storage at this recommended temperature. First, the pH falls because of platelet metabolism. Second, bacterial growth is possible, which could potentially lead to sepsis and death. To minimize these problems, platelet storage is limited to 5 days at 22° C (*Harmening: Modern Blood Banking and Transfusion Practices, ed 5, pp 15-17; Miller: Anesthesia, ed 6, pp 1822-1823*).

400.   **(A)**   Whole blood is rarely used today except in emergency cases where the rapid infusion of blood and volume is needed. Stored blood contains citrate, an anticoagulant that binds ionized calcium. When whole blood is rapidly transfused (i.e., >50 mL/70 kg/min) the citrate binds with calcium, producing transient decreases in ionized calcium. The abrupt decrease in ionized calcium can lead to prolonged QT intervals, an increase left ventricular end-diastolic pressure, and arterial hypotension. Within 5 minutes of stopping the transfusion, ionized calcium levels return to normal. The volume of an average unit of whole blood is 500 mL. This patient received 10 units of whole blood or 5000 mL over 30 minutes, then another 5 units in 15 minutes. This averages to a rate greater than 160 mL/min (*Miller: Anesthesia, ed 6, pp 1812-1813, 2466*).

401.   **(C)**   A 20-kg, 5-year-old child has an estimated blood volume of 70 mL/kg = 1400 mL. The acceptable blood loss can be determined using the following formula: Maximum allowable blood loss (in mL) = EBV × $(Hct_s - Hct_l)/Hct_s$
where EBV is the estimated blood volume (in mL), Hct_s is the starting hematocrit, and Hct_l is the lowest acceptable hematocrit. For this patient, the maximal allowable blood loss = 1400 × (40 – 30/40) = 1400 × (10/40) = 350 mL. This assumes the patient is getting volume expansion with crystalloid (3 mL per mL of blood lost). Also see explanation to question 393 (*Miller: Anesthesia, ed 6, pp 2389-2390*).

402.   **(B)**   The normal serum sodium concentration is 135 to 145 mEq/L. Hyponatremia occurs when the serum level is less than 135 mEq/L. Clinical symptoms correspond not only to the level of hyponatremia but also to how rapidly sodium levels are falling. Hyponatremia is most commonly not a deficiency in total body sodium but rather is an excess of total body water (e.g., absorption of irrigating fluids as seen in transurethral resection of the prostate syndrome, syndrome of inappropriate antidiuretic hormone secretion [SIADH]). It can also be caused by an excessive loss of sodium as seen in severe sweating, vomiting, diarrhea, burns, and the use of diuretics. With acute falls in serum sodium, neurologic symptoms (confusion, restlessness, drowsiness, seizures, coma) resulting from cerebral edema can be seen at serum levels below 120 mEq/L. Cardiac symptoms (ventricular tachycardia, ventricular fibrillation) can be seen at levels below 100 mEq/L. Therapy for severe hyponatremia includes water restriction, loop diuretics, and at times, the administration of hypertonic saline (3% NaCl). The dose of sodium needed for correction can be calculated by multiplying the total body water (TBW = Body weight × 0.6) times the increase in sodium desired, i.e.,

Dose of $[Na^+]$ = Bodyweight × 0.6 × (desired $[Na^+]$ level-current $[Na^+]$ level in mEq/L)

In this patient, the calculated dose of sodium would be 100 (weight in kg) × 0.6 × (120 mEq/L – 105 mEq/L) = 900 mEq. Three percent NaCl is infused no faster than 1 to 2 mL/Kg/hr. Too rapid a correction may lead to central pontine myelinolysis. Once the level reaches 120 mEq/L, further treatment is usually water restriction and diuretics (*Miller: Anesthesia, ed 6, pp 1764-1768*).

403.   **(C)**   See explanation to question 387.

404.   **(D)**   Abrupt discontinuation of total parenteral nutrition that contains 10% to 20% dextrose may result in profound rebound hypoglycemia. Tachycardia in this patient may signify hypoglycemia. Prompt diagnosis and treatment of severe hypoglycemia is essential if neurologic damage is to be avoided. Whenever a central line is placed for total parenteral nutrition (TPN) it should be properly checked before starting the hypertonic infusion (*Miller: Anesthesia, ed 6, pp 2910-2917; Stoelting: Pharmacology and Physiology in Anesthetic Practice, ed 4, pp 637-639*).

405. (E)   In an emergency when massive amounts of blood are immediately required and the supply of O-negative RBCs in the blood bank is low, it is acceptable to transfuse O-positive RBCs into male patients or into female patients past the age of childbirth before the patient's blood typing is known. This is because delaying blood transfusion for blood typing may be more hazardous to the patient than the risk of a significant transfusion reaction based on Rh type for these patients. However, for the female patient who has the potential for pregnancy, administration of Rh-positive RBCs is not recommended (unless no Rh-negative RBCs are available). This is because an Rh-negative patient who receives Rh-positive RBCs would develop isoimmunization. For these women, future pregnancies with Rh-positive fetuses could be associated with erythroblastosis fetalis. Note: RBCs are preferred over whole blood because Rh-negative whole blood contains a large quantity of anti-A and anti-B antibodies in the plasma (*Harmening: Modern Blood Banking and Transfusion Practices, ed 5, pp 273, 284; Miller: Anesthesia, ed 6, p 2465*).

406. (B)   Hydroxyethyl starch (Hetastarch) is a synthetic colloid. One liter of a 6% solution (Hespan) reduces factor VIII: C levels by 50% and will prolong the partial thromboplastin time (PTT) (*Miller: Anesthesia, ed 6, p 1787*).

407. (D)   RBCs are cooled to about 4° C to decrease cellular metabolism. CPDA-1 is a preservative anticoagulant solution often added to blood. It contains citrate, phosphate, dextrose, and adenine. The citrate is used to bind calcium and acts as an anticoagulant. Phosphate acts as a buffer. Dextrose is added, as an energy source for cellular metabolism, the day of donation to raise the blood sugar to greater than 400 mg/dL. At 35 days, the glucose level drops below 100 mg/dL. Adenine is added as a substrate source so that the cells can produce adenosine triphosphate (ATP). Other biochemical changes include a fall in pH to about 6.7 and a rise in plasma potassium from around 4 mEq/L on the day of donation to 76 mEq/L at 35 days. Concentrations of 2,3-DPG fall below 1 μM/mL, which causes a leftward shift in the oxyhemoglobin dissociation curve that allows for an increased oxygen affinity for the hemoglobin. This leftward shift produces a P_{50} value less than the normal 26 mm Hg (*Miller: Anesthesia, ed 6, pp 1804-1806*).

408. (B)   There are many preservation solutions used for whole blood and RBCs. Acid citrate dextrose (ACD), CPD, and citrate phosphate double dextrose (CP2D) each allows blood to have a shelf life of 21 days. In 1978, the FDA approved the additive adenine to CPD. This extended the shelf life of blood by 2 weeks. CPDA-1 has a shelf life of 35 days. These solutions were used mainly for whole blood. However, when component therapy became more widespread, it was noted that packing the RBCs by removing the plasma removed a significant amount of adenine and glucose as well. By using an additive solution (which contains primarily adenine, glucose, and saline) to the CPD or CP2D whole blood that has the plasma removed, the "packed" RBCs can now be stored for 42 days. The three different additive solutions currently used in the United States are Adsol (AS-1), Nutricel (AS-3), and Optisol (AS-5) (*Harmening: Modern Blood Banking and Transfusion Practices, ed 5, pp 8-10, Miller: Anesthesia, ed 6, pp 1804-1805*).

409. (D)   See explanation to question 408.

410. (E)   Low molecular weight heparin (LMWH) is produced by the fractionation or cleaving of "unfractionated heparin (UFH)" into shorter fragments. The anticoagulant properties of UFH and LMWH are complex and somewhat different. UFH binds to and activates antithrombin (more effectively than LMWH) and can be monitored easily with the activated partial thromboplastin time or aPTT. At the usual clinical doses of LMWH, aPTT is not prolonged. LMWH, on the other hand, is more effective in inactivating factor Xa and can be monitored by anti-Xa levels (although commonly this is not performed because of the more predictable action of prophylactic dosing of LMWH). At high doses of LMWH, antifactor Xa values are more commonly measured. Thrombin time is a measure of the ability of thrombin to convert fibrinogen to fibrin. It is prolonged with low amount of fibrinogen, heparin and fibrin degradation products (FDP). A reptilase test is done by adding reptilase to plasma and waiting for a clot to form and is prolonged in the presence of lupus anticoagulant, FDP, fibrinogen deficiency or abnormal fibrinogen. It is not prolonged in the presence of heparin (*Barash: Clinical Anesthesia, ed 5, p 229; Fleisher: Anesthesia and Uncommon Diseases, ed 5, pp 570-574; Stoelting: Basics of Anesthesia ed 5, pp 340-341*).

411.   **(D)**   The five selections to this question are the five major hereditary conditions associated with hypercoagulation. They cause an increased likelihood of clot formation by either increasing prothrombotic proteins (e.g., Factor V Leiden mutation, Prothrombin *G20210A* gene mutation), or decreasing endogenous antithrombotic proteins (e.g., antithrombin deficiency, Protein C deficiency, Protein S deficiency). Clot may also develop if heparin resistance occurs (usual doses produces less than the expected prolongation of the partial thromboplastin time or the activated clotting time) and is not recognized, as during cardiopulmonary bypass. It may occur as a result of excessive binding of heparin to plasma proteins or an insufficient amount of antithrombin. Because heparin binds to and potentiates antithrombin's activity, conditions with low amounts of antithrombin show resistance. Treatment of AT3 deficiency is replacement of AT3 with either specific AT III concentrate (Thrombate III) or fresh frozen plasma. Replacement of antithrombin to 100% activity is recommended before cardiac surgery in patients with congenital AT3 deficiency. (*Fleischer: Anesthesia and Uncommon Diseases, ed 5, pp 371-372; Hines: Stoelting's Anesthesia and Co-Existing Disease, ed 5, pp 430-431; Stoelting: Basics of Anesthesia, ed 5, pp 333-335, 340-341*).

412.   **(D)**   von Willebrand's disease (vWD) is the most common inherited abnormality affecting platelet function and is caused by a quantitative or qualitative deficiency of a protein called von Willebrand factor (vWF). Factor vWF is produced by endothelial cells and platelets and appears to have two main functions: it acts as an adhesion protein that diverts platelets to sites of vascular injury, and it helps protect Factor VIII from inactivation and clearance. Patients with vWD have prolonged bleeding times and a reduced amount of factor VIII. Patient's with hemophilia A also have a decrease in Factor VIII, but normal bleeding times. Type 1 vWD is the most common type (60%-80%) and is associated with a quantitative decrease in circulating plasma vWF caused by a decrease in release of available vWF. Type 2 vWD (20%-30%) has several subtypes and is associated with qualitative deficiency of vWF. Type 3 vWD is the least frequent (1%-5%) and the most severe form where there is almost no vWF and very low Factor VIII levels (3%-10% of normal). Treatment of vWD includes desmopressin (DDAVP), which increases the release of available vWF or blood products that contain vWF and Factor VIII (e.g., cryoprecipitate, fresh frozen plasma or Factor VIII concentrates). Recombinant Factor VIII is not used because it does not contain vWF. (*Stoelting: Basics of Anesthesia, ed 5, pp 336-337; Hines: Stoelting's Anesthesia and Co-Existing Disease, ed 5, pp 427-429*).

413.   **(A)**   Although allergic reactions after blood transfusions are common (up to 3%), true non-hemolytic anaphylactic reactions are rare. When anaphylactic reactions develop (often with only a few mL of blood or plasma transfused), the signs and symptoms may include dyspnea, bronchospasm, laryngeal edema, chest pain, hypotension and shock. These reactions are caused by the transfusion of "foreign" IgA protein to patients who have hereditary IgA deficiency and have formed anti-IgA as a result of previous transfusions or from earlier pregnancies. Treatment includes stopping the transfusion, administering epinephrine and steroids. If further transfusion is needed, washed RBC's or red cells from IgA deficient donors should be used (*Barash: Clinical Anesthesia, ed 5, p 212; Miller: Anesthesia, ed 6, p 1817*).

414.   **(E)**   For the years 2005 to 2006, there were 125 confirmed transfusion-related fatalities listed by the FDA in the United States. The most common cause was TRALI (51%), followed by non-ABO hemolytic transfusion reaction (20%), microbial infection (12%), ABO hemolytic transfusion reaction (7%), TACO (7%), and other (2%). Since March 2004, when voluntary bacterial detection testing was implemented for platelet transfusions, there has been a decrease in fatalities associated with transfusion of bacterially contaminated apheresis platelets. Considering there are about 29 million components transfused a year (2004 calendar year) in the United States, the reported incidence of death is quite small. (*www.fda.gov/cber/blood/fatal0506.htm; Barash Clinical Anesthesia, ed 5, p 212; Stoelting: Basics of Anesthesia, ed 5, p 359*).

415.   **(E)**   There is controversy not only as to which intravenous fluid is the best but also how much to give. Most would suggest that isotonic crystalloids should be the initial resuscitative fluids to any trauma patients and are certainly less expensive than 5% albumin, 6% hydroxyethyl starch and dextran 70. Clear advantages of one fluid over another are hard to find (*Miller: Anesthesia, ed 6, pp 1783-1788, 2460-2469*).

416.   **(B)**   Transmission of CMV to patients who have normal immune mechanisms is benign and self-limiting, but in patients who are immunocompromised (e.g., premature newborns, solid organ and bone marrow transplant patients, AIDS patients) CMV infection can be serious and life threatening. Leukocyte reduction can reduce CMV transmission but restriction of blood products from seronegative donors is preferred (*Barash: Clinical Anesthesia, ed 5, p 210*).

417. **(C)** Graft-versus-host disease (GVHD) is an often fatal condition that occurs in patients who are immunocompromised. It occurs when donor lymphocytes (graft) establish an immune response against the recipient (host). Blood products that have a significant amount of lymphocytes include RBCs and platelets. Fresh frozen plasma and cryoprecipitate appear to be safe. Although directed donor units from first degree relatives and leukoreduction may reduce the incidence of GVHD, only irradiated products (which inactivates donor lymphocytes) can prevent GVHD (*Barash: Clinical Anesthesia, ed 5, p 212*).

Chapter 6

General Anesthesia

DIRECTIONS (Questions 418 through 546): Each of the questions or incomplete statements in this section is followed by answers or by completions of the statement, respectively. Select the ONE BEST answer or completion for each item.

418. A 78-year-old patient with a history of hypertension and adult-onset diabetes for which she takes chlorpropamide (Diabinese) is admitted for elective cholecystectomy. On the day of admission, blood glucose is noted to be 270 mg/dL, and the patient is treated with 15 units of regular insulin subcutaneously (SQ) in addition to her regular dose of chlorpropamide. Twenty-four hours later after overnight fasting, the patient is brought to the operating room (OR) without her daily dose of chlorpropamide and is anesthetized. A serum glucose is measured and found to be 35 mg/dL. The most likely explanation for this is
  A. Insulin
  B. Chlorpropamide
  C. Hypovolemia
  D. Effect of general anesthesia
  E. It is a normal finding in fasting patients

419. Select the true statement.
  A. Dibucaine is an ester-type local anesthetic
  B. A dibucaine number of 20 is normal
  C. The dibucaine number represents the quantity of normal pseudocholinesterase
  D. Neuromuscular blockade with succinylcholine would last several hours in a patient with a dibucaine number of 80
  E. None of the above

420. A 56-year-old patient with a history of liver disease and osteomyelitis is anesthetized for tibial débridement. After induction and intubation, the wound is inspected and débrided with a total blood loss of 300 mL. The patient is transported intubated to the recovery room, at which time the systolic blood pressure falls to 50 mm Hg. Heart rate is 120 beats/min, arterial blood gases (ABGs) are Pao_2 103, $Paco_2$ 45, pH 7.3, with 97% O_2 saturation with 100% Fio_2. Mixed venous blood gases are Pvo_2 60, $Paco_2$ 50, pH 7.25, with 90% O_2 saturation. Which of the following diagnoses is most consistent with this clinical picture?
  A. Myocardial infarction
  B. Congestive heart failure
  C. Cardiac tamponade
  D. Sepsis with acute respiratory distress syndrome
  E. Hypovolemia

421. Normal tracheal capillary pressure is
  A. 5 to 15 mm Hg
  B. 15 to 25 mm Hg
  C. 25 to 35 mm Hg
  D. 35 to 45 mm Hg
  E. 45 to 55 mm Hg

422.   How many hours should elapse before performing a single-shot spinal anesthetic in a patient who is receiving 1 mg/kg enoxaparin twice a day for the treatment of a deep vein thrombosis?
   A. 2 hours
   B. 6 hours
   C. 12 hours
   D. 18 hours
   E. 24 hours

423.   Which of the following peripheral nerves is most likely to become injured in patients who are under general anesthesia?
   A. Ulnar nerve
   B. Median nerve
   C. Radial nerve
   D. Common peroneal nerve
   E. Sciatic and peroneal nerve

424.   Renal failure associated with fluoride toxicity anesthesia most closely resembles
   A. Papillary necrosis
   B. Acute tubule necrosis
   C. Hepatorenal syndrome
   D. Central diabetes insipidus
   E. Nephrogenic diabetes insipidus

425.   A 45-year-old obese male is in the intensive care unit (ICU) after an elective open lung biopsy. Which of the following would provide the best prophylaxis against deep vein thrombosis in this patient?
   A. Pneumatic compression boots
   B. Heparin 5000 units SQ every 8 hours
   C. Early ambulation
   D. Dextran 10 mL/kg IV during surgery
   E. Incentive spirometry

426.   A patient with which of the following eye diseases would be at greatest risk for retinal damage from hypotension during surgery?
   A. Strabismus
   B. Cataract
   C. Glaucoma
   D. Severe myopia
   E. Open eye injury

427.   Naltrexone is
   A. A narcotic with local anesthetic properties
   B. An opioid agonist-antagonist similar to nalbuphine
   C. A pure opioid antagonist with a shorter duration of action than naloxone
   D. An opioid antagonist used for treatment of previously detoxified heroin addicts
   E. A synthetic opioid derived from oxymorphone

428.   Which of the following mechanisms is most frequently responsible for hypoxia in the recovery room?
   A. Ventilation/perfusion mismatch
   B. Hypoventilation
   C. Hypoxic gas mixture
   D. Intracardiac shunt
   E. Abnormal gas diffusion

429. Hypoparathyroidism secondary to the inadvertent surgical resection of the parathyroid glands during total thyroidectomy typically results in symptoms of hypocalcemia how many hours postoperatively?
   A. 1 to 2 hours
   B. 3 to 12 hours
   C. 12 to 24 hours
   D. 24 to 72 hours
   E. Greater than 72 hours

430. Damage to which nerve may lead to wrist drop?
   A. Radial
   B. Axillary
   C. Median
   D. Musculocutaneous
   E. Ulnar

431. The most common cause of bronchiectasis is
   A. Cigarette smoking
   B. Air pollution
   C. α_1-Antitrypsin deficiency
   D. Recurrent bronchial infections
   E. Squamous cell carcinoma

432. A 6-year-old child is transported to the recovery room after a tonsillectomy. The patient was anesthetized with isoflurane, fentanyl, and N_2O. Twenty minutes before emergence and tracheal extubation, droperidol was administered. The anesthesiologist is called to the recovery room because the patient is "making strange eye movements." The patient's eyes are rolled back into his head, and his neck is twisted and rigid. The most appropriate drug for treatment of these symptoms is
   A. Dantrolene
   B. Thiopental
   C. Glycopyrrolate
   D. Chlorpromazine
   E. Diphenhydramine

433. A 32-year-old military officer is unable to oppose the left thumb and left little finger after an 8-hour exploratory laparotomy under general anesthesia. He had an IV induction through a peripheral IV and had a second IV placed in the antecubital fossa after he was asleep. Damage to which of the following nerves would most likely account for this deficit?
   A. Radial
   B. Ulnar
   C. Median
   D. Musculocutaneous
   E. Median antebrachial cutaneous nerve

434. Pheochromocytoma would be most likely to coexist with which of the following?
   A. Insulinoma
   B. Pituitary adenoma
   C. Primary hyperaldosteronism (Conn's syndrome)
   D. Medullary carcinoma of the thyroid
   E. Carcinoid tumor

435. The plasma concentration of which of the following liver enzymes is increased in patients with biliary obstruction?
   A. Serum glutamic-oxaloacetic transaminase
   B. Serum glutamic-pyruvic transaminase
   C. Lactate dehydrogenase
   D. Alkaline phosphatase
   E. Alcoholic dehydrogenase

436. The onset of delirium tremens after abstinence from alcohol usually occurs in
  A. 8 to 24 hours
  B. 24 to 48 hours
  C. 2 to 4 days
  D. 4 to 7 days
  E. Greater than 7 days

437. A 78-year-old retired coal miner with an intraluminal tracheal tumor is scheduled for tracheal resection. Which of the following is a relative contraindication for tracheal resection?
  A. Need for postoperative mechanical ventilation for underlying lung disease
  B. Tumor located at the carina
  C. Documented liver metastases
  D. Ischemic heart disease with a history of congestive heart failure
  E. Tracheal diameter of 0.5 cm at the level of the tumor

438. A 78-year-old patient with multiple myeloma is admitted to the ICU for treatment of hypercalcemia. The primary risk associated with anesthetizing patients with hypercalcemia (levels of 14 to 16 mg/dL) is
  A. Coagulopathy
  B. Cardiac dysrhythmias
  C. Hypotension
  D. Laryngospasm
  E. Fluid imbalance

439. Just before induction of general anesthesia for an 85-year-old demented male with an ischemic bowel, he mentions to you that he forgot to take his green capped eye drops. He states that not taking it daily will result in blindness. The green capped eye drops are
  A. NaCl drops used to prevent his eye from drying out
  B. Antibiotic drops
  C. Steroids
  D. Used to produce miosis
  E. Any of a number of eye medication and surgery should be delayed until the eye drops are identified

440. A normal healthy 3-year-old child was involved in a motor vehicle accident. He is coming emergently to the OR. Drug doses need to be calculated, but his weight is not known. What value should be used to estimate the 3-year-old child's weight?
  A. 8 kg
  B. 10 kg
  C. 12 kg
  D. 14 kg
  E. 16 kg

441. A 62-year-old male undergoes an emergency craniotomy for subdural hematoma. Two years earlier, a VVI pacemaker was placed for third-degree heart block. The patient received vancomycin 1 g IV, before arriving in the OR. General anesthesia is induced with thiopental 300 mg IV and the lungs are hyperventilated to a $Paco_2$ of 25 mm Hg by mask. Just before tracheal intubation, the patient's heart rate decreases from 70 to 40 beats/min and the pacemaker spikes that were previously present in lead II of the electrocardiogram disappear. The most likely cause of bradycardia in this patient is
  A. Hypocarbia
  B. Vancomycin allergy
  C. Acute increase in intracranial pressure
  D. A side effect of thiopental
  E. Pacemaker battery failure

442. A 28-year-old obese patient has diminished breath sounds bilaterally at the lung bases 18 hours after an emergency appendectomy under general anesthesia. Which of the following maneuvers would be **LEAST** effective in preventing postoperative pulmonary complications in this patient?
    A. Coughing
    B. Voluntary deep breathing
    C. Performing a forced vital capacity
    D. Use of incentive spirometry
    E. Sitting up in bed

443. Below what value of cerebral blood flow (CBF) will signs of cerebral ischemia first begin to appear on the electroencephalogram (EEG)?
    A. 6 mL/100 g/min
    B. 15 mL/100 g/min
    C. 22 mL/100 g/min
    D. 31 mL/100 g/min
    E. 40 mL/100 g/min

444. A 67-year-old patient is mechanically ventilated in the ICU 2 days after repair of a ruptured abdominal aortic aneurysm. To maintain Pao_2 in the 60 to 65 range, 10 cm H_2O positive end-expiratory pressure (PEEP) is added to the ventilator cycle. The patient's blood pressure has averaged 110/65 before addition of PEEP. After addition of PEEP, the blood pressure is noted to slowly fall to an average of approximately 95/50. The best explanation for this decrease in blood pressure is
    A. Tension pneumothorax
    B. Decreased venous return to the heart
    C. Increased afterload on the right side of the heart
    D. Increased afterload on the left side of the heart
    E. Decreased cardiac output from global myocardial ischemia

445. A 64-year-old male undergoes an elective cholecystectomy. Other than essential hypertension, for which he takes propranolol, he is in good health. The patient is anesthetized with isoflurane, N_2O, and fentanyl, and paralyzed with d-tubocurarine. At the end of the operation, neuromuscular blockade is antagonized with pyridostigmine and atropine, the trachea is suctioned, and the patient is extubated and taken to the recovery room. Oxymorphone is administered IV for analgesia. One hour after arrival in the recovery room, the patient's heart rate decreases from 70 to 40 beats/min. Which of the following would most likely account for bradycardia in this patient?
    A. Recurarization
    B. Oxymorphone
    C. Pyridostigmine
    D. Propranolol
    E. Paradoxical effect of atropine

446. Which of the following is most closely associated with minimum alveolar concentration (MAC)?
    A. Blood/gas partition coefficient
    B. Oil/gas partition coefficient
    C. Vapor pressure
    D. Brain/blood partition coefficient
    E. Molecular weight

447. A 15-year-old, 65-kg patient with Cushing's disease is to undergo a transsphenoidal hypophysectomy to remove a pituitary adenoma. General anesthesia is induced with thiopental IV and tracheal intubation is facilitated with vecuronium 0.25 mg/kg IV. Anesthesia is maintained with isoflurane, N_2O and O_2. Mannitol 1 g/kg is administered IV to reduce intracranial pressure. At the end of the operation, the patient is extubated and taken to the ICU. Over the next 6 hours the patient has a total urine output of 8.3 L. Serum sodium concentration is 154 mEq/L, serum potassium concentration is 4.8 mEq/L, and serum glucose concentration is 160 mg/dL. Urine specific gravity is 1.002 and urine osmolality is 125 mOsm/L. The most likely cause of the large urine output is
    A. Osmotic diuresis from mannitol
    B. Excess mineralocorticoid activity
    C. Hyperglycemia
    D. Nephrogenic diabetes insipidus
    E. Central diabetes insipidus

448. Scopolamine should not be given as a premedication in patients with which of the following neurologic diseases?
A. Parkinson's disease
B. Alzheimer's disease
C. Multiple sclerosis
D. Narcolepsy
E. Amyotrophic lateral sclerosis

449. A 63-year-old male patient is scheduled to undergo a right hemicolectomy under general anesthesia. Anesthesia is induced with thiopental 4 mg/kg IV and fentanyl 100 μg IV. Succinylcholine 1.5 mg/kg IV is administered to facilitate tracheal intubation. Anesthesia is maintained with isoflurane and N_2O. After all four twitches of the train-of-four stimulus return to baseline values, pancuronium 5 mg IV is administered. Gentamicin 80 mg and cefazolin 1 g are administered IV as a prophylactic treatment. At the end of surgery, two of four thumb twitches can be elicited to train-of-four stimulation of the ulnar nerve and neuromuscular blockade is antagonized with neostigmine 0.05 mg/kg IV and atropine 0.015 mg/kg IV. The patient, however, begins to move before the incision is completely closed, and succinylcholine 40 mg IV is given. Fifteen minutes later, all anesthetics are discontinued and the patient is ventilated with 100% O_2, but the patient remains apneic. The most likely cause of apnea is
A. Fentanyl
B. Recurarization
C. Succinylcholine
D. Thiopental
E. Gentamicin

450. A 53-year-old female with endometrial cancer is undergoing an abdominal hysterectomy under general anesthesia with enflurane. During the first hour of anesthesia, urine output is 100 mL. Blood loss is minimal. When the patient is placed in the Trendelenburg position, the urine output declines to virtually zero. The most likely explanation for this sudden decrease in urine output in this patient is
A. Pooling of urine in the dome of the bladder
B. Kinking of the urinary catheter
C. Fluoride toxicity from enflurane
D. Increased antidiuretic hormone (ADH) production from surgical stimulation
E. Hypovolemia

451. Which of the following diseases is not associated with a decrease in DLCO?
A. Emphysema
B. Lung resection
C. Pulmonary emboli
D. Anemia
E. Obesity

452. Each of the following postoperative complications of thyroid surgery can result in upper airway obstruction **EXCEPT**
A. Tracheomalacia
B. Tetany
C. Cervical hematoma
D. Bilateral recurrent laryngeal nerve injury
E. Bilateral superior laryngeal nerve injury

453. The most sensitive early sign of MH during general anesthesia is
A. Tachycardia
B. Hypertension
C. Fever
D. Hypoxia
E. Increased end-expiratory CO_2 tension (P_{ECO_2})

454. A 78-year-old female is anesthetized for a right hemicolectomy for 3 hours. At the end of the operation the patient's blood pressure is 130/85 mm Hg, heart rate is 84 beats/min, core body temperature is 35.4° C, and P_{ECO_2} on mass spectrometer is 38 mm Hg. Which of the following would be the **LEAST** plausible reason for prolonged apnea in this patient?
    A. Residual neuromuscular blockade
    B. Narcotic overdose
    C. Cerebral hemorrhage
    D. Unrecognized obstructive pulmonary disease and high baseline Pa_{CO_2}
    E. Persistent intraoperative hyperventilation

455. A 68-year-old woman with severe rheumatoid arthritis undergoes pulmonary function evaluation before an elective abdominal surgery. Forced expiratory volume in one second (FEV_1) and forced vital capacity (FVC) are within normal limits; however, the maximum voluntary ventilation (MVV) is only 40% of predicted. The next step in the pulmonary function evaluation of this patient should be to
    A. Obtain ABGs on room air
    B. Obtain a flow-volume loop
    C. Obtain a measurement of peak flow
    D. Obtain a ventilation/perfusion scan
    E. Assume, in the face of normal FEV_1, poor effort on the part of the patient and proceed

456. Which of the following is **NOT** a component of the post-anesthetic discharge scoring system (PADSS) used to evaluate the suitability of a patient to be discharged from an ambulatory surgical facility?
    A. Drinking
    B. Ambulation
    C. Nausea and vomiting
    D. Pain
    E. Surgical bleeding

457. During emergency repair of a mandibular jaw fracture in an otherwise healthy 19-year-old male, the patient's temperature is noted to rise from 37° C on induction to 38° C after 2 hours of surgery. Which of the following informational items would be **LEAST** useful in ruling out MH in this patient?
    A. Normal heart rate and blood pressure
    B. History of negative caffeine-halothane contracture test carried out 6 months earlier
    C. History of a uncomplicated general anesthetic at age 16 years with halothane and succinylcholine
    D. Normal ABGs drawn when the patient's temperature reached 38° C
    E. No increase in respiration rate with spontaneous breathing

458. Which of the following drugs is useful in the treatment of asthma by specifically interfering with the leukotriene pathway?
    A. Fluticasone (Flovent)
    B. Ipratropium bromide (Atrovent)
    C. Triamcinolone (Azmacort)
    D. Montelukast (Singulair)
    E. Salmeterol (Serevent)

459. A 68-year-old, 100-kg patient is undergoing a transurethral resection of the prostate gland under general anesthesia. Upon arrival in the recovery room, the patient appears restless and confused. Serum sodium is checked and found to be 110 mEq/L. How many mEq of sodium are needed to raise the serum $[Na^+]$ to 120 mEq/L?
    A. 300 mEq
    B. 400 mEq
    C. 500 mEq
    D. 600 mEq
    E. 700 mEq

460. Trismus after administration of succinylcholine IV signals the onset of MH in what percentage of patients?

A. Less than 50%

B. 50%

C. 75%

D. 80%

E. Greater than 80%

461. A 45-year-old male is brought to the OR emergently for repair of a ruptured abdominal aortic aneurysm. The patient is pretreated with d-tubocurarine 3 mg, anesthesia is induced with ketamine 2 mg/kg IV, and tracheal intubation is facilitated with succinylcholine 1.5 mg/kg IV. Immediately after tracheal intubation, the patient's blood pressure falls from 110/80 to 50/20 mm Hg. What is the most likely cause of the sudden severe hypotension in this patient?

A. Hypovolemia

B. Direct myocardial depression from ketamine

C. Vasovagal response to direct laryngoscopy

D. Arteriolar vasodilation from succinylcholine-mediated histamine release

E. Ganglionic blockade from d-tubocurarine

462. Malignant hyperthermia is believed to involve a generalized disorder of membrane permeability to

A. Sodium

B. Potassium

C. Calcium

D. Magnesium

E. Phosphate

463. A 25-year-old male with a history of testicular cancer is scheduled to undergo an exploratory laparotomy under general anesthesia. He has received bleomycin for metastatic disease. Which of the following is an important consideration concerning the pulmonary toxicity of bleomycin?

A. N_2O should not be used

B. Preoperative pulmonary function tests should be obtained

C. The patient should be ventilated at a slow rate and inspiratory-to-expiratory (I:E) ratio of 1:3

D. Aminophylline should be started preoperatively

E. F_{IO_2} should be less than 0.3

464. A 39-year-old obese female undergoes an abdominal hysterectomy under general anesthesia. Induction of anesthesia is uneventful. Sa_{O_2} is 98% during the first 15 minutes of the operation. However, when her head is flexed and she is placed in the Trendelenburg position to improve surgical exposure, Sa_{O_2} falls to 90%. The most likely explanation for this desaturation is

A. Diffusion hypoxia

B. Decreased functional residual capacity (FRC)

C. Mainstem intubation

D. Decreased cardiac output

E. Venous air embolism

465. How long after intravitreal injection of sulfur hexafluoride and air can N_2O be used without risk of increasing intra-ocular pressure?

A. 1 hour

B. 24 hours

C. 10 days

D. 1 month

E. Never

466. A 54-year-old female is undergoing a total thyroidectomy under general anesthesia. The patient is awakened in the OR, the mouth and pharynx are suctioned, and after intact laryngeal reflexes are demonstrated, the endotracheal tube is removed. Two days later, the anesthesiologist is consulted because the patient has severe stridor and upper airway obstruction. The most likely cause of airway obstruction in this patient is
      A. Damage to the recurrent laryngeal nerve
      B. Damage to the superior laryngeal nerve
      C. Tracheomalacia
      D. Hypocalcemia
      E. Hematoma

467. A 27-year-old obese woman is scheduled to undergo foot surgery under general anesthesia. She underwent a subtotal thyroidectomy 3 years ago and takes levothyroxine (Synthroid). Which of the following laboratory tests would be the most useful in evaluating whether this patient is euthyroid?
      A. Total plasma thyroxine (T_4)
      B. Total plasma triiodothyronine (T_3)
      C. Thyroid-stimulating hormone (TSH)
      D. Resin triiodothyronine uptake
      E. Radioactive iodine uptake

468. An 85-year-old male with no previous medical history except for cataracts is undergoing a transurethral resection of the prostate gland under spinal anesthesia. Twenty minutes into the procedure the patient becomes restless. Over the next 20 minutes his blood pressure increases from 110/70 to 140/90 mm Hg and his heart rate slows from 90 to 50 beats/min. The patient is noted to have some difficulty breathing. The most likely cause of these symptoms in this patient is
      A. Volume overload
      B. Hyponatremia
      C. High spinal
      D. Bladder perforation
      E. Autonomic hyperreflexia

469. A 17-year-old patient with third-degree burns over 30% of his body is scheduled for débridement and skin grafting 12 days after sustaining a thermal injury. Select the true statement regarding the use of depolarizing and nondepolarizing muscle relaxants in this patient, compared with normal patients.
      A. Sensitivity to both depolarizing and nondepolarizing muscle relaxants is increased
      B. Sensitivity to both depolarizing and nondepolarizing muscle relaxants is decreased
      C. Sensitivity to depolarizing muscle relaxants is increased while sensitivity to nondepolarizing muscle relaxants is decreased
      D. Sensitivity to depolarizing muscle relaxants is decreased while sensitivity to nondepolarizing muscle relaxants is increased
      E. Sensitivity to nondepolarizing is unchanged while sensitivity to depolarizing muscle relaxants is increased

470. A nervous 57-year-old woman with morbid fear of intramuscular injections is scheduled for breast biopsy and is given a premedication in the waiting area before surgery. The anesthesiologist is summoned 45 minutes later because the patient is complaining of dry mouth and has a heart rate of 45 beats/min. Which of the following premedications is most likely responsible for these side effects?
      A. Scopolamine
      B. Meperidine
      C. Midazolam
      D. Clonidine
      E. Droperidol

471. A 65-year-old patient with a history of chronic obstructive pulmonary disease and coronary artery disease (CAD) undergoes an appendectomy uneventfully under general anesthesia. In the recovery room, ABGs are as follows: Pao_2 60 mm Hg, $Paco_2$ 50 mm Hg, pH 7.35, and hemoglobin 8.1 g/dL. Which of the following steps would produce the greatest increase in O_2 delivery to the myocardium?
- **A.** Administration of 100% O_2 with a close-fitting mask
- **B.** Administration of 35% O_2 with a Venturi mask
- **C.** Withhold narcotics
- **D.** Transfuse with 2 units of packed red blood cells (RBCs)
- **E.** Administer 1 ampule of HCO_3

472. Allergic reactions occurring during the immediate perioperative period are most commonly attributable to administration of
- **A.** Muscle relaxants
- **B.** Local anesthetics
- **C.** Antibiotics
- **D.** Opioids
- **E.** β-Blockers

473. Caution is advised when using succinylcholine in patients with Huntington's chorea because
- **A.** They are at increased risk for MH
- **B.** Potassium release may be excessive
- **C.** They may have a decreased concentration of pseudocholinesterase
- **D.** There may be adverse interactions between succinylcholine and phenothiazine
- **E.** Succinylcholine increases intracranial pressure

474. Which of the following would not result in an increase in intraocular pressure?
- **A.** Increase in $Paco_2$ from 35 to 40 mm Hg
- **B.** Arterial hypoxemia
- **C.** 100 mg IM succinylcholine
- **D.** Acute rise in venous pressure from coughing
- **E.** 100 mg IV succinylcholine in patient in whom eye muscles have been detached from the globe

475. An apnea hypopnea index of 30 means?
- **A.** Episodes of hypopnea are 30 times more common than apnea
- **B.** Episodes of apnea are 30 times more common than hypopnea
- **C.** Episodes of apnea and hypopnea occur at a rate of 30 per hour
- **D.** Apnea/hypopnea episodes last 30 seconds
- **E.** Apnea/hypopnea episodes occur at rate of 30 per sleep cycle

476. Which of the following preoperative pulmonary function tests is **NOT** associated with an increased operative risk for pneumonectomy?
- **A.** FEV_1 less than 50% of the FVC
- **B.** FEV_1 less than 2 L
- **C.** Maximum breathing capacity less than 50% of predicted
- **D.** Residual volume/total lung capacity less than 50%
- **E.** Hypercarbia on room air ABGs

477. A 26-year-old male patient is undergoing an emergency exploratory laparotomy under general anesthesia with isoflurane. Sao_2 is 89% on the pulse oximeter. Pao_2 on ABGs is 77 mm Hg. The patient's core body temperature is 35° C. What is the corrected Pao_2?
- **A.** 68 mm Hg
- **B.** 72 mm Hg
- **C.** 77 mm Hg
- **D.** 86 mm Hg
- **E.** 92 mm Hg

478. A 27-year-old patient with a 10-year history of Crohn's disease is scheduled to undergo drainage of a rectal abscess under general anesthesia. His preoperative medications include prednisone, sulfasalazine, and cyanocobalamin. He has no known allergies and is otherwise healthy. Before induction of anesthesia the patient is noted to have central cyanosis and the pulse oximeter shows a SaO_2 of 89%, which does not increase after the administration of 100% O_2 for 2 minutes. ABGs are as follows: PaO_2 490 mm Hg, $PaCO_2$ 32 Hg, pH 7.43, SaO_2 89%. The most likely cause of these findings is
    A. Presence of sulfhemoglobin
    B. Presence of methemoglobin
    C. Presence of cyanhemoglobin
    D. Presence of carboxyhemoglobin
    E. Blood gas error

479. The muscle relaxant of choice (i.e., minimal cardiovascular changes) during resection of a pheochromocytoma is
    A. Mivacurium
    B. Pancuronium
    C. Curare
    D. Atracurium
    E. Vecuronium

480. In a given patient, if a creatinine of 1.0 corresponds to a glomerular filtration rate (GFR) of 120 mL/min, a creatinine of 4.0 would correspond to
    A. 20 mL/min
    B. 30 mL/min
    C. 40 mL/min
    D. 50 mL/min
    E. 60 mL/min

481. The incidence of each of the following is increased in patients with Down syndrome (trisomy 21) **EXCEPT**
    A. Malignant hyperthermia
    B. Hypothyroidism
    C. Smaller trachea
    D. Occipito-atlantoaxial instability
    E. Congenital heart disease

482. A 55-year-old male is to undergo a transurethral resection of the prostate gland under general anesthesia. The patient has a 40-pack-per-year smoking history and a history of congestive heart failure. The patient receives metoclopramide and scopolamine preoperatively. General anesthesia is induced with ketamine and the patient undergoes the procedure uneventfully. However, in the recovery room the patient complains of not being able to see objects "up close." Which of the following would be the most likely cause of this complaint?
    A. Emergence delirium from ketamine anesthesia
    B. Effect of scopolamine
    C. Effect of glycine in the irrigating solution
    D. Corneal abrasion
    E. Hyponatremia

483. Malignant hyperthermia and neuroleptic malignant syndrome share each of the following characteristics **EXCEPT**
    A. Generalized muscular rigidity
    B. Hyperthermia
    C. Effectively treated with dantrolene
    D. Tachycardia
    E. Flaccid paralysis after administration of vecuronium

484. A 23-year-old male involved in a motor vehicle accident is brought to the OR for open reduction and internal fixation of bilateral leg fractures under general anesthesia. During the surgery the patient is transfused with 7 units of type AB, Rh-negative packed RBCs and 3 units of platelets. At the end of the procedure the endotracheal tube is removed and the patient is taken to the ICU. Postoperatively the patient complains of shortness of breath and arterial hypoxemia is noted. His temperature is 38° C, heart rate is 146 beats/min, blood pressure is 105/69 mm Hg, and respiratory rate is 36 breaths/min. In addition, the patient is noted to have a fine petechial rash on his neck, chest and shoulders. Which of the following is the most likely cause of these signs and symptoms?

   A. Pulmonary embolism
   B. Transfusion reaction from packed RBCs
   C. Transfusion reaction from platelets
   D. Fat embolism
   E. Sepsis

485. Remifentanil is metabolized primarily by

   A. Kidneys
   B. Liver
   C. Hoffman elimination
   D. Pseudocholinesterase
   E. Nonspecific esterases

486. A 3-year-old child is brought to the OR after aspiration of a peanut. After an inhalation induction the trachea is intubated. The peanut is extracted through a rigid bronchoscope but then is lost in the upper airway. The anesthesiologist notes that he can no longer ventilate the patient's lungs. What should be the next step in the management of this problem?

   A. Needle cricothyroidotomy
   B. Emergency tracheotomy
   C. Placement of a chest tube
   D. Push the peanut more distally
   E. Attempt jet ventilation

487. Patients who undergo extracorporeal shock-wave lithotripsy are at increased risk for

   A. Venous air embolism
   B. Pneumothorax
   C. Peripheral neuropathies
   D. Postdural puncture headache with spinal anesthesia
   E. Hypotension with regional anesthesia at the end of the procedure

488. The most common reason for admitting outpatients to the hospital following general anesthesia is

   A. Angina
   B. Inability to void
   C. Inability to ambulate
   D. Surgical pain
   E. Nausea and vomiting

489. A 37-year-old male with myasthenia gravis arrives in the emergency room confused and agitated after a 2-day history of weakness and increased difficulty breathing. ABGs on room air are Pao_2 60 mm Hg, $Paco_2$ 51 mm Hg, HCO_3^- 25 mEq/L, pH 7.3, Sao_2 of 90%. His respiratory rate is 30 breaths/min and tidal volume (V_T) is 4 mL/kg. After administration of edrophonium 2 mg IV, his V_T declines to 2 mL/kg. What should be the most appropriate step in the management of this patient at this time?

   A. Tracheal intubation and mechanical ventilation
   B. Repeat the test dose of edrophonium
   C. Administer neostigmine 1 mg IV
   D. Administer atropine 0.4 mg IV
   E. Emergency tracheostomy and mechanical ventilation

490. Select the **FALSE** statement regarding tramadol (Ultram).
  A. Ondansetron may interfere with part of tramadol's analgesia
  B. Tramadol is associated with seizures in patients taking selective serotonin reuptake inhibitors (SSRIs)
  C. It exhibits monoamine oxidase (MAO) inhibiting effects
  D. Its analgesic effects are partially antagonized by naloxone
  E. It is relatively safe in patients whose pain makes them suicidal

491. Which of the following patients would not be a good candidate for outpatient inguinal hernia repair under general anesthesia?
  A. A 62-year-old pharmacist who lives 10 miles away
  B. A 20-year-old healthy college student who had a renal transplant 3 years earlier
  C. A 38-year-old housewife with a hiatal hernia
  D. A premature infant who is 43 weeks postconceptual age
  E. A 29-year-old diabetic who is well controlled on insulin

492. A 72-year-old male undergoes emergency repair of an abdominal aortic aneurysm. In the first hour after release of the suprarenal cross-clamp, urine output is only 10 mL. After administration of furosemide 20 mg IV, urine output increases to 100 mL/hr. Urine $[Na^+]$ is 43 mEq/L and urine osmolality is 210 mOsm/L. The most likely cause of the initial oliguria is
  A. Fluoride toxicity
  B. Renal hypoperfusion
  C. Acute tubular necrosis
  D. Increased ADH
  E. Impossible to differentiate

493. A healthy 25-year-old man is anesthetized for a sagittal split osteotomy. Anesthesia is induced with propofol, morphine, and vecuronium and maintained with 1.5% isoflurane and 50% N_2O. After induction, the nose is prepped with 4% lidocaine and 1% phenylephrine, and the patient is intubated through the right naris. Before emergence, the surgeon performs a bilateral inferior alveolar nerve block. The patient is reversed with neostigmine and glycopyrrolate. When the patient awakens he is noted to have an 8-mm pupil on the right and a 3-mm pupil on the left. Results of physical examination are otherwise unremarkable. The most likely explanation for the dilated pupil is
  A. Right stellate ganglion block
  B. Accidental introduction of lidocaine into right eye
  C. Accidental introduction of phenylephrine into right eye
  D. Right ciliary ganglion block
  E. Glycopyrrolate

494. A 40-year-old male is undergoing a left inguinal hernia repair under general anesthesia in San Diego, Calif. N_2O is administered at 3 L/min, O_2 at 1 L/min, and isoflurane at 0.85%. What minimum alveolar concentration (MAC) is this patient receiving?
  A. 0.8
  B. 1.25
  C. 1.50
  D. 1.75
  E. 2.0

495. An otherwise healthy 140-kg, 24-year-old male is scheduled for thyroid surgery under general anesthesia. Which of the following statements concerning his cardiac output at 140 kg compared with his cardiac output at his ideal body weight (70 kg) is correct?
  A. Cardiac output is diminished by factor of 2
  B. Cardiac output is diminished by 10%
  C. Cardiac output is the same
  D. Cardiac output is increased by 10%
  E. Cardiac output is doubled

496. Fenoldopam may be used as an alternative to which of the following?
   A. Epinephrine
   B. Phenylephrine
   C. Dopexamine
   D. Dopamine
   E. Sodium nitroprusside

497. A 58-year-old hemophiliac is scheduled for total knee arthroplasty. His factor VIII levels are 35% of normal. Which of the following would be the most appropriate therapy before surgery?
   A. Administer sufficient cryoprecipitate to raise factor VIII levels to 50% normal
   B. Administer sufficient factor VIII concentrate and platelets to raise levels to 50% normal
   C. Transfuse fresh frozen plasma until factor VIII levels are 100% normal
   D. Administer factor VIII concentrates until levels are 100% normal
   E. None of the above

498. A 16-year-old boy whose maternal uncle has hemophilia A is scheduled for wisdom tooth extraction. Which test below would be the best screening test for hemophilia A?
   A. Partial thromboplastin time (PTT)
   B. Prothrombin time (PT)
   C. Thrombin time
   D. Platelet count
   E. Bleeding time

499. The reason four twitches are used in the train-of-four to determine degree of neuromuscular blockade versus five (or more) is
   A. Comparison of greater than four twitches is too difficult
   B. Four twitches informs the user of the degree of blockade in the useful clinical range (i.e., 75% to 100% blockade)
   C. Post-tetanic facilitation will begin to appear after four twitches
   D. Additional twitches may damage the nerve by overstimulation
   E. There would be no additional decrement in twitch height after four twitches

500. A 57-year-old male is undergoing a right hemicolectomy under general anesthesia. The patient has no history of cardiac disease. During the operation 5-mm ST-segment elevation is noted on lead II and the patient develops complete heart block. The coronary artery most likely affected is
   A. Circumflex coronary artery
   B. Right coronary artery
   C. Left main coronary artery
   D. Left anterior descending coronary artery
   E. Branch to obtuse margin

501. Each of the following may increase MAC for volatile anesthetics **EXCEPT**
   A. Cocaine
   B. Hyperthyroidism
   C. Monoamine oxidase (MAO) inhibitor therapy
   D. Tricyclic antidepressants
   E. Hypernatremia

502. A 37-year-old patient with history of manic-depressive illness is scheduled to undergo surgery for removal of an intramedullary rod in the left tibia. Which of the following statements regarding potential untoward effects of lithium therapy is **NOT** true?
   A. Long-term administration may be associated with nephrogenic diabetes insipidus
   B. Administration of succinylcholine to patients treated with lithium may result in hyperkalemia
   C. Long-term therapy may be associated with hypothyroidism
   D. Duration of action of pancuronium may be prolonged
   E. Administration of thiazide diuretics may increase plasma lithium concentrations

503. Treatment of hypotension in a patient anesthetized for resection of metastatic carcinoid would be best accomplished with
    A. Epinephrine
    B. Ephedrine
    C. Vasopressin (DDAVP)
    D. Angiotensin
    E. Octreotide

504. A 75-year-old male patient is scheduled to undergo elective orchiectomy for prostate cancer. The patient has selected spinal anesthesia. What is the minimum dermatomal level that must be achieved to carry out this operation?
    A. T1
    B. T4
    C. T10
    D. L3
    E. S1

505. A 31-year-old patient has been in the ICU on a ventilator for 24 hours after a motor vehicle accident. The patient does not open his eyes to any stimulus and has no verbal or motor response. The Glasgow Coma Scale corresponding to this patient would be
    A. 0
    B. 1
    C. 2
    D. 3
    E. 4

506. Hypoglycemia is more likely to occur in the diabetic surgical patient with which of the following diseases?
    A. Renal disease
    B. Rheumatoid arthritis requiring high-dosage prednisone
    C. Chronic obstructive lung disease treated with a terbutaline inhaler and aminophylline
    D. Manic-depressive disorder treated with lithium
    E. Congestive heart failure

507. Which of the following is most likely to be associated with a falsely elevated SaO_2 as measured by pulse oximetry?
    A. Hemoglobin F
    B. Carboxyhemoglobin
    C. Bilirubin
    D. Fluorescein dye
    E. Methylene blue dye

508. The most sensitive test for detecting primary hypothyroidism in the preoperative evaluation of a patient in whom hypothyroidism is suspected is
    A. Thyroid-stimulating hormone (TSH) level
    B. Total plasma T_3 level
    C. Total plasma T_4 level
    D. Resin T_3 uptake
    E. Antithyroid antibodies

509. Gabapentin (Neurontin) as used in the treatment of chronic pain belongs to the same broad class of drugs as
    A. Carbamazepine
    B. Imipramine
    C. Clonidine
    D. Aspirin
    E. Fluoxetine (Prozac)

510. Which of the following medical conditions would not prompt the administration of prophylactic antibiotics for this 67-year-old patient scheduled to undergo a right hemicolectomy?
- **A.** A prosthetic cardiac valve
- **B.** Mitral valve prolapse
- **C.** Cardiac transplant recipient with cardiac valvulopathy
- **D.** Previous history of treated infective endocarditis
- **E.** All need prophylactic antibiotics

511. A 47-year-old morbidly obese patient develops bilateral blindness (only able to perceive light) after a 6 hour, 3 segment laminectomy and fusion. The patient received 6 units of blood and 5 L of Lactated Ringer's solution. A mean arterial blood pressure was maintained at 50 to 60 mm Hg. The most likely structure involved in this visual loss is
- **A.** Central retinal artery
- **B.** Optic nerve
- **C.** Retina
- **D.** Cerebral cortex
- **E.** Central retinal vein

512. All of the following concerning postoperative shivering are true **EXCEPT**
- **A.** May increase metabolism and oxygen consumption significantly
- **B.** May be treated with meperidine
- **C.** May be treated with droperidol
- **D.** May be treated with clonidine
- **E.** Does not occur in the absence of hypothermia

513. Electrocardiographic (ECG) changes associated with hyperkalemia include
- **A.** Increased P wave amplitude
- **B.** Shortened PR interval
- **C.** Narrowed QRS complex
- **D.** Narrowed and peaked T waves
- **E.** Increase in U-wave amplitude

514. A 24 year old is undergoing open reduction of an ankle fracture under general anesthesia with sevoflurane, N_2O and O_2 through an laryngeal mask airway (LMA). Just after the vaporizer dial is turned up to 2% the patient begins spontaneously breathing, but the inspiratory valve is not fully closing. The likely result of this (malfunctioning valve) is an increased in the inspired concentration of
- **A.** N_2O
- **B.** CO_2
- **C.** O_2
- **D.** Sevoflurane
- **E.** All of the above

515. All of the following are associated with acromegalic patients undergoing transsphenoidal hypophysectomy **EXCEPT**
- **A.** Enlargement of the tongue and epiglottis
- **B.** Narrowing of the glottic opening
- **C.** Nasal turbinate enlargement
- **D.** 20% to 30% incidence of difficult intubation
- **E.** Continuous positive airway pressure (CPAP) should be used postoperatively since obstructive sleep apnea (OSA) is very common

516. Evidence of an anaphylactic reaction to atracurium 1 to 2 hours after the episode could be best established by measuring blood levels of
- **A.** Tryptase
- **B.** Laudanosine
- **C.** Histamine
- **D.** Bradykinin
- **E.** Cortisol

517. Which of the following findings is **NOT** consistent with a diagnosis of malignant hyperthermia?
  A. $Paco_2$ 150 mm Hg
  B. MVo_2 50 mm Hg
  C. pH 6.9
  D. Arterial oxygen saturation 85% on 100% Fio_2
  E. Onset of symptoms an hour after end of operation

518. A 52-year-old business executive undergoes a radical retropubic prostatectomy uneventfully under general isoflurane anesthesia. He takes fluoxetine (Prozac) for depression. Upon discharge, which of the following analgesics would be the best choice for post-operative pain management in this patient?
  A. Oxycodone plus aspirin (Percodan)
  B. Hydrocodone with acetaminophen (Vicodin)
  C. Codeine with acetaminophen (Tylenol #3)
  D. Hydromorphone (Dilaudid)
  E. All would be equally effective

519. Anesthesia is induced in a 50-year-old, 125-kg man for anterior cervical fusion. The patient is placed on a ventilator. Peak airway pressure is noted to be 20 cm H_2O with O_2 saturation 99% on pulse oximeter. An hour later, the peak airway pressure rises to 40 cm H_2O, $Paco_2$ is 38 mm Hg on mass spectrometer, on O_2 saturation falls to 88%. Blood pressure and heart rate are unchanged. The most likely cause of these findings is?
  A. Mainstem intubation
  B. Thrombotic pulmonary embolism
  C. Tension pneumothorax
  D. Venous air embolism
  E. Laboratory error

520. The phase of liver transplantation where the greatest degree of hemodynamic instability is expected is
  A. Induction
  B. Dissection phase
  C. Anhepatic phase
  D. Reperfusion phase
  E. Emergence

521. Which of the following drugs is (are) likely to prolong nondepolarizing neuromuscular blockade?
  A. Prednisone
  B. Diltiazem
  C. Clindamycin
  D. Dantrolene
  E. All of the above

522. Drugs considered suitable for patients who are susceptible to malignant hyperthermia MH include all **EXCEPT**
  A. Etomidate
  B. N_2O
  C. Calcium chloride
  D. Ketamine
  E. All of the above are safe

523. Near the end of a three-hour colectomy the surgeon complains that the patient is not relaxed. Two twitch monitor placed at different locations show only one twitch of a train of four. Blood gases are reported to be pH 6.9, CO_2 82, K 4.6 and acetate 4.6. Most appropriate action would be
  A. Administer more vecuronium
  B. Administer bicarbonate
  C. Administer succinylcholine
  D. Increase minute ventilation
  E. Administer dantrolene

524. A 22-year-old parturient is anesthetized for an emergency laparoscopic cholecystectomy. She is in the 24th week of gestation and receives general sevoflurane anesthesia and has received rocuronium for muscle relaxation. Just prior to emergence, muscle relaxation is reversed with glycopyrrolate and neostigmine. Three minutes later, the fetal heart rate falls to 88 beats per minute. The most likely cause of this is
   A. Fetal head compression
   B. Maternal hypoxia
   C. Fetal hypoxia
   D. Uteroplacental insufficiency
   E. Reversal agents

525. Each of the following is associated with an increased risk of nausea and vomiting with anesthesia **EXCEPT**
   A. Smoking
   B. Female gender
   C. History of motion sickness
   D. History of postoperative nausea and vomiting
   E. Postoperative codeine

526. Ketorolac is contraindicated in patients undergoing scoliosis surgery because of
   A. Renal effects
   B. Risk of postoperative hemorrhage
   C. Effects on bone healing
   D. Effects on pulmonary function
   E. Paradoxical effect with bone pain

527. Causes of sickling in patients with sickle-cell anemia include all of the following **EXCEPT**
   A. Inhaled nitric oxide
   B. Dehydration
   C. Metabolic acidosis
   D. Hypothermia
   E. Hypoxemia

528. Which of the following factors is the greatest predictor of sleep apneas in an adult?
   A. Neck circumference
   B. Edentulousness
   C. Weight
   D. Body mass index
   E. Micrognathia

529. Greatest number of malpractice claims made against anesthesiologists (according to the ASA closed claims task force) is associated with which adverse outcome?
   A. Airway trauma
   B. Brain damage
   C. Nerve damage
   D. Death
   E. Eye injury

530. Resynchronization therapy
   A. Is indicated for short QRS complexes
   B. Synchronizes QRS with breathing
   C. Requires pacemaker implantation
   D. Is usually accomplished with biphasic defibrillator
   E. Is contraindicated in patients with coronary artery disease

531.   The underlying feature in patients with syndrome X is
   A.   Hypertension
   B.   Coronary artery disease
   C.   Hypoglycemia
   D.   Insulin resistance
   E.   Morbid obesity

532.   A 65-year-old hospitalized patient is being treated for pain from pancreatic cancer and is well-controlled on 30 mg IV morphine per day. What is the equivalent total oral daily dosage of morphine in this patient for discharge planning?
   A.   10 mg
   B.   30 mg
   C.   90 mg
   D.   120 mg
   E.   150 mg

533.   The effect of inhaled anesthetics is determined by
   A.   The partial pressure of the anesthetic
   B.   The percent of the anesthetic in the inspired gas
   C.   Partial pressure for N_2O and percent of inspired gas for volatiles
   D.   Partial pressure for N_2O and desflurane and percent inspired gas for all others
   E.   Partial pressure only for agents with vapor pressure less than or equal to 250

534.   Hazards of O_2 administration include
   A.   Retinopathy of prematurity
   B.   Retention of CO_2
   C.   Adsorption atelectasis
   D.   Bronchopulmonary dysplasia
   E.   All of the above

535.   Which of the following nerves is **NOT** derived from a cranial nerve?
   A.   Great auricular
   B.   Infraorbital
   C.   Supratrochlear
   D.   Supraorbital
   E.   Mental

536.   A 45-year-old female is experiencing progressive mental deterioration over a 6 hour period, 5 days after emergency evacuation of a large subarachnoid hemorrhage and clipping of a middle cerebral artery aneurysm. The most likely cause for deterioration is:
   A.   Cerebral edema
   B.   Hyponatremia
   C.   Recurrent cerebral hemorrhage
   D.   Vasospasm
   E.   Improper placement of the aneurysm clip

537.   Which of the following treatments should not be used in the management of thyrotoxicosis?
   A.   Aspirin
   B.   Cold crystalloid
   C.   Cholestyramine
   D.   Dexamethasone
   E.   Esmolol

538.   The most common adverse cardiac event in the pediatric population is
   A.   Hypotension
   B.   Bradycardia
   C.   Premature ventricular contraction (PVC) salvos
   D.   Bigeminy
   E.   Tachycardia

539. Each of the following is a predictor of difficulty with mask ventilation **EXCEPT**
    A. Presence of beard
    B. BMI greater than 26
    C. Presence of teeth
    D. Age greater than 55
    E. History of snoring

540. In a patient with compartment syndrome, which of the following signs would be the last to appear?
    A. Pulselessness
    B. Pain
    C. Swelling
    D. Paralysis
    E. Paresthesia

541. Select the **TRUE** statement regarding the dose and duration, respectively, of local anesthetics for spinals in infants compared with adults
    A. Greater dose and longer duration
    B. Greater dose and shorter duration
    C. Greater dose and duration is the same
    D. Smaller dose and longer duration
    E. Smaller dose and shorter duration

542. A No. 6 endotracheal tube indicates which size?
    A. 6 mm internal diameter
    B. 6 mm external diameter
    C. 6 mm external circumference
    D. 6 mm internal circumference
    E. 6 cm external radius

543. If a patient were to become trapped in the MRI scanner by a metal object and the engineers decided to quench the magnet, the greatest hazard to the patient would be
    A. Heat
    B. Cold
    C. Fire
    D. Explosion
    E. Noise

544. A 25-year-old black male is brought to the emergency room unconscious. Supplemental oxygen is administered and a pulse oximeter is placed on his finger and a reading of 98% is recorded. Arterial gas sampling at the same time shows Pao_2 of 190 mm Hg, pH 7.2 and O_2 saturation of 90%. Presence of which of the following could explain the discrepancies between these two readings?
    A. Methemoglobin (Hb Met)
    B. Sickle cell hemoglobin
    C. Carboxyhemoglobin (HbCO)
    D. Hemoglobin shifted to right
    E. Pulse oximeter error

545. During surgery for correction of scoliosis, somatosensory evoked potential (SSEP) monitoring is employed. An increase in SSEP latency and decrease in amplitude could be explained by each of the following **EXCEPT**
    A. Anterior spinal artery syndrome
    B. Ischemia of posterior tibial nerve
    C. Hypotension
    D. 2 MAC isoflurane anesthesia
    E. Propofol infusion (200 µg/kg/min)

546. In which of the following conditions would the response to atropine be most pronounced?
- **A.** Diabetic autonomic neuropathy
- **B.** Brain death
- **C.** Status post heart transplant
- **D.** High (C8) spinal anesthesia
- **E.** A patient with chronic atrial fibrillation, complete heart block with VVI pacemaker

DIRECTIONS (Questions 547 through 566): Each group of questions consists of several numbered statements followed by lettered headings. For each numbered statement, select the ONE lettered heading that is most closely associated with it. Each lettered heading may be selected once, more than once, or not at all.

547. Skin lesions all appear at the same stage and at the same time

548. Ciprofloxacin for 60 days is prophylaxis for exposed patients

549. Not contagious

550. Treatment may include streptomycin, gentamicin or tetracycline

551. Treatment includes trivalent equine antitoxin

552. Three primary types: cutaneous, gastrointestinal and inhalation

553. Vaccine may prevent or greatly attenuate symptoms if given within 4 days of exposure

554. Hemorrhagic fever
- **A.** Smallpox
- **B.** Anthrax
- **C.** Plague
- **D.** Botulism
- **E.** Ebola virus

555. Decreased FEV_1/FVC ratio

556. Decreased total pulmonary compliance

557. Increased total lung capacity

558. Decreased FRC

559. Decreased FEV_1, normal FEV_1/FVC ratio

560. Increased lung compliance due to loss of elastic recoil of the lung
- **A.** Pulmonary emphysema
- **B.** Chronic bronchitis
- **C.** Restrictive pulmonary disease
- **D.** Pulmonary emphysema and chronic bronchitis
- **E.** Pulmonary emphysema and restrictive pulmonary disease

561.   Weakness of all muscles below the knee

562.   Foot drop; loss of dorsal extension of the toes

563.   Weakness of the muscles that extend the knee

564.   Inability to adduct the leg; diminished sensation over the medial side of the thigh

565.   Most commonly caused by placement of patient into the lithotomy position

566.   Numbness over the lateral aspect of the thigh
    A. Sciatic nerve injury
    B. Common peroneal nerve injury
    C. Femoral nerve injury
    D. Obturator nerve injury
    E. Lateral femoral cutaneous nerve injury

General Anesthesia

Answers, References, and Explanations

418. (B) Patients with insulin-dependent diabetes and noninsulin-dependent diabetes require special consideration when presenting for surgery. Geriatric age patients come to the OR in the fasting state and without having taken their morning dose of their oral diabetic agent. Chlorpropamide is the longest-acting sulfonylurea and has a duration of action up to 72 hours. Accordingly, it is prudent to measure serum glucose before inducing anesthesia and periodically during the course of the anesthetic and surgery. Regular insulin has a peak effect 2 to 3 hours after SQ administration and a duration of action approximately 6 to 8 hours and would therefore not cause a serum glucose of 35 mg/dL 24 hours after it was administered (*Stoelting: Pharmacology and Physiology in Anesthetic Practice, ed 4, pp 479, 483-484*).

419. (E) Dibucaine is an amide-type local anesthetic that inhibits normal pseudocholinesterase by approximately 80%. In patients who are heterozygous for atypical pseudocholinesterase, enzyme activity is inhibited by 40% to 60%. In patients who are homozygous for atypical pseudocholinesterase, enzyme activity is inhibited by only 20%. The dibucaine number is a qualitative assessment of pseudocholinesterase. Quantitative as well as qualitative determination of enzyme activity should be carried out in any patient who is suspected of having a pseudocholinesterase abnormality (*Stoelting: Basics of Anesthesia, ed 5, p 140*).

420. (D) All hypotension can be broadly broken down into two main categories: decreased cardiac output and decreased systemic vascular resistance. Flow or cardiac output can be further subdivided into problems related to decreased heart rate (i.e., bradycardia versus problems related to decreases in stroke volume). Normal Po_2 in mixed venous blood is 40 mm Hg. Increased mixed venous arterial oxygen levels can be due to many conditions including high cardiac output, sepsis, left-to-right cardiac shunts, impaired peripheral uptake (e.g., cyanide), decreased oxygen consumption (e.g., hypothermia) as well as sampling error. The other choices in this question all represent conditions whereby cardiac output is diminished and consequently would not be consistent with the data given in the question (*Morgan: Clinical Anesthesiology, ed 4, pp 560-561*).

421. (C) Tracheal capillary arteriolar pressure (25-35 mm Hg) is important to keep in mind in patients who are intubated with cuffed endotracheal tubes. If the endotracheal tube cuff exerts a pressure greater than capillary arteriolar pressure, tissue ischemia may result. Persistent ischemia may lead to destruction of tracheal rings and tracheomalacia. Endotracheal tubes with low-pressure cuffs are recommended in patients who are to be intubated for periods longer than 48 hours because this will minimize the chances for development of tissue ischemia (*Miller: Anesthesia, ed 6, p 1630*).

422. (E) Enoxaparin, dalteparin, and ardeparin are low-molecular-weight heparins (LMWH). Because of the possibility of spinal and epidural hematoma in the anticoagulated patient with neuraxial blockade, caution is advised. The plasma half-life of LMWH is two to four times longer than standard heparin. These drugs are commonly used for prophylaxis for deep vein thrombosis. These drugs are also used at high doses for treatment of deep vein thrombosis and (off label) as "bridge therapy" for patients chronically anticoagulated with Coumadin. In these patients who are being prepared for surgery, Coumadin is discontinued and LMWH started. With high-dose enoxaparin administration (1 mg/kg twice daily) it is recommended to wait at least 24 hours before administration of a single-shot spinal anesthetic (*Barash: Clinical Anesthesia, ed 5, p 713; Miller: Anesthesia, ed 6, pp 1677, 2742-2743; Second Consensus Conference on Neuraxial Anesthesia and Anticoagulation, April 25-28, 2002 www.asra.com/consensus-statements/2.html*).

423. (A) The principal mechanism of peripheral nerve injury is ischemia caused by stretching or compression of the nerves. Anesthetized patients are at increased risk for peripheral nerve injuries because they are unconscious and unable to complain about uncomfortable positions that an awake patient would not tolerate and because of reduced muscle tone that facilitates placement of patients into awkward positions. The ulnar nerve in particular is vulnerable because it passes around the posterior aspect of the medial epicondyle of the humerus. The ulnar nerve may become compressed between the medial epicondyle and the sharp edge of the operating table, leading to ischemia and possible nerve injury which may be transient or permanent (*Stoelting: Basics of Anesthesia, ed 5, pp 299-300*).

424. (E) Methoxyflurane is extensively metabolized resulting in the liberation of the fluoride anion. When the inorganic fluoride levels are less than 50 μmol/L no evidence of renal injury is seen. With levels of 50 to 80 μmol/L (which develops with 2.5-3 MAC hours of methoxyflurane use) moderate injury occurs and with levels of 80 to 120 μmol/L severe injury develops. Several patients have died when levels were above 120 μmol/L. Fluoride in appropriate concentrations is capable of making the kidney unresponsive to ADH. This condition is known as nephrogenic diabetes insipidus and is the reason why methoxyflurane was withdrawn from clinical practice. Enflurane (now obsolete in the United States) also is capable of yielding free fluoride ions, but at levels much less than with methoxyflurane. Sevoflurane is defluorinated through oxidative metabolism and can produce serum fluoride levels that can peak above 50 μmol/L, although typically levels are commonly around 30 μmol/L. Renal failure has not been clinically seen with sevoflurane use, possibly because the drug is rapidly excreted via the lungs (methoxyflurane is very slowly excreted via the lungs). Very small amounts of free fluoride ions are produced through the metabolism of isoflurane and halothane. Desflurane is very resistant to defluorination and is not associated with nephrotoxicity (*Miller: Anesthesia, ed 6, pp 248-251*).

425. (C) The incidence of deep vein thrombosis can be reduced from 30% to less than 10% in patients undergoing thoracoabdominal surgery if low-dose heparin (5000 units) is administered 2 hours before surgery and every 8 to 12 hours thereafter (until the patient is able to walk). Although the reduction in deep vein thrombosis in these patients is clear, it is not certain if this therapy prevents pulmonary embolism or reduces mortality. Aspirin, Coumadin, dextran, and compression boots may be of benefit in specific clinical situations. Early ambulation, however, is the best prophylaxis against deep vein thrombosis. Coughing does nothing to prevent deep vein thromboses (*Hines: Stoelting's Anesthesia and Co-Existing Disease, ed 5, pp 155-157*).

426. (C) Blood flow to the retina can be decreased by either a decrease in mean arterial pressure or an increase in intraocular pressure. Decreased blood flow and stasis are more likely in patients with glaucoma because of their elevated intraocular pressure. During periods of prolonged hypotension, the incidence of retinal artery thrombosis increases in these patients (*Hines: Stoelting's Anesthesia and Co-Existing Disease, ed 5, p 235; Stoelting: Basics of Anesthesia, ed 5, pp 463-469*).

427. (D) Naloxone (Narcan) is a competitive inhibitor at all opioid receptors but has the greatest affinity for μ-receptors. Its duration of action is relatively short (elimination half-life of about 1 hour). For this reason, one must be vigilant for the possibility of renarcotization when reversing long acting narcotics. Naltrexone (ReVia) is the N-cyclopropylmethyl derivative of oxymorphone with a long elimination half-life of 8 to 12 hours. It is currently only available as an oral preparation and is used to block the euphoric effects of injected heroin in addicts who have been previously detoxified. Nalmefene (Revex) is another opioid antagonist that can be administered orally or parenterally and has an extremely long duration of action (elimination terminal half life of 8.5 hours) (*Longnecker: Principles and Practice of Anesthesiology, ed 2, pp 1251-1252; Miller: Anesthesia, ed 6, p 421; Morgan: Clinical Anesthesiology, ed 4, p 285*).

428. (A) In the recovery room, the most common cause of postoperative hypoxemia is a uneven ventilation/perfusion distribution caused by loss of lung volume resulting from small airway collapse and atelectasis. Risk factors for ventilation/perfusion mismatch in the postoperative period include old age, obstructive lung disease, obesity, increased intraabdominal pressure, and immobility. Supplemental oxygen should be administered to keep the Pao_2 in the 80 to 100 mm Hg range, which is associated with a 95% saturation of hemoglobin. Other measures can be taken to restore lung volume, which include recovering obese patients in the sitting position, coughing, and deep breathing (*Barash: Clinical Anesthesia, ed 5, pp 1391-1395*).

429. (D) Airway obstruction after total thyroidectomy may be caused by a postoperative hematoma, compression of the trachea, tracheomalacia, bilateral recurrent laryngeal nerve damage, or hypocalcemia resulting from inadvertent removal of the parathyroid glands. Although the airway symptoms of hypocalcemia can develop as early as 1 to 3 hours after surgery, they typically do not develop until 24 to 72 hours postoperatively. Because the laryngeal muscles are particularly sensitive to hypocalcemia, early symptoms may include inspiratory stridor, labored breathing, and eventual laryngospasm. Therapy consists of IV administration of calcium gluconate or calcium chloride (*Stoelting: Basics of Anesthesia, ed 5, pp 443-444*).

430.   **(A)**   Damage to the radial nerve is manifested by weakness in abduction of the thumb, inability to extend the meta-carpophalangeal joints, wrist drop, and numbness in the webbed space between the thumb and index fingers. The radial nerve passes around the humerus between the middle and lower portions in the spiral groove posteriorly. As it wraps around the bone, the radial nerve can become compressed between it and the OR table, resulting in nerve injury (*Barash: Clinical Anesthesia, ed 5, p 650*).

431.   **(D)**   Bronchiectasis is one of several obstructive lung diseases characterized by a diminished FEV_1 when pulmonary function is evaluated. It is characterized by permanently dilated bronchi that frequently contain purulent secretions. The affected bronchi are often highly vascularized, giving rise to the possibility of hemoptysis. Collateral circulation through the intercostal and bronchial arteries is also possible in these patients. If these vessels connect with the pulmonary circulation, pulmonary hypertension and eventual cor pulmonale are possible sequelae. Any patient with chronic bronchial infections may develop bronchiectasis (*Hines: Stoelting's Anesthesia and Co-Existing Disease, ed 5, p 175*).

432.   **(E)**   Drugs that block dopamine receptors may cause acute dystonic reactions in some patients. The incidence with droperidol is about 1%. Treatment is the administration of a drug that crosses the blood brain-barrier with anticholinergic properties such as diphenhydramine or benztropine. Although glycopyrrolate is an anticholinergic drug, it would not be useful in this setting because it does not cross the blood-brain barrier (*Hines: Stoelting's Anesthesia and Co-Existing Disease, ed 5, p 644; Stoelting: Pharmacology and Physiology in Anesthetic Practice, ed 4, p 414*).

433.   **(C)**   The median nerve is most frequently injured at the antecubital fossa by extravasation of IV drugs (e.g., thiopental) that are toxic to neural tissue, or by direct injury caused by the needle during attempts to cannulate the medial cubital or basilic veins. The median nerve provides sensory innervation to the palmar surface of the lateral three and one-half fingers and adjacent palm, and motor function to the abductor pollicis brevis, flexor pollicis brevis, and opponens pollicis muscles (*Stoelting: Basics of Anesthesia, ed 5, p 301*).

434.   **(D)**   Pheochromocytoma is an endocrine tumor (with release of catecholamines) in which 90% of patients are hypertensive, 90% of the tumors originate in one adrenal medulla, and 90% of all pheochromocytomas are benign. This disease is rare (<0.1% of hypertension in adults), but when it occurs, it is often seen with a triad of diaphoresis, tachycardia, and headache in patients with hypertension. Other symptoms include palpitations, tremulousness, weight loss, hyperglycemia, hypovolemia, and in some cases dilated cardiomyopathy and congestive heart failure. Death as a result of pheochromocytoma is due to cardiac conditions (e.g., myocardial infarction, congestive heart failure) or an intracranial bleed. In about 5% of cases, pheochromocytomas show an autosomal dominant pattern and may coexist with other endocrine diseases such as medullary carcinoma of the thyroid and hyperparathyroidism. This combination is called multiple endocrine neoplasia or MEN type II or IIA (Sipple's syndrome). MEN type IIB consists of pheochromocytoma, medullary carcinoma of the thyroid, and neuromas of the oral mucosa. The von Hippel-Lindau disease consists of hemangiomas of the nervous system (i.e., retina or cerebellum) and 10% to 25% of these patients also have a pheochromocytoma. The average sized pheochromocytoma contains 100 to 800 mg of norepinephrine (*Barash: Clinical Anesthesia, ed 5, p 1142; Hines: Stoelting's Anesthesia and Co-Existing Disease, ed 5, pp 388-393*).

435.   **(D)**   Serum glutamic-oxaloacetic transaminase (aspartate aminotransferase), serum glutamic-pyruvic transaminase (alanine aminotransferase), and lactate dehydrogenase all are elevated in patients with liver disease. The serum level of alkaline phosphatase may be a specific indicator of biliary obstruction. Because this enzyme is also produced in the intestines, bone, and placenta, other serum tests must be ordered to differentiate among these potential sources. Concurrent measurement of the serum γ-glutaryl transferase (GGT), leucine aminopeptidase, or 5′-nucleotidase levels can be measured simultaneously with alkaline phosphatase to determine the origin of the latter (*Miller: Anesthesia, ed 6, pp 754-755*).

436.   **(C)**   Although early mild symptoms of alcohol withdrawal can be seen within 6 to 8 hours after a substantial drop in the serum alcohol levels, delirium tremens (DTs) which is seen in about 5% of patients, is a life-threatening medical emergency which develops 2 to 4 days after the cessation of alcohol in alcoholics. Symptoms of DT's include hallucinations, combativeness, hyperthermia, tachycardia, hypertension or hypotension, and grand mal seizures. Treatment of severe alcohol withdrawal consists of fluid replacement, electrolyte replacement, and IV vitamin administration with particular attention paid to thiamine. Aggressive administration of benzodiazepines is indicated to prevent seizures (5 to 10 mg of diazepam every 5 minutes until the patient becomes sedated but not unconscious). β-Blockers are used to suppress overactivity of the sympathetic nervous system, and lidocaine may be effective in the treatment of cardiac dysrhythmias (*Hines: Stoelting's Anesthesia and Co-Existing Disease, ed 5, p 543*).

437. (A) Operations on the trachea may be indicated in patients who have tracheal tumors or patients who had a previous trauma to the trachea resulting in tracheal stenosis or tracheomalacia. Eighty percent of the operations on the trachea involve segmental resection with primary anastomosis, 10% involve resection with prosthetic reconstruction, and another 10% involve insertion of a T-tube stent. These operations frequently are very complicated and require constant communication between the surgeon and the anesthesiologist. Preoperative pulmonary function tests are indicated in all patients who are to undergo elective tracheal resection. Severe lung disease necessitating postoperative mechanical ventilation is a relative contraindication for tracheal resection because positive airway pressure may cause wound dehiscence (*Miller: Anesthesia, ed 6, pp 1912-1913*).

438. (B) Hypercalcemia is associated with a number of signs and symptoms, including hypertension, dysrhythmias, shortening of QT interval, kidney stones, seizure, nausea and vomiting, weakness, depression, personality changes, psychosis, and even coma. Generally patients with total serum calcium levels of 12 mg/dL or less do not require any intervention, with the possible exception of rehydration with saline. Higher calcium levels may be associated with clinical symptoms and should be treated before anesthetizing the patient. Caution should be taken with digitalis administration to any patient who is hypercalcemic because some patients may exhibit extreme digitalis sensitivity (*Fleisher: Anesthesia and Uncommon Diseases, ed 5, pp 414-415; Longnecker: Principles and Practice of Anesthesiology, ed 2, pp 309-310*).

NORMAL CALCIUM LEVELS

	Serum Calcium	Serum Ionized Calcium
Conventional units (mEq/L)	4.5-5.5 mEq/L	2.1-2.6 mEq/L (mEq/L)
Conventional units mg/dL	9.0-11.0 mg/dL	4.25-5.25 mg/dL (mg/dL)
SI units (mmol/L)	2.25-2.75 mmol/L	1.05-1.30 mmol/L

439. (D) Red-top eye drops cause mydriasis and should be used with caution in patients with closed angle glaucoma. Green top eye drops cause miosis and the pupillary constriction helps keep the drainage route open in patients with glaucoma and helps prevent an acute attack of glaucoma. Clear or white top eye drops do not change pupillary size.

440. (D) When reviewing growth curves, the normal 40-week term newborn weighs about 3.5 kg. Children then double their birthweight by 5 months and triple their weight by 1 year. Therefore, the average 1-year-old weighs 10 kg (22 pounds). From the age of 1 to 6 years, children gain about 2 kg per year. Thus, an average 2-year-old weighs 12 kg, 3-year-old weighs 14 kg, 4-year-old weighs 16 kg, 5-year-old weighs 18 kg, and 6-year-old weighs 20 kg. From age 6 to 10 years, children gain about 3 kg per year (*Motoyama: Smith's Anesthesia for Infants and Children, ed 7, pp 1203-1205*).

441. (A) Causes for acute pacemaker malfunction in the OR are numerous and include threshold changes, inhibition, generator failure, and lead or electrode dislodgement or breakage. A VVI pacemaker may be inhibited by myopotentials. In this regard, administration of succinylcholine could actually inhibit a VVI pacemaker. Similarly, electrocautery can inhibit a VVI pacemaker through electromagnetic interference. Should this occur, a magnet should be placed over the pacemaker to convert it into a VOO pacemaker, eliminating the possibility of further inhibition. Pacemakers should be evaluated preoperatively to eliminate the possibility of generator failure. Lead breakage or dislodgement is an unlikely cause of pacemaker failure unless the surgeon is working in the vicinity of the electrodes. Acute threshold changes are almost always associated with changes in the serum potassium concentration. In this particular patient, hyperventilation causes a respiratory alkalosis that results in the intracellular shifting of serum potassium. The net result is that the electrical threshold for the pacemaker is raised, preventing ventricular capture (*Miller: Anesthesia, ed 6, pp 1426-1427; Thomas: Manual of Cardiac Anesthesia, ed 2, pp 382-383*).

442. (C) Therapies aimed at increasing functional residual capacity (FRC) of the lungs are useful in reducing the incidence of post-operative pulmonary complications. Forced expiratory maneuvers may lead to airway closure, which would be of no benefit for this patient (*Miller: Anesthesia, ed 6, pp 2713, 2818-2819*).

443. **(C)** The human brain is able to maintain neuronal function in the face of decreasing CBF below the normal level of 50 mL/100 g/min. Because O_2 delivery is directly related to CBF, EEG evidence of cerebral ischemia will appear if CBF is diminished sufficiently. The CBF reserve, however, is substantial and the first signs of cerebral ischemia do not appear on EEG until CBF has fallen to approximately 22 mL/100 g/min. When CBF has fallen to 15/100 g/min, the EEG becomes isoelectric. Irreversible membrane damage and cellular death do not occur, however, until CBF falls to 6 mL/100 g/min. Areas of the brain in which CBF falls in the 6 to 15 mL/100 g/min range are referred to as zones of ischemic penumbra. Several hours may elapse in these areas of the brain before irreversible membrane damage occurs (*Miller: Anesthesia, ed 6, pp 833-834*).

444. **(B)** Positive end-expiratory pressure (PEEP) is the maintenance of positive airway pressure during the entire ventilator cycle. The addition of PEEP to the ventilator cycle is often recommended when Pao_2 is not maintained above 60 mm Hg, when breathing an Fio_2 of 0.50 or greater. Although not completely understood, PEEP is thought to increase arterial oxygenation, pulmonary compliance, and FRC by expanding previously collapsed but perfused alveoli, thereby decreasing shunt and improving ventilation/perfusion matching. An important adverse effect of PEEP is a decrease in arterial blood pressure caused by a decrease in venous return, left ventricular filling and stroke volume, and cardiac output. These effects are exaggerated in patients with decreased intravascular fluid volume. Other potential adverse effects of PEEP include pneumothorax, pneumomediastinum, and subcutaneous emphysema (*Miller Anesthesia, ed 6, pp 2820-2821; Stoelting: Basics of Anesthesia, ed 5, p 596*).

445. **(C)** Reversal of neuromuscular blockade with an anticholinesterase drug requires coadministration of an anticholinergic drug to prevent the muscarinic side effects (e.g., bradycardia and salivation) from the neuromuscular reversal agent. The onset of neuromuscular reversal activity is most rapid with edrophonium, followed by neostigmine and pyridostigmine. The durations of action of edrophonium and neostigmine are similar, but pyridostigmine has a longer duration of action. Of the anticholinergic drugs, glycopyrrolate has a longer duration of action than atropine and for this reason should be coadministered with pyridostigmine. In this question, the patient received long-acting pyridostigmine in combination with short-acting atropine. After the effects of atropine wore off, the antimuscarinic effects of pyridostigmine became evident, resulting in bradycardia (*Stoelting: Pharmacology and Physiology in Anesthetic Practice, ed 4, pp 258-259*).

446. **(B)** As a rough approximation, if one divides 150 by the MAC for any given volatile anesthetic, the quotient will be approximately equal to the oil/gas partition coefficient. For example, if one were to divide the MAC of halothane (0.75) into 150, the quotient would be 200, which is very close to the actual oil/gas partition coefficient for halothane (224). Similarly, if one were to divide the MAC of enflurane (1.68) into 150, the quotient would be 89, which is very similar to the oil/gas partition coefficient for enflurane (98). The fact that anesthetics with a high oil/gas partition coefficient (i.e., lipid-soluble agents) have lower MACs supports the Meyer-Overton theory (critical volume hypothesis) (*Stoelting: Pharmacology and Physiology in Anesthetic Practice, ed 4, p 29*).

447. **(E)** Diabetes insipidus is characterized by hypernatremia, serum hyperosmolality, polyuria, and urine hypo-osmolality. Diabetes insipidus may occur after any intracranial procedure, but it is particularly common in surgery involving the pituitary gland. It may develop intraoperatively, but it commonly develops 4 to 12 hours postoperatively. Intravenous half normal saline and dextrose 5% in water are started as replacement fluids. The pharmacologic treatment for diabetes insipidus is synthetic ADH, 1-(3-mercaptoproprionic acid)-D-arginine vasopressin (DDAVP) commonly started when the urine output is greater than 350-400 mL/hr. In a conscious patient it is not essential to administer DDAVP because the patient may increase his oral intake to compensate for polyuria. In the unconscious patient, however, administration of DDAVP is necessary. Vasopressin (DDAVP) may be administered SQ, IV, or intranasally. Fortunately, diabetes insipidus related to surgery and head trauma usually is transient (*Hines: Stoelting's Anesthesia and Co-Existing Disease, ed 5, pp 403-404; Miller: Anesthesia, ed 6, p 2159*).

448. **(B)** The principal feature of Alzheimer's disease is progressive dementia. The onset typically occurs after age 60 years and may affect as many as 20% of patients more than age 80 years. In addition to age, other risk factors include history of serious head trauma (e.g., boxing), Down syndrome, and presence of the disease in a parent or sibling. One biochemical feature of this disease is a decrease in the enzyme choline acetyltransferase in the brain. There is a strong correlation between reduced enzyme activity and decreased cognitive function. Interestingly, administration of the anticholinergic drugs scopolamine or atropine (but not glycopyrrolate which does not cross the blood-brain barrier) causes confusion similar to that seen in the early stages of Alzheimer's disease. Conversely, administration of anticholinesterase drugs capable of penetrating the blood-brain barrier, such as donepezil

(Aricept), galantamine, rivastigmine (Exelon), and tacrine are used to treat patients with Alzheimer's disease. Physostigmine may have beneficial effects in some patients as well. Scopolamine is therefore a poor choice for premedication in patients with Alzheimer's disease (*Hines: Stoelting's Anesthesia and Co-Existing Disease, ed 5, p 227; Morgan: Clinical Anesthesiology, ed 4, p 652*).

449. (C) At the end of any general anesthetic, spontaneous ventilation must be restored before the patient can be extubated. The differential diagnosis for persistent apnea includes muscle relaxants (inadequate reversal or pseudocholinesterase deficiency), volatile anesthetics, narcotics, hypocarbia, damage to the phrenic nerves bilaterally, and the possibility of a central nervous system (CNS) event. Succinylcholine is hydrolyzed by pseudocholinesterase to succinylmonocholine and choline. This is further hydrolyzed by plasma cholinesterase to succinic acid and choline. All of the anticholinesterase agents used to reverse nondepolarizing neuromuscular blockade also inhibit pseudocholinesterase. Administration of succinylcholine to any patient who has already received an anticholinesterase will result in a prolonged block from the succinylcholine because it can no longer be easily hydrolyzed. In this patient, therefore, succinylcholine would be by far the most likely cause of apnea at the end of the operation (*Stoelting: Pharmacology and Physiology in Anesthetic Practice, ed 4, p 218*).

450. (A) Pooling of urine in the dome of the bladder should be considered as a possible cause of oliguria in a patient in the Trendelenburg position. Acute hypovolemia is an unlikely cause of oliguria in this patient in the absence of bleeding. Fluoride toxicity from the metabolism of enflurane is extremely rare and is associated with nonoliguric renal failure. See also the answer to question 424 (*Morgan: Clinical Anesthesiology, ed 4, pp 739-741*).

451. (E) D_L is defined as the diffusing capacity of the lung. When a nontoxic low concentration of carbon monoxide is used for the measurement it is called D_{LCO}. The normal value of D_{LCO} is 20 to 30 mL/min/mm Hg and is influenced by the volume of blood (hemoglobin) within the pulmonary circulation. Thus, diseases associated with a decrease in pulmonary blood volume (i.e., anemia, emphysema, hypovolemia, pulmonary hypertension) will be reflected by a decrease in the D_{LCO}. D_{LCO} is also decreased with oxygen toxicity as well as pulmonary edema. Conditions associated with an increased D_{LCO} include the supine position, exercise, obesity and left-to-right cardiac shunts (*Barash: Clinical Anesthesia, ed 5, pp 806-807; Miller: Anesthesia, ed 6, p 1011*).

452. (E) Patients undergoing thyroid surgery are at risk for airway obstruction from a number of causes. Postoperative hemorrhage sufficient to cause a large hematoma could compress the trachea and cause airway obstruction because of the close proximity of the thyroid gland to the trachea. Permanent hypoparathyroidism is a rare complication that may cause hypocalcemia leading to progressive stridor followed by laryngospasm. The most common nerve injury after thyroid surgery is damage to the abductor fibers of the recurrent laryngeal nerve. Unilaterally, this is manifested as hoarseness. Bilateral recurrent laryngeal nerve damage, however, may lead to airway obstruction during inspiration. Selective injury of the adductor fibers of the recurrent laryngeal nerve is a possible complication of thyroid surgery. This injury would leave the vocal cords open because the abductor fibers would be unopposed, placing the patient at great risk for aspiration. The superior laryngeal nerve has an extrinsic branch that innervates the cricothyroid muscle (which tenses the vocal cords), and an internal branch that provides sensory innervation to the pharynx above the vocal cords. Bilateral damage to this nerve would result in hoarseness and would predispose the patient to aspiration but would not lead to airway obstruction per se (*Stoelting: Basics of Anesthesia, ed 5, pp 443-444*).

453. (E) Malignant hyperthermia is a clinical syndrome that may develop rapidly or take hours to manifest, sometimes not occurring until the patient is in the recovery room. Clinical signs include hypertension, tachycardia, respiratory acidosis, metabolic acidosis, muscle rigidity, myoglobinuria, and fever. The diagnosis of MH is unlikely, however, if only one of these signs is manifested. Because MH is a metabolic disorder, one of the first sensitive signs is an increase in the production of CO_2 and concomitant respiratory acidosis. This is the most reliable early sign of the syndrome (*Miller: Anesthesia, ed 6, p 1178*).

454. (E) Hyperventilation to $Paco_2$ of 20 mm Hg or higher for more than 2 hours will result in active transport of HCO_3 out of the CNS. This results in spontaneous breathing at a lower (not higher) $Paco_2$. The other choices should be included in the differential diagnosis of apnea (*Hines: Stoelting's Anesthesia and Co-Existing Disease, ed 5, pp 359-361; Miller: Anesthesia, ed 6, p 718*).

455. (B) Maximum voluntary ventilation (MVV) is a nonspecific pulmonary function test that measures the endurance of the ventilatory muscles and indirectly reflects the compliance of the lung and thorax as well as airway resistance. A decreased MVV may be caused by impairment to inspiration or expiration. In this patient, FEV_1 is normal, which strongly suggests that the ventilatory impairment is during inspiration. A flow-volume loop would be a very useful confirmatory test (*Barash: Clinical Anesthesia, ed 5, pp 805-808, 815-817*).

456.   **(A)**   Guidelines for safe discharge of patients from ambulatory surgical centers include stable vital signs, ability to walk without dizziness, controlled pain, absence of nausea and vomiting, and minimal surgical bleeding. The PADSS is a tool for objectively assessing a patient's readiness for discharge from the surgical center and includes these five criteria. Requirements to drink fluids and to void before home discharge are controversial and are not parameters included in the PADSS (*Barash: Clinical Anesthesia, ed 5, pp 1242-1243; Miller: Anesthesia, ed 6, pp 2708-2709*).

457.   **(C)**   Malignant hyperthermia is a difficult diagnosis to make on clinical grounds alone. Signs of MH may be fulminant or very subtle. They may occur immediately after induction or may not be manifested until the patient has reached the recovery room or even later. Malignant hyperthermia is a disorder of metabolism and is associated with hypertension, tachycardia, dysrhythmias, respiratory acidosis, metabolic acidosis, muscular rigidity, rhabdomyolysis, and fever. Contrary to what one might believe based on the name of this disease, fever is typically a late finding. Other diseases that may mimic MH include alcohol withdrawal, acute cocaine toxicity, bacteremia, pheochromocytoma, hyperthyroidism, and neuroleptic malignant syndrome. An elevation in temperature alone with normal blood gases, heart rate, and blood pressure, and no evidence of muscle breakdown would very likely not be due to MH. If a patient had been previously subjected to muscle biopsy and caffeine-halothane contracture testing with negative results, MH would be exceedingly rare, although a false-negative result is possible. A history of a previous anesthetic without MH triggering would be of little reassurance in a patient in whom a MH episode is suspected. It is not uncommon for MH-susceptible individuals to not trigger when a triggering anesthetic is administered initially but develop fulminant MH with a subsequent anesthetic (*Miller: Anesthesia, ed 6, pp 1180-1186*).

458.   **(D)**   Asthma is an inflammatory illness that has bronchial hyperreactivity and bronchospasm as a result. Treatment is first directed at the inflammatory component as the underlying problem, reserving bronchodilators for symptomatic use. Because leukotrienes may function as inflammatory mediators, the leukotriene pathway inhibitors such as zileuton and the leukotriene receptor antagonist montelukast (Singulair) are being used for treatment of asthma. Zileuton and montelukast are only available as oral preparations, whereas the other drugs listed are given by inhalation. Fluticasone and triamcinolone are anti-inflammatory corticosteroids. Ipratropium is a quaternary ammonium compound formed by the introduction of an isopropyl group to the N atom of atropine and produces effects similar to those of atropine. One unexpected finding is a relative lack of effect on mucociliary clearance, which makes it useful in patients with airway disease, especially if parasympathetic tone of the airways is increased. Salmeterol is a β_2-selective adrenergic drug (*Hardman: Goodman & Gilman's The Pharmacological Basis of Therapeutics, ed 11, pp 721-725, 730-731*).

459.   **(D)**   Acute decreases in serum sodium, due to absorption of bladder irrigating fluids, rarely cause symptoms unless the sodium level drops below 120 mEq/L. At this level, tissue edema may develop and clinical neurologic signs (e.g., restlessness, nausea, confusion, seizures, coma) or ECG changes (e.g., widening of the QRS complex, elevation of the ST segment, ventricular tachycardia, or ventricular fibrillation) may be manifested. Treatment of mild decreases in serum sodium (i.e., 120 to 135 mEq/L with no neurologic or ECG changes) is by fluid restriction and/or administration of a diuretic such as furosemide. When the sodium levels drops below 120 mEq/L and neurologic symptoms or changes in the ECG develop, sodium chloride administration is needed. To calculate the amount needed, one multiplies the patient's total body water (i.e., $0.6 \times$ body weight = TBW) by the change in sodium desired. In this case, the TBW is 60 L (0.6×100 kg) and the change of sodium is 10 mEq (120 mEq/L – 110 mEq/L), thus 60 L $\times$ 10 mEq/L = 600 mEq. Caution is advised in administering sodium because too rapid administration may lead to demyelinating CNS lesions. The recommended rate of 3% sodium chloride (513 mEq/L) is 1 to 2 mL/kg/hour. Serum sodium levels should be checked at least every hour until the sodium level increases above 120 mEq/L (*Barash: Clinical Anesthesia, ed 5, pp 188-192, 1026-1028*).

460.   **(A)**   Trismus (masseter spasm) is characterized by rigidity of the jaw muscles while the limb muscles remain flaccid after administration of succinylcholine. Trismus may herald the onset of MH in some patients, but may be due to a number of other causes and may occur in normal patients. It previously had been believed that 50% of patients who experience trismus after administration of succinylcholine would go on to develop MH. Recent evidence suggests, however, that the incidence is less. If masseter spasm occurs in a patient after administration of succinylcholine, the most conservative course would be to cancel the operation. If cancellation of the operation is not feasible, then a nontriggering anesthetic should be used and the anesthesiologist should pay close attention for any signs of MH (*Miller: Anesthesia, ed 6, pp 1180-1181*).

461. (B) Ketamine is unique among the IV induction agents in that it usually produces cardiac stimulation manifested by increased heart rate, mean arterial pressure, and cardiac output. Ketamine is believed to have a centrally mediated sympathetic nervous system-stimulating effect. This effect is, however, not related to dose. In isolated rabbit and canine hearts and in intact dogs, ketamine has been demonstrated to produce myocardial depression. Clinically, however, the myocardial depressant properties of ketamine are overridden by its sympathetic nervous system stimulating properties. When systemic catecholamines have been depleted or when the patient is under deep anesthesia, the myocardial depressant properties of ketamine may predominate (*Stoelting: Pharmacology and Physiology in Anesthetic Practice, ed 4, p 172*).

462. (C) In the normal muscle cell, depolarization results in release of calcium from the sarcoplasmic reticulum. The increased intracellular calcium concentration results in muscle contraction. The calcium then is rapidly taken up via calcium pumps back into the sarcoplasmic reticulum, resulting in relaxation. Both the release and reuptake of calcium are energy-requiring processes, i.e., result in the hydrolysis of adenosine triphosphate (ATP). Dantrolene, the pharmacologic treatment for MH, blocks release of calcium from the sarcoplasmic reticulum without affecting the reuptake process. The defect in MH is thought to be decreased control of intracellular calcium stores preventing muscle relaxation (*Miller: Anesthesia, ed 6, pp 1170-1179*).

463. (E) Approximately 4% of patients treated with bleomycin develop pulmonary toxicity, which manifests as severe pulmonary fibrosis and hypoxemia. Death from severe pulmonary toxicity occurs in approximately 1% to 2% of patients treated with bleomycin. Patients who are at greater risk for bleomycin-induced pulmonary toxicity include elderly patients, those receiving more than 200 to 400 mg, those with coexisting lung disease, and those recently exposed to bleomycin. In addition, there is evidence that prior radiotherapy and possibly receipt of enriched concentrations of O_2 (i.e., inspired oxygen > 30%) during surgery increase risk of pulmonary toxicity. Clinically, patients gradually develop dyspnea, a nonproductive cough, and hypoxemia, and pulmonary function tests typically demonstrate changes in gas flow and lung volumes consistent with restrictive pulmonary disease. If radiographic evidence such as bilateral diffuse interstitial infiltrates appears, pulmonary fibrosis usually is irreversible (*Stoelting: Pharmacology and Physiology in Anesthetic Practice, ed 4, pp 564-565*).

464. (C) Head flexion can advance the tube up to 1.9 cm toward the carina and in some cases convert an endotracheal intubation into an endobronchial intubation. Extension of the head has the opposite effect and can withdraw the tube up to 1.9 cm, resulting in extubation of some patients. Turning the head laterally can move the distal tip of the endotracheal tube about 0.7 cm away from the carina. The Trendelenburg position causes a cephalad shift of the mediastinum and can cause the endotracheal tube to migrate distally as well (*Lobato: Complications in Anesthesiology, p 834; Stoelting: Basics of Anesthesia, ed 5, p 232*).

465. (C) Sulfur hexafluoride is sometimes injected in the vitreous in patients with a detached retina to mechanically facilitate reattachment. To prevent changes in the size of the gas bubble, the patients should be given 100% O_2 15 minutes before injection of sulfur hexafluoride. If these patients are anesthetized with general anesthesia within 10 days, N_2O should not be given because N_2O can diffuse into the gas bubble, increasing intraocular pressure, and may result in blindness (*Barash: Clinical Anesthesia, ed 5, p 982*).

466. (D) The symptoms of hypocalcemia, which may be manifested as laryngospasm or laryngeal stridor, usually develop within the first 24 to 96 hours after total thyroidectomy. After the airway is established and secured, the patient should be treated with IV calcium in the form of either calcium gluconate or calcium chloride (*Barash: Clinical Anesthesia, ed 5, pp 199, 1133*).

467. (C) Because the circulating levels of T_3 and T_4 regulate TSH release from the anterior pituitary gland by a negative feedback mechanism, a normal plasma concentration of TSH confirms an euthyroid state. The pharmacologic treatment of choice for patients with hypothyroidism is sodium levothyroxine (T_4). Sodium levothyronine (triiodothyronine, T_3) and desiccated thyroid are alternate therapeutic agents (*Barash: Clinical Anesthesia, ed 5, pp 1130-1134; Hines: Stoelting's Anesthesia and Co-Existing Disease, ed 5, pp 378-381*).

468. **(A)** Large quantities of irrigating fluid can be absorbed during transurethral resection of the prostate gland because the open venous sinuses in the prostate allow the irrigation fluid to be absorbed. From 10 to 30 mL of fluid per minute are absorbed on the average. During long cases, this can amount to several liters, causing hypertension, reflex bradycardia, and pulmonary congestion. Treatment consists of fluid restriction and a loop diuretic (e.g., furosemide) when the [Na$^+$] level is greater than 120 mEq/L. Rarely does the amount of fluid absorbed cause significant hyponatremia (i.e., <120 mEq/L). In these cases of significant hyponatremia, 3% sodium chloride may be infused slowly intravenously (in addition to the loop diuretic and fluid restriction) until the sodium level reaches 120 mEq/L (*Barash: Clinical Anesthesia, ed 5, pp 1027-1028*).

469. **(C)** Patients who have sustained thermal injuries are at risk for massive potassium release and potential cardiac arrest if succinylcholine is administered 24 hours or more after they sustain the burn, and they remain at risk until the burn has healed. This increased sensitivity to succinylcholine is thought to be related to proliferation of extrajunctional receptors. These same receptors are thought to be related to the increased requirement for nondepolarizing neuromuscular blocking agents in these patients (*Barash: Clinical Anesthesia, ed 5, p 1288*).

470. **(D)** Scopolamine, an anticholinergic, has stronger antisialagogue effects than glycopyrrolate or atropine. Scopolamine has better sedative and amnesic effects than atropine. Glycopyrrolate, which does not cross the blood-brain barrier, has no CNS or bradycardiac effects. Although heart rate may decrease with atropine and scopolamine, these effects are minimal (i.e., about 4 to 8 beats/min). These anticholinergics usually are administered parenterally; however, a scopolamine patch could be applied topically. Meperidine may produce a dry mouth in some patients, but it is much more likely to increase the heart rate rather than lower it because of its modest atropine-like effects. Meperidine is well absorbed from the gastrointestinal tract but is usually administered parenterally. Midazolam, which is usually administered parenterally, may produce bradycardia or tachycardia in selected patients but does not cause a dry mouth and may produce excessive salivation. Droperidol can produce tachycardia is some patients and is usually given parenterally. Clonidine is the most likely agent to cause bradycardia, hypotension and dry mouth. The oral dose is 5 μg/kg (*Stoelting: Basics of Anesthesia, ed 5, pp 170-172; Stoelting: Pharmacology and Physiology in Anesthetic Practice, ed 4, pp 340-344*).

471. **(D)** One gram of hemoglobin can combine with 1.34 mL of O$_2$. None of the other choices in this question will do as much to increase the O$_2$-carrying capacity of this patient's blood as a transfusion (*Stoelting: Pharmacology and Physiology in Anesthetic Practice, ed 4, p 849*).

472. **(A)** Many of the drugs commonly administered during surgery and anesthesia have the potential to evoke allergic reactions (e.g., pentothal, propofol, local anesthetics, antibiotics, and protamine, as well as other materials used during surgery, such as vascular graft material, chymopapain, and latex). Virtually all drugs administered IV have been reported to cause allergic reactions. Possible exceptions include benzodiazepines and ketamine. An allergic reaction should be considered when there is an abrupt fall in blood pressure accompanied by increases in heart rate that exceed 30% of the control values. Greater than 60% of all drug-induced allergic reactions observed during the perioperative period are attributable to muscle relaxants. Latex allergy is thought to be responsible for 15% of allergic reactions under anesthesia, sometimes including reactions originally attributed to other substances. Patients at risk for latex allergy include health care workers and patients with spina bifida. Although most drug-induced allergic reactions develop within 5 to 10 minutes of exposure, latex signs typically take more than 30 minutes to develop (*Hines: Stoelting's Anesthesia and Co-Existing Disease, ed 5, pp 527-530; Miller: Anesthesia, ed 6, p 1092*).

473. **(C)** Decreased levels of pseudocholinesterase have been reported in patients with Huntington's chorea. For this reason, the effects of succinylcholine may be prolonged in some of these patients. It has been suggested that the sensitivity to nondepolarizing muscle relaxants is also increased (*Hines: Stoelting's Anesthesia and Co-Existing Disease, ed 5, p 229*).

474. **(A)** Normal intraocular pressure is 10 to 22 mm Hg. In general, IV anesthetics, with the possible exception of ketamine, decrease intraocular pressure. In addition, nondepolarizing neuromuscular blockers, inhaled anesthetics, narcotics, carbonic anhydrase inhibitors, osmotic diuretics, and hypothermia decrease intraocular pressure. However, elevation of Paco$_2$ out of the physiologic range, as seen with hypoventilation as well as arterial hypoxemia, will increase intraocular pressure. Depolarizing neuromuscular blockers, such as succinylcholine, also increase intraocular pressure. This increase in intraocular pressure occurs when succinylcholine is administered IM or IV. Pretreatment with a nondepolarizing muscle relaxant before administering succinylcholine may attenuate the rise in intraocular pressure. The mechanism for the increase in intraocular pressure after succinylcholine use is related to drug-induced cycloplegia rather than contraction of extraocular muscles, as this increase in intraocular pressure will occur even if the intraocular muscles are cut. The greatest increase in intraocular pressure occurs with coughing or vomiting, where the intraocular pressure may increase as much as 35 to 50 mm Hg. The proposed mechanism for the acute increase in intraocular pressure is an increase in venous pressure. There does not appear to be a change in intraocular pressure with changes within normal physiologic ranges in arterial blood pressure or $Paco_2$ (*Barash: Clinical Anesthesia, ed 5, pp 978-980; Stoelting: Basics of Anesthesia, ed 5, pp 464-465*).

475. (C) The apnea-hypopnea index (AHI) is used to quantify the number of apnea or hypopnea episodes that occur per hour. Apnea is defined as no ventilation for periods of 10 seconds or more. Hypopnea is defined as a 50% decrease in airflow or a decrease sufficient to cause a decrease in oxygen saturation of 4%. An apnea-hypopnea index of greater than 30 signifies severe OSA (*Barash: Clinical Anesthesia, ed 5, p 1042; Lobato: Complications in Anesthesiology, p 625*).

476. (D) Any patient who is scheduled for a pneumonectomy should undergo a series of preoperative pulmonary function tests. These tests are generally conducted in three phases. The tests listed in this question pertain to the first battery of pulmonary function tests, which are whole-lung tests. Residual volume to total lung capacity greater than 50% (not <50%) is associated with an increased operative risk. If the results of any of the initial whole-lung tests are below the acceptable limits, a second phase of testing should be carried out in which the function of each lung is evaluated separately. The predicted postoperative FEV_1 after the second phase of pulmonary function testing is carried out should be greater than 0.85 L. If the criteria for the second level of pulmonary function testing cannot be met and pneumonectomy is still desired, then a third level of testing should be carried out. During the third phase of testing, postoperative conditions mimicking pneumonectomy are produced by occluding the pulmonary artery with a balloon on the side that is to be resected. Results of this test that are consistent with poor outcome after pneumonectomy include mean pulmonary artery pressure greater than 40 mm Hg, $Paco_2$ greater than 60 mm Hg, or Pao_2 less than 45 mm Hg (*Miller: Anesthesia, ed 6, pp 1852-1854*).

477. (A) Measured Pao_2 should be decreased about 6% for each degree Celsius cooler the patient's temperature is than the electrode (37° C). Because the patient is 2° C cooler than the electrode, a 12% decrease (9 mm Hg) would be expected in this patient (77 mm Hg – 9 mm Hg = 68 mm Hg) (*Stoelting: Basics of Anesthesia, ed 5, p 325*).

478. (A) The two main causes of central cyanosis are decreased arterial oxygen saturation and hemoglobin abnormalities (e.g., methemoglobinemia and sulfhemoglobinemia). Sulfasalazine (Azulfidine) can cause the formation of sulfhemoglobin. Sulfhemoglobin, like methemoglobin, may cause low O_2 saturation in the face of high Pao_2. There is no treatment for sulfhemoglobinemia except to wait for the destruction of the erythrocytes (*Hines: Stoelting's Anesthesia and Co-Existing Disease, ed 5, pp 287-288; Kasper: Harrison's Principles of Internal Medicine, ed 16, pp 210-211*).

479. (E) Muscle relaxants that stimulate histamine release or cause increased sympathetic outflow should not be given to patients with pheochromocytoma. Vecuronium has no histamine-releasing properties and does not stimulate the sympathetic nervous system. Mivacurium, curare, and metocurine and atracurium all release histamine to some degree. Pancuronium is associated with tachycardia and should be avoided in patients with pheochromocytoma. Of the listed relaxants in this question, vecuronium is the best choice; however, cisatracurium and rocuronium also have minimal effects on the cardiovascular system and would be good choices in patients with pheochromocytomas as well (*Hines: Stoelting's Anesthesia and Co-Existing Disease, ed 5, p 392; Stoelting: Pharmacology and Physiology in Anesthetic Practice, ed 4, pp 223-241*).

480. (B) Serum creatinine is inversely proportional to the GFR. With the increase in creatinine by a factor of 4, the GFR is divided by 4; i.e., 120/4 = 30 mL/min. (*Lobato: Complications in Anesthesiology, p 433; Miller: Anesthesia, ed 6, pp 786-788*).

481. (A) Trisomy 21 or Down syndrome is the most common human chromosomal syndrome seen. An increase incidence of congenital hypothyroidism occurs. About one fourth of children with Down syndrome and many adults have smaller tracheas than predicted and require an endotracheal tube that is one or two sizes smaller. One should avoid unnecessary flexion or extension of the neck during intubation because occipito-atlantoaxial instability occurs in about 15% to 20% of patients. Because subluxation is relatively uncommon, routine neck radiographs for all Down patients are excessive. More than 40% of Down syndrome children have congenital heart disease, (e.g., endocardial cushion defects, ventricular septal defects, tetralogy of Fallot, patent ductus arteriosus). Although some children have hypotonia, an increased incidence of MH has not been reported in these patients (*Baum: Anesthesia for Genetic, Metabolic, and Dysmorphic Syndromes of Childhood, ed 2, pp 105-107; Hines: Stoelting's Anesthesia and Co-Existing Disease, ed 5, pp 611-612; Miller: Anesthesia, ed 6, p 1099*).

482. (B) Scopolamine is an anticholinergic that may produce mydriasis and cycloplegia. This can result in the inability of patient's eyes to accommodate (*Stoelting: Basics of Anesthesia, ed 5, p 172*).

483. (E) Neuroleptic malignant syndrome is a potentially fatal disease that affects 0.5% to 1% of all patients being treated with neuroleptic (antipsychotic) drugs. The syndrome develops gradually over 1 to 3 days in young males and is characterized by the following: (1) hyperthermia, (2) skeletal muscle rigidity, (3) autonomic instability manifested by changes in blood pressure and heart rate, and (4) fluctuating levels of consciousness. The mortality from neuroleptic malignant syndrome is 20% to 30%. Liver transaminases and creatine phosphokinase levels are often elevated in these patients. Treatment includes supportive care and administration of dantrolene. This disease may mimic MH because of its many similarities. One difference between neuroleptic malignant syndrome and MH is the fact that nondepolarizing muscle relaxants such as vecuronium or cisatracurium will cause flaccid paralysis in patients with neuroleptic malignant syndrome but not in patients with MH (*Stoelting: Pharmacology and Physiology in Anesthetic Practice, ed 4, p 412*).

484. (D) The classic signs of fat embolism include tachycardia, dyspnea, mental confusion, and fever, and frequently there may be a petechial rash on the upper part of the body. Fat embolism is more common after long bone fractures (e.g., femur and tibia) and usually occurs between 12 and 72 hours after long bone fractures (*Hines: Stoelting's Anesthesia and Co-Existing Disease, ed 5, p 193*).

485. (E) Remifentanil is an ultrashort-acting narcotic. Chemically it is a derivative of piperidine (like fentanyl), but remifentanil has an ester linkage and is rapidly broken down by nonspecific plasma as well as tissue esterases. The elimination half-life is less than 20 minutes and is best administered by a continuous infusion. Pseudocholinesterase deficiency or renal or hepatic failure does not affect remifentanil's rapid metabolism (*Barash: Clinical Anesthesia, ed 5, pp 371, 374; Stoelting: Pharmacology and Physiology in Anesthetic Practice, ed 4, p 114*).

486. (D) If a peanut or other foreign body becomes lost in the upper airway such that ventilation of the patient is impossible and retrieval is not feasible, the person performing the bronchoscopy should push the foreign body distally past the carina so that gas exchange can take place. Once the patient is stabilized, another attempt to retrieve the foreign body can be made (*Motoyama: Smith's Anesthesia for Infants and Children, ed 7, pp 815-818*).

487. (E) Anesthesia for extracorporeal shock wave lithotripsy may be accomplished with either general anesthesia or epidural anesthesia. When a patient is submerged in the stainless steel tub, the peripheral vasculature becomes compressed by the hydrostatic pressure, resulting in an increase in preload. Removing the patient from the tank has the opposite effect. In patients who have received epidural anesthesia, there is an increased incidence of hypotension caused by epidural-induced sympathectomy after they emerge from the bath (*Barash: Clinical Anesthesia, ed 5, pp 1030-1032*).

488. (E) The most common reason for unexpected hospital admission after outpatient general anesthesia, as well as a prolonged recovery-room stay (for both adults and children), is nausea and vomiting. Two other reasons for a prolonged recovery-room stay are pain and drowsiness (*Barash: Clinical Anesthesia, ed 5, p 1242*).

489. (A) Cholinergic crisis can be differentiated from myasthenic crisis by administering small IV doses of anticholinesterases. With a cholinergic crisis, there are significant muscarinic effects (e.g., salivation, bradycardia, miosis) and an accentuated muscle weakness. Because this patient's V_T decreased with the administration of edrophonium, the diagnosis of cholinergic crisis is made. Although atropine may be needed to treat the cholinergic symptoms, muscle weakness will be worse and these patients need to be intubated until the muscle strength returns (*Hines: Stoelting's Anesthesia and Co-Existing Disease, ed 5, p 452*).

490. (E) Tramadol, a synthetic codeine analogue, is a centrally acting analgesic. It can be used for mild to moderate pain but is not as effective as morphine or meperidine for severe or chronic pain. One drawback for tramadol's perioperative use is its high incidence of nausea and vomiting. Its mechanism of action for analgesia is complex.

It is a weak μ-receptor agonist, it inhibits serotonin and norepinephrine reuptake, and it enhances serotonin release. Tramadol-induced analgesia is not entirely reversed with naloxone, however, the respiratory depression and sedation can be reversed. Ondansetron, a serotonin antagonist, may interfere with part of tramadol's analgesic action. Because of its low μ-receptor agonist activity, it may be less likely to produce physical dependence than other stronger narcotics. Seizures have been reported in patients receiving tramadol alone. The drug should be used with caution in patients taking drugs that lower the seizure threshold, such as tricyclic antidepressants and SSRIs. It has some MAO inhibiting activity and should not be used in patients taking MAO inhibitors. Another warning is its use in patients who are depressed or suicidal. Tramadol is not recommended in depressed or suicidal patients since excessive doses, either alone or with other CNS depressants including alcohol, are a major cause of drug-related deaths with fatalities reported within the first hour of overdosage. Patients who are depressed or suicidal are better managed with non-narcotic analgesics (*Hardman: Goodman and Gilman's The Pharmacological Basis of Therapeutics ed 10, p 590; Physicians Desk Reference-2009, ed 63, pp 2428-2431; Stoelting: Pharmacology and Physiology in Anesthetic Practice, ed 4, p 117*).

491. (D) Premature infants are at increased risk for development of apnea until they have reached 60 weeks postconceptual age (PCA), which is defined as gestational age at birth (GA) plus chronologic age. Apnea in these patients is central apnea, that is, apnea associated with the absence of respiratory effort related to immaturity of the CNS. Infants with a history of apnea as well as anemia (Hct <30) are especially at risk. Because postoperative apnea is highest in the first 4 to 6 hours and may present up to 12 hours after surgery, monitoring of all infants (<60 weeks PCA) for apnea and bradycardia for at least 12 hours is recommended. In our practice, healthy full term infants (>38 weeks GA) that have not yet reached 44 weeks PCA and healthy preterm infants (<38 weeks) that have not reached 50 weeks PCA are admitted for overnight monitoring. See also question 631 (*Motoyama: Smith's Anesthesia for Infants and Children, ed 7, pp 24-25, 562-563, 875-876, 1163-1164*).

492. (E) In the absence of diuretics, oliguria associated with urine sodium concentration greater than 40 mEq/L and urine osmolality less than 400 mOsm/L is strongly suggestive of intrinsic renal disease (e.g., acute tubule necrosis) whereas prerenal causes have urine sodium concentration less than 20 mEq/L and urine osmolality greater than 400 mOsm/L. Furosemide, mannitol and dopamine, however, obscures the accurate diagnosis (*Hines: Stoelting's Anesthesia and Co-Existing Disease, ed 5, pp 325-327; Stoelting: Basics of Anesthesia, ed 5, pp 430-431*).

493. (C) In an unconscious patient, a unilateral dilated pupil would be a matter of grave concern. In an awake patient with a normal neurologic examination, however, it is less worrisome. An inferior alveolar nerve block involves injection of about 2 mL of 2% lidocaine around the inferior alveolar nerve just behind the molars in the lower jaw. Even a grossly misdirected needle probably could not reach the stellate ganglion, but were it possible, the result would be a Horner's syndrome (miosis, not mydriasis, ptosis, anhidrosis, and vasodilation over the face). Blockade of the ciliary ganglion could cause mydriasis on the ipsilateral side, but reaching the ciliary ganglion, located between the optic nerve and lateral rectus muscle about 1 cm from the posterior limit of the orbit, would be almost impossible with a needle directed toward the mandible. Glycopyrrolate administered systemically does not cause mydriasis, as it is not capable of crossing the blood-brain barrier. Lidocaine instilled directly into the eye does not produce mydriasis, but phenylephrine does. Care must be taken not to spray local anesthetic (with or without vasoconstrictor) into the eyes while applying topical anesthesia to the nares (*Stoelting: Pharmacology and Physiology in Anesthetic Practice, ed 4, p 304*).

494. (C) MAC is the minimum alveolar concentration of anesthetic that will prevent movement of 50% of patients when a skin incision is made at sea level (e.g., San Diego). MAC × 1.3 will prevent movement in 95% of patients. In this question, total gas flow is 4 L/min (1 L/min + 3 L/min). Roughly 75% of the total gas is N_2O. The MAC of N_2O is 104%. The patient is receiving about 0.75 MAC N_2O. The MAC for isoflurane is 1.15. A concentration of 0.85% would represent 0.75 MAC. Because MACs are additive, the total MAC would be 1.5 (*Barash: Clinical Anesthesia, ed 5, pp 397-398; Stoelting: Basics of Anesthesia, ed 5, p 82*).

495. (E) Cardiac output increases by about 100 mL/min for each kilogram of weight gained. It is estimated that every kilogram of adipose tissue contains nearly 3000 m of additional blood vessels. The additional cardiac output is due to ventricular dilation and increased stroke volume, as resting heart rates are not increased in obese patients (*Hines: Stoelting's Anesthesia and Co-Existing Disease, ed 5, p 302; Stoelting: Basics of Anesthesia, ed 5, p 448*).

496. (E) Fenoldopam (Corlopam) is a selective dopamine-1 receptor agonist with significant vasodilating properties. It has moderate affinity for α_2-receptors but has no affinity for dopamine-2, α_1, β, $5\text{-}HT_1$, or $5\text{-}HT_2$ receptors.

It is used for treatment of patients with severe hypertension (especially with reduced renal function) and is administered as an IV infusion. It can be used as an alternative to sodium nitroprusside and has the advantage of no thiocyanate toxicity, rebound effect, or "coronary steal" effect, but it does contain sodium bisulfite and is contraindicated in patients with a known sulfite sensitivity. Dopexamine (Dopacard) is a synthetic analogue related to dopamine with intrinsic activity at dopamine as well as β_2-receptors and is used as an inotropic agent (*Hardman: Goodman & Gilman's The Pharmacologic Basis of Therapeutics, ed 10, p 227; Miller: Anesthesia, ed 6, pp 649-650; Stoelting: Pharmacology and Physiology in Anesthetic Practice, ed 4, p 495*).

497. (D) Ideally, factor VIII levels should be raised to 100% predicted before elective surgery to ensure that the levels will not fall below 30% intraoperatively. Thirty percent of the normal factor VIII concentration or greater is thought to be necessary for a patient who is to undergo major surgery. Elimination half-time of factor VIII is 12 hours. This may be accomplished with factor VIII concentrate or cryoprecipitate. Fresh frozen plasma is no longer considered therapy for hemophilia (*Hines: Stoelting's Anesthesia and Co-Existing Disease, ed 5, pp 419-420*).

498. (A) Hemophilia A is associated with decreased levels of factor VIII. PTT tests the intrinsic coagulation cascade and would be abnormally elevated in all but the most mild disease. A normal PTT is 25 to 35 seconds. Platelet count PT and bleeding times are normal (*Hines: Stoelting's Anesthesia and Co-Existing Disease, ed 5, p 420; Kasper: Harrison's Principles of Internal Medicine, ed 16, pp 680-681*).

499. (E) Conventional peripheral nerve stimulators deliver four twitches at 2 Hz spaced 0.5 second apart. These devices were designed with the knowledge that successive twitches deplete acetylcholine stores. After the fourth twitch, there is no additional decrement in twitch height (*Stoelting: Basics of Anesthesia, ed 5, p 150*).

500. (B) Inferior ischemia is associated with blockage or spasm of the right coronary artery. The right coronary artery supplies blood to the atrioventricular node in 90% of patients. Complete heart block therefore is not unexpected in patients with severe CAD involving the right coronary artery (*Hines: Stoelting's Anesthesia and Co-Existing Disease, ed 5, p 19*).

501. (B) Minimum alveolar concentration (MAC) is influenced by a variety of disease states, conditions, drugs, and other factors. Drugs that increase CNS catecholamines, such as MAO inhibitors, tricyclic antidepressants, acute amphetamine ingestion, and cocaine, increase MAC. Other factors that increase MAC include hyperthermia, hypernatremia, patients with natural red hair, and infancy. It is interesting that MAC values are higher for infants than for neonates or older children and adults. Thyroid gland dysfunction including hyperthyroidism does not affect the MAC. Factors that lower MAC include narcotics, IV anesthetics, local anesthetics (except cocaine) and other sedatives, age (6% per decade), hypothermia, hypoxia, severe anemia (e.g., Hgb < 5). The following table modified from the references in this question summarizes the impact of various factors on MAC (*Barash: Clinical Anesthesia, ed, 5 pp 397-398; Morgan: Clinical Anesthesiology, ed 4, p 165; Stoelting: Basics of Anesthesia, ed 5, p 83*

IMPACT OF PHYSIOLOGIC AND PHARMACOLOGIC FACTORS ON MINIMUM ALVEOLAR CONCENTRATION

No Change in MAC	Increase in MAC	Decrease in MAC
Duration of anesthesia	Drugs that increase CNS catecholamines (MAO inhibitors, tricyclic antidepressants acute amphetamine use, cocaine, ephedrine)	CNS depressants (narcotics, IV anesthetics, chronic amphetamine use)
Type of surgery	Chronic ethanol abuse	Acute ethanol use
Hyperthyroidism	Hyperthermia	Hypothermia
Hypothyroidism	Hypernatremia	Hyponatremia
Gender	Infants	Increasing age
Hyperkalemia	Patients with natural red hair	Pregnancy
		Hypoxia

502. (B) Long-term lithium therapy in patients with manic-depressive illness may be associated with nephrogenic diabetes insipidus. Hypothyroidism may develop in about 5% of patients because lithium can inhibit the release of thyroid hormones. Lithium is almost 100% renally excreted. Reabsorption occurs at the proximal convoluted tubule and is inversely related to the concentration of sodium in the glomerular filtrate. Consequently, administration of diuretics (mainly thiazide, but to a lesser extend loop diuretics) may lead to the development of toxic lithium levels. Lithium has sedative properties and may reduce the need for IV and inhalational anesthetic agents. It may prolong the duration of action of both pancuronium and succinylcholine, but it is not associated with an exaggerated release of potassium when succinylcholine is administered (*Hardman: Goodman & Gilman's The Pharmacological Basis of Therapeutics, ed 10, pp 508-509; Hines: Stoelting's Anesthesia and Co-Existing Disease, ed 5, p 539*).

503. (E) Carcinoid tumors can arise wherever enterochromaffin cells are present. Most (>70%) originate in the intestine and about 20% originate in the lung. Of those that originate in the gastrointestinal tract, 50% occur in the appendix, 25% in the ileum, and 20% in the rectum. These interesting tumors were called carcinoid because they were originally believed not to metastasize. We now know this is not true. The hormones released by the nonmetastatic tumors reach the liver by the portal vein and are rapidly inactivated. However, once metastases reach the liver, the released hormones reach the systemic circulation and produce signs and symptoms of the "carcinoid syndrome." Symptoms include cutaneous flushing, abdominal pain, vomiting, diarrhea, hypotension or hypertension, bronchospasm, and hyperglycemia. The natural hormone somatostatin suppresses the release of serotonin and other vasoactive substances from the tumor. Because the half-life is about 3 minutes, somatostatin is given by infusion. Octreotide is a synthetic somatostatin analogue with a half-life of 2.5 hours and is given SQ or IV for the prevention and treatment of carcinoid symptoms (e.g., hypotension, hypertension, bronchospasm). However, the treatment of hypotension in patients with carcinoid disease is different because ephedrine, epinephrine, and norepinephrine can release vasoactive hormones from the tumor and make the hypotension worse. Hypotension is best treated with fluids and IV octreotide or somatostatin. Hypertension is treated with deepening the anesthetic and administering octreotide, somatostatin or labetalol. Bronchospasm is treated with IV octreotide, somatostatin or nebulized ipratropium. When giving anesthesia to these patients it is probably wise to avoid drugs that release histamine and other vasoactive hormones that may precipitate symptoms. Propofol or etomidate are good induction agents, followed by maintenance anesthesia with a volatile anesthetic (e.g., isoflurane, sevoflurane or desflurane) and/or nitrous oxide with oxygen. Vecuronium, cisatracurium and rocuronium appear to be safe muscle relaxants. Fentanyl, sufentanil, alfentanil and remifentanil and benzodiazepines are also safe to use. The serotonin antagonist ondansetron is a useful antiemetic (*Barash: Clinical Anesthesia, ed 5, pp 1058-1059; Hines: Stoelting's Anesthesia and Co-Existing Disease, ed 5, pp 289-291; Physicians Desk Reference-2009, ed 63, pp 2300-2306*).

504. (C) Testicular innervation can be traced up to the T10 dermatomal level. For this reason, any operation that involves manipulation or traction on the testicles must have adequate anesthesia to prevent pain. This can be achieved with spinal or epidural anesthesia, which is associated with a T10 level of blockade (*Barash: Clinical Anesthesia, ed 5, p 701*).

505. (D) The Glasgow Coma Scale has three categories: eye opening for which a maximum of 4 points can be received; best verbal response for a maximum of 5 points; and best motor response for a maximum of 6 points. The higher the score the better the response, the minimal score for each category is 1. Mild head injury scores are 13 to 15, moderate are 9 to 12 and severe are 3 to 8. This severe head injured patient is totally unresponsive and would receive a score of 3 (*Barash: Clinical Anesthesia, ed 5, p 782*).

506. (A) Insulin metabolism involves both the liver and kidneys. Renal dysfunction, however, has a greater impact on insulin metabolism than does hepatic dysfunction. In fact, unexpected prolonged effects of insulin sometimes are seen in patients with renal disease (*Stoelting: Pharmacology and Physiology in Anesthetic Practice, ed 4, p 478*).

507. (B) Most pulse oximeters illuminate tissue with two wavelengths of light; 660-nm red light and 940-nm infrared light. Since carboxyhemoglobin has an absorbance at 660 nm, very similar to O_2 hemoglobin, it produces a falsely elevated Sao_2 when present in the blood. Hemoglobin F, bilirubin, and fluorescein dye have no effect on pulse oximetry. Methylene blue, as well as indigo carmine and indocyanine green, lowers the Sao_2 as measured by pulse oximetry. Methemoglobin absorbs red and infrared light equally well and gives saturation readings of 85% (*Barash: Clinical Anesthesia, ed 5, pp 672, 1280; Stoelting: Basics of Anesthesia, ed 5, pp 312-313*).

508. (A) Hypothyroidism occurs when there is a decreased amount of the circulating thyroid hormones (T_4, T_3, or both). It is estimated to occur in about 0.5% to 0.8% of the adult population. There are many causes of hypothyroidism, and they are classified into two main groups. The most common group (95% of cases) is primary hypothyroidism, where the thyroid gland is not capable of making enough hormones despite an adequate amount of TSH (thyrotropin). Secondary hypothyroidism (5% of cases) occurs when there is CNS dysfunction, i.e., hypothalamic or pituitary disease and low levels of TSH. It is the free and not total T_3 or T_4 level that parallels thyroid status. The T_3 or T_4 resin uptake test is used to measure free amounts of T_3 or T_4, but it is the TSH level that is used to differentiate primary from secondary hypothyroidism. Although antithyroid antibodies such as thyroid antimicrosomal antibody are seen in 95% of patients with multinodular diffuse goiter of Graves' disease, the most common type of hyperthyroidism, it also is seen in about 10% of adults with no thyroid disease (*Barash: Clinical Anesthesia, ed 5, pp 1130-1131; Hines: Stoelting's Anesthesia and Co-Existing Disease ed 5, pp 384-386; Miller: Anesthesia, ed 6, pp 1047-1048*).

509. (A) Gabapentin, an anticonvulsant, was developed to be a centrally active GABA agonist but does not appear to interact with GABA receptors. Its mechanism for producing analgesia is unclear, but it may involve inhibition of voltage-activated calcium channels as well as potentiating GABA release. Carbamazepine slows the recovery rate of voltage-gated sodium channels, but it also is an anticonvulsant. Carbamazepine is indicated in the treatment of trigeminal neuralgia (*Stoelting: Pharmacology and Physiology in Anesthetic Practice, ed 4, pp 571-575; Loeser: Bonica's Management of Pain, ed 3, pp 106, 1728-1730*).

510. (B) In 2007, the American Heart Association revised the guidelines for "Prevention of Infective Endocarditis." Patients with mitral valve prolapse (MVP) do not need prophylaxis. Only patients in the highest risk groups, such as prosthetic cardiac valves, previous infective endocarditis, several types of congenital heart disease and cardiac transplantation recipients who develop cardiac valvulopathy need prophylactic antibiotics for elective GI or GU procedures (see also question 915) (*Wilson W, Taubert KA, Gewitz, et al.; Prevention of infective endocarditis - Guidelines from the American Heart Association. Circulation, 2007; 115:1736-1754. (http://circ.ahajournals.org)*).

511. (B) Perioperative visual loss associated with non-ocular surgery is rare and may result from corneal trauma, retinal artery occlusion, retinal vein occlusion, optic nerve ischemia or cortical disease. Although overall a rare problem, it may develop in up to 1% of prone spinal surgical cases and is most commonly due to ischemic optic neuropathy. The cause is unknown and multifactorial. Associated factors include prolong intraoperative hypotension, anemia (Hgb < 8), large intraoperative blood loss, prolonged surgery and facial edema. It is more common in males and in patients with peripheral vascular disease, diabetes mellitus, and tobacco users (*Lobato: Complications in Anesthesiology pp 418-422; Miller: Anesthesia, ed 6, pp 3005-3011*).

512. (E) Postoperative shivering or postanesthetic tremor can occur during recovery from all types of general anesthesia. If profound, shivering can increase metabolic rate and O_2 consumption (100%-200%) with an associated increase in cardiac output and minute ventilation. Although shivering usually occurs in patients with decreased body temperature, it also may occur in patients with normal body temperature after anesthesia. Postanesthesia shivering is best treated by a combination of supplemental oxygen, rewarming the patient and/or administering IV meperidine. Other less frequently used pharmacologic treatments include clonidine, magnesium sulfate, calcium chloride, chlorpromazine, droperidol, and other opioids (e.g., butorphanol). Application of radiant heat to the face, head, neck, chest, and abdomen has been shown to eliminate shivering within minutes in postoperative patients, despite low core body temperatures (*Longnecker: Principles and Practice of Anesthesiology, ed 2, pp 2318-2319; Morgan Clinical Anesthesiology, ed 4, pp 771-772; Stoelting: Basics of Anesthesia, ed 5, pp 574-575*).

513. (D) The ECG signs of hyperkalemia include narrowed and peaked T waves (earliest manifestation of hyperkalemia), decrease in P wave amplitude, prolonged PR interval, and a widened QRS interval. In extreme cases, the ECG can appear as a sine wave as well as cardiac arrhythmias (e.g., sinus arrest, supraventricular tachycardia, atrial fibrillation, PVCs, ventricular tachycardia and ventricular fibrillation). These changes are potentiated by hypocalcemia and intravenous calcium can rapidly correct some of these ECG changes. An increase in U-wave amplitude suggests hypokalemia, not hyperkalemia (*Miller: Anesthesia, ed 6, p 1106*).

514. (B) If the inspiratory valve becomes stuck in the open position, it will "malfunction" only during exhalation since, during inhalation, it is supposed to be open. During the exhalation phase of breathing, exhaled gases will exit through the expiratory valve into the expiratory limb of the circuit and beyond (proper path) as well as through the inspiratory valve into the inspiratory limb of the circuit (errant path). Gases traveling into the inspiratory limb (old gas) will be returned to the patient with next breath. The volume of recently exhaled gas is now drawn back into the patient's lungs along with the "new" gas that would be inspired in a fully functional breathing circuit. The net effect is that oxygen, sevoflurane, and N_2O will all be diluted, but the patient rebreathes CO_2, thus it will be the only gas with an increased inspired concentration (normal inspired CO_2 is zero) as a result of the stuck inspiratory valve (*Barash: Clinical Anesthesia, ed 5, p 580*).

515. (E) Enlargement of the tongue and epiglottis predisposes the patient to upper airway obstruction and makes visualization of the vocal cords more difficult. The vocal cords are enlarged, making the glottic opening narrower. In addition, subglottic narrowing may be present as well as tracheal compression from an enlarged thyroid (seen in about 25% of acromegalic patients). This often necessitates the use of a narrower endotracheal tube than one might choose based on the facial enlargement. The placement of nasal airways may be more difficult due to the enlarged nasal turbinates. The use of CPAP is contraindicated after transsphenoidal hypophysectomy (*Barash: Clinical Anesthesia, ed 5, pp 776, 1149; Fleisher: Anesthesia and Uncommon Diseases, ed 5, pp 21-22; Hines: Stoelting's Anesthesia and Co-Existing Disease, ed 5, pp 402-403*).

516. (A) There are four types of immune mediated allergic reactions. Anaphylaxis is a Type I IgE mediated reaction that involves mast cells and basophils. Anaphylactoid reactions appear like anaphylaxis but are not immune mediated. Tryptase is a neutral protease normally stored in mast cells but is released into systemic circulation during anaphylactic but not anaphylactoid reactions. Tryptase levels would need to be measured within 1 to 2 hours of the suspected allergic reaction. Plasma histamine levels return to baseline within 30 to 60 minutes of an anaphylactic reaction. Laudanosine is a normal metabolic product of atracurium metabolism (*Hines: Stoelting's Anesthesia and Co-Existing Disease, ed 5, p 526; Morgan: Clinical Anesthesiology, ed 4, p 972*).

517. (B) Signs of MH reflect the hypermetabolic state (up to 10 times normal) that develops. Clinical signs include tachycardia, tachypnea, arterial hypoxemia, hypercarbia (e.g., $Paco_2$ 100-200 mm Hg), metabolic and respiratory acidosis (e.g., pH 6.80-7.15), hyperkalemia, hypotension, muscle rigidity, trismus after succinylcholine administration, and increased body temperature. Mixed venous oxygen tension would be very low. The clinical presentations are quite variable and some reactions may not develop until the postoperative period (*Hines: Stoelting's Anesthesia and Co-Existing Disease, ed 5, pp 620-622*).

518. (D) The selective serotonin reuptake inhibitor (SSRI) fluoxetine, is one of the most potent inhibitors of the cytochrome P-450 enzymes CYP3A4 and CYP2D6. CYP2D6 facilitates the conversion of codeine to morphine, meaning the response from a "normal" dose would be less than expected because of decreased conversion. Oxycodone and hydrocodone are metabolized by CYP2D6 to their active form as well and a "normal" dose of these would give less response than expected. Thus, codeine, oxycodone and hydrocodone would be poor analgesic choices for patients taking SSRIs. CYP3A4 is responsible for the metabolism of fentanyl, sufentanil and alfentanil. Remifentanil is metabolized by non-specific plasma esterases (*Miller: Anesthesia, ed 6, p 101*).

519. (A) Symptoms of a mainstem or bronchial intubation include asymmetric chest expansion, unilateral breath sounds, elevation of peak airway pressures, and arterial blood gas abnormalities (e.g., hypoxemia). Frequently, bronchial intubation is intentional (e.g., thoracic surgery with double lumen endotracheal tubes) but if undetected with a single lumen tube, atelectasis, hypoxia and pulmonary edema may result in time. Peak airway pressures can also increase with many conditions such as airway obstruction (e.g., kinked endotracheal tube, secretions, overinflated cuffs), bronchospasm, increasing V_T, increase in chest wall muscle tone (rigid chest with narcotics, coughing), and tension pneumothorax. If a tension pneumothorax develops, associated hypotension usually is present. Pulmonary embolism would not cause the peak airway pressure to rise as in this case (*Lobato: Complications in Anesthesiology, pp 101-102*).

520. (D) Although hemodynamic instability can occur at any time during liver transplantation, it is during the initial part of the reperfusion phase, when the vascular clamps are removed from the liver graft, when cardiovascular instability is most marked. At this time there can be profound hypotension, reduced cardiac contractility, cardiac arrhythmias as well as hyperkalemic cardiac arrest. Epinephrine, atropine, calcium, and sodium bicarbonate should be available, as well as blood products, during this critical part of the surgery (*Miller: Anesthesia, ed 6, pp 2249-2252; Stoelting: Basics of Anesthesia, ed 5, p 534*).

521. **(E)**   Metabolic and physiologic conditions as well as certain medications can contribute to a prolonged duration of action of nondepolarizing neuromuscular blockade. Metabolic and physiologic conditions include respiratory acidosis, myasthenia syndromes, hepatic/renal failure, hypocalcemia, hypothermia, and hypermagnesemia. Both inhaled and local anesthetics as well as corticosteroids, many antibiotics (e.g., polymyxins, aminoglycosides, lincosamines [e.g., clindamycin], metronidazole [Flagyl]), calcium channel blockers, dantrolene and furosemide can prolong nondepolarizing neuromuscular blockade (*Stoelting: Basics of Anesthesia, ed 5, p 566*).

522. **(E)**   Drugs considered unsafe for patients susceptible to MH include all of the volatile anesthetics and the depolarizing muscle relaxant succinylcholine. All local anesthetics (both amide and ester), N_2O, opiates, barbiturates, ketamine, propofol, vasoactive drugs, calcium salts, antibiotics, antihistamines, nondepolarizing muscle relaxants, as well as drugs used to reverse nondepolarizing muscle relaxants, are safe (i.e., nontriggering) in patients susceptible to MH (*Barash: Clinical Anesthesia, ed 5, pp 533-534; Miller: Anesthesia, ed 6, p 1182*).

523. **(E)**   Rare muscle diseases can have dramatic anesthetic implications. Malignant hyperthermia (MH) is among the most important manifestations of a muscular disorder. Malignant hyperthermia is thought to be caused by alterations in calcium control in muscle sarcoplasmic reticulum in response to succinylcholine or potent volatile anesthetics (most likely mediated by mutations of the ryanodine receptor). Because MH is a disorder in muscle metabolism, rigidity during administration of a volatile anesthetic or after succinylcholine use may be the presenting sign. Additionally, administration of any muscle relaxant would not provide muscle relaxation and succinylcholine would be contraindicated. The patient does have a respiratory and metabolic acidosis and significantly increasing minute ventilation with 100% oxygen and the use of sodium bicarbonate would be needed; however, stopping the triggering agent and administration of dantrolene is most important (*Hines: Stoelting's Anesthesia and Co-Existing Disease, ed 5, pp 620-623*).

524. **(E)**   Atropine and scopolamine cross the placenta easily, whereas glycopyrrolate is poorly transferred across the placenta. Although neostigmine crosses the placenta poorly, enough does cross the placenta and can cause fetal bradycardia in utero. That is why it is better to reverse muscle relaxants in pregnant patients for non-delivery surgery with neostigmine and atropine (*Chestnut: Obstetric Anesthesia, ed 3, p 60*).

525. **(A)**   The overall estimated incidence of postoperative nausea and vomiting (PONV) for all surgical procedures is 25% to 30%. Several factors are associated with an increased risk of PONV including patient related factors (e.g., a previous history of PONV, history of motion sickness, nonsmoking, female gender, pregnancy, obesity), certain surgical procedures (e.g., eye muscle surgery, ear, nose, and throat (ENT), dental), as well as postoperative pain and narcotic use (*Lobato: Complications in Anesthesiology pp 571-573; Stoelting: Basics of Anesthesia, ed 5 p 575*).

526. **(C)**   Ketorolac is one of the few nonsteroidal anti-inflammatory drugs (NSAIDs) approved for parenteral use. Although NSAIDs have analgesic and anti-inflammatory effects without ventilatory depression; they also inhibit platelet aggregation, can produce gastric ulceration, are associated with renal dysfunction and may impair bone healing. Nonsteroidal anti-inflammatory drugs are contraindicated in patients undergoing spinal fusion, where bone healing is essential to a successful surgical procedure (*Stoelting: Pharmacology and Physiology in Anesthesia Practice, ed 4, pp 276-282, 2872-2888*).

527. **(A)**   Sickle-cell anemia is an inherited disease that affects approximately 0.3% to 1% of the black population in the United States. Affected patients are homozygous for hemoglobin S such that 70% to 98% of the hemoglobin found in their RBCs is of the unstable S type, resulting in severe hemolytic anemia. Factors that favor the formation of sickle cells include arterial hypoxemia, acidosis, dehydration, and reductions in body temperature. Inhaled nitric oxide and other new investigational drugs may help reduce the sickling process and may even unsickle cells (*Fleisher: Anesthesia and Uncommon Diseases, ed 5, pp 362-363; Hines: Stoeling's Anesthesia and Co-Existing Disease, ed 5, pp 411-412*).

528. **(C)**   Although many books suggest that obesity is the most common cause of OSA, more recent data suggests that a large neck circumference (>44 cm) reflects pharyngeal fat deposition and is more strongly correlated with OSA than obesity (BMI >30). Other risk factors include male gender, middle age, evening alcohol consumption or sleep-inducing medications (*Hines: Stoelting's Anesthesia and Co-Existing Disease, ed 5, pp 299-301; Miller: Anesthesia, ed 6, p 1030; Stoelting: Basics of Anesthesia, ed 5, pp 411-412*).

529. **(D)** The ASA closed claims task force lists the leading causes of malpractice claims against anesthesiologists in the 1990s to be death (22%), followed by nerve damage (21%), and brain damage (10%) (*Barash: Clinical Anesthesia, ed 5, p 101*).

530. **(C)** Cardiac resynchronization therapy (CRT) is used in patients with heart failure (EF < 35%) and ventricular conductive delay (prolonged QRS complex usually is 120-150 msec). The conduction delay creates a mechanical dyssynchrony and worsens the heart failure. Cardiac resynchronization therapy requires biventricular pacing with one lead in the coronary sinus to activate the LV. Cardiac resynchronization therapy has nothing to do with breathing. Although CRT has nothing to do with an ICD, many patients may require both as the typical scenario is a patient with poor LV function is also at risk for sudden death. Most of these patients also have underlying CAD (*Hines: Stoelting's Anesthesia and Co-Existing Disease, ed 5, p 112; Miller: Anesthesia, ed 6, pp 1418-1419, 1427-1428*).

531. **(D)** Patients with syndrome X (also called metabolic syndrome X) have insulin resistance that leads to elevated levels of insulin and the metabolic changes that occur with elevated insulin levels, except that hypoglycemia does not develop. Associated with it are low levels of high-density lipoproteins, hypertension, and increased plasminogen activator inhibitor-1 levels, which are associated with coronary artery disease. Many of these patients are obese (*Miller: Anesthesia, ed 6, p 1777*).

532. **(C)** The parenteral to oral conversion for morphine sulfate is 1:3, thus 30 mg morphine parenterally would be similar to 30 mg × 3 = 90 mg of morphine orally. The parenteral to oral conversion for methadone is 1:2 (*Hardman: Goodman & Gilman's The Pharmacological Basis of Therapeutics, ed 11, p 606*).

533. **(A)** It is the partial pressure of the inhalation anesthetic in the brain (Pbr) that determines activity (*Stoelting: Basics of Anesthesia, ed 5, pp 82-83*).

534. **(E)** Retinopathy of prematurity (retrolental fibroplasia) is a hazard associated with O_2 administration to neonates up to 44 weeks (gestational age + life age). It is especially a hazard in the extremely premature (birth weight less than 1000 g and gestational age less than 28 weeks). Bronchopulmonary dysplasia is a chronic lung disorder that afflicts infants who required mechanical ventilation at birth to treat respiratory distress syndrome. CO_2 retention is a hazard in patients with chronic obstructive lung disease. Adsorption atelectasis is a potential hazard of oxygen administration in any patient receiving oxygen concentrations greater than 50%. It results from rapid uptake of oxygen into the circulation greater than the delivery of oxygen by ventilation. Normally, the presence of nitrogen serves as an internal splint, protecting the alveoli from collapse. Prolonged high concentration of oxygen can damage "normal lungs" if given for prolonged periods of time and may lead from mild irritation to tracheobronchitis to pulmonary interstitial edema to pulmonary fibrosis (*Miller: Anesthesia, ed 6, pp 711, 716, 717, 2853; Morgan: Clinical Anesthesiology, ed 4, pp 1028-1029*).

535. **(A)** All of the nerves listed in this question are derived from the fifth cranial nerve (trigeminal nerve) except the great auricular nerve. The ophthalmic nerve (V1 branch of trigeminal nerve) gives rise to the supratrochlear, infratrochlear, and supraorbital nerves. The infraorbital nerve is a branch of V2 (maxillary branch of the trigeminal nerve). The mental nerve is a branch of V3 (mandibular nerve). The great auricular nerve arises from branches of C2 and C3 spinal nerves and innervates the skin of the outer ear, the mastoid process and the parotid gland (*Miller: Anesthesia, ed 6, pp 1706-1707, 2518*).

536. **(D)** Cerebral vasospasm is often associated in patients who have suffered a subarachnoid bleed. Angiographic evidence of vasospasm can be noted in up to 70% of patients, however, clinical vasospasm with detectable ischemia (e.g., mental confusion, lethargy, focal motor and speech impairments) is detected in about 30% of patients. When clinical vasospasm develops, it usually occurs between 4 and 12 days after the bleed. Although it may resolve spontaneously, it may also progress to coma and death within a few hours or days. Rebleeding tends to occur earlier, i.e., within 24 hours (*Barash: Clinical Anesthesia, ed 5, p 778*).

537. **(A)** Thyroid storm (thyrotoxicosis) is a medical emergency with a 10% to 75% mortality rate. It usually occurs in poorly controlled or undiagnosed Graves' disease patients. It may develop intraoperatively but more likely develops 6 to 18 hours after surgery. Symptoms include mental status changes, tachycardia, fever, cardiac arrhythmias. Treatment includes large doses of dexamethasone, which inhibits the synthesis, release and conversion of T_4 to T_3. Propylthiouracil inhibits thyroid hormone production. Sodium iodine is used to inhibit release of thyroid hormone from the thyroid gland. Propranolol helps to control the tachycardiac response and may inhibit conversion of T_4 in the periphery. Acetaminophen is used to help control the temperature. Aspirin is contraindicated since it displaces thyroid hormones from thyroglobin and could aggravate the disease (*Morgan: Clinical Anesthesiology, ed 4, pp 1016, 1017; Stoelting: Basics of Anesthesia, ed 5, p 443*).

538. (B.) The most common adverse cardiac event in pediatric population is bradycardia. An outcome study from the Medical College of Virginia examined the incidence of bradycardia in nearly 8000 children younger than 4 years old. The most common causes of bradycardia are cardiac disease or surgery and inhalation anesthesia, followed by hypoxemia. Of those children who had bradycardia, hypotension occurred in 30%, asystole or ventricular fibrillation in 10%, and death in 8%. Tachycardia, which is common, is not an adverse event (*Motoyama: Smith's Anesthesia for Infants and Children, ed 7, p 1161*).

539. (C) Mask ventilation, one of the most basic anesthesia techniques, can be challenging in some patients. Patients who are prone to airway obstruction can be more difficult due to extra airway tissue (i.e. obese patients with a BMI > 26), patients without teeth (i.e., tongue is closer to the roof of the mouth and face conformity may not fit the mask well), patients who snore (i.e., already have reason for airway obstruction). Mask ventilation can also be more difficult in patients who have a beard (i.e., harder to get a good mask seal), patients whose age is greater than 55, patients with facial tumors and patients with facial trauma. Use of an oral airway may be needed in many of these patients (*Stoelting: Basics of Anesthesia, ed 5, p 215; Miller: Anesthesia, ed 6, pp 1623-1625*).

540. (A) Whenever perfusion to an extremity is inadequate (e.g., trauma or poor perfusion), hypoxic edema develops, producing swelling. When this occurs in a compartment, tissue pressures rise, decreasing capillary perfusion. Symptoms of compartment syndrome include extreme pain unrelieved by analgesics, paresthesias, paralysis and pallor. Extensive rhabdomyolysis may develop as well as permanent nerve and muscle injury in the compartment. Because the problem is at the tissue level, pulses and capillary refill may still be present. Treatment includes fasciotomy to relieve the elevated pressure (*Barash: Clinical Anesthesia, ed 5, pp 652-653, 1279; Miller: Anesthesia, ed 6, pp 2478-2479*).

541. (B) The amount and distribution of CSF is different in neonates compared with adults. The neonate has about 4 mL/kg of CSF compared to the adult's 2 mL/kg. In addition, almost half of the neonate's CSF is in the spinal subarachnoid space, compared with about a quarter of the adult's CSF in the spinal subarachnoid space. These factors help explain why the dose is greater in neonates and infants and of shorter duration compared to adults (*Motoyama: Smith's Anesthesia for Infants and Children, ed 7, p 467*).

542. (A) Endotracheal tube sizes are measured according to the internal diameter (ID). They are available in 0.5 mm ID increments (*Stoelting: Basics of Anesthesia, ed 5, p 218*).

543. (B) Magnetic resonance imaging (MRI) scanners have superconducting electrical currents that produce large magnetic fields (up to 6 m) and are always "on". The presence of any ferromagnetic objects in the room may cause a missile-type injury when the objects are strongly attracted to the scanner. If a patient is pinned into the scanner by a magnetic object that flew into the scanner, the MRI technicians may have to turn off the superconducting magnet. During magnetic shutdown (quench) the scanner will become extremely cold (*Stoelting: Basics of Anesthesia, ed 5, pp 553-554*).

544. (C) Carbon monoxide is a colorless, odorless gas which binds to hemoglobin with an affinity over 200 times stronger than oxygen. Inhalation of CO is a major cause of morbidity and mortality in the United States. A dual wave (660 nm and 940 nm) pulse oximeter is incapable of distinguishing CO hemoglobin from oxyhemoglobin, but the distinction is easily made in the clinical laboratory with a co-oximeter. Significant quantities of methemoglobin would result in a saturation of 85% of the pulse oximeter. The slight right shift from a mild acidemia would be insufficient to account for 90% saturation in the face of a Pao_2 of 190. Furthermore, the pulse oximeter reading would be nearly the same as the co-oximeter value (*Miller: Anesthesia, ed 6, pp 1450-1451; Hines: Stoelting's Anesthesia and Co-Existing Disease, ed 5, p 552*).

545. (A) The pathway for SSEP monitoring of the lower extremity starts with a stimulus of the posterior tibial nerve, which generates an impulse that passes through the dorsal root ganglion into the dorsal (posterior) columns and then to the dorsal column nuclei. Second order nerves carry the impulse across the midline to the thalamus and the impulse travels over third order nerves to the sensory cortex of the brain. Electrodes in the scalp record the electrical activity in the brain. Severe hypotension or ischemia in any portion of the pathway along which the induced signal is conducted can result in a reduced evoked potential amplitude or increased latency. Volatile anesthetic administration in MAC values greater than 0.5 to 0.75 can produce a similar effect. Barbiturates, benzodiazepines, propofol and other sedative drugs can likewise interfere with SSEP monitoring. Anterior spinal artery syndrome affects the anterior (motor) portion of the spinal cord and does not interfere with SSEP monitoring (*Stoelting: Basics of Anesthesia, ed 5, pp 313-314*).

546. (D) Diabetic autonomic neuropathy can affect the autonomic nervous system to such an extent that atropine and propranolol would have little effect (because there would be nothing to block). After heart transplantation, the new heart (donor heart) is denervated and will not respond to autonomic nervous system blocking drugs. Brain death by definition is associated with absence of autonomic function. A high spinal would be associated with total sympathectomy and propranolol would have no effect on heart rate, but the vagus nerve would be unaffected. Atropine would have no effect on a patient with atrial fibrillation and complete heart block (*Hines: Stoelting's Anesthesia and Co-Existing Disease, ed 5, pp 22, 213, 375; Stoelting: Basics of Anesthesia, ed 5, pp 260, 438-439*).

547. (A)   548. (B)   549. (D)   550. (C)   551. (D)   552. (B)

553. (A)   554. (E)

There are three categories of biological weapons (A,B,C). All of the diseases in this question are in the highly contagious Category A agents.

Smallpox is caused by a virus *(Variola major)* and in 1980 was declared extinct by the World Health Organization. The incubation period was 7 to 14 days and patients with the disease presented with malaise, headache, fever. Two to 4 days later a characteristic rash develops where all lesions are at the same stage (papules, vesicles, pustules and scabs). Exposed patients and health care workers who received a vaccination within 4 days of exposure had greatly attenuated symptoms. Unvaccinated patients who were untreated had a mortality rate of greater than 30%. Patients who previously had been vaccinated had a lower mortality rate. Treatment includes the drug cidofovir.

Anthrax is caused by an aerobic Gram-positive spore forming bacillus *(Bacillus anthracis)* and has three primary forms (cutaneous, gastrointestinal, inhalational). Weaponized anthrax is mainly an inhalational disease. Inhalational anthrax symptoms occur within 1 to 7 days of exposure and initially looks like viral flu (fever, chills, myalgia, and a non-productive cough). Later on, the patient's mediastinal lymph nodes, where the spores germinate, enlarge, producing a widened mediastinum that can be seen on a chest x-ray film. Treatment is primarily with ciprofloxacin, prophylaxis to exposed personnel includes 60 days of ciprofloxacin. Mortality rate for inhaled anthrax is greater than 80%.

Plague is caused by a Gram-negative coccobacillus *(Yersinia pestis)* and has two forms, bubonic and pneumonic. With the more common bubonic plague there is painful swelling of the lymph nodes (buboes) that can grow to 5 to 10 cm in diameter. The patients develop cyanosis, shock and gangrene in peripheral tissues (black death). If the lungs become infected, pneumonic plague develops, which if untreated has 100% mortality. Treatment is primarily with streptomycin, although gentamicin, tetracycline and chloramphenicol have been used.

Botulism is caused by the toxin from *Clostridium botulinum*. Because this disease is due to a neurotoxin, it is not contagious. The neurotoxin affects cholinergic neurons and prevents the release of acetylcholine. Symptoms typically develop within 12 to 36 hours of exposure and include acute flaccid paralysis, decrease salivation, ileus and urinary retention. There are no sensory deficits. With appropriate supportive care and trivalent equine antitoxin, the mortality rate is less than 5%. Without the use of antitoxin, patients may take 2 to 8 weeks to recover. Mortality rate is 5% to 10%.

There are more than 18 hemorrhagic fever viruses including the Ebola virus. The incubation period is 2 to 21 days and the patients present with fever, myalgias, headaches, thrombocytopenia and hemorrhagic complications (petechiae, ecchymosis). Untreated, the mortality rate for Ebola is 90%. Treatment includes the drug ribavirin (*Barash: Clinical Anesthesia, ed 5, pp 1529-1533; Miller: Anesthesia, ed 6, pp 2516-2523; Stoelting: Basics of Anesthesia, ed 5, pp 621-626*).

555. (D)   556. (C)   557. (D)   558. (C)   559. (C)   560. (A)

Pulmonary function tests can be used to classify patients with chronic pulmonary disease into those with obstructive airway diseases (e.g., asthma, pulmonary emphysema, and chronic bronchitis) and those with restrictive pulmonary diseases (e.g., pulmonary fibrosis, scoliosis). The forced expiratory volume in 1 second or FEV_1 is the amount of air expired in 1 second and commonly is expressed as a percentage of the forced vital capacity, or FEV_1/FVC. The normal FEV_1/FVC is 75% to 80%. In the presence of obstructive airway disease, FEV_1 of less than 70% has mild obstruction, less than 60% has moderate obstruction and less than 50% has severe obstruction. Patients with obstructive lung disease also have a normal (asthma) or increase in (bronchitis, emphysema) total lung capacity and functional residual capacity or FRC. In the presence of restrictive pulmonary disease, FEV_1 is reduced but because FVC is also reduced, the FEV_1/FVC is normal. Patients with restrictive disease have a total lung capacity (TLC), FRC, and total pulmonary compliance that are reduced. In patients with pulmonary emphysema, lung compliance is increased because the elastic recoil of the lungs is decreased (*Miller: Anesthesia, ed 6, pp 999-1010; Stoelting: Basics of Anesthesia, ed 5, pp 406-411*).

561. (A)   562. (B)   563. (C)   564. (D)   565. (B)   566. (E)

In many cases of peripheral nerve injuries the mechanism of injury is largely unknown; however, stretching or compression of the nerves can lead to nerve ischemia and damage. In the lithotomy position, hyperflexion of the hips and/or extension of the knees can aggravate stretch of the sciatic nerve. Also in the lithotomy position, compression of the common peroneal nerve between the head of the fibula and the metal supporting frame can occur. The common peroneal nerve is the most common nerve injured in the lithotomy position. Proper padding between the metal leg braces and positioning of the legs will limit the occurrence of these injuries. The sciatic nerve provides motor function for all the skeletal muscles below the knees and sensory innervation for the lateral half of the leg and most of the foot. Injury to the common peroneal nerve, a branch of the sciatic nerve, causes a foot drop from the impaired ankle dorsiflexion and the loss of foot eversion and toe extension. Injury to the femoral or obturator nerves can occur with excessive retraction during lower abdominal surgery. The obturator nerve can also be injured during a difficult forceps vaginal delivery or by excessive flexion of the thigh to the groin. Injury to the femoral nerve will manifest as decreased extension of the knee (paresis of the quadriceps femoris muscle) and numbness over the anterior aspect of the thigh and medial/anteromedial side of the leg. The inability to adduct the leg and thigh as well as numbness over the medial side of the thigh are clinical manifestations consistent with damage to the obturator nerve. Excessive flexion of the hip on the abdomen can cause a neuropathy of the lateral femoral cutaneous nerve (sensory only) resulting in numbness of the lateral aspect of the thigh (*Miller: Anesthesia, ed 6, pp 1155-1159; Stoelting: Basics of Anesthesia, ed 5, pp 292, 294, 301*).

Chapter 7

Pediatric Physiology and Anesthesia

567. A 1-month-old infant with a strong family history of sickle-cell anemia is brought to the emergency room with an incarcerated inguinal hernia. Which of the following should be carried out before surgery?
    A. Sickle cell prep
    B. Hemoglobin electrophoresis
    C. Peripheral smear
    D. Hematology consultation
    E. None of the above

568. In the newborn, the cricoid cartilage is at which level relative to the cervical spine?
    A. C3
    B. C4
    C. C5
    D. C6
    E. C7

569. A 5-month-old infant is scheduled for an elective operative reduction of a right inguinal hernia. Spinal anesthesia is performed. The first sign of a high spinal in this patient would be
    A. Hypotension
    B. Tachycardia
    C. Hypoxia
    D. Bradycardia
    E. Asystole

570. What percentage of a term newborn's total body weight consists of water?
    A. 25%
    B. 40%
    C. 60%
    D. 75%
    E. 90%

571. What is the maximum F_{IO_2} that can be administered to the mother without increasing the risk of retinopathy of prematurity in the fetus in utero?
    A. 0.35
    B. 0.50
    C. 0.65
    D. 0.80
    E. 1.0

572.   Which of the following patients is **LEAST** likely to develop retinopathy of prematurity?
   A. A term infant, 46 weeks postconceptual age, exposed to 100% oxygen for 6 hours
   B. A premature infant 29 weeks postconceptual age exposed to a Pao₂ of 150 mm Hg for 1 hour
   C. A premature infant 28 weeks postconceptual age never exposed to supplemental oxygen
   D. A cyanotic infant with tetralogy of Fallot, 34 weeks postconceptual age, receiving supplemental oxygen
   E. A term infant at 39 weeks postconceptual age receiving 100% oxygen for 2 hours after birth

573.   A 5-week-old male infant is brought to the emergency room with projectile vomiting. At the time of admission the patient is lethargic with a respiratory rate of 12 breaths/min and has had no urine output in the preceding 3 hours. A diagnosis of pyloric stenosis is made and the patient is brought to the operating room (OR) for pyloromyotomy. The most appropriate anesthetic management would be
   A. Induction with IM ketamine, glycopyrrolate, and succinylcholine with cricoid pressure followed by immediate intubation
   B. Inhalation induction with halothane with cricoid pressure
   C. Awake intubation
   D. Awake saphenous IV catheter followed by rapid sequence induction with ketamine, atropine, and succinylcholine
   E. Postpone surgery

574.   Which figure of esophageal atresia or tracheoesophageal fistula is the most common?

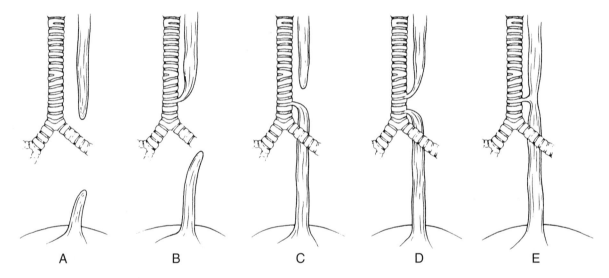

   A   B   C   D   E

575.   A 4-year-old boy is scheduled for completion of a hypospadias repair. The child is anxious. He has a history of a viral illness with a cough 2 weeks before surgery that has resolved. Anesthesia is induced with halothane, nitrous oxide, and oxygen. During the inhalation induction the patient's rhythm changes from sinus tachycardia to multifocal ventricular ectopy. The most likely explanation for this patient's heart rhythm is
   A. Undiagnosed viral myocarditis
   B. Hypoxia
   C. Halothane irritability
   D. Pheochromocytoma
   E. Prolonged QT syndrome

576.   Preterm neonates are at an increased risk for retinopathy of prematurity until what postconceptual age?
   A. 36 weeks
   B. 38 weeks
   C. 42 weeks
   D. 44 weeks
   E. 60 weeks

577. Reasons for selecting a cuffed endotracheal tube over an uncuffed endotracheal tube include all of the following **EXCEPT**
   A. Fewer intubations and endotracheal tubes are needed
   B. Lower gas flows can be used
   C. Less chance for airway fires
   D. Spontaneous breathing is easier
   E. Aspiration of gastric contents is less likely

578. An otherwise healthy 4-year-old male patient is undergoing elective tonsillectomy. Before induction of general anesthesia, the patient is breathing at a rate of 20 breaths/min. An inhalation induction is begun with sevoflurane, nitrous oxide, and oxygen. Sixty seconds later, the patient is noted to breathe at a rate of 40 breaths/min. This rapid respiratory rate most likely represents
   A. Hypoxia
   B. Hypercarbia
   C. The excitement stage of anesthesia
   D. Malignant hyperthermia
   E. Pulmonary embolism

579. A healthy 1-month-old neonate is anesthetized for an inguinal hernia repair. An inhalation induction with sevoflurane is carried out and the patient is intubated. Before making the surgical incision the systolic blood pressure is noted to be 65 mm Hg and the heart rate is 130 beats/min. The most appropriate intervention for this patient's blood pressure would be
   A. Administration of ephedrine
   B. Administration of phenylephrine
   C. 50-mL fluid bolus
   D. Administration of epinephrine
   E. None of the above

580. A 5-year-old boy is anesthetized for elective repair of an umbilical hernia. General anesthesia is induced and maintained with sevoflurane, nitrous oxide, and oxygen via an anesthesia mask. At the conclusion of the operation, the patient is taken to the recovery room and subsequently discharged to the outpatient ward. Before discharge, the patient's mother noted that the urine was dark brown in appearance. The most appropriate action at this time would be
   A. Discharge the patient with instructions to return if urine color does not normalize
   B. Discharge the patient in 3 hours if no other signs or symptoms are manifested
   C. Obtain serum creatinine and blood urea nitrogen (BUN) levels and discharge the patient if they are normal
   D. Admit the patient to rule out acute tubular necrosis
   E. Evaluate the patient for malignant hyperthermia

581. At what inspiratory pressure should an endotracheal tube leak in an infant?
   A. 5 to 15 cm H_2O
   B. 15 to 25 cm H_2O
   C. 25 to 35 cm H_2O
   D. 35 to 45 cm H_2O
   E. 45 to 55 cm H_2O

582. A premature newborn delivered at 32 weeks of gestation is brought to the OR for repair of a left-sided congenital diaphragmatic hernia. After awake tracheal intubation, general anesthesia is maintained with halothane, O_2, and fentanyl. Shortly thereafter, the anesthesiologist notes difficulty with ventilation. The Sao_2 subsequently falls to 65% and the heart rate decreases to 50 beats/min. What would be the most appropriate step to take at this time?
   A. Pull the endotracheal tube from the right mainstem bronchus
   B. Ventilate with positive end-expiratory pressure (PEEP) and administer furosemide
   C. Pass an oral gastric tube to decompress the stomach
   D. Place a chest tube on the right side
   E. Pull out the endotracheal tube and reintubate the patient

583. Symptoms of infantile pyloric stenosis occur most frequently between the ages of
    A. 1 and 2 weeks
    B. 2 and 6 weeks
    C. 6 and 12 weeks
    D. 3 and 6 months
    E. 6 and 12 months

584. In a 12-year-old child, the length of an oral endotracheal tube (from the lips to the midtrachea) should be
    A. 12 cm
    B. 14 cm
    C. 16 cm
    D. 18 cm
    E. 20 cm

585. In which of the following conditions would a preoperative evaluation of the heart with echocardiogram be indicated before anesthesia and surgery?
    A. Necrotizing enterocolitis
    B. Pyloric stenosis
    C. Gastroschisis
    D. Omphalocele
    E. Hypospadias

586. An otherwise healthy 14-day-old neonate is transported to the OR well hydrated for surgery for a bowel obstruction. A rapid sequence induction is planned. Compared with the adult dose, the dose of succinylcholine administered to this patient should be
    A. Diminished because of the immature nervous system
    B. The same as the adult dose
    C. Increased because of increased acetylcholine receptors
    D. Decreased because of decreased acetylcholine receptors
    E. Increased because of a greater volume of distribution

587. The most common cause of neonatal bradycardia (heart rate less than 100 beats/min) is
    A. Congenital heart disease
    B. Maternal drug intoxication (narcotics, alcohol, magnesium, barbiturates, digitoxin)
    C. Fever
    D. Postpartum cold stress
    E. Hypoxemia

588. A 10-week-old infant born at 31 weeks of gestation is anesthetized for repair of an inguinal hernia. General anesthesia is induced by mask with sevoflurane, an endotracheal tube is placed, and anesthesia is maintained with isoflurane, nitrous oxide, and oxygen. At the end of the procedure, the endotracheal tube is removed and the patient is transported to the recovery room. What is the best postoperative pain management for this patient?
    A. Ilioinguinal-iliohypogastric nerve block and discharge home with instructions to parents
    B. Caudal block with 0.25% bupivacaine, 1 mL/kg, and admit to a pediatric ward for overnight observation
    C. Caudal block with 0.25% bupivacaine, 2 mL/kg, and admit to a pediatric ward for overnight observation
    D. Oral pain medication and discharge home with instructions to the parent
    E. Fentanyl, 1 mL IV, and admit to a pediatric ward for overnight observation

589. A 6-year-old, 20-kg girl develops pulseless ventricular tachycardia after induction of anesthesia with halothane, nitrous oxide, and oxygen for a tonsillectomy. The anesthesiologist intubates the child, administers 100% oxygen, and starts chest compressions. When the defibrillator quickly arrives in the OR the defibrillator should be charged to what energy level for the initial shock?
    A. 20 joules (J)
    B. 40 joules (J)
    C. 60 joules (J)
    D. 80 joules (J)
    E. 120 joules (J)

590. The spinal cord of newborns extends to the
- **A.** L1 vertebra
- **B.** L2 vertebra
- **C.** L3 vertebra
- **D.** L5 vertebra
- **E.** S1 vertebra

591. The most common initial symptom of esophageal atresia (EA) and tracheoesophageal fistula (TEF) is
- **A.** Respiratory distress at delivery (e.g., retractions, tachypnea)
- **B.** Pneumonia
- **C.** Hypoxia
- **D.** Regurgitation during feeding
- **E.** Projectile vomiting

592. A 4-kg, 3-hour-old newborn with macrosomia and large fontanelles is scheduled for surgical repair of an omphalocele. Physical examination reveals macroglossia but no other anomalies are found. Which of the following is likely to occur in this patient?
- **A.** Hypokalemia
- **B.** Hyperkalemia
- **C.** Metabolic acidosis
- **D.** Hypoxemia
- **E.** Hypoglycemia

593. Which of the following is the **LEAST** appropriate technique for induction of general anesthesia in a newborn for surgical repair of TEF?
- **A.** Awake tracheal intubation
- **B.** Inhalation induction with spontaneous ventilation and tracheal intubation
- **C.** Inhalation induction using positive-pressure bag and mask ventilation and tracheal intubation
- **D.** Rapid IV induction and tracheal intubation
- **E.** Intramuscular induction with high-dose ketamine and tracheal intubation

594. Each of the following statements concerning side effects of succinylcholine when used to paralyze neonates is true **EXCEPT**
- **A.** It seldom causes muscle fasciculation
- **B.** It can cause bradycardia
- **C.** Dysrhythmias frequently occur following intramuscular injections
- **D.** It can cause myoglobinuria
- **E.** It can cause hyperkalemia

595. The predicted blood volume in a 4-kg neonate is
- **A.** 240 mL
- **B.** 280 mL
- **C.** 340 mL
- **D.** 400 mL
- **E.** 440 mL

596. The pulmonary vascular resistance in newborns decreases to that of adults by age
- **A.** 1 day
- **B.** 1 week
- **C.** 2 months
- **D.** 2 years
- **E.** 5 years

597. A 10-month-old infant is undergoing elective repair of a left testicular hydrocele under general anesthesia with isoflurane, nitrous oxide, oxygen, and fentanyl. All of following are effective and reasonable means of preventing hypothermia in this patient **EXCEPT**
  A. Placement of an infrared heater over the operating table and prewarming the OR
  B. Covering the OR table with a heating blanket
  C. Wrapping the extremities with sheet wadding and covering the head with a cloth cap
  D. Ventilating the patient with a Mapleson D circuit at low gas flows (e.g., 50 mL/kg/min)
  E. Warming and humidifying the inspired anesthetic gases

598. Central postoperative depression of ventilation in a full-term neonate is most likely to occur after surgery for which of the following?
  A. Gastroschisis
  B. Omphalocele
  C. Tracheoesophageal fistula
  D. Diaphragmatic hernia
  E. Pyloric stenosis

599. A premature male neonate born at 32 weeks of gestation is scheduled to undergo emergency repair of a left-sided diaphragmatic hernia. Which of the following vessels could be cannulated for preductal arterial blood sampling?
  A. Femoral artery
  B. Umbilical artery
  C. Dorsalis pedis artery
  D. Right radial artery
  E. Left radial artery

600. In which of the following patients would the minimum alveolar concentration (MAC) for halothane or isoflurane be the greatest?
  A. A premature infant 30 weeks postconceptual age
  B. Full-term neonate
  C. 3-month-old infant
  D. 19-year-old male bodybuilder
  E. 35-year-old woman with hyperthyroidism

601. A 40-kg, 10-year-old child sustains a thermal injury to his legs, buttocks, and back. The estimated area involved is 50%. How much fluid should be administered during the first 24 hours?
  A. 2.5 L
  B. 4.0 L
  C. 5.5 L
  D. 8.0 L
  E. 10.0 L

602. An otherwise healthy 3-month-old black female infant with a hemoglobin of 19 mg/dL at birth presents for elective repair of an inguinal hernia. Her preoperative hemoglobin is 10 mg/dL. Her father has a history of polycystic kidney disease. The most likely explanation for this patient's anemia is
  A. Sickle cell trait
  B. Sickle-cell anemia
  C. Iron deficiency
  D. Undiagnosed polycystic kidney disease
  E. It is a normal finding

603. The anesthesiologist is called to the emergency room by the pediatrician to help manage a 3-year-old boy with a high fever and upper airway obstruction. His mother states that earlier that afternoon, he complained of a sore throat and hoarseness. The patient is sitting erect and leaning forward, has inspiratory stridor, tachypnea, and sternal retractions, and is drooling. Which of the following is the most appropriate management of airway obstruction in this patient?
   A. Aerosolized racemic epinephrine
   B. Awake tracheal intubation in the emergency room
   C. Transfer to the OR and awake tracheal intubation
   D. Transfer to the OR, inhalation induction, and tracheal intubation
   E. Transfer to the OR, IV induction, paralysis with succinylcholine, and tracheal intubation

604. A 2-year-old child with cerebral palsy and known severe gastroesophageal reflux (with frequent nightly aspiration) is scheduled to undergo iliopsoas release under general anesthesia. Which of the following would be the most appropriate technique for inducing general anesthesia in this patient?
   A. Inhalation induction with sevoflurane followed by mask anesthesia with cricoid pressure
   B. Inhalation induction with sevoflurane followed by tracheal intubation
   C. IV induction with propofol followed by laryngeal mask airway
   D. IV induction with propofol followed by tracheal intubation
   E. Rapid-sequence induction with thiopental and succinylcholine followed by tracheal intubation

605. A 7-week-old male infant is admitted to the pediatric intensive care unit (ICU) with a bowel obstruction. His laboratory values are sodium 120 mEq/L, chloride 85 mEq/L, glucose 85 mg/dL, and potassium 2.0 mEq/L. Respiratory rate is 20 breaths/min, and according to the patient's mother, urine output has been 0 for the last 4 hours. The most appropriate fluid for resuscitation of this patient would be
   A. D_5W
   B. D_5W with 0.45 sodium chloride and 20 mEq/L potassium chloride
   C. 0.45% sodium chloride
   D. 0.9% sodium chloride with 30 mEq/L potassium chloride
   E. 0.9% sodium chloride

606. An 8-hour-old, 1600-g neonate, 30 weeks postgestational age, is noted in the ICU to begin making twitching movements. Blood pressure is 45 mm Hg systolic, blood glucose 50 mg/dL, and urine output 10 mL/hr. The O_2 saturation on pulse oximeter is 88%. The most appropriate course of action to take at this point would be
   A. Administer calcium gluconate 250 mg (2.5 mL of 10% solution)
   B. Glucose 10 mg IV over 5 minutes (2 mL of D_5W)
   C. Hyperventilate with 100% O_2
   D. Administer a 20-mL bolus of 5% albumin
   E. Begin a dopamine infusion

607. An Eutectic Mixture of the Local Anesthetics (EMLA) cream is a mixture of which local anesthetics?
   A. Lidocaine and prilocaine
   B. Lidocaine and benzocaine
   C. Prilocaine and benzocaine
   D. Mepivacaine and lidocaine
   E. Prilocaine, benzocaine, and lidocaine

608. Advantages of catheterization of the umbilical artery versus the umbilical vein in a newborn include all of the following **EXCEPT**
   A. It allows assessment of oxygenation
   B. Hepatic damage from hypertonic infusion is avoided
   C. It permits assessment of systemic blood pressure
   D. It is easier to cannulate
   E. There are two vessels to choose from

609. The true statement concerning thermoregulation in neonates is which of the following?
- **A.** A significant proportion of their heat loss can be accounted for by their small surface area-to-weight ratio
- **B.** They compensate for hypothermia by shivering
- **C.** The principal method of heat production is metabolism of brown fat
- **D.** Heat loss through conduction can be reduced by humidification of inspired gases
- **E.** Heat loss by convection is reduced with the use of a warming blanket

610. Normal values for a healthy 6-month-old, 7-kg infant include
- **A.** Hemoglobin 17 g/dL
- **B.** Heart rate 90 beats/min
- **C.** Respiratory rate 20 breaths/min
- **D.** O_2 consumption at rest 35 mL/min
- **E.** Systolic blood pressure of 70

611. A 5-year-old child undergoing strabismus surgery under general anesthesia suddenly develops sinus bradycardia and intermittent ventricular escape beats, but is hemodynamically stable. Which therapy is appropriate for treating this arrhythmia?
- **A.** Tell the surgeon to stop pulling on the eye muscle
- **B.** Tell the surgeon to do a retrobulbar block
- **C.** Change from halothane to sevoflurane
- **D.** Decrease the depth of the volatile anesthetic
- **E.** Administer atropine

612. Which of the following respiratory indices is increased in neonates compared with adults?
- **A.** Tidal volume (V_T) (mL/kg)
- **B.** pH
- **C.** Alveolar ventilation (mL/kg/min)
- **D.** Functional residual capacity (mL/kg)
- **E.** $Paco_2$

613. A 14-year-old girl with neurofibromatosis is anesthetized for resection of an acoustic neuroma. Each of the following may potentially complicate the anesthetic management of this patient **EXCEPT**
- **A.** Presence of a pheochromocytoma
- **B.** Upper airway obstruction from a laryngeal neurofibroma
- **C.** Intracranial hypertension
- **D.** Increased risk for malignant hyperthermia
- **E.** Abnormal response to neuromuscular blocking agents

614. Retinopathy of prematurity
- **A.** Occurs only after exposure to high concentrations of O_2 for 12 or more hours
- **B.** Cannot occur in patients who have never received supplemental O_2
- **C.** Is caused by obliteration of immature retinal arteries
- **D.** Is most commonly seen in newborns younger than 44 weeks postconceptual age
- **E.** Is more common in newborns when anesthesia is administered for non-ophthalmologic procedures

615. The most reliable method of determining mild dehydration in a child is by the observation of
- **A.** Dryness of mucous membrane
- **B.** Skin turgor
- **C.** Urine output
- **D.** Fontanelles
- **E.** Blood pressure

616. Postoperative bleeding following tonsillectomy occurs most commonly
- **A.** By the first 6 hours
- **B.** 6-24 hours postop
- **C.** On third postoperative day
- **D.** On seventh postoperative day
- **E.** On tenth postoperative day

617. A 9 year old undergoing sinus surgery is treated with an unmeasured amount of 0.5% phenylephrine by the surgeon and the patient develops a blood pressure of 250/150. The most appropriate treatment for this would be
  A. Administer verapamil
  B. Administer esmolol
  C. Administer labetalol
  D. Administer atropine
  E. Administer phentolamine

618. A 6-kg, 3-month-old male infant undergoes a left inguinal herniorrhaphy with a spinal anesthetic. How long would 0.5 mL of a 0.5% bupivacaine solution be expected to last?
  A. Less than 30 minutes
  B. 30 to 60 minutes
  C. 60 to 90 minutes
  D. 90 minutes to 2 hours
  E. Cannot be predicted

619. In addition to inspiratory stridor, which sign or symptom is consistent with epiglottitis?
  A. Rapid onset in less than 24 hours
  B. Mild temperature elevation (<39° C)
  C. Age younger than 2 years
  D. Rhinorrhea
  E. Lymphocytosis

620. Which technique for resuscitation of a 6-month-old by a lay single rescuer is correct
  A. Mouth-to-mouth or mouth-to-nose ventilation at a rate of 12 to 20 breaths/min with good chest expansion
  B. Chest compressions with two fingers on the upper half of the sternum just above the intermammary line
  C. Sternal compression depth of no more than ½ cm
  D. Lay rescuer should check the carotid pulse every minute
  E. Compression to ventilation ratio of 5:1

621. All of the following are true statements concerning physiology of newborns compared with that in adults **EXCEPT**
  A. Newborns have a greater percentage of total body water compared with adults
  B. Newborns have a prolonged effect with thiopental
  C. Newborns have a higher glomerular filtration rate than adults
  D. Newborn hearts are relatively non-compliant compared with adults
  E. Newborn diaphragms have a lower proportion of type I muscle fibers (i.e., fatigue resistant, highly oxidative fibers)

622. Which of the following statements concerning the anatomy of the infant airway compared with the adult airway is true?
  A. The larynx is at the C5-C6 level in infants and C6-C7 in adults
  B. The epiglottis is relatively small in infants compared with adults
  C. The glottic opening is more anterior in infants than in adults
  D. The vocal cords are in a more horizontal position within the larynx in infants than in adults
  E. The vocal cords are the narrowest part of the larynx in infants, whereas the cricoid cartilage is the narrowest part of the larynx in adults

623. Which of the following operations would be associated with the **LEAST** incidence of postoperative nausea and vomiting (PONV) in a 5-year-old boy?
  A. Tonsillectomy
  B. Strabismus surgery
  C. Myringotomy tube placement
  D. Orchiopexy
  E. Inguinal herniorrhaphy

624. Anomalies and features associated with Down syndrome include
    A. Smaller tracheas
    B. Atlanto-occipital instability
    C. Thyroid hypofunction
    D. Endocardial cushion defect
    E. All of the above are correct

625. Congenital syndromes frequently associated with cardiac abnormalities include all of the following **EXCEPT**
    A. Tracheoesophageal fistula
    B. Meningomyelocele
    C. Omphalocele
    D. Gastroschisis
    E. Congenital diaphragmatic hernia

626. Appropriate management of a neonate born with congenital diaphragmatic hernia (CDH) should include
    A. Ventilation of the lungs with a bag and mask to keep saturation greater than 95%
    B. Insertion of an orogastric tube
    C. Expansion of the hypoplastic lung with positive-pressure ventilation
    D. Hyperventilation to keep the $PaCO_2$ below 40 and pH greater than 7.40
    E. Rapid transport to the operating room for surgical correction

627. Factors associated with an increased incidence of laryngospasm include all of the following **EXCEPT**
    A. Younger age (<5 years of age)
    B. Presence of an airway anomaly
    C. Presence of an active upper respiratory infection (URI)
    D. Use of a laryngeal mask airway
    E. All are correct

628. Which of the following statements regarding perioperative cardiac arrest in children is **NOT CORRECT?**
    A. Cardiac arrest is more common in neonates than infants or older children
    B. "Equipment related" causes occur in more than 25% of cardiac arrests
    C. Resuscitation is more often successful if the cause is anesthesia-related rather than non-anesthesia related
    D. Many cases of cardiac arrest occur in children with concomitant congenital heart disease
    E. Emergency surgery is associated with greater than 5 times the chance of a cardiac arrest

629. Klippel-Feil syndrome is associated with
    A. Kyphoscoliosis
    B. Renal anomalies
    C. Congenital heart abnormalities
    D. Cervical spine instability
    E. All are correct

630. Which of the following statements regarding the Mapleson D breathing circuit is **FALSE?**
    A. It is an semi-open breathing system
    B. It has a proximal fresh gas inflow and a distal overflow valve
    C. With an inspiratory to expiratory (I:E) breathing ratio of 1:2, rebreathing is eliminated with spontaneous ventilation when the fresh gas flow is 3 times the minute ventilation
    D. To eliminate rebreathing, higher fresh gas flows are needed with controlled ventilation than with spontaneous ventilation
    E. The Mapleson D circuit is the most widely used of the Mapleson circuits for pediatric anesthesia

631. Which of the following is **LEAST** likely to reduce the incidence of postoperative apnea in preterm infants undergoing surgery for inguinal hernia repair?
   A. Delaying operation until 60 weeks post conception
   B. Preoperative correction of anemia
   C. Caffeine administration
   D. Ketamine administration
   E. Spinal anesthetic without sedation

632. Air should not be used to identify the epidural space in children because of the risk of
   A. Venous air embolism
   B. Infection
   C. Epidural hematoma
   D. Subcutaneous emphysema
   E. Neurologic complications

633. Induction of general anesthesia for an elective operation should be delayed how many hours after breast feeding?
   A. 2 hours
   B. 4 hours
   C. 6 hours
   D. 8 hours
   E. No fasting needed because breast milk is OK

634. In the infant, hypothermia can be manifested as
   A. Metabolic acidosis
   B. Prolonged duration of action of nondepolarizing muscle relaxants
   C. Hypoglycemia
   D. Respiratory depression
   E. All are correct

635. Necrotizing enterocolitis has all of the following characteristics **EXCEPT**
   A. Most have thrombocytopenia (<75,000/mm3)
   B. A potential complication of umbilical artery catheterization
   C. Commonly associated with decreased cardiac output in the presence of fetal asphyxia or postnatal respiratory complications
   D. Umbilical artery catheters are useful to assess acid base status
   E. Occurs in 10% to 20% of newborns weighing less than 1500 g

636. The **LEAST** useful analgesic for prevention/treatment of tonsillar pain
   A. Acetaminophen
   B. Ropivacaine infiltration
   C. Dexmedetomidine
   D. Codeine
   E. Ketorolac

637. Which of the following statements concerning sudden infant death syndrome (SIDS) is true
   A. SIDS most frequently occurs from 1 to 3 years of age
   B. Risk of SIDS is the same with lower birth weight infants as with normal birth weight infants
   C. Maternal smoking is associated with a higher incidence of SIDS
   D. The risk of SIDS is increased with a recent general anesthetic
   E. Sleeping in the prone position has a lower frequency of SIDS than sleeping in the supine position

638. A 5-year-old girl with hemolytic-uremic syndrome is brought to the OR for placement of a dialysis catheter. Medical issues typical for this disease include
    A. Anemia
    B. Thrombocytopenia
    C. Increased intracranial pressure
    D. Pancreatitis
    E. All are correct

639. A 3-year-old child status postresection of Wilms' tumor at age 2 years is receiving doxorubicin (Adriamycin) and cyclophosphamide for metastatic disease. The patient is scheduled for placement of a Hickman catheter for continued chemotherapy. Anesthetic concerns related to this patient's chemotherapeutic treatment include all of the following **EXCEPT**
    A. Thrombocytopenia
    B. Inhibition of plasma cholinesterase
    C. Cardiac depression
    D. Pulmonary fibrosis
    E. Hypertension

640. Preoperatively, hypotension (i.e., decompensated shock) is characterized by a systolic blood pressure (SBP)
    A. Less than 60 mm Hg for the term neonate (0 to 28 days old)
    B. Less than 70 mm Hg for infants 1 to 12 months old
    C. Less than 70 mm Hg + (2 × age in years) for children 1 to 10 years old
    D. Less than 90 mm Hg for children 10 years or older
    E. All of the above are correct

641. During peanut retrieval from the left mainstem bronchus, the foreign body becomes lodged in the trachea and is pushed back, but goes now into right mainstem bronchus. Air movement is impossible with bag and mask and the patient's heart rate falls to 30 beats per minute. The most appropriate next step would be to
    A. Intubate the left mainstem
    B. Intubate the right mainstem
    C. Attempt the Heimlich maneuver
    D. Institute cardiopulmonary bypass
    E. Perform an emergent tracheostomy

642. Each of the following results in a reduction of the incidence of nausea and vomiting in children undergoing strabismus surgery **EXCEPT**
    A. Withholding oral intake
    B. Premedication with clonidine 4 mg/kg orally
    C. Dexamethasone 0.15-1 mg/kg IV
    D. Ondansetron 50-200 μg/kg IV
    E. Gastric content evacuation before emergence from anesthesia

Pediatric Physiology and Anesthesia

Answers, References, and Explanations

567. **(E)** At birth, the concentration of hemoglobin F (fetal hemoglobin) is about 80% and reaches its lowest level by 2 to 3 months of age. Sickle-cell anemia (hemoglobin SS) is an inherited disorder of the β-chain of the adult hemoglobin molecule caused by a single amino acid substitution. It has an incidence of about 0.2% in the African-American population, in contrast to the relatively benign heterozygous condition, sickle cell trait (hemoglobin AS), which affects 8% to 10% of the same group. Sickling can occur in homozygous patients who become hypoxic, acidotic, hypothermic, or dehydrated. The predominant hemoglobin in this 1-month-old infant is hemoglobin F, which would temporarily protect the infant from the manifestations of sickle-cell anemia were he or she homozygous for hemoglobin S. The patient should, however, be worked up for sickle-cell anemia at some point in early life, but such a workup is not a prerequisite for surgery at 1 month of age (*Miller: Anesthesia, ed 6, pp 1112-1113; Motoyama: Smith's Anesthesia for Infants and Children, ed 7, pp 49, 397-398; Stoelting: Anesthesia and Co-Existing Disease, ed 5, pp 411-412*).

568. **(B)** The anatomy of the oropharynx and larynx of the newborn is different from that of the adult in many aspects. These differences may make it more difficult for a successful direct laryngoscopy and tracheal intubation. Newborns have larger arytenoids and tongue, and the lower border of the cricoid cartilage is at the level of the fourth cervical vertebra. (At age 6 years the cricoid cartilage is opposite the fifth cervical vertebra and in adults the cricoid cartilage is opposite the sixth cervical vertebra.) Additionally, the epiglottis of the infant is relatively larger and stiffer compared with the adult (*Barash: Clinical Anesthesia ed 5, p 1186; Miller: Anesthesia, ed 6, pp 1646-1647; Motoyama: Smith's Anesthesia for Infants and Children, ed 7, p 339*).

569. **(C)** Spinal anesthesia can be administered safely to children of all ages. Hypotension secondary to a loss of sympathetic tone, common in the adult, is rare in the child younger than 5 years even with levels of T-3. Because of this hemodynamic stability, some pediatric anesthesiologists start an IV line after the spinal anesthetic is administered to the infant. Respiratory depression including apnea and hypoxia will likely be the initial symptom associated with a high spinal anesthetic in the infant (*Barash: Clinical Anesthesia, ed 5, pp 1191-1192; Motoyama: Smith's Anesthesia for Infants and Children, ed 7, pp 465-468*).

570. **(D)** The body compartment volumes change with age. Muscle contains about 75% water, whereas adipose tissue contains only 10% water. Total body water (TBW) decreases with age as muscle and fat content increases. The fraction of total body weight that consists of water is 80% to 85% in premature newborns, 75% in term newborns, and 60% in 6-month-old infants and in adults. These alterations in body composition have implications on the volume of distribution and redistribution of drugs (*Miller: Anesthesia, ed 6, pp 1764, 2371; Motoyama: Smith's Anesthesia for Infants and Children, ed 7, pp 115-116*).

571. **(E)** The fetal Pao_2 does not increase above 45 mm Hg when 100% O_2 is administered to the mother because of the high O_2 consumption of the placenta and uneven distribution of the maternal and fetal blood flow in the placenta. For these reasons, the Fio_2 administered to the mother is not a factor in the etiology of retinopathy of prematurity in utero (*Hughes: Shnider and Levinson's Anesthesia for Obstetrics, ed 4, p 222*).

572. **(A)** Retinopathy of prematurity (ROP), formally called retrolental fibroplasia, typically occurs in newborns who are born at less than 35 weeks of gestational age. The risk of ROP is inversely related to age and birth weight, with a significant risk occurring in infants weighing less than 1500 g. The risk is negligible after 44 weeks postconceptional age. The mechanism for retrolental fibroplasia is complex and is related to the complicated process of retinal development and maturation. Under normal circumstances, retinal vasculature develops from the optic disk toward the periphery of the retina. This process is typically complete by 40 to 44 weeks of gestation. Hyperoxia causes constriction of the retinal arterioles, resulting in swelling and degeneration of the endothelium that disrupts normal retinal development. Vascularization of the retina resumes in an abnormal fashion when normoxic conditions return, resulting in neovascularization and scarring of the retina. In the worst-case scenario, this process can lead to retinal detachment and blindness. Consequently, hyperoxia should be avoided when anesthetizing preterm infants. Exposure of preterm infants to Pao$_2$ greater than 80 mm Hg for prolonged periods may be associated with increased incidence and severity of retinopathy. To reduce this risk, it is recommended that the oxygen saturation be maintained between 93% and 95% (about Pao$_2$ of 70 mm Hg) during anesthesia. On the other hand, one must never compromise O$_2$ delivery to the neonate's brain to protect the eyes. Although oxygen has been associated with ROP, other factors are also important. In fact, newborns with cyanotic congenital heart disease who have not been exposed to supplemental oxygen therapy have also developed ROP (*Barash: Clinical Anesthesia, ed 5, p 1193; Hines: Stoelting's Anesthesia and Co-Existing Disease, ed 5, pp 588-589; Motoyama: Smith's Anesthesia for Infants and Children, ed 7, pp 781-782*).

573. (E) This patient has signs consistent with severe dehydration and needs resuscitation with fluid and electrolytes before surgery. Surgery should be delayed until there is thorough evaluation and treatment of the fluid and electrolyte imbalances. Pyloric stenosis occurs in approximately 1 in every 500 live births, making it the most common cause of gastrointestinal obstruction in pediatric patients. Pyloric stenosis occurs as frequently in preterm as in term neonates and there is a predilection for male infants. Persistent vomiting usually manifests itself between the second and sixth weeks of age and can result in dehydration, hypokalemia, hypochloremia, and metabolic alkalosis. Fluid resuscitation should be initiated with isotonic saline. If an IV line catheter cannot be established, an intraosseous needle should be placed. After the patient voids, potassium then can be safely added to the IV fluids. Once there has been adequate hydration and correction of the electrolyte and acid-base abnormalities, the patient can undergo surgery. Although several days may be required to restore normal fluid and electrolyte balance in some children, most respond within 12 to 48 hours (*Hines: Stoelting's Anesthesia and Co-Existing Disease, ed 5, pp 599-600; Motoyama: Smith's Anesthesia for Infants and Children, ed 7, pp 690-691*).

574. (C) Esophageal atresia (EA) and tracheoesophageal fistulas (TEFs) result from failure of the esophagus and the trachea to completely separate during development. This lesion occurs with an incidence of approximately 1 in 4000 live births. Although each of the listed answers is possible, the most common type is esophageal atresia with the lower segment of the esophagus communicating with the back of the trachea. This occurs in about 90% of all TEFs. In the delivery room, one is unable to pass a suction catheter into the stomach and if an x-ray is taken, the presence of air in the stomach suggests a fistula between the trachea and the stomach. If it is not detected in the delivery room, the newborn tends to have excessive oral secretions and is unable to feed. Note: 20% to 25% of patients with EA or TEF have associated cardiovascular anomalies (e.g., ventricular septal defect (VSD), atrial septal defect (ASD), tetralogy of Fallot, atrioventricular (AV) canal, coarctation of the aorta) (*Hines: Stoelting's Anesthesia and Co-Existing Disease, ed 5, pp 595-596; Motoyama: Smith's Anesthesia for Infants and Children, ed 7, pp 550-552*).

575. (C) Volatile anesthetics, particularly halothane, can have significant adverse effects on cardiac heart rate and rhythm. Halothane may cause direct depression of the sinoatrial node and has been shown to increase the refractory period of the atrioventricular conduction system. Both bradydysrhythmias and tachydysrhythmias have been reported during inhalation induction of anesthesia with halothane. These include sinus bradycardia, nodal or junctional rhythms, and ventricular dysrhythmias. Whereas cardiac dysrhythmias after inhalation induction with halothane are common in children, they are usually benign and do not represent a disease state. Halothane "sensitizes" the myocardium to catecholamines, particularly in the presence of hypoxia, acute hypercarbia, and acidosis. Under these conditions, ventricular rhythms such as bigeminy, multifocal ventricular ectopic beats, and even ventricular tachycardia may occur (*Miller: Anesthesia, ed 6, pp 2373-2374*).

576. (D) The risk of developing ROP is negligible after 44 weeks postconceptional age. Thus, a preterm neonate born at 36 weeks gestational age remains at risk until after 8 weeks of age. See also explanation to question 572 (*Hines: Stoelting's Anesthesia and Co-Existing Disease, ed 5, pp 588-589; Motoyama: Smith's Anesthesia for Infants and Children, ed 7, pp 781-782*).

577. (D) Since cuffed endotracheal tubes are often chosen to be a size smaller (i.e., 0.5 mm) than uncuffed endotracheal tubes, the lumen is narrower and therefore spontaneous breathing is more difficult. Because a smaller endotracheal tube can be used with a cuff, fewer intubations are needed to select the correct tube size. Also because of the cuff, less leakage of gas exists from the trachea into the pharynx, allowing administration of lower gas flows with potential cost savings as well as less environmental pollution. The gases are less likely to leak into the pharynx and should decrease the chance of an airway fire if high oxygen or nitrous oxide concentrations are used and cautery is used in the oral cavity. The chance of aspiration of gastric contents should also be less likely (*Motoyama: Smith's Anesthesia for Infants and Children, ed 7, pp 334-336, 343-346*).

578. (C) Inhalation agents are respiratory depressants. In general, they increase the respiratory rate and decrease the V_T of respirations and are associated with an increase in $Paco_2$. When inducing a child with an inhalation agent, especially below the MAC level, the respiratory pattern can vary and include breath holding, excessive hyperventilation and laryngospasm. Although the stages of inhalation anesthesia were classically described with ether, similar stages are seen with the newer inhalation agents, but because the signs are less pronounced they are rarely described anymore. The classic stages of depth of ether anesthesia include the first stage of anesthesia (analgesia). Patients in the first stage can respond to verbal stimulation, have an intact lid reflex, have normal respiratory patterns, and intact airway reflexes and have some analgesia. The second stage of anesthesia (delirium or excitement stage) is associated with unconsciousness, irregular and unpredictable respiratory patterns (including hyperventilation), nonpurposeful muscle movements, and the risk of clinically important reflex activity (e.g., laryngospasm, vomiting, cardiac arrhythmias). The third stage of anesthesia (surgical anesthesia) is associated with a return to more regular periodic respirations and is the level associated with the achievement of MAC. MAC is noted by the absence of movement (in 50% of patients) in response to a surgical incision. As anesthesia is deepened, stage four (respiratory paralysis) is associated with respiratory and cardiovascular arrest. In the case cited in this question, the second stage of anesthesia is demonstrated. Note: Malignant hyperthermia triggered by the sole use of volatile anesthetics (especially halothane) produces an elevation of carbon dioxide levels with tachypnea and tachycardia, but this is rare during the first 20 minutes of an anesthetic (*Miller: Anesthesia, ed 6, p 706; Morgan: Clinical Anesthesiology, ed 4, pp 934-935*).

579. (E) The hemodynamic indices described in this question are normal for healthy 1-month-old neonates (*Motoyama: Smith's Anesthesia for Infants and Children, ed 7, pp 89-91; Stoelting: Basics of Anesthesia, ed 5, pp 508-509*).

COMPARISON OF CARDIOVASCULAR VARIABLES

	Neonate	Infant	5 years of Age	Adult
Weight (kg)	3	4-10	18	70
Oxygen consumption (mL/kg/min)	6	5	4	3
Systolic blood pressure (mm Hg)	65	90-95	95	120
Heart rate (beats/min)	130	120	90	80

(*Stoelting: Basics of Anesthesia, ed 5, p 509.*)

580. (E) The presence of dark brown urine (i.e., myoglobinemia) may be caused by rhabdomyolysis, a possible sign of malignant hyperthermia. More typical signs and symptoms include tachycardia, tachypnea, acidosis, increased sympathetic activity, and increased temperature. Accordingly, this patient should be evaluated for malignant hyperthermia. Supportive laboratory tests for malignant hyperthermia include elevated serum creatine phosphokinase (CPK); myoglobin in the serum and urine; increased serum potassium, calcium, and lactate levels; and a metabolic/respiratory acidosis on an arterial blood gas. If the presumed diagnosis is malignant hyperthermia, therapy should be initiated (*Barash: Clinical Anesthesia, ed 5, pp 531-532; Hines: Stoelting's Anesthesia and Co-Existing Disease, ed 5, pp 620-622*).

581. (B) In infants and young children, there should be a small air leak around the endotracheal tube at peak inflation pressures of approximately 15 to 25 cm H_2O. This test can be performed by slowly increasing the airway pressure and listening with a stethoscope over the larynx to hear when a leak develops. An air leak within this pressure range allows for adequate ventilation and reduces the incidence of postintubation croup (*Motoyama: Smith's Anesthesia for Infants and Children, ed 7, pp 335-337*).

582. (D) A congenital diaphragmatic hernia (CDH) is the herniation of abdominal viscera into the chest cavity through a defect in the diaphragm and occurs in approximately 1 in every 4000 live births. Approximately 90% of CDHs occur through a defect in the left side of the diaphragm. Symptoms depend upon the degree of herniation and the amount of respiratory compromise. Some newborns deteriorate in the delivery room whereas others deteriorate hours later. Immediate intubation of the trachea and decompression of the stomach are needed. Because CDH is associated with hypoplastic lungs, current ventilatory support aims at maintaining a preductal oxygen saturation above 90% using airway pressure below 35 cm H_2O and allowing the $Paco_2$ to rise to 60 to 65 mm Hg. If a patient experiences sudden oxygen desaturation during positive-pressure ventilation, a tension pneumothorax should be suspected and, if confirmed, a chest tube should be placed on the side contralateral to the congenital diaphragmatic hernia. Despite intensive treatments, about 40% to 50% of these newborns will die in the newborn period (*Hines: Stoelting's Anesthesia and Co-Existing Disease, ed 5, pp 593-594; Miller: Anesthesia, ed 6, pp 2396-2397; Motoyama: Smith's Anesthesia for Infants and Children, ed 7, pp 545-550*).

583. (B) Infantile pyloric stenosis is one of the most common surgical diseases of neonates and infants. It occurs in about 1 of every 500 live births. Symptoms usually appear between 2 and 6 weeks of age, but they have been diagnosed as early as the first week and as late as the fifth month of life (*Miller: Anesthesia, ed 6, p 2395; Motoyama: Smith's Anesthesia for Infants and Children, ed 7, pp 690-691; Stoelting: Anesthesia and Co-Existing Disease, ed 5, pp 599-600*).

584. (D) The depth of insertion of an oral endotracheal tube from the lips to the midtrachea is approximately 7 cm for a 1-kg newborn, 8 cm for a 2-kg, 9 cm for 3-kg and 10 cm for a typical 3.5-kg term newborn. There are many ways to estimate the appropriate depth of insertion of an oral endotracheal tube (in cm) for infants and children.

One method is age (>3 years):   (Age in years)/2 + 12 = tube length

In this 12-year-old child: 12/2 + 12 = 18 cm.

Another way is to multiply the tube size by 3. For example when you use a size 4.0 ID endotracheal tube, insert it 12 cm; a size 6.0 endotracheal tube is inserted 18 cm (*Motoyama: Smith's Anesthesia for Infants and Children, ed 7, pp 337-338*).

585. (D) The preanesthetic assessment of neonates with an omphalocele or an imperforate anus should include an assessment for other abnormalities including congenital heart disease. Omphalocele is associated with a 20% incidence of congenital heart disease, as well as several other congenital anomalies. Conversely, the other conditions in this question are rarely associated with other congenital anomalies. Recall that children with tracheal esophageal fistulas also have a 20% incidence of major cardiovascular anomalies (see answer 574) (*Miller: Anesthesia, ed 6, pp 2395-2396, 2864*).

586. (E) Neonates and infants (<2 years of age) require more succinylcholine per body weight than do older children and adults to produce neuromuscular blockade, because the extracellular fluid volume is much greater in neonates and infants. Because the volume of distribution of succinylcholine is greater, the recommended dose of succinylcholine in neonates and infants to provide optimal conditions for tracheal intubation is 2 mg/kg instead of the 1 mg/kg used for adults (*Miller: Anesthesia, ed 6, pp 2378-2379; Motoyama: Smith's Anesthesia for Infants and Children, ed 7, pp 217-219, 537*).

587. (E) Heart rates less than 100 beats/min are poorly tolerated in the neonate because of the reduced cardiac output and poor tissue perfusion that develops. Congenital heart disease, such as congenital heart block or congenital heart failure, is rare and can be diagnosed by neonatal electrocardiogram and echocardiogram. Maternal medications during labor and delivery rarely cause bradycardia, however, fetal distress as a result of hypoxia may. Fever tends to cause tachycardia. Cold stress of the neonate may lead to hypoxemia, which will promote persistence of the fetal circulation, which is why a neutral thermal environment to minimize heat loss is important. However, the most common cause of neonatal bradycardia in the delivery room is respiratory failure resulting in hypoxia and acidosis. In the operating room, bradycardia results from hypoxia, vagal stimulation and the depressant effects of anesthetic agents (e.g., halothane), which can lead to cardiac arrest (*Motoyama: Smith's Anesthesia for Infants and Children, ed 7, pp 1128-1131*).

588. (B) Apnea spells are defined as cessation of breathing for at least 20 seconds and are often accompanied by bradycardia and/or cyanosis. Infants (especially former premature newborns) younger than 60 weeks postconceptual age are at risk for apnea after general anesthesia. These patients should be admitted to the hospital and have at least 12 apnea-free hours of monitoring before discharge. This child was born at 31 weeks estimated gestational age and is now 10 weeks old or is 41 weeks postconceptual age and needs to be admitted. Of the postoperative analgesia plans listed with overnight observation, answer B is the most appropriate. Answers C and E include analgesic doses that are too high (*Barash: Clinical Anesthesia, ed 5, pp 1192-1193; Miller: Anesthesia, ed 6, pp 1732-1736, 2397-2399*).

589. (B) The treatment for documented ventricular fibrillation or pulseless ventricular tachycardia is electrical defibrillation as soon as possible. Cardiopulmonary resuscitation is performed until the defibrillator arrives, then defibrillation is attempted. With manual defibrillators (monophasic or biphasic) the initial dose should be 2 J/kg, increasing to 4 J/kg for subsequent shocks. In this 20-kg child the initial dose is 20 × 2 J/kg = 40 J. Automated external defibrillators (AEDs) can be safely used in children 1 to 8 years of age. If using an AED, it is best to use one with a pediatric attenuator system, which decreases the delivered energy to doses appropriate for children (*2005 American Heart Association Guidelines for Cardiopulmonary Resuscitation and Emergency Cardiovascular Care. Circulation 112, pp IV 172-IV 175*).

590. (C)

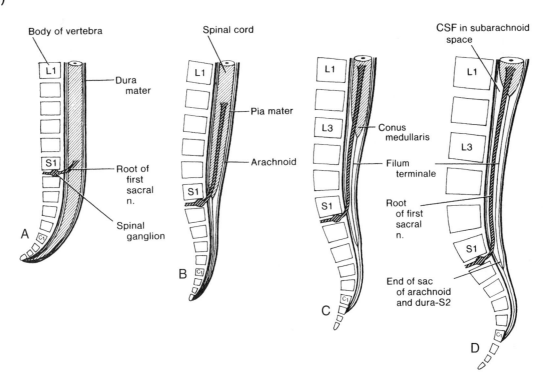

The position of the inferior end of the spinal cord in relation to the vertebral column and meninges at various stages of development: A, Eight weeks; B, 24 weeks; C, newborn; D, 8-year-old child and adult. The spinal cord of newborns can extend as far down as L3. Therefore, lumbar puncture should be performed in these patients no higher than the L4-L5 interspace (*Motoyama: Smith's Anesthesia for Infants and Children, ed 7, pp 465-468*).

591. (D) Esophageal atresia (EA) and TEF are frequently suspected soon after birth when excessive oral secretions, drooling, or coughing are noted and an oral suction catheter cannot be passed into the stomach. Because passage of an oral gastric tube is not routine in many centers, the first manifestation of esophageal atresia occurs when the newborn has trouble breathing (e.g., coughing) and regurgitates with the first feeding. After the diagnosis is made, these patients should be placed in the head-up position and the blind upper pouch of the esophagus should be decompressed with a suction tube immediately to reduce pulmonary aspiration of secretions. Other abnormalities associated with EA and TEF include VACTERL (Vertebral abnormalities, imperforate Anus, Congenital heart disease, Tracheoesophageal fistula, Renal abnormalities, Limb abnormalities) (*Hines: Stoelting's Anesthesia and Co-Existing Disease, ed 5, pp 595-596; Miller: Anesthesia, ed 6, p 2396*).

592. (E) Omphalocele is the external herniation of abdominal viscera through the base of the umbilical cord. It occurs in about 1 of 5000 cases. Thirty percent of these newborns will die in the neonatal period, primarily from cardiac defects or prematurity. Some of these newborns with omphalocele have a syndrome called Beckwith-Wiedemann syndrome. This syndrome is characterized by omphalocele, organomegaly, macrosomia, large fontanelles, macroglossia, polycythemia, and hypoglycemia. These patients may be very difficult to intubate because of their significant macroglossia (*Hines: Stoelting's Anesthesia and Co-Existing Disease, ed 5, p 596; Motoyama: Smith's Anesthesia for Infants and Children, ed 7, p 1215*).

593. (C) Anesthesia for patients with EA and TEF can be safely induced with either an intravenous or volatile anesthetic. However, positive-pressure bag and mask ventilation will force gas into the stomach, potentially making ventilation of the lungs more difficult and should be avoided. A frequently used technique to facilitate correct placement of the endotracheal tube is to advance the tube into a bronchus. While listening over the stomach, slowly withdraw the tube until breath sounds are heard over the stomach. Advance the tube until these sounds become diminished (*Hines: Stoelting's Anesthesia and Co-Existing Disease, ed 5, p 596; Motoyama: Smith's Anesthesia for Infants and Children, ed 7, pp 551-552*).

594.   (C)   Unlike adults, neonates and infants seldom have muscle fasciculations with succinylcholine. The most frequently encountered side effect associated with succinylcholine in neonates and infants is bradycardia, especially when succinylcholine is given intravenously. The incidence of bradydysrhythmias is significantly decreased when the succinylcholine is administered intramuscularly. Other side effects include rhabdomyolysis, myoglobinuria, hyperkalemia, and malignant hyperthermia (*Miller: Anesthesia, ed 6, pp 2378-2379; Motoyama: Smith's Anesthesia for Infants and Children, ed 7, pp 219-220*).

595.   (C)   The estimated blood volume (EBV) of healthy full-term neonates is approximately 80 to 90 mL/kg. For this 4-kg neonate the volume is 320 to 360 mL. Premature newborns have an EBV of 90 to 100 mL/kg, whereas the 3- to 12-month-old infant has an EBV of 75 to 80 mL/kg (*Motoyama: Smith's Anesthesia for Infants and Children, ed 7, p 367; Stoelting: Basics of Anesthesia, ed 5, p 510*).

596.   (C)   In the fetus, pulmonary vascular resistance is extremely high. Most of the right ventricular output in utero bypasses the lungs and flows into the descending aorta through the ductus arteriosus. With the onset of ventilation at birth the pulmonary vascular resistance suddenly decreases, enabling blood to flow more easily through the lungs. Pulmonary vascular resistance continues to decrease after birth reaching adult levels by 2 to 3 months of life. This is when children with left-to-right cardiac shunts increase their shunts making symptoms of congestive heart failure (CHF) more apparent. The increase in Pao_2 not only acts as a pulmonary artery vasodilator (along with the lowering of the $Paco_2$) but also acts as a vasoconstrictor to the ductus arteriosus (thus further assisting the change from the fetal to the adult circulation) (*Miller: Anesthesia, ed 6, pp 2833-2834; Motoyama: Smith's Anesthesia for Infants and Children, ed 7, p 73*).

597.   (D)   A comprehensive understanding of thermoregulation and meticulous attention to details during the anesthetic care of infants are necessary to minimize intraoperative heat loss. In anesthetized infants, the heat loss occurs through the transfer of heat from the patient to the environment in one of four ways: radiation, conduction, convection and evaporation. For this reason, placement of an infrared heater over the OR table and prewarming the OR atmosphere are the most effective means of preventing hypothermia in these patients. Covering the OR table with a heating blanket; ventilating the patient with warm, humidified anesthetic gases; wrapping the extremities of the patient with sheet wadding; and covering the patient's head with a cloth or plastic cap can also reduce heat loss and prevent hypothermia. Convective forced-air warmers can help prevent a decrease in body temperature and also have been effective in rewarming hypothermic patients. A Mapleson D breathing circuit is not a circle system and does not preserve heat or moisture. To prevent rebreathing of expired gases spontaneous breathing flow rates need to be 2 to 3 times the minute ventilation and for controlled ventilation fresh gas flows need to be greater than 90 mL/kg/min. Low flows such as 50 mL/kg/min with Mapleson circuits are inadequate and will result in respiratory acidosis (*Miller: Anesthesia, ed 6, pp 1584-1586; Motoyama: Smith's Anesthesia for Infants and Children, ed 7, pp 170-173*).

598.   (E)   Although all of the conditions can produce ventilatory depression in the postoperative period, only pyloric stenosis produces central nervous system (CNS) depression of respiration. Patients with pyloric stenosis have protracted vomiting that leads to dehydration, hypokalemia, hyponatremia, hypochloremia, and metabolic alkalosis. Postoperative ventilatory depression frequently occurs in infants with pyloric stenosis, thought to be related to cerebrospinal fluid (CSF) alkalosis that is worsened by intraoperative hyperventilation of the lungs. Thus, these patients should be fully awake with a normal rate and pattern of respiration before extubation is considered. This is one reason infants with pyloric stenosis should be stabilized and hydrated before coming to the OR. The other conditions listed can lead to mechanical, not central, causes of respiratory difficulty in the postoperative period (*Hines: Stoelting's Anesthesia and Co-Existing Disease, ed 5, pp 599-600*).

599.   (D)   Newborns with diaphragmatic hernia have significant respiratory difficulty. In addition to their hypoplastic lungs, persistent pulmonary hypertension is present, producing right-to-left shunting through the patent ductus arteriosus. To more appropriately administer the anesthetic, a preductal (ductus arteriosus) artery should be cannulated to monitor arterial blood gases and blood pressure. The right radial or temporal arteries arise from vessels that originate from the aorta proximal to the ductus arteriosus. The oxygen saturation monitors should be placed on the right arm as well (*Hines: Stoelting's Anesthesia and Co-Existing Disease, ed 5, pp 593-594*).

600.   (C)   The MAC for halothane and isoflurane is greatest at age 3 months. The MAC is lower in preterm neonates compared with term neonates. The low MAC in the newborns may be related to the immaturity of the CNS and/or related to the elevated levels of progesterone and β-endorphins. The increase in MAC in the first few weeks after birth seems to be related to the falling progesterone levels. After age 3 months, the MAC of these volatile anesthetics steadily declines with aging except for a slight increase at puberty. For reasons that are unclear, the MAC for sevoflurane is similar in neonates and infants younger than 6 months (3.2%). The MAC of sevoflurane then decreases with age, 6 months to 12 years (2.5%) (*Hines: Stoelting's Anesthesia and Co-Existing Disease, ed 5, p 584; Motoyama: Smith's Anesthesia for Infants and Children, ed 7, p 211*).

601. (D) Intravascular fluid-volume deficits in patients with burn injuries are roughly proportional to the extent and depth of the burn. For reasons that are unclear, the vascular compartment, particularly in the area of the burn, becomes hyperpermeable to plasma proteins, such as fibrinogen and albumin. These proteins subsequently exert an osmotic pressure gradient that favors the translocation of intravascular fluid into the extravascular third space. Therefore, during this period (approximately first 24 hours), administration of colloid solutions would be of no benefit to the patient and might exacerbate third-space translocation of fluids. As a rule of thumb, an estimated 4 mL/kg of fluid is lost for each percent of body surface area burned. Thus, in this case: 4 × 40 (kg) × 50 (%) = 8000 mL. Approximately two thirds of this fluid should be replaced with isotonic crystalloid solutions during the first 8 hours after the injury. This estimate is modified clinically by the patient's clinical response as noted by the vital signs and urine output (*Hines: Stoelting's Anesthesia and Co-Existing Disease, ed 5, pp 630-635*).

602. (E) The most likely explanation for the "falling" hemoglobin level in this patient is that this is a normal physiologic finding. At birth, a full-term infant has a hemoglobin level of approximately 15 to 20 g/dL. A physiologic anemia occurs by age 2 to 3 months, resulting in hemoglobin concentrations of approximately 10 to 12 g/dL. After 3 months, there is a progressive increase in hemoglobin concentration, which reaches levels similar to that of adults by age 6 to 9 months (*Hines: Stoelting's Anesthesia and Co-Existing Disease, ed 5, p 583; Motoyama: Smith's Anesthesia for Infants and Children, ed 7, p 397*).

603. (D) This history is consistent with an acute life-threatening cause of upper airway obstruction called epiglottitis (or more appropriately supraglottitis because other supraglottic structures are involved as well). In the past it was caused most often by *Haemophilus influenzae*. With widespread immunization against *H. influenzae* this condition has become much less frequent and the primary causes now are *Neisseria meningitidis*, group A Streptococcus, and *Candida albicans*. This condition is a medical emergency that can progress to respiratory obstruction in just a few hours. When suspected, the anesthesiologist and otolaryngologist should be notified and the child immediately transferred to the OR (with the parent if appropriate) before complete upper airway obstruction ensues. In the OR, anesthesia should be induced with halothane or sevoflurane and oxygen with the child in a sitting position. Halothane or sevoflurane are less likely to induce laryngospasm than isoflurane, or desflurane. IV access should be established as soon as the child is deeply anesthetized. Atropine should be administered to block vagally mediated bradycardia induced by direct laryngoscopy. Muscle relaxants are contraindicated because they can cause complete obstruction of the upper airway in these patients. The trachea should be intubated under direct laryngoscopy when the depth of anesthesia is sufficient to blunt laryngeal reflexes (*Hines: Stoelting's Anesthesia and Co-Existing Disease, ed 5, pp 614-616; Motoyama: Smith's Anesthesia for Infants and Children, ed 7, pp 810-812*).

604. (E) Cerebral palsy is a CNS symptom complex. The most common clinical manifestation is skeletal muscle spasticity. It is usually classified according to the extremity affected (e.g., monoplegia, hemiplegia, diplegia, or quadriplegia) and the characteristics of the neurologic dysfunction (spastic, hypotonic, dystonic, athetotic). Other manifestations include cerebellar ataxia, seizure disorders, varying degrees of mental retardation, and speech deficits. Gastroesophageal reflux is also common. For this reason, the preferred induction of general anesthesia in these patients should include a rapid-sequence IV induction followed by immediate tracheal intubation. Even though these patients have skeletal muscle spasticity, there have been no reports of succinylcholine-induced hyperkalemia. The response to nondepolarizing muscle relaxants is normal (*Hines: Stoelting's Anesthesia and Co-Existing Disease, ed 5, p 603*).

605. (E) The symptoms described in this patient are consistent with severe dehydration. Thus, the vascular volume should be expanded initially with an isotonic saline solution or a colloid solution until the patient voids. When the urine output increases, potassium can be added to the IV fluids. Although glucose administration for long procedures may prevent hypoglycemia, D_5W alone or with a crystalloid solution should not be used to replace fluid deficits (*Motoyama: Smith's Anesthesia for Infants and Children, ed 7, pp 119-121*).

606.   **(A)**   Preterm infants have very limited calcium reserves and are very susceptible to hypocalcemia. Hypocalcemia (serum ionized calcium level less than 1.5 mEq/L) manifests itself in a number of nonspecific ways, including irritability, twitching, hypotension, and seizure. A dose of 100 to 200 mg/kg of calcium gluconate administered over 2 to 3 minutes will be appropriate and repeated every 6 to 8 hours until the calcium levels stabilize. Some of the signs of hypoglycemia are similar to those of hypocalcemia and include seizure, irritability, hypotension, and sometimes bradycardia and apnea. In the patient described in this question, the glucose has already been measured at 50 mg/dL, which is acceptable for a preterm infant. An O_2 saturation of 88% is also acceptable because the patient is at risk for retinopathy of prematurity (i.e., younger than 44 weeks postconceptual age). Hyperventilation would cause alkalosis, which would decrease the unbound fraction of calcium and make the patient more susceptible to seizures. Furthermore, calcium binds to albumin, which would further reduce the free calcium. Because the urine output is more than adequate, it is unlikely that the patient needs a fluid bolus to correct hypotension (*Hines: Stoelting's Anesthesia and Co-Existing Disease, ed 5, pp 590-592*).

607.   **(A)**   An Eutectic Mixture of the Local Anesthetics (EMLA) cream is lidocaine (2.5%) and prilocaine (2.5%). When the 5% EMLA cream is applied to dry intact skin and covered with an occlusive dressing for at least 1 hour, topical anesthesia to a depth of 5 mm is obtained. Eutectic mixture of the local anesthetics (EMLA) appears to be relatively safe in neonates, and methemoglobinemia is exceeding rare (*Miller: Anesthesia ed 6, pp 589-590; Motoyama: Smith's Anesthesia for Infants and Children, ed 7, p 500*).

608.   **(D)**   Although the umbilical vein (UV) is larger and easier to cannulate than the umbilical artery (UA), the UV will not allow for adequate assessment of arterial blood gases or systemic blood pressure. Additionally, administration of drugs or hypertonic solutions into the umbilical vein may be hazardous, because the catheter can become wedged in a portal radicle and may lead to hepatic necrosis or portal vein thrombosis. To prevent this, the umbilical vein catheter tip is advanced only 2 to 3 cm into the umbilical vein (to a point where blood can first be aspirated). Careful placement of an umbilical artery catheter is equally important. The tip of the umbilical artery catheter should be placed just above the bifurcation of the aorta and below the celiac, renal, and mesenteric arteries (i.e., ideally between L3 and L4). Dislocation may be hazardous because improper placement may be associated with thrombosis or embolism in these major vessels. As there are two arteries and only one vein, difficulty with one artery gives another artery to use (*Miller: Anesthesia, ed 6, pp 2356-2357, 2843-2844*).

609.   **(C)**   Because of the large surface-area-to-weight ratio, the thin layer of insulating subcutaneous fat, and the limited ability to compensate for cold stress, neonates and infants are at greater risk for intraoperative hypothermia than adults. Infants younger than 3 months do not produce heat by shivering; their principle method of thermogenesis is metabolism of brown fat. Heat loss can occur by radiation, conduction, convection and evaporation. Heat loss through evaporation (not conduction) can be reduced by humidification of inspired gases. Heat loss by conduction (not convection) is reduced with the use of a warming blanket (*Miller: Anesthesia, ed 6, pp 1576, 2371*).

610.   **(D)**   In a 6-month-old infant, a normal hemoglobin value is approximately 11 to 12 gm/dL. The normal heart rate is about 120 beats/min, systolic blood pressure is 90 to 95, and the respiratory rate is about 24 to 30 breaths/min. O_2 consumption in infants is 5 mL/kg/min (5 mL/kg × 7 kg = 35 mL/min), approximately two times that of adults (*Stoelting: Basics of Anesthesia, ed 5, pp 508-510*).

611.   **(A)**   The oculocardiac reflex (OCR) is commonly defined as a 10% to 20% decrease in heart rate that is sustained for more than 5 seconds. It can be induced by traction on extraocular muscles, pressure on the eye, orbital hematoma, ocular trauma, or eye pain. It is commonly seen with strabismus operations and may produce a wide variety of cardiac arrhythmias, including sinus bradycardia, nodal bradycardia, ectopic beats, ventricular fibrillation, and, rarely, asystole (1 in 2200 strabismus operations). The initial treatment of this is to stop the stimulus (i.e., tell the surgeon to stop what he or she is doing). This reflex quickly responds and future similar stimulation typically gives less of a response. In many cases no further treatment is necessary. Other manipulations that can be done include increasing the depth of general anesthesia, changing from halothane to sevoflurane (which has a lower incidence of the reflex), and reassessing the adequacy of ventilation (as hypercarbia decreases the threshold to elicit the OCR). A retrobulbar block with prevent the reflex. Infiltrating lidocaine locally into the recti muscles may be effective in preventing and treating the OCR. Atropine or glycopyrrolate can be administered if the arrhythmia persists. Some advocate the prophylactic use of atropine or glycopyrrolate during strabismus surgery, especially in children (*Miller: Anesthesia, ed 6, pp 2535-2536; Motoyama: Smith's Anesthesia for Infants and Children, ed 7, pp 778-780*).

612. (C) There is no difference in Vt between neonates and adults. Neonates have a high O_2 consumption (about twice the adult). To compensate for the increased oxygen demand alveolar ventilation is increased (also about twice the adult). The increase in alveolar ventilation explains the slightly lower $Paco_2$. Of note, however, is that the pH is slightly lower as well. The reduced functional residual capacity with the increased O_2 consumption places the neonate at an increased risk for hypoxia during general anesthesia if there is any difficulty with ventilation (*Hines: Stoelting's Anesthesia and Co-Existing Disease, ed 5, pp 582-583; Stoelting: Basics of Anesthesia, ed 5, pp 508-509*).

PHYSIOLOGIC VARIABLES

	Neonate	Infant	5 year old	Adult
Weight (kg)	3	4-10	18	70
Respiratory rate (breaths/min)	35	24-30	20	15
Alveolar ventilation (mL/kg/min)	130			60
Tidal volume (mL/kg)	6	6	6	6
Vital capacity (mL/kg)	35			70
Functional residual capacity (mL/kg)	30			35
Oxygen consumption (mL/kg/min)	6	5	4	3
Carbon dioxide production (mL/kg/min)	6			3
Pao_2 (room air, mm Hg)	65-85			85-95
$Paco_2$ (room air, mm Hg)	30-36			36-44
pH	7.34-7.40			7.36-7.44

(Stoelting: Basics of Anesthesia, ed 5, pp 508-509; Hines: Stoelting's Anesthesia and Co-Existing Diseases, ed 5, p 583.)

613. (D) Neurofibromatosis (von Recklinghausen's disease) is an autosomal dominant genetic disorder characterized by multiple neurofibromas involving the skin and peripheral and central nervous systems. The clinical features of this disease are diverse and always progress with time. The anesthetic management of patients with neurofibromatosis can be complicated by the associated clinical manifestations of this disease. For example, a pheochromocytoma may be present in approximately 1% of patients. If this is unrecognized, severe hypertension can occur during anesthesia. Intracranial tumors occur in 5% to 10% of patients and signs and symptoms of intracranial hypertension may develop. If intracranial pressure is elevated, efforts to reduce intracranial pressure should be initiated. Finally, airway patency may become compromised by an enlarging laryngeal neurofibroma. Abnormal responses to both depolarizing neuromuscular blocking agents (sensitive or resistant) and nondepolarizing neuromuscular blocking agents (sensitive) have been described. There is no evidence that these patients are at increased risk for malignant hyperthermia (*Motoyama: Smith's Anesthesia for Infants and Children, ed 7, p 1221; Hines: Stoelting's: Anesthesia and Co-Existing Disease, ed 5, pp 226-227*).

614. (D) Retinopathy of prematurity (ROP) is an abnormal proliferation of immature retinal vessels, which usually occurs after exposure to hyperoxia. The most significant risk factor for ROP is prematurity and is inversely related to birth weight. More than 50% of premature infants who weigh 750 to 1000 g and survive develop ROP; fortunately, many of these infants have spontaneous regression of the retinal changes. The most recognized risk of ROP in premature infants is elevated oxygen concentrations (i.e., Pao_2 > 80 to 90 mm Hg for prolonged periods) in neonates younger than 44 weeks postconceptual age. It is possible to develop ROP with exposures as short as 1 to 2 hours to a Pao_2 of 150 mm Hg. However, ROP has also occurred in patients who have never received supplemental oxygen and in some newborns who have cyanotic heart disease, making the etiology a bit unclear. Other associated factors include hypoxia, hypercarbia, hypocarbia, sepsis, and apnea. Retinopathy of prematurity (ROP) is clearly a multifactorial disease that cannot be explained simply by exposure to high concentrations of oxygen. At one time, the administration of anesthesia for non-ophthalmologic procedures was believed to cause an increase incidence of ROP, but further studies have revealed no increased incidence. When administering anesthesia to infants younger than 44 weeks postconceptual age, the goal of oxygen therapy is to maintain a Pao_2 of 60 to 90 mm Hg (oxygen saturation of 90% to 95%) (*Miller: Anesthesia, ed 6, pp 2534-3535; Motoyama: Smith's Anesthesia for Infants and Children, ed 7, pp 781-782*).

615. (C) The amount of dehydration that children have can be assessed by a variety of observations. For mild dehydration (5% weight loss) the only abnormal finding of the listed answers is urine output which would be less than 2 mL/kg/hr. With moderate dehydration (10% weight loss) mucous membranes would be dry, skin turgor would be decreased, urine output would be less than 1mL/kg/hr, the anterior fontanel would be depressed and blood pressure would be normal to low. With severe dehydration (15% weight loss) mucous membranes would be very dry, skin turgor would be greatly decreased, urine output would be less than 0.5 mL/kg/hr, the anterior fontanel would be markedly depressed and blood pressure would be reduced and orthostatic (*Motoyama: Smith's Anesthesia for Infants and Children, ed 7, pp 119-120*).

616.   **(A)**   Postoperative bleeding after a tonsillectomy occurs in 0.1% to 8% of cases. The bleeding is defined as primary if it occurs within 24 hours and secondary if more than 24 hours after surgery. Most fatal cases are due to primary bleeding. Because of the risk of significant bleeding most often occurs within the first 6 hours after the surgery (75% of bleeding cases), most units keep patients for at least 6 to 8 hours after the surgery is completed. Sixty-seven percent of bleeding occurs in the tonsillar fossa alone, 27% in the nasopharynx alone, and the rest in both the tonsillar fossa and the nasopharynx (*Barash: Clinical Anesthesia, ed 5, pp 998-1001; Motoyama: Smith's Anesthesia for Infants and Children, ed 7, pp 798-799*).

617.   **(E)**   Ear, nose and throat surgeons often use vasoconstrictors (e.g., phenylephrine, cocaine or oxymetazoline) to control bleeding in pharyngeal and nasal surgery. For adults, the initial dose of phenylephrine is up to 0.5 mg (4 drops of a 0.25% solution). For children, the initial dose is up to 0.20 μg/kg. When excessive doses are used, severe hypertension and cardiovascular decompensation may develop due to the marked increase in peripheral vascular resistance. This also shifts blood from the peripheral site into the pulmonary vasculature (which is less sensitive to vasoconstrictors) and increases left ventricular filling pressure. In this case, the use of labetalol and deepening the anesthesia has been associated with severe pulmonary edema, cardiac arrest, and death. If labetalol or a β blocker (e.g., esmolol) is used and CHF develops, consider using high dose glucagon (5-10 mg) to counteract the loss of cardiac contractility. This may also occur with the use of calcium channel blockers. Baroreceptor-induced bradycardia may not occur in the pediatric patient who has been pretreated with atropine or glycopyrrolate during the anesthetic. The hypertension may be short lived and deepening the inhalation anesthetic may help; however, treatment of severe hypertension is best with direct vasodilators or α adrenergic receptor antagonists (*Miller: Anesthesia, ed 6, pp 2547-2548; Groudine SB et al. New York State Guidelines on the topical use of phenylephrine in the operating room. Anesthesiology, 92:859-864, 2000*).

618.   **(C)**   Tetracaine and bupivacaine are the most commonly used drugs for spinal anesthesia in infants. For infants who weigh 5 to 15 kg, a dose of 0.4 mg/kg of 1% tetracaine will last about 80 minutes, 0.4 mg/kg of 0.5% bupivacaine would last about 70 to 80 minutes. For infants less than 5 kg, the dose is larger, i.e., 0.5 mg/kg for tetracaine and 0.5 mg/kg for bupivacaine, and the duration of the anesthetic is about 5 minutes shorter. If epinephrine is added, the duration of a tetracaine spinal anesthetic is about 30% to 50% longer. Epinephrine added to bupivacaine has little effect (*Miller: Anesthesia, ed 6, pp 1737-1738*).

619.   **(A)**   About 80% of children with inspiratory stridor have laryngotracheobronchitis (croup) and about 5% have epiglottitis (also called acute supraglottitis). All of the answers listed except A, as well as a "barking cough," refer to signs and symptoms of laryngotracheobronchitis, a viral illness that usually presents in children between 6 months and 6 years of age. Patients with acute epiglottitis (or supraglottitis) are usually 2 to 7 years of age. The onset of signs and symptoms of acute epiglottitis is typically rapid, less than 24-hours. They present with difficulty swallowing, a high fever (often > 39° C), and inspiratory stridor. Other signs and symptoms include drooling, lethargy, cyanosis, tachypnea, neutrophilia, and a propensity to sit up and lean forward (in an attempt to maintain their airway). Total upper airway obstruction can occur in these children at any time because of the rapid progression of the disease. For this reason, attempts to visualize the epiglottis should not be undertaken until the patient is in the OR and appropriate preparations are completed for direct laryngoscopy and tracheal intubation, and possible emergency tracheostomy. The definitive treatment of acute epiglottitis includes appropriate antibiotic therapy and a secured airway. Also see explanation to question 603 (*Motoyama: Smith's Anesthesia for Infants and Children, ed 7, pp 810-812; Hines: Stoelting's: Anesthesia and Co-Existing Disease, ed 5, pp 614-617*).

620.   **(A)**   The technique for cardiopulmonary resuscitation of infants (younger than 1 year) and children (ages 1 to 8 years) is different from that of adults. Ventilation is begun for adults at a rate of 10 to 12 breaths/min, whereas for children and infants, the rate is 12 to 20 breaths/min. For adults, sternal compressions should be performed with the heel of one hand placed on top of the other hand and compressing the lower half of the sternum 4 to 5 cm (1.5 to 2 inches). For children, sternal compressions should be performed with the heel of one hand compressing the lower half of the sternum 2.5 to 4 cm (1 to 1.5 inches; or about one third to one half the depth of the chest). For infants, sternal compressions should be performed by depressing the lower half of the sternum just below the intermammary line. This is done with either two or three fingers or by encircling the chest with both hands and depressing the sternum with the thumbs. Sternal compressions are performed to a depth of 1 to 2.5 cm (0.5 to 1 inch; or about one third to one half the depth of the chest). The compression rate is the same for adults, children and infants, approximately 100 compressions/min. Lay rescuers should not check for pulses in infants or children as they often feel a pulse that is not present. When health care providers palpate for pulses, the brachial artery is preferred in the infant and the carotid or femoral is preferred in the child. A universal compression to ventilation ratio of 30:2 is used for (infants, children and adults) by single rescuers. Earlier it was taught to use a 5:1 ratio, but more recent evidence shows 30:2 to be more effective. For newborns however, a ratio of 3:1 (90 compressions and 30 ventilations/minute) is used (*2005 American Heart Association Guidelines for cardiopulmonary resuscitation and emergency cardiovascular care. Circulation 112: IV15, IV157-IV161, IV 192, 2005*).

621. **(C)**   Body composition changes dramatically during the first year of life. Total body water is about 80% for a term newborn compared with 55% for an adult woman and 60% for an adult man. Drugs that are water soluble (such as many antibiotics) will need to have higher mg/kg dose to achieve the desired blood concentrations. With the corresponding lower fat content of the preterm newborn (<5%) term newborn (10%) compared with the adult (15+%), fat soluble drugs that depend on redistribution such as thiopental will have a longer clinical effect. The glomerular filtration rate (GFR) of newborns is low at birth and doubles or triples over the first 3 months of life, with a slower rise until adult values are reached by 1 to 2 years of age. This decrease in renal function can delay excretion of drugs that are dependent on renal clearance for elimination. The relatively noncompliant heart of a newborn gives it a limited capacity to deal with a volume load, compared with the adult. The preterm newborn has 10%, the term newborn has 25% and the adult has 55% of type I muscle fibers (i.e., fatigue resistant, highly oxidative fibers). The lower proportion of type I fibers predisposes the newborn's primary respiratory muscle fibers to fatigue (*Miller: Anesthesia, ed 6, p 2371; Stoelting: Basics of Anesthesia, ed 5, pp 505-509*).

622. **(C)**

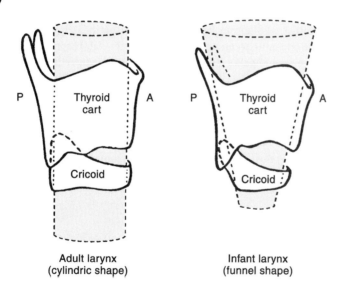

The anatomy of the infant's airway is different from the adult's anatomy in several respects. The head and tongue are relatively larger in the newborn. The larynx and glottic opening are more anterior and cephalad in the infant (infant's C3-C4, adult's C4-C5). The infant's larynx is funnel shaped compared with the adult's. The narrowest part of the adult larynx is at the vocal cord level, whereas in the child (younger than 10 years) the narrowest part is at the cricoid ring. The infant's epiglottis is relatively large, stubby and "U" shaped. The vocal cords of the infant are in a diagonal (not horizontal) position within the larynx. This diagonal position makes it more likely to have the endotracheal tube lodge in the anterior commissure rather than slide down the trachea (*Miller: Anesthesia, ed 6, pp 2369-2370; Stoelting: Basics of Anesthesia, ed 5, p 507*).

623. **(C)**   Children at the highest risk for PONV include patients with a history of previous PONV and/or motion sickness, strabismus corrections and cases where narcotics are routinely needed, such as tonsillectomy, orchiopexy and herniorrhaphy. Brief procedures with minimal pain such as myringotomy tube placements have a low incidence of PONV. In cases where PONV is likely, prophylaxis is recommended (*Motoyama: Smith's Anesthesia for Infants and Children, ed 7, p 867*).

624. **(E)** Down syndrome (trisomy 21) occurs in 1 in 700 to 1000 live births. There are many significant associated conditions. Congenital cardiac lesions are seen in about 40% of these patients (about one half are endocardial cushion defects; one fourth are ventricular septal defects; other lesions include patent ductus arteriosus, atrial septal defects, tetralogy of Fallot) and commonly necessitate prophylactic antibiotics. Other findings include short neck, small mouth, narrow nasopharynx, large tongue, thyroid hypofunction (50%), atlanto-occipital instability (15% to 20% that is most often asymptomatic), and smaller airways. Despite these abnormalities, tracheal intubation is usually not difficult in the hands of an experienced anesthesiologist. The size of the endotracheal tube used to create an air "leak" with increasing airway pressure should be one to two sizes smaller because of the smaller trachea (e.g., in children age 18 months to 8 years the endotracheal tube size is 1 mm smaller) (*Miller: Anesthesia, ed 6, p 1099; Shott, SR: Down syndrome: Analysis of airway size and a guide for appropriate intubation, Laryngoscope, 110:585-592, 2000; Hines: Stoelting's: Anesthesia and Co-Existing Disease, ed 5, pp 611-612*).

625. **(D)** Congenital cardiac abnormalities frequently occur in association with congenital diaphragmatic hernias, tracheoesophageal fistulas, meningomyeloceles, and omphaloceles. Gastroschisis is rarely associated with other congenital anomalies (*Hines: Stoelting's: Anesthesia and Co-Existing Disease, ed 5, pp 593-598, 608-609*).

626. **(B)** Newborns with CDH present with respiratory distress immediately after birth. They often have a flat (scaphoid) abdomen because some of the intestines herniate into the chest and are therefore not in the abdomen. Immediate care includes endotracheal intubation for ventilatory support and placement of an orogastric or nasogastric tube to evacuate the stomach. Ventilation of the lungs with a bag and mask may cause more respiratory compromise by producing gastric and intestinal distention and is contraindicated. When ventilating the newborn with an endotracheal tube, you must remember not to try to expand the lungs to normal size because the lungs are hypoplastic and prone to rupturing and producing a pneumothorax. Although at one time hyperventilation was recommended, more recently better outcomes have been found when permissive hypercarbia has been used ($Paco_2$ 45-55 mm Hg range). Associated congenital anomalies include CNS anomalies (e.g., spina bifida, hydrocephalus, anencephaly), cardiovascular (e.g., hypoplastic left heart syndrome, atrial and ventricular septal defects, coarctation, tetralogy of Fallot), gastrointestinal (e.g., malrotation, atresia), and genitourinary (e.g., hypospadias). Rushing the child to the operating room does not increase survival. It appears better to stabilize the child and look for associated congenital anomalies (seen in up to 50% of these children) before proceeding with surgery (*Fleisher: Anesthesia and Uncommon Diseases, ed 5, pp 626-630; Hines: Stoelting's: Anesthesia and Co-Existing Disease, ed 5, pp 593-594*).

627. **(E)** Respiratory adverse events (RAE) are common in children undergoing noncardiac surgeries. They are more often associated with younger children (<5 years of age compared with >5 years of age), in children with a recent URI (although a few studies question this), in children with airway anomalies (e.g., cleft palate, subglottic stenosis, Pierre Robin syndrome), and when a laryngeal mask airway is used, compared with the use of mask anesthesia (*Flick et al. Risk factors for laryngospasm in children during general anesthesia. Pediatric Anesthesia, 18:289-296, 2008; Motoyama: Smith's Anesthesia for Infants and Children, ed 7, pp 1161-1162*).

628. **(B)** Perioperative cardiac arrest is often defined as the need for cardiopulmonary resuscitation or death during anesthesia care (OR and postanesthesia care unit [PACU]). It is more than 4 times greater in neonates (0-30 days) than infants or children. Causes of cardiac arrest vary from study to study and often include medication related (e.g., inhalation or intravenous overdosage, succinylcholine-induced dysrhythmia, medication "swaps"), drug related (e.g., high spinal anesthesia, local anesthetic toxicity, opioid-induced respiratory depression, inadequate reversal of muscle relaxants), cardiovascular related (e.g., hemorrhage, hyperkalemia, vagal reflexes, embolism, sepsis), respiratory related (e.g., inadequate ventilation, loss of the airway, aspiration, pneumothorax), and equipment related (e.g., disconnects, stuck valves). Equipment-related causes are relatively rare causes of cardiac arrest (about 4% of cases). About 90% of cardiac arrests due to anesthesia-related episodes are reversed (adequate native heartbeat and blood pressure for at least 20 minutes after the arrest). If the cardiac arrest is not anesthesia-related, outcome is worse (only about 50%-60% are reversed). Regardless of surgical procedure, children with congenital heart disease have a greater chance of a cardiac arrest. Emergency surgery is associated with a six times greater incidence of cardiac arrest than elective surgery (*Flick et al: Perioperative cardiac arrests in children between 1988 and 2005 at a tertiary referral center. Anesthesiology, 106:226-237, 2007; Motoyama: Smith's Anesthesia for Infants and Children, ed 7, pp 1110-1116*).

629. **(E)** Klippel-Feil syndrome (1 in 42,000 births) is characterized by musculoskeletal abnormalities (short neck which results from reduction in the number of cervical vertebra due to cervical vertebral fusion, kyphoscoliosis in 50%

of patients, micrognathia, spinal canal stenosis), renal anomalies (33%), congenital heart disease (most commonly VSD), and hearing impairment. The most important consideration in the anesthetic management of these patients is a possibility of cervical spine instability, which can result in neurologic damage during direct laryngoscopy. Lateral and anteroposterior flexion-extension neck radiographs should be performed to assist in the evaluation of the stability of the cervical spine. Cervical MRI should be considered to assess neurologic function. Evaluation for congenital heart disease, as well as assessment of current respiratory and renal function should be done (*Fleisher: Anesthesia and Uncommon Diseases, ed 5, pp 294-296; Hines: Stoelting's: Anesthesia and Co-Existing Disease, ed 5, p 465*).

630. (D) All of the statements are correct except for D. To eliminate rebreathing, higher fresh gas flows are needed with spontaneous ventilation than with controlled ventilation (*Motoyama: Smith's Anesthesia for Infants and Children, ed 7, pp 276-278*).

631. (D) At birth, the respiratory center of newborns is not fully developed. Newborns not uncommonly show two types of pauses in respiration. Periodic breathing exists if the pauses are short (i.e., 5-10 seconds) and not associated with a decrease in heart rate or oxygen saturation. Episodes of central apnea of infancy, also called apnea and bradycardia (A&B) spells, are longer and more significant. With A&B spells, the respiratory pauses are usually greater than 15 to 20 seconds and are associated with a decrease in heart rate (<100), a decrease in oxygen saturation, cyanosis and/or pallor. Treatment is usually tactile stimulation for A&B spells whereas periodic breathing patterns do not need treatment. Untreated A&B spells can be lethal. Postoperative apnea is inversely correlated with both gestational age at birth (GA) and postconceptual age (PCA) (PCA = GA + chronologic age) up to 60 weeks PCA. Postoperative apnea is highest in the first 4 to 6 hours, but can present up to 12 hours after surgery. Postoperative apnea is also associated with infants who have had a history of A&B spells as well as anemia (Hct <30). Caffeine has been used as a respiratory stimulant to decrease the incidence and severity of postoperative apnea. Although spinal anesthesia with no sedation has a lower incidence of apnea, compared with general anesthesia, the addition of any sedation such as ketamine increases the incidence of apnea more than that observed with general anesthesia. Some controversy exists as to when young infants can be treated as outpatients due to this risk of postoperative apnea. In our practice, healthy full term infants (>38 weeks GA) who have not reached 44 weeks PCA and healthy preterm infants (<38 weeks GA) who have not reached 50 weeks are admitted for overnight monitoring (*Motoyama: Smith's Anesthesia for Infants and Children, ed 7, pp 24-25, 562-563, 875-876, 1163-1164*).

632. (A) The loss of resistance technique used when placing an epidural needle into the epidural space of a child should be done with saline and not air to decrease the risk of an air embolism. Note that the loss of resistance is much more subtle in the child, compared with the adult, when the epidural space is located (*Motoyama: Smith's Anesthesia for Infants and Children, ed 7, p 476*).

633. (B) The fasting recommendations to reduce the risk of pulmonary aspiration is commonly called the 2-4-6-8 rule.

MINIMUM FASTING PERIODS

Ingested Material	Minimum Fasting Period
Clear fluids (water, Jello, apple or grape juice)	2 hours
Breast milk	4 hours
Infant formula, non-human milk, orange juice	6 hours
Solid food (toast or cereal) or high-fat meals	8 hours

(*ASA task force on preoperative fasting: Practice guidelines for preoperative fasting and the use of pharmacologic agents to reduce the risk of pulmonary aspiration: Application to healthy patients undergoing elective procedures, Anesthesiology 90:896-905, 1999; Motoyama: Smith's Anesthesia for Infants and Children, ed 7, pp 265, 321, 882*).

634. (E) In neonates or infants, hypothermia can result in increased total body O_2 consumption, metabolic acidosis, hypoglycemia, delayed awakening, prolonged duration of action of nondepolarizing muscle relaxants, and depression of ventilation. Therefore, monitoring the body temperature and maneuvers to minimize or eliminate significant loss of body heat during anesthesia for neonates and small infants are essential during the perioperative period (*Miller: Anesthesia, ed 6, pp 516, 2371, 2862; Morgan: Clinical Anesthesiology, ed 4, p 924*).

635. (D) Necrotizing enterocolitis (NEC) classically occurs in premature infants and in infants with low birth weight (typically less than 2500 g) and carries a high mortality rate (10%-30% and higher in severely affected very low birth weight infants). In newborns less than 1500 g, the incidence is 10% to 20%. These children may be acidotic, hypoxic, and in shock. Most have thrombocytopenia (50,000-70,000/mm^3) and prolonged prothrombin time (PT) and activated partial thromboplastin time (aPPT). Necrotizing enterocolitis (NEC) follows intestinal mucosal injury from ischemia. It is most commonly associated with decreased cardiac output in the presence of fetal asphyxia or postnatal respiratory complications in the early postnatal period. Other factors associated with the pathogenesis of necrotizing enterocolitis include a history of umbilical artery catheterization, enteral feeding of small preterm infants, bacterial infection, polycythemia, and gram-negative endotoxemia. Although umbilical artery catheters are often used in the newborn period, these should be removed if NEC develops, because they may compromise mesenteric blood flow. Unless there is evidence of intestinal necrosis or perforation, nonoperative therapy should be instituted. This includes cessation of enteral feeding, decompression of the stomach, administration of broad-spectrum antibiotics, fluid and electrolyte therapy, parenteral nutrition, and correction of hematologic abnormalities. Inotropic drugs may be needed in the presence of shock (*Hines: Stoelting's Anesthesia and Co-Existing Disease, ed 5, pp 600-601; Motoyama: Smith's Anesthesia for Infants and Children, ed 7, pp 552-555*).

636. (C) For the treatment of postoperative pain, regional anesthesia including local infiltration, narcotics and nonopioid analgesics such as acetaminophen and ketorolac are useful. Ketorolac should not be given to patients when you are concerned about postoperative bleeding, such as after a tonsillectomy. Although dexmedetomidine could provide analgesia, it is not commonly used for postoperative analgesia because of its expense and the need for an IV (See also answer to question 616) (*Motoyama: Smith's Anesthesia for Infants and Children, ed 7, pp 866-867*).

637. (C) Sudden infant death syndrome (SIDS) is the unexplained death of an infant that is younger than 1 year of age. The peak age of SIDS is 3 to 4 months and is rare during the first month of life. Epidemiologic studies show an increased chance of SIDS with low birth weight infants, maternal smoking, maternal cocaine use, low socioeconomic status, and with African Americans. There is no association with general anesthesia. Recently it has been noted that infants that sleep in the supine position have a lower rate of SIDS than infants who sleep in the prone position (*Barash: Clinical Anesthesia, ed 5, pp 1193-1194*).

638. (E) Hemolytic-uremic syndrome (HUS) is a commonly acquired cause of acute renal failure in children. Patients present with abdominal cramping, bloody diarrhea and vomiting; it is often caused by the toxin from *Escherichia coli* O157. About 10% of children with bloody diarrhea caused by *E. coli* O157 progress to HUS. Hemolytic-uremic syndrome (HUS) is characterized by a triad of microangiopathic hemolytic anemia (Hgb levels around 4-5 g/dL), thrombocytopenia (platelet destruction as well as sequestration of platelets in the liver and spleen), and acute nephropathy. Although the age of children most frequently affected by this disease is between 6 months and 4 years, HUS can occur from the neonatal period through adulthood. Occasionally CNS abnormalities develop (e.g., decreased levels of consciousness, seizures, and at times cerebral edema and increased intracranial pressure [ICP]). Pancreatitis is common and CHF may develop as a result of fluid overload, hypertension and myocardial depression from the toxins. Treatment is supportive and many of these children will require dialysis. The mortality rate is less than 5% (*Hines: Stoelting's Anesthesia and Co-Existing Disease, ed 5, p 424; Miller: Anesthesia, ed 6, pp 2859-2861*).

639. (D) Wilms' tumor, also called nephroblastoma, is a common malignant abdominal malignancy of children. Children commonly present with increasing abdominal girth and have a palpable mass. Peak age of diagnosis is 1 to 3 years of age. Renal function is usually preserved but hypertension, often mild, is common (60%). Treatment consists of surgery, radiation, and chemotherapy. Chemotherapeutic drugs used in this tumor include actinomycin, doxorubicin (Adriamycin), vincristine, and cyclophosphamide (Cytoxan). Bone marrow suppression (e.g., anemia, thrombocytopenia) can occur with all cytotoxic drugs. Because cardiomyopathy can occur with cyclophosphamide (>100 mg/m^2) and with doxorubicin (>220 mg/m^2), preoperative echocardiography should be considered even in asymptomatic patients. Late cardiac dysfunction may develop 7 to 14 years after treatment. Alkylating agents, such as cyclophosphamide, inhibit plasma cholinesterases, which may affect the metabolism of succinylcholine. Pulmonary fibrosis and/or pneumonitis can occur in patients who have received bleomycin (the patient in this case did not receive bleomycin). This pulmonary toxicity may be related to high inspired oxygen concentrations and excessive fluid administration. Vincristine has several CNS side effects, including peripheral neuropathy, impaired sensorium, and encephalopathy and renal toxicity (*Hines: Stoelting's Anesthesia and Co-Existing Disease, ed 5, pp 628-629; Motoyama: Smith's Anesthesia for Infants and Children, ed 7, pp 691-692, 1064-1067*).

640. **(E)** Shock occurs when perfusion to vital organs is inadequate to meet the organ's metabolic demands. When shock is developing, cardiac output is initially well maintained by increasing the heart rate and myocardial contractility. When cardiac output falls, blood pressure can only be maintained by a compensatory vasoconstriction. Shock is classified as compensated shock (systolic blood pressure in the normal range) or decompensated shock (systolic blood pressure less than the fifth percentile for age). If hypotension is present, one must be vigorous in treatment. Treatment is often begun with volume expansion; however, other causes of hypotension must be considered and treated as necessary (e.g., tension pneumothorax, pericardial tamponade, neurologic injury). The median (50th percentile) systolic blood pressure in children 1 to 10 years old is approximated by the formula: 90 mm Hg + (2 × age in years). Hypotension (i.e., decompensated shock) is based on systolic blood pressures and is correctly described in each of the choices in the question (*2005 American Heart Association Guidelines for cardiopulmonary resuscitation and emergency cardiovascular care. Circulation, 112:167, 2005*).

641. **(A)** In this life-threatening situation, the anesthesiologist should intubate the child immediately and advance the endotracheal tube into the left mainstem bronchus. Bradycardia is the most common antecedent rhythm to cardiac arrest in the pediatric population. The most common cause of bradycardia in infants and children is hypoxia, vagal stimuli, or a side effect of medication. In the present case, the child is bradycardic from severe hypoxia, caused by a complete obstruction of the airway. The mucosa in the left mainstem bronchus where the peanut was originally embedded most likely became sufficiently edematous to completely obstruct the lumen of the left mainstem bronchus. The patient might not have become hypoxic from this alone, but after attempting retrieval, the foreign became lodged in the trachea and had to be pushed back. Unfortunately, the peanut made its way into the right mainstem bronchus, effectively obstructing all airflow to the lungs.

To avoid the problem of losing a foreign body before retrieval is complete, the forceps and the bronchoscope should be withdrawn simultaneously. Performing an emergency tracheostomy would not bypass the distal airway obstructions in the left mainstem bronchus or the peanut in the right mainstem bronchus and is thus a useless measure. Attempting the Heimlich maneuver would only bring the peanut into the trachea, where it could again become trapped and create more airway obstruction and irritation. Intubating the right mainstem will not relieve the airway obstruction from the peanut, but intubating the left mainstem and using a smaller sized tube to get past the swollen portion would be the most rapid and effective way of rescuing the child. Instituting cardiopulmonary bypass might be an option; however, it would take considerable time and would increase the child's morbidity if not mortality (*Motoyama: Smith's Anesthesia for Infants and Children, ed 7, pp 816-817, 1128*).

642. **(E)** Prophylaxis for PONV is recommended for patients undergoing strabismus surgery, because untreated, the incidence is 40% to 90% of patients. No benefit was demonstrated with the use of anticholinergic medications or with gastric content evacuation before emergency from anesthesia. Benefits were demonstrated with all of the other answers and with the use of droperidol, metoclopramide and by avoiding narcotic analgesics. Avoiding the maintenance use of nitrous oxide is controversial (*Motoyama: Smith's Anesthesia for Infants and Children, ed 7, pp 780-781*).

643. Uterine blood flow is consistently decreased after the administration of
   A. Thiopental 4 mg/kg bolus and 1 mg/kg succinylcholine followed by intubation
   B. 0.5-1.5 minimum alveolar concentration (MAC) of desflurane
   C. Epidural fentanyl, uncomplicated by hypotension
   D. Clonidine 300 μg epidurally, uncomplicated by hypotension
   E. Epidural loaded with local anesthetic, uncomplicated by hypotension

644. An 38-year-old obese patient is receiving subcutaneous low molecular weight heparin (LMWH) for thromboprophylaxis. She received her epidural 14 hours after the heparin was stopped and develops a Horner's syndrome on the left side 30 minutes after placement of an epidural for an elective cesarean section. On physical examination, a T4 anesthetic level is noted, but aside from the Horner's syndrome no other findings are revealed. The most appropriate course of action at this time would be
   A. Remove the epidural
   B. Consult a neurosurgeon
   C. Obtain a computed tomographic scan
   D. Secure the airway
   E. None of the above

645. What percentage of all pregnancies are affected by preeclampsia?
   A. 2%
   B. 7%
   C. 12%
   D. 17%
   E. 22%

646. An 18-year-old patient preeclamptic patient develops back pain after the placement of an epidural for labor analgesia. The pain is severe and the patient has more weakness of the legs than expected. The most appropriate course of action at this time would be
   A. Inject a higher concentration of a local anesthetic
   B. Add IV narcotics
   C. Replace the epidural and use epidural narcotics to decrease the motor weakness
   D. Consult a neurosurgeon
   E. None of the above

647. Magnesium sulfate ($MgSO_4$) is used as an anticonvulsant in patients with preeclampsia as well as a tocolytic to prevent preterm delivery. $MgSO_4$ may produce any of the following effects **EXCEPT**
   A. Sedation
   B. Respiratory paralysis
   C. Inhibition of acetylcholine release at the myoneural junction
   D. Antagonism of α-adrenergic agonists
   E. Stimulation of NMDA receptors

648. Normal fetal heart rate (FHR) is
   A. 60 to 100 beats/min
   B. 100 to 140 beats/min
   C. 120 to 160 beats/min
   D. 150 to 200 beats/min
   E. None of the above

649. The leading direct cause of pregnancy related deaths in the United States is
   A. General anesthesia (failed intubation or aspiration)
   B. Hemorrhage
   C. Thromboembolism
   D. Hypetensive disorders of pregnancy
   E. Infection

650. Drugs useful in the treatment of uterine atony in an asthmatic with severe preeclampsia include
   A. Oxytocin, 15-methyl prostaglandin F_{2a} (PGF_{2a}) and ergonovine
   B. Oxytocin and 15-methyl PGF_{2a}
   C. Oxytocin and ergonovine
   D. 15-methyl PGF_{2a} only
   E. Oxytocin only

651. What is the P_{50} of fetal hemoglobin at term?
   A. 15
   B. 20
   C. 27
   D. 30
   E. 37

652. Side effects of ritodrine include all of the following **EXCEPT**
   A. Tachycardia
   B. Hypertension
   C. Hyperglycemia
   D. Pulmonary edema
   E. Hypokalemia

653. Cardiac output increases dramatically during pregnancy and delivery. The cardiac output returns to nonpregnant values by how long postpartum?
   A. 12 hours
   B. 1 day
   C. 2 weeks
   D. 1 month
   E. 2 months

654. A 32-year-old parturient with a history of spinal fusion, severe asthma and pregnancy-induced hypertension is brought to the operating room (OR) wheezing and needs an emergency cesarean section under general anesthesia for a prolapsed umbilical cord. Which of the following induction agents would be most appropriate for this induction?
   A. Sevoflurane
   B. Midazolam
   C. Ketamine
   D. Thiopental
   E. Propofol

655. Uterine blood flow at term pregnancy is
   A. 50 mL/min
   B. 250 mL/min
   C. 700 mL/min
   D. 1100 mL/min
   E. 1500 mL/min

656. Which one of the following statements is true regarding human immunodeficiency virus (HIV) infected parturients?
   A. Central neurologic blockade increases the chance of neurologic complications
   B. Ninety percent of newborns of untreated HIV seropositive mothers become infected in-utero, during vaginal delivery or with breastfeeding
   C. The pharmacologic effects of benzodiazepines are prolonged in patients taking protease inhibitors
   D. The risk of seroconversion after percutaneous exposure to HIV infected blood is about 5%
   E. Epidural blood patch is contraindicated for the treatment of post-dural puncture headaches

657. Which of the following cardiovascular parameters is decreased at term?
   A. Central venous pressure (CVP)
   B. Pulmonary capillary wedge pressure
   C. Systemic vascular resistance
   D. Left ventricular end-systolic volume
   E. Ejection fraction

658. Which of the following signs and symptoms is **NOT** associated with amniotic fluid embolism?
   A. Cardiopulmonary arrest
   B. Hypertension
   C. Bleeding (disseminated intravascular coagulation)
   D. Pulmonary edema or acute respiratory distress syndrome (ARDS)
   E. Seizures

659. When is the fetus most susceptible to the effects of teratogenic agents?
   A. 1 to 2 weeks of gestation
   B. 3 to 8 weeks of gestation
   C. 9 to 14 weeks of gestation
   D. 15 to 20 weeks of gestation
   E. Greater than 20 weeks of gestation

660. A 28-week estimated gestational age (EGA), 1000-g male infant is born to a 24-year-old mother who is addicted to heroin. The mother admits taking an extra "hit" of heroin before coming to the hospital because she was nervous. The infant's respiratory depression would be best managed by
   A. 0.1 mg naloxone IV through an umbilical artery catheter
   B. 0.1 mg naloxone IM in the newborn's thigh muscle
   C. 0.1 mg naloxone down the endotracheal tube
   D. 0.4 mg naloxone IM to the mother during the second stage of labor
   E. None of the above

661. Cardiac output is greatest
   A. During the first trimester of pregnancy
   B. During the second trimester of pregnancy
   C. During the third trimester of pregnancy
   D. During labor
   E. Immediately after delivery of the newborn

662. A 1000-g, 27-week EGA boy is born with a heart rate of 60. He is completely limp, shows no respiratory effort, and has no initial response to stimulation. He is totally cyanotic. The umbilical cord has only two vessels. The 1-minute Apgar score would be
   A. 0
   B. 1
   C. 2
   D. 3
   E. 4

663. Which of the following respiratory parameters is **NOT** increased in the parturient?
      A. Minute ventilation
      B. Tidal volume (VT)
      C. Arterial Pao$_2$
      D. Oxygen consumption
      E. Serum bicarbonate

664. A lumbar epidural catheter is placed in a healthy 23-year-old gravida 1, para 0 parturient for an elective cesarean section. Twenty-five minutes after the full dose of local anesthetic is administered, the patient states that she has difficulty breathing through her nose. The most likely explanation for this is
      A. A total spinal from inadvertent subarachnoid injection of local anesthetic
      B. A total sympathectomy and nasal congestion from a high level of blockade
      C. Volume overload
      D. Amniotic fluid embolism
      E. Intravascular injection of local anesthetic

665. Which of the following pharmacologic agents decreases uterine contraction in a dose-dependent fashion?
      A. Barbiturates
      B. Diazepam
      C. Ketamine
      D. Nitrous oxide
      E. Local anesthetics

666. In a normal sized term fetus, the normal oxygen consumption is approximately
      A. 7 mL/min
      B. 14 mL/min
      C. 21 mL/min
      D. 32 mL/min
      E. 45 mL/min

667. A 24-year-old gravida 2, para 1 parturient is anesthetized for emergency cesarean section. On emergence from general anesthesia, the endotracheal tube is removed and the patient becomes cyanotic. Oxygen is administered by positive-pressure mask-bag ventilation. High airway pressures are necessary to ventilate the patient, and wheezing is noted over both lung fields. The patient's blood pressure falls from 120/80 to 60/30 mm Hg, and heart rate increases from 105 to 180 beats/min. The most likely cause of these manifestations is
      A. Venous air embolism
      B. Amniotic fluid embolism
      C. Mucous plug in trachea
      D. Pneumothorax
      E. Aspiration

668. A 29-year-old gravida 1, para 0 parturient at 10 weeks of gestation is to undergo an emergency appendectomy under general anesthesia with isoflurane, N$_2$O, and O$_2$. Which of the following is a proven untoward consequence of general anesthesia in the unborn fetus?
      A. Nephroblastoma
      B. Cleft palate
      C. Mental retardation
      D. Behavioral defects
      E. None of the above

669. A lumbar epidural is placed in a 24-year-old gravida 1, para 0 parturient with myasthenia gravis for labor. Select the true statement regarding neonatal myasthenia gravis.
      A. The newborn is usually affected
      B. The newborn is affected by maternal immunoglobulin M (IgM) antibodies
      C. The newborn may require anticholinesterase therapy for up to 4 weeks
      D. The newborn will need lifelong treatment
      E. Only female newborns are affected

670. A patient having which of the following conditions is **LEAST** likely to develop disseminated intravascular coagulation?
   A. Pregnancy-induced hypertension
   B. Placenta abruption
   C. Placenta previa (bleeding)
   D. Amniotic fluid embolism
   E. Dead fetus syndrome

671. A 28-year-old gravida 1, para 0 parturient with Eisenmenger's syndrome (pulmonary hypertension with an intracardiac right-to-left or bidirectional shunt) is to undergo placement of a lumbar epidural for analgesia during labor. It may be wise to avoid a local anesthetic with epinephrine in this patient because it
   A. Lowers pulmonary vascular resistance
   B. Lowers systemic vascular resistance
   C. Increases heart rate
   D. Acts as a tocolytic agent
   E. Causes excessive increases in systolic blood pressure

672. Which of the following patients is most likely to need an emergency hysterectomy for uncontrolled bleeding at the time of delivery?
   A. Patient with placenta abruption
   B. Patient undergoing a vaginal birth after a cesarean section
   C. Patient with quadruplets
   D. Patient with a placenta previa (not bleeding) for an elective repeat cesarean section
   E. Patient with an abdominal pregnancy

673. The most common injury recorded in the ASA - Closed Claim Project regarding obstetric anesthetic claims is
   A. Headache
   B. Pain during anesthesia
   C. Neonatal brain damage
   D. Maternal brain damage
   E. Aspiration pneumonitis

674. Morphine is not used routinely for labor epidurals because it
   A. Increases uterine tone
   B. Causes excessive neonatal respiratory depression
   C. Has a slow onset
   D. Decreases uterine blood flow
   E. Adversely affects FHR variability

675. Which of the following statements regarding newborns with thick meconium-stained amniotic fluid is **TRUE?**
   A. Routine intrapartum oropharyngeal and nasopharyngeal suction is not recommended
   B. Intubation is required for all such newborns
   C. Antibiotics are needed to treat the infection
   D. Steroids are needed to treat the inflammation
   E. Respiratory distress syndrome is common

676. A 38-year-old primiparous patient with placenta previa and active vaginal bleeding arrives in the OR with a systolic blood pressure of 85 mm Hg. A cesarean section is planned. The patient is lightheaded and scared. Which of the following anesthetic induction plans would be most appropriate for this patient?
   A. Spinal anesthetic with 12 to 15 mg bupivacaine
   B. Epidural anesthetic with 20 to 25 mL 3% 2-chloroprocaine
   C. General anesthetic induction with 3 to 4 mg/kg thiopental, intubation with 1 to 1.5 mg/kg succinylcholine
   D. General anesthesia induction with 0.5 to 1 mg/kg ketamine, intubation with 1 to 1.5 mg/kg succinylcholine
   E. Replace lost blood volume first, then use any anesthetic the patient wishes

677. Which of the following lung volumes or capacities change the **LEAST** during pregnancy?
   A. Tidal volume (V_T)
   B. Functional residual capacity (FRC)
   C. Expiratory reserve volume (ERV)
   D. Residual volume (RV)
   E. Vital capacity (VC)

678. General anesthesia is induced in a 35-year-old patient for elective cesarean section. No part of the glottic apparatus is visible after two unsuccessful attempts to intubate, but mask ventilation is adequate. The most appropriate step at this point would be
   A. Wake up the patient
   B. Use an esophageal-tracheal Combitube
   C. Attempt a blind nasal intubation
   D. Continue mask ventilation and cricoid pressure
   E. Use a laryngeal mask airway

679. If 2-chloroprocaine is accidentally injected into maternal blood, it will be rapidly hydrolyzed by pseudocholinesterase. In a patient who is homozygous for atypical cholinesterase, the half-life for this drug in the blood would be expected to be
   A. Approximately 2 minutes
   B. Approximately 5 minutes
   C. Approximately 15 minutes
   D. Approximately 30 minutes
   E. Greater than 1 hour

680. Which of the following properties of epidurally administered local anesthetics determines the extent to which epinephrine will prolong the duration of blockade?
   A. Molecular weight
   B. Lipid solubility
   C. pKa
   D. Amide versus ester structure
   E. Concentration

681. Which of the following opioids is unique in that it has both local anesthetic and narcotic properties?
   A. Morphine
   B. Nalbuphine
   C. Hydrocodone
   D. Meperidine
   E. Oxymorphone

682. A 23-year-old parturient in the first trimester is brought to the OR for emergency appendectomy. General anesthesia is planned. An increased risk of congenital malformation associated with which drug has been suggested (but not proven) that almost always should be avoided?
   A. Thiopental
   B. Nitrous oxide
   C. Isoflurane
   D. Diazepam
   E. None of the above

683. True statements regarding inclusion of intrathecal morphine, fentanyl, or sufentanil in obstetric anesthesia practice include each of the following **EXCEPT**
   A. The chief site of action is the substantia gelatinosa of the dorsal horn of the spinal column
   B. There is no motor blockade
   C. There is no sympathetic blockade
   D. Pain relief is adequate for the second stage of labor
   E. Lipophilic narcotics are associated with less respiratory depression than nonlipophilic narcotics

684. The most common side effect of intraspinal narcotics in the obstetric population is
   A. Pruritus
   B. Nausea and vomiting
   C. Respiratory depression
   D. Urinary retention
   E. Headache

685. A 110-kg (242-pound), gravida 1, para 0 woman has a blood pressure of 180/95 during an office visit at the 18th week of gestation and 170/95 one week later. She has some ankle but no facial edema, and no protein detected in her urine. These findings would be classified as
   A. Preeclampsia
   B. Chronic hypertension
   C. Chronic hypertension with superimposed preeclampsia
   D. Gestational hypertension
   E. A normal finding

686. An epidural is placed into a 32-year-old parturient receiving magnesium therapy for preeclampsia. Five minutes after administration of the test dose, the bolus infusion is interrupted because of a contraction. After the contraction subsides, a slow epidural injection of the loading dose of bupivacaine and fentanyl is resumed. At the same time, the patient complains of shortness of breath. She is panic-stricken and wrestles violently with the nurses who are trying to reassure her. She repeats that she cannot breathe, becomes cyanotic, and loses consciousness. During resuscitation, blood is oozing from the IV sites and a pink froth is noted in the endotracheal tube. The most likely diagnosis is
   A. Amniotic fluid embolism
   B. High spinal
   C. Intravascular bupivacaine injection
   D. Magnesium overdose
   E. Eclampsia

687. Which of the following intraspinal opioid dose(s) would **NOT** be acceptable to administer in combination with 12 mg bupivacaine to a 60 kg parturient about to undergo a cesarean section?
   A. 25 μg fentanyl
   B. 5 μg sufentanil
   C. 0.25 mg morphine
   D. 15 μg fentanyl and 0.1 mg morphine
   E. 60 mg meperidine

688. Which of the following is not increased during pregnancy?
   A. Kidney size
   B. Renal plasma flow
   C. Creatinine clearance
   D. Blood urea nitrogen (BUN)
   E. Glucose excretion

689. Which inhalation anesthetic does **NOT** produce uterine relaxation
   A. Desflurane
   B. Isoflurane
   C. Sevoflurane
   D. Nitrous oxide
   E. All produce uterine relaxation

690. Passive diffusion of substances across the placenta is enhanced by all of the following **EXCEPT**
   A. Decreased maternal protein binding
   B. Low molecular weight of the substance
   C. High water solubility of the substance
   D. Low degree of ionization of the substance
   E. Large concentration gradient of the drug

691. Cesarean delivery is associated with a blood loss of about
      A. 100 mL
      B. 250 mL
      C. 500 mL
      D. 750 mL
      E. 1000 mL

692. Which of the following statements is correct in describing differences between fetal and maternal blood during labor?
      A. Fetal blood has a lower hemoglobin concentration than does maternal blood
      B. Fetal placental blood flow is twice maternal placental blood flow
      C. Fetal hemoglobin has a greater affinity for O_2 than does maternal hemoglobin
      D. The fetal oxyhemoglobin dissociation curve is shifted to the right of the maternal oxyhemoglobin dissociation curve
      E. Fetal blood has a higher pH than does maternal blood

693. Which of the following antihypertensive drugs used to treat used to treat severe pregnancy-induced hypertension is not capable of causing increased postpartum hemorrhage?
      A. Nitroprusside
      B. Nifedipine
      C. Nitroglycerin
      D. Labetalol
      E. Diazoxide

694. Which of the following is not a sign of "severe preeclampsia"
      A. Proteinuria greater than 5 g/24 hours
      B. Visual disturbances
      C. Urine output less than 500 mL/24 hours
      D. White blood cell count greater than 15,000
      E. All are signs of "severe preeclampsia"

695. Which condition best describes the maternal condition with the following signs and symptoms; new onset vaginal bleeding that stops, no pain, no fetal distress?
      A. Vasa previa
      B. Placenta abruption
      C. Ectopic pregnancy
      D. Uterine rupture
      E. Placenta previa

696. During the second stage of labor, complete pain relief can be obtained with
      A. Paracervical block
      B. Neuraxial block with fentanyl and morphine
      C. Pudendal nerve block
      D. Lumbar epidural block with bupivacaine and no narcotic
      E. Bilateral lumbar paravertebral sympathetic blocks with bupivacaine

697. Which of the following drugs should **NOT** be used as a tocolytic for preterm labor
      A. Magnesium sulfate
      B. Nifedipine
      C. Ketorolac
      D. Indomethacin
      E. Captopril

698. 15-Methyl PGF_{2a} is administered directly into the myometrium to treat uterine atony in a 28-year-old mother. Possible effects from treatment with this drug include
      A. Nausea and vomiting
      B. Bronchospasm
      C. Fever
      D. Hypoxemia
      E. All of the above

699. Which of the following statements regarding $MgSO_4$ therapy for preeclampsia is true?
  A. The therapeutic range for serum magnesium is 10 to 15 mEq/L
  B. High serum magnesium levels can be estimated by changes in deep tendon patellar reflexes in a patient with an epidural anesthetic loaded for a cesarean section
  C. Excessive serum magnesium levels cause widening of the QRS complex
  D. The antidote for magnesium toxicity is neostigmine
  E. As soon as delivery occurs, the chance for eclampsia no longer exists and the magnesium should be reversed so that postpartum bleeding is less likely to occur

700. While moving a parturient from the birthing room to the operating room for an emergency cesarean section for a prolapsed umbilical cord, the parturient develops cough, wheezing, stridor, and becomes cyanotic. The trachea is intubated and food is noted in the pharynx. Appropriate treatment in this patient should consist of
  A. Intravenous lidocaine to suppress the cough
  B. Glucocorticoids
  C. 100% oxygen and positive end-expiratory pressure (PEEP)
  D. Saline lavage
  E. Sodium bicarbonate lavage

701. Aortocaval compression starts to become significant in a normal pregnancy at how many weeks EGA?
  A. 5 weeks
  B. 10 weeks
  C. 15 weeks
  D. 20 weeks
  E. 25 weeks

702. Which agent is the most useful for raising the gastric pH just before induction of general anesthesia for emergency cesarean section?
  A. Cimetidine
  B. Metoclopramide
  C. Ranitidine
  D. Sodium citrate
  E. Magnesium hydroxide and aluminum hydroxide

703. Causes of fetal bradycardia include all of the following **EXCEPT?**
  A. Hypoxemia
  B. Acidosis
  C. Neostigmine and glycopyrrolate reversal of neuromuscular blockers
  D. Maternal smoking
  E. Umbilical cord compression

704. Etiology of cerebral palsy occurs most frequently
  A. Antepartum
  B. During the first stage of labor
  C. During the second stage of labor
  D. Immediately after delivery
  E. In the first 30 days of life

705. All of the following statements regarding pregnant diabetic patients are true **EXCEPT** for
  A. 2% to 5% of all pregnancies are associated with gestational diabetes mellitus (GDM)
  B. Insulin requirements increase during pregnancy
  C. Preeclampsia is more common in diabetics
  D. Insulin readily crosses the placenta and causes larger babies
  E. Diabetic ketoacidosis (DKA) occurs in 8% to 9% of type I DM pregnancies

706. In addition to the postural component of a postdural puncture headache (PDPH), signs and symptoms may include any of the following **EXCEPT**
    A. Double vision
    B. Nausea and vomiting
    C. Hearing changes
    D. Neck stiffness
    E. Fever

707. Variable decelerations may occur in response to
    A. Fetal head compression
    B. Uteroplacental insufficiency
    C. Maternal hypotension
    D. Umbilical cord compression
    E. Severe fetal anemia

708. Agents that are useful for decreasing the incidence of shivering during cesarean section under epidural analgesia include all of the following **EXCEPT**
    A. Administration of epidural sufentanil
    B. Warming of IV fluids
    C. Administration of epidural meperidine
    D. Warming the epidural anesthetic solutions to body temperature
    E. Intravenous meperidine

709. An umbilical arterial blood gas sample at the time of a STAT cesarean delivery shows a Po_2 of 20 mm Hg, a Pco_2 of 50 mm of Hg, a bicarbonate value of 22 mEq/L and a pH of 7.25. This shows
    A. Severe hypoxemia
    B. Respiratory acidosis
    C. Metabolic acidosis
    D. Mixed respiratory and metabolic acidosis
    E. Normal values

710. Which condition most frequently requires blood transfusions during or after a cesarean delivery?
    A. Multiple gestations
    B. Preeclampsia
    C. Intrauterine fetal demise
    D. Placenta abruption
    E. Placenta previa

711. All of the following are appropriate techniques or drug doses and may be needed to resuscitate a severely depressed 3 kg term newborn **EXCEPT**
    A. 30 breaths with 90 chest compressions per minute
    B. 0.1 to 0.3 mL/kg of 1:1000 solution of epinephrine IV
    C. 10 mL/kg of normal saline, Ringer's lactate or type O Rh negative blood given IV
    D. 0.1 mg/kg (1 mg/mL or 0.4 mg/mL solution) of naloxone given IV or IM
    E. 4 mL/kg of 4.2% sodium bicarbonate solution given IV

712. Failed intubation is how many times greater in the obstetric population than the general population?
    A. The incidence is the same
    B. Double
    C. Four times
    D. Eight times
    E. Twenty times

713. Compared with a healthy 25-year-old primigravida, which of the following conditions is **NOT** associated with a significantly higher incidence of pregnancy-induced hypertension (PIH)?
    A. Young primigravida (<20 years of age)
    B. Multiple gestation
    C. Diabetes mellitus type I
    D. Obesity (BMI >35)
    E. Smoking (>1 pack/day)

714. Adverse effects (on the mother) associated with aortocaval compression by the gravid uterus include
    A. Nausea and vomiting
    B. Pallor
    C. Changes in cerebration
    D. Decreases in uterine blood flow
    E. All of the above

715. Which of the following statements regarding a pregnant patient abusing cocaine is **TRUE?**
    A. Hypotension is common with the rapid sequence induction of general anesthesia in the acutely intoxicated patient
    B. The MAC for general anesthetics is increased in chronic cocaine addicts
    C. Hypertension is common with the induction of epidural anesthesia for labor
    D. Some states consider in utero drug exposure to be a form of child abuse and require physicians to report these patients
    E. If a vasopressor is needed to treat hypotension, ephedrine is preferred over phenylephrine

716. Each of the following is correct when advising the surgeon to perform infiltration anesthesia for an emergency cesarean delivery when general and neuraxial anesthesias are contraindicated **EXCEPT**
    A. A midline incision is most desirable
    B. The rectus muscle should be injected to provide good skin analgesia
    C. The skin incision is the most painful part of the surgery
    D. Bupivacaine with bicarbonate is the local anesthetic of choice
    E. Mild sedation with ketamine and midazolam is permissible

717. A 24-year-old primiparous woman is undergoing an elective cesarean section (breech position). After prehydration with 1500 mL of saline, a spinal anesthetic is performed and 5 minutes later the blood pressure is noted to be 80/40 and the heart rate is 100. The best treatment (best fetal pH) after assuring that adequate left uterine displacement is performed would be
    A. Phenylephrine
    B. Ephedrine
    C. Epinephrine
    D. 1000 mL D5LR
    E. 1000 mL hetastarch

718. A woman has been admitted for a dilation and evacuation (D&E) at 10 weeks estimated gestational age. She has some persistent bleeding and cramping after the expulsion of some tissue. Her obstetric condition is called
    A. A threatened abortion
    B. An inevitable abortion
    C. A complete abortion
    D. An incomplete abortion
    E. A habitual abortion

719. The action of epidural narcotics is antagonized by the prior or concomitant administration of which of the following epidurally administered local anesthetics?
    A. Lidocaine
    B. Bupivacaine
    C. Ropivacaine
    D. Chloroprocaine
    E. None of the above

720. Factors associated with advanced molar pregnancy (i.e., >14-16 week size uterus) include all of the following **EXCEPT**
    A. Pregnancy-induced hypertension
    B. Hypothyroidism
    C. Acute cardiopulmonary distress
    D. Hyperemesis gravidarum
    E. Malignant sequelae (metastasis)

721. Refractory cardiac arrest is most likely after the rapid unintentional IV injection of which of the following local anesthetics
    A. Lidocaine
    B. Bupivacaine
    C. Ropivacaine
    D. Levobupivacaine
    E. Chloroprocaine

722. Transient neurologic syndrome (TNS) is most commonly seen after the spinal anesthetic injection of which local anesthetic?
    A. Lidocaine
    B. Bupivacaine
    C. Prilocaine
    D. Tetracaine
    E. Procaine

723. Chloroprocaine-induced severe back pain is associated with epidural anesthesia and
    A. Metabisulfite
    B. Methylparaben
    C. Pregnancy
    D. Disodium ethylenediaminetetraacetic acid (EDTA)
    E. High concentrations such as 3%

724. Which of the following local anesthetics is associated with methemoglobinemia
    A. Lidocaine
    B. Bupivacaine
    C. Prilocaine
    D. Levobupivacaine
    E. Chloroprocaine

725. Which local anesthetic has the most rapid metabolism in maternal and fetal blood?
    A. Lidocaine
    B. Bupivacaine
    C. Prilocaine
    D. Levobupivacaine
    E. Chloroprocaine

Obstetric Physiology and Anesthesia

Answers, References, and Explanations

643. (A) Thiopental followed by succinylcholine and tracheal intubation causes a transient but consistent 20% to 40% reduction in uterine blood flow (UBF). This appears to be related to the sympathetic response to tracheal intubation. Uterine blood flow is unchanged with 0.5-1.5 MAC of a volatile anesthetic (i.e., halothane, isoflurane, sevoflurane or desflurane), a propofol bolus (2 mg/kg) or with an infusion of propofol (<450 μg/kg/min), epidural fentanyl or morphine, epidural clonidine, or a local anesthetic epidural uncomplicated with hypotension. IV-administered clonidine decreases UBF by uterine artery vasoconstriction, however, epidurally clonidine does not (providing hypotension does not develop). The unintentional intravenous injection of a local anesthetic can decrease UBF by increasing intrauterine pressure and/or by a direct vasoconstricting affect on the uterine arteries (epidurally injected local anesthetics have low blood concentrations and a minimal direct affects on UBF). Although based on uterine blood studies, propofol appears better than thiopental as an induction agent for cesarean deliveries, propofol has been associated with severe bradycardia when used with succinylcholine in pregnant patients, thus, thiopental is more commonly used. This observation needs further study (*Chestnut: Obstetric Anesthesia, ed 3, pp 44-45; Hughes: Anesthesia for Obstetrics, ed 4, pp 26-31, 220*).

644. (E) After low dose prophylaxis with LMWH, a time of at least 12 hours should elapse prior to performing neuraxial techniques to decrease the likelihood of an epidural hematoma forming (you should wait at least 24 hours after high dose LMWH used for therapeutic anticoagulation). If the patient has back pain and unexpected neurologic paralysis, a workup for a hematoma should be performed. This case is a benign condition that occasionally develops after a lumbar epidural anesthetic even when the highest dermatome level blocked is below T5. It may be related to the superficial anatomic location of the descending spinal sympathetic fibers that lie just below the spinal pia of the dorsolateral funiculus (which is within diffusion range of subanesthetic concentrations of local anesthetics in the cerebrospinal fluid) as well as increased sensitivity of local anesthetics during pregnancy (*Chestnut: Obstetric Anesthesia, ed 3, pp 685-688; Hughes: Anesthesia for Obstetrics, ed 4, pp 134, 417; Second Consensus Conference on Neuraxial Anesthesia and Anticoagulation, April 25-28, 2002. www.asra.com/consensus-statements/2.html*).

645. (B) Preeclampsia is a hypertensive disorder of pregnancy (sustained systolic blood pressure [BP] >140 mm Hg or a sustained diastolic BP >90 mm Hg) associated with proteinuria (>300 mg protein per 24 hour urine collection). It rarely occurs before the 24th week of gestation (unless a hydatidiform mole is present). It occurs with an overall incidence of approximately 5% to 9% of all pregnancies and is the third leading cause of maternal death in the United States. The incidence of preeclampsia is significantly higher in parturients with a hydatidiform mole, multiple gestations, obesity, polyhydramnios, or diabetes. Mothers with preeclampsia during their first pregnancy have a 33% chance of having preeclampsia in subsequent pregnancies. Preeclampsia can progress to eclampsia (preeclampsia accompanied by a seizure not related to other conditions). Sixty percent of eclamptic cases precede delivery. Of the rest, most occur within the first 24 hours after delivery. Approximately 5% of untreated parturients with preeclampsia will develop eclampsia (*Chestnut: Obstetric Anesthesia, ed 3, pp 794-795; Hughes: Anesthesia for Obstetrics, ed 4, pp 297-298*).

646. (D) The combination of severe unremitting back pain, more leg weakness than expected, tenderness over the spinal or paraspinal area, unexplained fever or a significant delay in normal recovery should alert you to the possibility of an expanding epidural hematoma forming that needs to be surgically removed quickly to decrease the chance of permanent neurologic deficits. A neurosurgeon should be contacted and if a magnetic resonance imaging (MRI) scan shows a hematoma, rapid delivery of the child should be performed followed by a neurosurgical removal of the hematoma. Rarely will an epidural hematoma form; however, a patient with a clotting disorder and perhaps marked difficulty in placing a block may lead to a hematoma formation. Because the preeclamptic patient may develop a coagulopathy, you should carefully evaluate her coagulation status prior to initiating a regional block. Most would evaluate a platelet count and look for any clinical signs for unexplained bleeding prior to initiating a regional block (*Chestnut: Obstetric Anesthesia, ed 3, pp 588-590, 688; Hughes: Anesthesia for Obstetrics, ed 4, pp 420-421*).

647. (E) The normal serum magnesium level is 1.5 to 2 mEq/L with a therapeutic range of 4 to 8 mEq/L. As magnesium sulfate is administered IV, patients often note a warm feeling in the vein as well as some sedation. With increasing serum levels, loss of deep tendon reflexes (10 mEq/L), respiratory paralysis (15 mEq/L), and cardiac arrest (>25 mEq/L) can occur. Note: Many labs report values in mg/dL (1 mEq/L = 1.2 mg/dL). Magnesium decreases the release of acetylcholine (ACh) at the myoneural junction and decreases the sensitivity of the motor endplate to ACh. This can produce marked potentiation of non-depolarizing muscle relaxants. The effect on depolarizing muscle relaxants is less clear and most clinicians use standard intubating doses of succinylcholine (i.e., 1 mg/kg) followed by a much reduced dose of a non-depolarizing relaxant if needed. Because magnesium antagonizes the effects of α-adrenergic agonists, ephedrine is preferred over phenylephrine if a vasopressor is needed to restore blood pressure, along with fluids, after a central neuraxial blockade. Magnesium acts as an antagonist at the N-methyl-D-aspartic acid (NMDA) receptors; however, clinically, labor analgesia is minimal (*Chestnut: Obstetric Anesthesia, ed 3, pp 295-296, 619-622, 808-809, 817-818; Hughes: Anesthesia for Obstetrics, ed 4, pp 304-306, 331-334*).

648. (C) Fetal monitors consist of a two-channel recorder for simultaneous recording of FHR and uterine activity. In looking at the FHR one assesses the baseline rate, the FHR variability, and the periodic changes (accelerations or decelerations) that occur with uterine contractions. The normal FHR varies between 120 and 160 beats/min. Some extend the lower limit of normal to 110 beats/min. See also answer 703 (*Chestnut: Obstetric Anesthesia, ed 3, pp 111-113; Hughes: Anesthesia for Obstetrics, ed 4, pp 625-630*).

649. (D) The leading direct cause of pregnancy related deaths in the United States is hypertensive disorders of pregnancy (16% or 1.83 deaths/100,000 live births) followed by infection, hemorrhage other than ectopic pregnancy related, thrombotic embolism, amniotic fluid embolism, cardiomyopathy, ruptured ectopic pregnancy, cerebral accidents and complications of anesthesia. (*Chestnut: Obstetric Anesthesia ed 4 pp 853-858*).

650. (E) Uterine atony is a common cause of postpartum hemorrhage (2%-5% of all vaginal deliveries). Treatment consists of uterine massage, drugs, and, in rare cases, hysterectomy. Drugs commonly used include oxytocin, ergot alkaloids (ergonovine, methylergonovine), and prostaglandins (PGE_2, PGF_{2a}, 15-methyl PGF_{2a}). The ergot alkaloids not infrequently cause elevations in blood pressure and are relatively contraindicated in patients with hypertension (such as preeclampsia). Ergot alkaloids have been associated with bronchospasm (rarely) and may not be appropriate in asthmatics. The prostaglandin 15-methyl PGF_{2a} (carboprost, Hemabate) is the only prostaglandin currently approved for uterine atony in the United States and may cause significant bronchospasm in susceptible patients (*Chestnut: Obstetric Anesthesia, ed 3, pp 428, 670-671; Hughes: Anesthesia for Obstetrics, ed 4, pp 367-369*).

651. (B) The term P_{50} denotes the blood oxygen tension (PaO_2) that produces 50% saturation of erythrocyte hemoglobin. The P_{50} value of fetal blood (75% to 85% of fetal blood is hemoglobin F) is around 19 to 21 mm Hg versus the adult value of 27 mm Hg. Thus, fetal hemoglobin has a higher affinity for oxygen than maternal hemoglobin (*Chestnut: Obstetric Anesthesia, ed 3, p 69; Hughes: Anesthesia for Obstetrics, ed 4, pp 24-25*).

652. (B) Ritodrine and terbutaline are β adrenergic agonists with tocolytic properties. Side effects are similar to those of other β adrenergic drugs and include tachycardia, hypotension, myocardial ischemia, pulmonary edema, hypoxemia (inhibition of hypoxic pulmonary vasoconstriction), hyperglycemia, metabolic (lactic) acidosis, hypokalemia (shift of potassium from extracellular to intracellular space), anxiety and nervousness. Electrocardiogram (ECG) changes of ST segment depression, T wave flattening or inversion may occur and typically resolve after stopping the β adrenergic therapy. Whether these ECG changes reflect myocardial ischemia or hypokalemia is unclear (*Chestnut: Obstetric Anesthesia, ed 3, pp 614-619; Hughes: Anesthesia for Obstetrics, ed 4, pp 323-331*).

653. (C) The numerous changes that take place in the cardiovascular system during pregnancy provide for the needs of the fetus and prepare the mother for labor and delivery. During the first trimester of pregnancy, cardiac output increases by approximately 30% to 40%. At term, the cardiac output is increased 50% over nonpregnant values. This increase in cardiac output is due to an increase in stroke volume and an increase in heart rate. During labor, the cardiac output increases another 10% to 15% during the latent phase, 25% to 30% during the active phase, and 40% to 45% during the expulsive stage. Each uterine contraction increases the cardiac output by about 10% to 25%. The greatest increase in cardiac output occurs immediately after delivery of the newborn when the cardiac output can increase to greater than 75% to 80% above prelabor values. This final increase in cardiac output is attributed primarily to autotransfusion and increased venous return associated with uterine involution. Cardiac output falls to prelabor values within 2 days after delivery. But it takes about 2 weeks time for the cardiac output to decrease to nonpregnant values (*Chestnut: Obstetric Anesthesia, ed 3, pp 18-21; Hughes: Anesthesia for Obstetrics, ed 4, pp 6-8*).

654. (E) Asthma occurs in about 4% of all pregnancies. Although sevoflurane is a good induction agent for asthmatics, a rapid sequence IV induction with endotracheal intubation to secure the airway is preferred. Because midazolam has a slow onset of action, it is not recommended for a rapid sequence induction. When inducing general anesthesia in an asthmatic patient, it is imperative to establish an adequate depth of anesthesia before placing an endotracheal tube. If the patient is "light," then severe bronchospasm may occur. In patients with mild asthma, induction may work with ketamine, thiopental, or propofol. Since thiopental can trigger histamine release in some patients it should not be used in patients with severe asthma. In a patient with severe asthma, ketamine or propofol is preferred. Because propofol does not stimulate the cardiovascular system as does ketamine, propofol would be preferred in this patient with pregnancy-induced hypertension. In patients with mild asthma who do not need the accessory muscles of respiration, regional anesthesia should be strongly considered if time permits, because it would eliminate the need for endotracheal intubation (*Chestnut: Obstetric Anesthesia, ed 3, pp 920-921; Hughes: Anesthesia for Obstetrics, ed 4, pp 487-493*).

655. (C) Uterine blood flow (UBF) increases dramatically from 50 to 100 mL/min before pregnancy to about 700 to 900 mL/min at term (i.e., >1 unit of blood per minute). Ninety percent of the uterine blood flow at term goes to the intervillous spaces. Uterine blood flow is related to the perfusion pressure (uterine arterial pressure minus uterine venous pressure) divided by the uterine vascular resistance. Thus, factors that decrease UBF include systemic hypotension, aortocaval compression, uterine contraction, and vasoconstriction (*Chestnut: Obstetric Anesthesia, ed 3, pp 37-41; Hughes: Anesthesia for Obstetrics, ed 4, pp 22-23*).

656. (C) Central neurologic blockade (i.e., epidural, spinal or combined spinal epidural) as well as epidural blood patches appear to be safe for the HIV infected parturients. Vertical transmission from the mother to the newborn can occur in 15% to 40% when the mother is untreated. With antiretroviral therapy and elective cesarean delivery, the rate of transmission is reduced to about 2%. The risk of developing HIV after a needlestick injury with HIV infected blood is 0.3%. (Risk of developing hepatitis B from a needlestick injury with hepatitis B infected blood is 30% and hepatitis C from a needlestick injury with hepatitic C infected blood is 2% to 4%.) Patients taking protease inhibitors as part of their drug therapy have inhibition of cytochrome P-450 and both benzodiazepines as well as narcotics have prolonged effects (*Chestnut: Obstetric Anesthesia, ed 3, pp 780-793; Hughes: Anesthesia for Obstetrics, ed 4, pp 583-595*).

657. (C) There is no change in central venous pressure, pulmonary capillary wedge pressure, pulmonary artery diastolic pressure or left ventricular end-systolic volume. Left ventricular end-diastolic volume is increased as is stroke volume, ejection fraction, heart rate and cardiac output. Systemic vascular resistance is decreased about 20% (*Chestnut: Obstetric Anesthesia, ed 3, pp 18-19*).

658. (B) Amniotic fluid embolism (AFE) is a very rare but serious complication of labor and delivery that results from the entrance of amniotic fluid and constituents of amniotic fluid into the maternal systemic circulation. About 10% of maternal deaths are caused by AFE and two thirds of these deaths occur within 5 hours. For AFE to occur, the placental membranes must be ruptured, and abnormal open sinusoids at the uteroplacental site or lacerations of endocervical veins must exist. The classic triad is acute hypoxemia, hemodynamic collapse (i.e., severe hypotension), and coagulopathy without an obvious cause. Pulmonary edema, cyanosis, cardiopulmonary arrest and disseminated intravascular coagulation (DIC) and fetal distress are common (>80% of cases), with seizures occurring about 50% of the time. Recently, AFE is believed to be a bit different from a pure embolic event, because findings of anaphylaxis and septic shock also are involved (*Chestnut: Obstetric Anesthesia, ed 3, pp 688-691; Hughes: Anesthesia for Obstetrics, ed 4, pp 355-360*).

659. (B) Organogenesis mainly occurs between the 15th to 56th days (3 to 8 weeks) of gestation in humans and is the time during which the fetus is most susceptible to teratogenic agents. Although all commonly used anesthetic drugs are teratogenic in some animal species, there is no conclusive evidence to implicate any currently used local anesthetics, IV induction agents or volatile anesthetic agents in the causation of human congenital anomalies (*Chestnut: Obstetric Anesthesia, ed 3, pp 257-263; Hughes: Anesthesia for Obstetrics, ed 4, pp 251-259*).

660. (E) Opioid abuse includes morphine, heroin, methadone, meperidine, and fentanyl. The problems associated with abuse are many and include the drug effect itself, substances mixed with the narcotics (e.g., talc, cornstarch), as well as infection and malnutrition. Newborn respiratory depression as manifested by a low respiratory rate is treated with controlled ventilation but not with naloxone. Naloxone can precipitate an acute withdrawal reaction and should not be administered to patients with chronic narcotic use (mother or newborn). The dose of naloxone to treat narcotic-induced respiratory depression in the nonaddicted newborn is 0.1 mg/kg (*Chestnut: Obstetric Anesthesia, ed 3, pp 134, 934-935; Hughes: Anesthesia for Obstetrics, ed 4, pp 602-604, 668*).

661. (E) Immediately after delivery, the cardiac output can increase up to 75% to 80% above prelabor values. This is thought to result from autotransfusion and increased venous return to the heart associated with involution of the uterus, as well as increased blood return as the result of the lithotomy position (*Chestnut: Obstetric Anesthesia, ed 3, pp 18-21; Hughes: Anesthesia for Obstetrics, ed 4, pp 7-8*).

662. (B) The Apgar score is a subjective scoring system used to evaluate the newborn and is commonly performed 1 and 5 minutes after delivery. If the score is less than 7, the scoring is also performed at 10, 15, and 20 minutes after delivery. A value of 0, 1, or 2 is given to each of five signs (heart rate, respiratory effort, reflex irritability, muscle tone, and color) and totaled. In this case the child gets 1 point for heart rate and 0 for each other sign.

THE APGAR SCORE

Sign	0	1	2	Total
1. Heart rate	Absent	<100	>100	_____
2. Respiratory effort	Absent	Slow, irregular	Good, crying	_____
3. Reflex irritability	No response	Grimace	Cough or sneeze	_____
4. Muscle tone	Flaccid	Some flexion	Active motion	_____
5. Color	Blue or pale	Pink body with blue extremities	Completely pink	_____
			Sum =	_____

A score of 7 to 10 is normal, 4 to 6 moderate depression, and 0 to 3 severe depression. Weight, gestational age, and sex are not factors included in the scoring system (*Chestnut: Obstetric Anesthesia, ed 3, pp 126-127; Hughes: Anesthesia for Obstetrics, ed 4, pp 639-642*).

663. (E) The respiratory system undergoes many changes during pregnancy with an increase in minute ventilation about 45% to 50%, V_T 40% to 45%, and arterial Pao_2 increases slightly due to a fall in $Paco_2$. Oxygen consumption increases about 20% to 60%. The serum bicarbonate level falls an average of 4 mEq/L to keep pH in the normal range because of the respiratory alkalosis ($Paco_2$ to approximately 30 to 32 mm Hg) that occurs (*Chestnut: Obstetric Anesthesia, ed 3, pp 15-17; Hughes: Anesthesia for Obstetrics, ed 4, pp 3-6*).

664. (B) The sympathetic nerve fibers exit the spinal cord through T1-L2. A high spinal or high epidural can block all of the sympathetic fibers, causing hypotension, bradycardia, and venodilation. Venodilation of the veins in the nasal mucosa causes nasal stuffiness and swelling. Because this patient can speak, the patient does not have a "total spinal." Acute volume overload, amniotic fluid embolism (see explanation to questions 658 and 686), and intravascular injection of local anesthetic do not lead to nasal stuffiness (*Hughes: Anesthesia for Obstetrics, ed 4, p 417*).

665. (A) Barbiturates cause a dose-dependent reduction in uterine contractions. Diazepam and nitrous oxide have no effect. Ketamine produces a dose-related oxytocic effect on uterine tone during the second trimester of pregnancy but no increase in tone at term. Local anesthetics injected intravenously cause an increase in uterine tone and at high levels can lead to tetanic contractions (*Hughes: Anesthesia for Obstetrics, ed 4, pp 41-44*).

666. (C) The normal term (approximately 3 kg) fetus has an oxygen consumption of 7 mL/kg/min or about 21 mL/min. Because the fetal store of oxygen is about 42 mL, in theory it would take 2 minutes to completely deplete it during an interruption in the normal blood supply of oxygen. In reality, the fetus has several compensatory mechanisms that allow it to survive for longer periods of time (e.g., 10 minutes) during periods of hypoxia, including a redistribution of blood flow to vital organs (*Chestnut: Obstetric Anesthesia, ed 3, p 66; Hughes: Anesthesia for Obstetrics, ed 4, p 24*).

667. (E) Many of the signs are consistent with the choices described in this question. From the temporal perspective, gastric acid aspiration is the most likely cause, because aspiration can develop not only on induction but on extubation as in this case. That is why it is so important to always empty the patient's stomach with an oral-gastric tube after an endotracheal tube is placed in any pregnant patient undergoing general anesthesia. Morbidity and mortality occurring after gastric acid aspiration is determined by both the amount and the pH of the aspirated material. Aspiration of a gastric volume greater than 0.4 mL/kg with a pH less than 2.5 causes severe pneumonitis with high morbidity and mortality. Using these values, 70% of women who fasted before elective cesarean section are "at risk for aspiration." Recently, it has been noted that the volume needed to cause aspiration in primates should be 0.8 mL/kg and the pH less than 3.5. Regardless of the definition of the "patient at risk," when aspiration occurs it can be lethal. Bronchospasm (often associated with higher airway pressures) and wheezing are suggestive of gastric acid aspiration and not amniotic fluid embolism. Other signs and symptoms of aspiration include sudden coughing or laryngospasm, dyspnea, tachypnea, the presence of foreign material in the mouth or posterior pharynx, chest wall retraction, cyanosis not relieved by oxygen supplementation, tachycardia, hypotension, and the development of pinky frothy exudates. The onset of these signs and symptoms is usually rapid. Early treatment consists of supplemental oxygen with positive-pressure ventilation, PEEP or continuous positive airway pressure (CPAP), and suctioning of the airway can decrease the incidence of mortality from acid aspiration. The use of prophylactic antibiotics and/or steroids has not been helpful (*Chestnut: Obstetric Anesthesia, ed 3, pp 523-534; Hughes: Anesthesia for Obstetrics, ed 4, pp 391-407*).

668. (E) The primary objectives in the anesthetic management of parturients undergoing general anesthesia for non-obstetric surgery are as follows: to (1) ensure maternal safety; (2) avoid teratogenic drugs; (3) avoid intrauterine fetal asphyxia; and (4) prevent the induction of preterm labor. Premature onset of labor is the most common complication associated with surgery during the second trimester of pregnancy. Performance of intra-abdominal procedures in which the uterus is manipulated is the most significant factor in causing premature labor in these patients. Neurosurgical, orthopedic, thoracic, or other surgical procedures that do not involve manipulation of the uterus do not cause preterm labor. No anesthetic agent or technique has been found to be significantly associated with a higher or lower incidence of preterm labor. Furthermore, there is no evidence that the risk of developing any of the conditions listed in this question is increased for the offspring of patients who receive general anesthesia during pregnancy (*Hughes: Anesthesia for Obstetrics, ed 4, pp 249-265*).

669. (C) Myasthenia gravis (MG) is an autoimmune neuromuscular disease in which immunoglobulin G (IgG) antibodies are directed against the ACh receptors in skeletal muscle, causing patients to present with general muscle weakness and easy fatigability. Smooth muscle and cardiac muscle are not affected. About 10% to 20% of newborns born to mothers with MG are transiently affected because the IgG antibody is transferred through the placenta. Neonatal MG is characterized by muscle weakness (e.g., hypotonia, respiratory difficulty) and may appear within the first 4 days of life (80% appear within the first 24 hours). Anticholinesterase therapy may be required for 2 to 4 weeks until the maternal IgG antibodies are metabolized (*Chestnut: Obstetric Anesthesia, ed 3, pp 877-878; Hughes: Anesthesia for Obstetrics, ed 4, pp 537-539*).

670. (C) Disseminated intravascular coagulation (DIC) is an acquired coagulopathy characterized by excessive fibrin deposition, depression of the normal coagulation inhibition mechanism and impaired fibrin degradation. The formation of clots causes a depletion of platelets and factors. Laboratory diagnosis of DIC is based on the demonstration of consumption of procoagulants (decrease in fibrinogen, decrease in platelet count, and prolongation of prothrombin time [PT] and activated partial thromboplastin time [aPTT]), demonstration of circulating fibrin-fibrinogen degradation products, and indirect evidence of obstruction of the microcirculation. Disseminated intravascular coagulation (DIC) is associated with the following obstetric conditions: placental abruption, dead fetus syndrome, amniotic fluid embolism, gram-negative sepsis, and severe pregnancy-induced hypertension. Placental abruption is the most common cause of DIC in pregnant patients. If you look at severe placenta abruptions (where the abruption is large enough to cause fetal death), about 30% of patients will develop DIC within 8 hours of the abruption. Patients with placenta previa who are bleeding do not develop DIC because the blood loss does not induce a coagulopathy (*Barash: Clinical Anesthesia, ed 5, pp 237-238; Chestnut: Obstetric Anesthesia, ed 3, p 665; Hughes: Anesthesia for Obstetrics, ed 4, pp 349, 356-357, 364-365*).

671. (B) Eisenmenger's syndrome may develop in patients with uncorrected left-to-right intracardiac shunting such as ventricular septal defect, atrial septal defect, or patent ductus arteriosus. In this syndrome, the pulmonary and vascular tone and right ventricular muscle undergo changes in response to the shunt, producing pulmonary hypertension and a change in the direction of the shunt to a right-to-left or bidirectional type with peripheral cyanosis. The maternal mortality rate is 30% to 50%. Approximately 3% of all newborns with congenital heart defects will develop this condition over time. Because the pulmonary vascular resistance is fixed in these patients, this condition is not amenable to surgical correction; thus, survival beyond age 40 years is uncommon. Any event or drug that increases pulmonary vascular resistance (e.g., hypercarbia, acidosis, hypoxia) or decreases systemic vascular resistance will worsen the right-to-left shunt, exacerbate peripheral cyanosis, and may precipitate right ventricular heart failure in these patients. Controversy exists regarding pain management for these patients because pain can elevate pulmonary artery pressures and cause more shunting. Many practitioners prefer a narcotic-based analgesic (spinal or epidural). Because these patients are very dependent upon preload and afterload, placing invasive monitors (CVP and arterial catheter), and using the pulse oximeter to evaluate amount of shunting, aggressive treatment of any fall in preload or peripheral vascular resistance can be performed. Recall that centrally administered local anesthetics reduce preload and afterload. Low-dose epinephrine, which can be used to decrease absorption of local anesthetics, should be used cautiously, if at all, because a further decrease in systemic vascular resistance may result from the β effect of absorbed epinephrine, and intravascular injection may elevate pulmonary pressures more, exacerbating the right-to-left shunt (*Chestnut: Obstetric Anesthesia, ed 3, pp 709-710; Fleisher: Anesthesia and Uncommon Diseases, ed 5, pp 118-119; Hughes: Anesthesia for Obstetrics, ed 4, pp 468-469*).

672. (D) The patient with placenta previa and a previous scar in the uterus has a very high chance of needing an emergency cesarean hysterectomy for uncontrolled bleeding at the time of delivery because of a placenta accreta (abnormally adherent placenta). The incidence of placenta accreta in a patient with placenta previa and no previous cesarean section is 5% to 7%, with one previous cesarean section is about 10% to 30%, and with two or more previous sections is 40% to 70%. About two thirds of patients with placenta accreta require a cesarean hysterectomy. The average blood loss during an emergency obstetric hysterectomy is 5 to 7 units of blood (*Chestnut: Obstetric Anesthesia, ed 3, pp 667-676; Hughes: Anesthesia for Obstetrics, ed 4, pp 363-364*).

673. (C) According to the ASA's Closed Claim Project (850 claims as of December 2003), neonatal brain damage (18%) and maternal death (15%) were the most frequent claims. Other causes include maternal nerve damage (15%), headache (14%), back pain (9%), emotional distress (8%), pain during anesthesia (7%), maternal brain damage (6%), neonatal death (6%) and aspiration pneumonitis (3%). (*Chestnut: Obstetric Anesthesia ed 4 pp 738-739*).

674. (C) The main reason morphine is not routinely used for labor epidurals is its long onset time (i.e., 30-60 minutes) despite the high doses needed for adequate first stage analgesia (e.g., 7.5 mg morphine), and the high incidence of pruritus, nausea, vomiting, as well as drowsiness. Morphine has little effect on uterine tone, UBF, or FHR. The doses used epidurally do not cause significant neonatal depression in term newborns but may cause some mild depression in preterm newborns (*Chestnut: Obstetric Anesthesia, ed 3, pp 350-353; Hughes: Anesthesia for Obstetrics, ed 4, pp 35, 162-163*).

675. (A) Meconium-stained amniotic fluid occurs in about 10% of all deliveries. Although intrapartum oropharyngeal and nasopharyngeal suction for all newborns born to mothers with meconium staining has been routine care for many years, current evidence shows no real benefit and it is no longer recommended. Intubation and tracheal suction should only be performed in newborns who are not vigorous and does not depend upon the consistency of the meconium-stained fluid as was once recommended. In newborns who are vigorous (i.e., strong respiratory efforts, good muscle tone, and heart rate >100 beats/min), no further treatment is needed. Because meconium is sterile, antibiotics are not needed. Steroids have not been necessary in the treatment of meconium-stained newborns. Respiratory distress syndrome (RDS) is a condition that occurs as a result of low levels of pulmonary surfactant in the alveoli. Respiratory distress syndrome (RDS) occurs in premature newborns, whereas meconium staining occurs typically in older, often postterm, newborns (*Chestnut: Obstetric Anesthesia, ed 3, pp 136-138; Hughes: Anesthesia for Obstetrics, ed 4, pp 666-668*).

676. (D) Placenta previa occurs when the placenta implants on the lower uterine segment so that all (total) or part of the placenta (partial) covers the internal cervical os. A marginal placenta previa occurs when the placenta lies close to but does not cover the internal cervical os. It occurs in about 0.5% of all pregnancies and has a maternal mortality less than 1% but a fetal mortality approaching 20% (primarily because of prematurity and intrauterine asphyxia). Patients typically present with painless vaginal bleeding that stops spontaneously (first bleed). Delivery is cesarean and is often made a few weeks after the "first" bleed when the baby's lungs are more mature (e.g., after 37 weeks EGA). A later bleed can be uncontrolled and may be accompanied by significant hypovolemia and hypotension. Regional anesthesia is contraindicated in severely hypovolemic patients. Replacing blood loss may not be practical because bleeding may be quicker than replacement is possible (i.e., may be greater than 1 unit per minute). A rapid-sequence general anesthetic (assuming acceptable airway) is preferred. Ketamine supports the cardiovascular system better than thiopental or propofol. In rare but severe cases of hypovolemic shock, all IV anesthetics may cause the blood pressure to fall further and succinylcholine alone may be all that is required. In these severe cases, maternal recall should be considered secondary to maternal safety. In cases where a difficult intubation is likely and the patient is hypovolemic, an infiltration local anesthetic may be best (*Chestnut: Obstetric Anesthesia, ed 3, pp 436, 662-665; Hughes: Anesthesia for Obstetrics, ed 4, pp 361-364*).

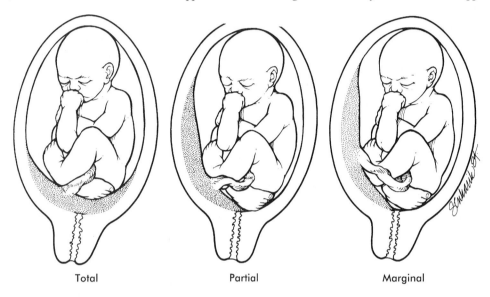

Total   Partial   Marginal

677. **(E)** At term pregnancy, V_T increases about 40% to 45% and the inspiratory reserve volume (IRV) increases about 5%. A decrease occurs in both the expiratory reserve volume (ERV) 20% to 25% and the residual volume (RV) 15% to 20%. A capacity is defined as two or more lung volumes. Functional residual capacity (FRC = ERV + RV) is decreased about 15% to 20% and is partly responsible for the rapid fall in maternal oxygenation that occurs with apnea during the induction of general anesthesia. Total lung capacity (TLC = V_T + IRV + ERV + RV) decreases about 5%, whereas vital capacity (VC = V_T + IRV + ERV) remains unchanged (*Chestnut: Obstetric Anesthesia, ed 3, pp 16-17; Hughes: Anesthesia for Obstetrics, ed 4, pp 3-4*).

678. **(A)** Evaluation of the airway should be performed before the induction of any general anesthetic. In cases where an unrecognized difficult airway exists (unable to perform endotracheal intubation in a reasonable period of time) the patient should be awakened if the procedure is purely elective and the fetus has minimal or no fetal distress (as in this elective case). A regional anesthetic or awake intubation then can be safely performed. In cases of fetal or maternal distress, other options for securing the airway may be necessary (*Chestnut: Obstetric Anesthesia, ed 3, pp 535-550; Hughes: Anesthesia for Obstetrics, ed 4, pp 217, 379-381*).

679. **(A)** Chloroprocaine is broken down rapidly in the blood by normal pseudocholinesterase. In vitro plasma half-life is 21 seconds in maternal blood and 43 seconds in fetal blood. In patients who are homozygous for the atypical cholinesterase, the half-life is prolonged to about 2 minutes (*Hughes: Anesthesia for Obstetrics, ed 4, p 75*).

680. **(B)** Epinephrine is primarily added to local anesthetics to check for the IV placement of an epidural catheter, to decrease the vascular uptake of local anesthetics, or to increase the intensity and duration of the block. By producing vasoconstriction of the epidural blood vessels, vascular uptake of the local anesthetic is reduced, allowing more of the drug to enter the nervous tissue. The more lipid-soluble the local anesthetic, the less effect epinephrine has (*Chestnut: Obstetric Anesthesia, ed 3, pp 200-201; Hughes: Anesthesia for Obstetrics, ed 4, p 87*).

681. **(D)** Meperidine demonstrates local anesthetic actions in addition to its narcotic effects (*Chestnut: Obstetric Anesthesia, ed 3, pp 354, 477-478; Hughes: Anesthesia for Obstetrics, ed 4, p 173*).

682. **(D)** An increased risk of congenital malformations has been suggested by several old studies with the use of minor tranquilizers such as diazepam, meprobamate, and chlordiazepoxide during the first trimester of pregnancy.

The cause-and-effect relationship has not been proven; in fact, several newer studies failed to show an association between minor tranquilizers and congenital malformations. Nevertheless, the U.S. Food and Drug Administration (FDA) recommends that diazepam (caution with midazolam) should not be used in the first trimester of pregnancy (*Chestnut: Obstetric Anesthesia, ed 3, p 216; Hughes: Anesthesia for Obstetrics, ed 4, p 253; Physicians Desk Reference - 2008, ed 62, p 2765*).

683. (D) Intrathecal opiates (e.g., morphine, fentanyl, sufentanil) are very effective in relieving the visceral pain during the first stage of labor. Intrathecal opiates administered alone (except for meperidine, which has local anesthetic properties) do not provide adequate pain relief for the second stage somatic pain (*Chestnut: Obstetric Anesthesia, ed 3, pp 349-365; Hughes: Anesthesia for Obstetrics, ed 4, pp 155-180*).

684. (A) The most common side effect of intraspinal narcotics is pruritus. The next most common side effects are nausea and vomiting, followed by urinary retention. Respiratory depression and headache may occur, but are relatively infrequent (*Chestnut: Obstetric Anesthesia, ed 3, pp 358-360; Hughes: Anesthesia for Obstetrics, ed 4, pp 170-178*).

685. (B) Hypertension (systolic blood pressure >140 or an increase >30 mm Hg over baseline; diastolic blood pressure >90 or an increase of 15 mm Hg over baseline) occurs in about 7% of all pregnancies. It is commonly classified by the American College of Obstetricians and Gynecologists as one of five types (preeclampsia-eclampsia, HELLP syndrome [*H*emolysis, *E*levated *L*iver enzymes, and *L*ow *P*latelet count], chronic hypertension, chronic hypertension with preeclampsia-eclampsia, or gestational hypertension). Preeclampsia rarely occurs before 24 weeks EGA except in patients with gestational trophoblastic neoplasms (e.g., molar pregnancy) and manifests as a triad of hypertension, generalized edema, and proteinuria. Chronic hypertension is persistent hypertension before, during, and after pregnancy (e.g., >6 weeks postpartum). Some patients develop gestational hypertension, which is an increase in blood pressure without generalized edema or proteinuria, which resolves by 2 to 6 weeks postpartum (*Chestnut: Obstetric Anesthesia, ed 3, pp 794-806; Hughes: Anesthesia for Obstetrics, ed 4, pp 297-299*).

686. (A) The four cardinal features of amniotic fluid embolism are dyspnea, hypoxemia, cardiovascular collapse, and coma. The patient may develop DIC, seizures, and pulmonary edema from left ventricular failure. Patients with a high spinal or epidural may complain of dyspnea, but they also have marked weakness and would certainly not be able to wrestle or struggle with their health care providers. Patients experiencing an intravascular injection of local anesthetic present with central nervous system (CNS) signs of toxicity (lightheadedness, visual or auditory disturbances, muscular twitching, convulsion, coma) or, at higher levels, cardiovascular collapse. Magnesium overdosage is also associated with muscle weakness. The typical eclamptic seizure is tonic-clonic. Patients with eclampsia do not complain of dyspnea, although an associated aspiration may produce similar symptoms (*Chestnut: Obstetric Anesthesia, ed 3, pp 688-691, 909-911; Hughes: Anesthesia for Obstetrics, ed 4, pp 355-359*).

687. (E) Intrathecal opioids are often mixed with local anesthetics to provide better intraoperative and postoperative pain control. Fentanyl is commonly used in doses of 10 to 25 μg, sufentanil in doses of 2.5 to 5.0 μg, and morphine in doses of 0.1 to 0.25 mg. Some anesthesiologists mix morphine with fentanyl because morphine is slow in onset but has a long duration of action and fentanyl is faster in onset but has a short duration of action. If you add meperidine to bupivacaine, the dose is 10 mg, however, if you use meperidine as a sole agent, the dose is 1 mg/kg. In this case we are adding meperidine to bupivacaine and 60 mg is too high a dose (*Chestnut: Obstetric Anesthesia, ed 3, pp 355-357, 429-430; Hughes: Anesthesia for Obstetrics, ed 4, pp 170-173, 205*).

688. (D) The renal system undergoes dramatic anatomical (increase in kidney size as well as dilation of the ureters) and functional changes in pregnancy. Renal plasma flow increases about 75% to 85%, glomerular filtration rate (GFR) increases about 50% and is reflected by an increase in clearance of urea, creatinine, and uric acid. Because of the increased clearance, we see a decrease in BUN to 8 to 9 mg/dL, serum creatinine to 0.5-0.6 mg/dL, as well as serum urate to 2 to 3 mg/dL. Glucosuria is common and is attributed to both the increase in GFR and a reduced renal tubular resorption of glucose (*Chestnut: Obstetric Anesthesia, ed 3, pp 24-25; Miller: Anesthesia, ed 6, p 2311*).

689. (D) All halogenated anesthetic agents (halothane, enflurane, isoflurane, desflurane, sevoflurane) cause a dose-related relaxation of uterine smooth muscle. With anesthetic concentrations of 0.2 MAC, the decrease in uterine activity is slight, and these agents have been used for inhalation analgesia during labor. At 0.5 MAC, uterine relaxation is more significant but the uterine response to oxytocin remains intact. Nitrous oxide does not affect uterine activity (*Chestnut: Obstetric Anesthesia, ed 3, pp 107, 320-321; Hughes: Anesthesia for Obstetrics, ed 4, pp 29-30, 41, 195*).

690. (C)   Passive diffusion is the primary means for the placental transfer of drugs. Factors that promote diffusion of drugs across placental membranes include decreased maternal protein binding (although some believe this is not very important because of rapid diffusion of drugs from protein), low molecular weight (<500 daltons), high lipid solubility, a low degree of ionization, and a large concentration gradient across the membranes. Highly water soluble drugs, such as neuromuscular drugs, do not pass the placental in significant amounts (*Chestnut: Obstetric Anesthesia, ed 3, pp 199-201; Hughes: Anesthesia for Obstetrics, ed 4, pp 61-64*).

691. (E)   The average blood loss associated with a vaginal delivery is about 600 mL and about 1000 mL after a cesarean delivery (*Chestnut: Obstetric Anesthesia, ed 3, pp 22-23*).

692. (C)   The fetus has several compensatory mechanisms for dealing with low O_2 pressures (umbilical vein Po_2 approximately equal to 30 mm Hg when mother is breathing room air) to which it is exposed. These include a higher hemoglobin concentration (15 to 20 g/dL) and the presence of fetal hemoglobin, which has a greater affinity for oxygen (the fetal oxyhemoglobin dissociation curve is shifted to the left of the maternal oxyhemoglobin dissociation curve). Fetal and maternal blood flow through the placenta are equal. Fetal blood has a lower pH than maternal blood, which may be related to the higher $Paco_2$ levels seen in fetal blood (*Hughes: Anesthesia for Obstetrics, ed 4, pp 24-25*).

693. (D)   Nitroprusside, nifedipine, and nitroglycerin are all used successfully in patients with pregnancy-induced hypertension (PIH), all have direct effects on smooth muscle (such as the uterus) and are associated with increased postpartum hemorrhage. Nitroprusside and nitroglycerin's effects are short lived after the drug is discontinued. Labetalol (adrenergic blocker) does not affect uterine contractions significantly and is often used in patients with PIH. Because diazoxide has been reported to cause sudden uncontrolled hypotension with decreased uterine blood flow and fetal distress, it is rarely used in obstetrics today. Diazoxide is also a very potent uterine relaxant and can lead to increased hemorrhage as well (*Hughes: Anesthesia for Obstetrics, ed 4, pp 306-307*).

694. (D)   Preeclampsia occurs in about 7% of all pregnancies and is associated with hypertension, proteinuria, and/or generalized edema. It usually occurs after the 24th week of gestation but patients may present earlier in cases of gestational trophoblastic disease (e.g., molar pregnancy). It is classified as either mild or severe. It becomes severe if any of the following conditions coexists: systolic BP greater than or equal to 160 mm Hg; diastolic BP greater than or equal to 110 mm Hg; proteinuria greater than or equal to 5 g/24 hr; elevated serum creatinine, urine output of less than 500 mL/24 hr; CNS disturbances (seizures, altered consciousness, headaches, visual disturbances); pulmonary edema; epigastric or right upper quadrant pain; hepatic rupture; impaired liver function; thrombocytopenia; or HELLP syndrome. Most patients have increased cardiac output, normal or increased systemic vascular resistance, and normal or decreased blood volumes and filling pressures. The white blood count is not part of the diagnosis of preeclampsia. In fact, the white blood count progressively rises during normal pregnancy from 6000/mm³ to 9000 to 11,000/mm³. During labor the white blood count increases to 13,000/mm³ and rises to an average of 15,000/mm³ on the first postpartum day (*Chestnut: Obstetric Anesthesia, ed 3, pp 794-817; Hughes: Anesthesia for Obstetrics, ed 4, pp 297-303*).

695. (E)   Placenta previa is classically described as painless vaginal bleeding during the second or third trimester and is not associated with maternal shock or fetal distress with the presentation of the first bleed (*Chestnut: Obstetric Anesthesia, ed 3, pp 662-663; Hughes: Anesthesia for Obstetrics, ed 4, p 361*).

696. (D)   The first stage of labor starts with the onset of labor and ends with complete cervical dilation (10 cm). It is visceral pain and is associated with uterine contractions and dilation of the cervix and is transmitted via the autonomic nervous system through the sympathetic fibers that pass through the paracervical region and enter the CNS at T10-L1 segments. The second stage of labor includes these pathways and adds the somatic fibers of the birth canal that are transmitted via the pudendal nerve entering the CNS at S2-S4. Neuraxial block (spinal and/or epidural) with only narcotics can be useful for first stage pain, however the somatic pain is not well treated with narcotics alone. A local anesthetic induced lumbar epidural block with or without narcotics can produce complete anesthesia during both first and second stage of labor pain. If a low spinal or saddle block is performed with local anesthetics (covering only sacral areas), the uterine contraction pain still will be felt. Paracervical blocks only block the first stage pain. Pudendal blocks block the somatic component during the second stage but not visceral pain

of contractions. Bilateral lumbar paravertebral sympathetic blocks were once used to treat first stage labor pain (no effect on second stage somatic birth canal pain) but are more of historical significance, because epidural and spinal blocks are much easier (*Chestnut: Obstetric Anesthesia, ed 3, pp 290-292, 335-336, 387, 391-392; Hughes: Anesthesia for Obstetrics, ed 4, pp 123-133*).

697. (E) There are several drugs that can be used for tocolytic therapy for preterm labor. Most commonly, $MgSO_4$ and/or β-adrenergic agonists (ritodrine, terbutaline) are used. Prostaglandin-synthetase inhibitors (indomethacin, ketorolac) and calcium entry blockers (nifedipine) have recently been used in selected cases. Ace inhibitors (captopril) can cause injury and even death to the developing fetus during the second and third trimester and should not be given during this part of pregnancy (*Chestnut: Obstetric Anesthesia, ed 3, pp 609-625; Hughes: Anesthesia for Obstetrics, ed 4, pp 323-337; Physicians' Desk Reference - 2008, ed 62, p 2169*).

698. (E) 15-Methyl PGF_{2a} (carboprost, Hemabate) is the preferred prostaglandin for use in the treatment of refractory uterine atony (after oxytocin). The dose is 250 μg IM, repeat as needed every 15 to 30 minutes with a maximum total dose of 2 mg. It has several important side effects, such as bronchospasm, ventilation-to-perfusion ($\dot{V}/\dot{Q}$) mismatch with an increase in intrapulmonary shunting, and hypoxemia. Other side effects include nausea, vomiting, fever, and diarrhea (*Chestnut: Obstetric Anesthesia, ed 3, pp 671, 919; Hughes: Anesthesia for Obstetrics, ed 4, pp 367-369*).

699. (C) Magnesium sulfate is the anticonvulsant of choice in the preeclamptic patient in North America and is more effective than phenytoin. In addition to its anticonvulsant effect, $MgSO_4$ exerts a peripheral effect at the neuromuscular junction. The therapeutic range for serum $MgSO_4$ is 4 to 8 mEq/L. (1 mEq/L = 1.22 mg/dL). In an unanesthetized patient, a loss of deep tendon reflexes occurs at 10 mEq/L, respiratory arrest occurs at 15 mEq/L. As long as deep tendon reflexes are present, significant toxicity is unlikely. In a patient with an epidural or spinal anesthetic loaded for a cesarean section. the patellar reflex is gone; estimation of deep tendon reflexes should be done with the biceps tendon (unless a total spinal develops). Electrocardiogram (ECG) changes including P-Q interval prolongation and QRS complex widening occurs at serum levels of 5 to 10 mEq/L; sinoatrial and atrioventricular block at 15 mEq/L and cardiac arrest at levels greater than 25 mEq/L. The treatment for magnesium toxicity is calcium. Patients with therapeutic $MgSO_4$ levels should not be reversed with calcium to decrease the chance for postpartum uterine atony and hemorrhage, since eclamptic seizures may develop. About 60% of eclamptic seizures occur before delivery. Most postpartum seizures develop in the first 24 hours after delivery but eclamptic seizures may occur as late as 22 days after delivery (*Chestnut: Obstetric Anesthesia, ed 3, pp 808-809, 825-827; Hughes: Anesthesia for Obstetrics, ed 4, pp 304-306*).

700. (C) Three different aspiration syndromes have been described in the general population: aspiration of particulate matter, aspiration of acid fluid (Mendelson's syndrome), and aspiration of fecal material. Aspiration of fecal material has the highest mortality rate but fortunately occurs only with an associated bowel obstruction, which is rarely a problem in obstetrics. Symptoms of aspiration include coughing, tachypnea, tachycardia, bronchospasm, and hypoxemia. Treatment is supportive and includes the Heimlich maneuver if a large foreign body is lodged in the oropharynx (which is unlikely in the fasting laboring patient), endotracheal intubation, suctioning the airway to remove particulate material, administration of increased concentrations of oxygen, and application of PEEP to achieve oxygenation goals as needed (prophylactic PEEP does not provide any benefit). Coughing is due to the airway irritation and is most effectively decreased with muscle paralysis. Intravenous lidocaine would not be effective. Use of saline or bicarbonate lavage does not decrease lung damage and can worsen hypoxemia. Glucocorticoids or other anti-inflammatory drugs have not been effective in limiting the inflammation and may increase the risk of secondary bacterial infection (*Chestnut: Obstetric Anesthesia, ed 3, pp 523-529; Hughes: Anesthesia for Obstetrics, ed 4, pp 393-397*).

701. (D) Aortocaval compression typically is not a problem until about 20 weeks' gestation when the uterus is large enough to compress the aorta and vena cava when the patient assumes the supine position (*Chestnut: Obstetric Anesthesia, ed 3, p 241; Hughes: Anesthesia for Obstetrics, ed 4, pp 8-10*).

702. (D) Cimetidine and ranitidine are H_2-receptor antagonists that will increase gastric pH but take at least 30 minutes to work. Metoclopramide is not an antacid but may be useful by increasing the lower esophageal sphincter tone. Only liquid antacids raise gastric pH quickly. Sodium citrate, a clear nonparticulate antacid (0.3 M sodium citrate) is preferred over particulate antacids (aluminum hydroxide, magnesium trisilicate, magnesium hydroxide) because clear nonparticulate antacids cause less pulmonary damage if aspirated. Sodium citrate 30 mL neutralizes 255 mL of HCl with a pH of 1.0. Neutralization of gastric acid occurs rapidly (i.e., <5 minutes) and will last up to an hour (*Chestnut: Obstetric Anesthesia, ed 3, pp 530-531; Hughes: Anesthesia for Obstetrics, ed 4, pp 401-402*).

703.   **(D)**   Causes of fetal bradycardia include hypoxemia, acidosis, complete heart block, and some drugs. Atropine readily crosses the placenta but at low doses does not seem to cause fetal tachycardia; at high doses, it may produce tachycardia. The combination of neostigmine, which crosses the placenta slightly, and glycopyrrolate, which does not cross the placenta well, has been associated with fetal bradycardia, which is why neostigmine with atropine is preferred when reversing neuromuscular blockers if a fetus is present. Bradycardias are associated with early decelerations (head compression with vagal stimulation), late decelerations (fetal hypoxemia with vagal stimulation or myocardial failure), variable decelerations (umbilical cord compressions with vagal stimulation). Causes of fetal tachycardia include infection, fever, maternal smoking, fetal paroxysmal supraventricular tachycardia, and some drugs (ritodrine, terbutaline, atropine) (*Chestnut: Obstetric Anesthesia, ed 3, pp 111-115, 264; Hughes: Anesthesia for Obstetrics, ed 4, pp 625-630*).

704.   **(A)**   Cerebral palsy (CP) is a nonprogressive disorder of the central nervous system and is associated with impairment of motor function. Mental retardation may or may not be present and is not an essential diagnostic criterion. The cause is unknown and most likely multifactorial. Associated conditions include maternal mental retardation, birth weight of less than 2000 grams and fetal malformations, but many other factors may play a role. It occurs in about 2 per 1000 live births. At one time, fetal heart rate monitoring was thought to be able to prevent CP but this has not happened. In fact, among patients with new onset late deceleration patterns the false positive rate is 99% if used to predict the development of CP. This is not to say that intrapartum asphyxial insults do not cause damage, they might, and probably account for about 6% of cases of CP. There is also a very weak association of low Apgar scores and CP, in fact most children who develop CP had a 5 minute Apgar score that was normal (*Chestnut: Obstetric Anesthesia, ed 3, pp 148-163; Hughes: Anesthesia for Obstetrics, ed 4, p 634*).

705.   **(D)**   Diabetes mellitus is the most common endocrine problem associated with pregnancy. Type I diabetes mellitus (due to a decrease in insulin secretion) occurs in one of every 700 to 1000 gestations. Gestational diabetes, which occurs only during pregnancy, is seen in about 2% to 5% of all pregnancies. Although substantial advances in the obstetric and anesthetic management of diabetic parturients has been made, maternal and fetal mortality are still higher in these patients than in parturients without diabetes. Diabetic ketoacidosis (DKA) occurs in 8% to 9% of type I DM pregnancies. One important goal of insulin therapy in these patients is to avoid both hyperglycemia and hypoglycemia. In general, insulin requirements are increased during pregnancy from 0.7 units/kg/day at 2 weeks of gestation to 0.8 units/kg/day at 18 weeks and 0.9 to 1.0 units/kg/day at 32 weeks and more of gestation. Insulin does not readily cross the placenta and therefore does not have any direct effects on glucose metabolism in the fetus. Glucose, however, readily crosses the placenta. Preeclampsia and large-for-gestational-age fetuses occur more frequently in parturients with diabetes. Because of fetal macrosomia, cesarean section is more common in diabetics than nondiabetics (*Chestnut: Obstetric Anesthesia, ed 3, pp 734-744; Hughes: Anesthesia for Obstetrics, ed 4, pp 497-505*).

706.   **(E)**   Postdural puncture headaches (PDPH) are positional headaches (exacerbated by sitting or standing and relieved with recumbency). They are bilateral and typically located in the fronto-occipital regions. In one prospective series of non-obstetric patients with PDPH, symptoms included nausea 60%, vomiting 24%, neck stiffness 43%, ocular changes (photophobia, diplopia, difficulty in accommodation) 13%, and auditory changes (hearing loss, hyperacusis, tinnitus), 12%. Although postpartum seizures have been associated with PDPH, other etiologies are more likely. Seizures, lethargy, fever, nuchal rigidity, focal neurologic deficits (other than listed above) and a unilateral location suggest other headache etiologies (*Chestnut: Obstetric Anesthesia, ed 3, pp 562-574; Hughes: Anesthesia for Obstetrics, ed 4, pp 414-415*).

707.   **(D)**   There are several periodic FHR patterns. Accelerations in FHR in response to fetal movement signify fetal well-being. Early decelerations are decreases in FHR usually less than 20 beats/min and occur concomitantly with uterine contractions. Typically they are smooth and are mirror images of the uterine contractions. They are not associated with fetal compromise and are caused by head compression, which produces a vagal slowing of the FHR. Late decelerations are decreases in FHR that occur 10 to 30 seconds after the onset of a contraction and end 10 to 30 seconds after the end of a contraction. They are due to uteroplacental insufficiency and can result whenever uterine blood flow decreases. The delayed onset is due to the time required to sense a low oxygen tension. The decrease in FHR may be a vagal reflex (mild cases) or due to direct myocardial depression from hypoxia (severe cases). Typically, in severe cases beat-to-beat variability is decreased or absent as well. Variable decelerations are decreases in FHR that vary in shape, depth, and duration from contraction to contraction. They are thought to be due to transient umbilical cord compression. A sinusoidal pattern is a regular smooth wavelike pattern with no short-term variability. It may be caused by severe fetal anemia or result from the maternal administration of narcotics (*Chestnut: Obstetric Anesthesia, ed 3, pp 114-115; Hughes: Anesthesia for Obstetrics, ed 4, pp 625-633*).

708. **(D)** Shivering occurs in 10% of all normal deliveries. The frequency increases from 20% to 70% of patients receiving epidural or spinal anesthesia for labor or cesarean deliveries. It is more common with spinal than epidural anesthesia. Use of epidural sufentanil (50 µg), fentanyl (100 µg), or meperidine (25 mg) with the local anesthetic and warming the IV fluid can help decrease the incidence of shivering. It is postulated that the greater efficacy of epidural meperidine may reside in its properties as both a µ- and a κ-receptor agonist within the spinal cord. Warming the epidural anesthesia solution to body temperature has no effect (*Chestnut: Obstetric Anesthesia, ed 3, p 487; Hughes: Anesthesia for Obstetrics, ed 4, p 417; Hughes: Anesthesia for Obstetrics, ed 3, pp 439-440*).

709. **(E)** These are normal umbilical cord values. Chart is modified from values listed in Chestnut's and Hughes' books.

NORMAL VALUES FOR UMBILICAL CORD BLOOD

Cord Blood	pH	P_{CO_2} (mm Hg)	P_{O_2} (mm Hg)	Bicarbonate (mEq/L)
Arterial	7.25	50	20	22
Venous	7.35	40	30	20

(*Chestnut: Obstetric Anesthesia, ed 3, pp 127-129; Hughes: Anesthesia for Obstetrics, ed 4, pp 659-660.*)

710. **(E)** Overall, the incidence of transfusion of blood for parturients (not including placenta previa) is 1%. However, about 3.5% of cesarean sections receive blood during or after cesarean section with the most frequent indication being placenta previa (*Chestnut: Obstetric Anesthesia, ed 3, p 676*).

711. **(B)** After clearing the airway, drying and stimulating the newborn, the apneic newborn receives positive pressure ventilation at a rate of 40 to 60 breaths/minute. After 30 seconds of assisted ventilation and if the heart rate is less than 60, chest compressions are started. At this point the newborn receives 30 breaths and 90 compressions/min (e.g., one and two and three and breath). If after another 30 seconds the newborn is not improving, epinephrine is administered. The correct dose is 0.1 to 0.3 mL/kg of a 1:10,000 (not 1:1000) solution. Intubation can be performed any time during resuscitation based on the skill level of the resuscitation team and equipment availability. If the newborn is intubated and IV access has not yet been achieved, consider administering a higher dose of epinephrine such as 0.3 to 1.0 mL/kg of a 1:10,000 solution down the endotracheal tube (the higher dose is used since blood levels are unpredictable after endotracheal instillation). If volume expansion is needed, normal saline, Ringer's lactate or, if severe fetal anemia is suspected or documented, type O Rh negative blood is administered IV at an initial dose of 10 mL/kg given over 5 to 10 minutes and repeated as needed. If the newborn has depressed respirations that are thought to be due to narcotic administration, naloxone at a dose of 0.1 mg/kg (1 mg/mL or 0.4 mg/mL solution) IV or IM is given. Recall that naloxone is not given to a newborn if the mother is addicted to narcotics or is on a methadone maintenance program or else the newborn could withdraw suddenly and develop seizures. With severe metabolic acidosis and adequate lung ventilation, a dilute solution of sodium bicarbonate (4.2% or 0.5 mEq/mL) at a dose of 2 mEq/kg is given slowly, no faster than 1 mEq/kg/min. Drugs used in newborn resuscitation that can be given down the endotracheal tube include *O*xygen, *N*aloxone, and *E*pinephrine (ONE) (*Kattwinkel: Textbook of Neonatal Resuscitation, ed 5, pp 1-11, 3-22, 4-10, 6-7, 6-10, 7-10, 7-14*).

712. **(D)** The incidence of failed intubation is 8 times higher in the obstetric population than the general population with an estimated rate of 1 in 280 obstetric patients (*Chestnut: Obstetric Anesthesia, ed 3, p 535*).

713. **(E)** Although the cause of PIH is not known, several associated factors are noted. Pregnancy-induced hypertension (PIH) is 5 times more common in primigravidas younger than 20 years of age compared with primigravidas older than 20 years of age. When there is rapid growth of the uterus, PIH is significantly more common (e.g., twins, type 1 DM, polyhydramnios, hydatidiform mole). The incidence of PIH is progressive with increasing body mass index (BMI) (4.3% with BMI <19.8, 13.3% with BMI >35). Although smoking is associated with many adverse pregnancy outcomes, there appears to be a lower incidence of PIH (*Cunningham: Williams Obstetrics, ed 22 pp 765, 1181; Hughes: Anesthesia for Obstetrics, ed 4, pp 297-298*).

714. (E)   Aortocaval compression can occur in up to 15% of pregnant patients at term. Compression of the vena cava reduces venous return, producing symptoms of hypotension, nausea and vomiting, pallor, and changes in cerebration. Compression of the aorta decreases uterine blood flow (*Hughes: Anesthesia for Obstetrics, ed 4, pp 8-10*).

715. (D)   Cocaine can produce life-threatening complications that are usually related to the accumulation of catecholamines and patients may present with the classic signs of toxemia (i.e., hypertension, proteinuria and edema). Because some states consider in utero cocaine exposure a form of child abuse that requires physicians to report positive drug tests in pregnant women, many cocaine abusing patients have no prenatal care. Urine tests may be positive for 24 to 72 hours after cocaine use (depending on the amount used). Life-threatening events are more common with general than regional anesthesia. The most frequent problem with induction of general anesthesia is severe hypertension. The MAC is increased in patients who are acutely intoxicated, whereas chronic abusing cocaine addicts have a lower MAC (depletion of catecholamines). These patients are at risk of having hypotension commonly seen after induction of regional anesthesia for cesarean section. Ephedrine may not be an effective vasopressor in these catecholamine depleted patients. Phenylephrine, a direct acting drug is a better vasopressor (*Chestnut: Obstetric Anesthesia, ed 3, pp 929-933; Hughes: Anesthesia for Obstetrics, ed 4, pp 604-608*).

716. (D)   In cases of emergency cesarean section when general anesthesia is contraindicated (e.g., poor airway when you question your ability to intubate and/or ventilate the patient), and neuraxial anesthesia is contraindicated (e.g., severe hypovolemia or coagulopathy), emergency infiltration anesthesia is acceptable. All of the choices are correct except the choice of local anesthetic. As the surgeon will be injecting a fair volume of local anesthetic (often 100 mL) and bupivacaine has a slow onset and potentially dangerous cardiac toxicity with large doses, bupivacaine is a poor choice. A dose of 0.5% lidocaine (plasma half-life of 90 minutes) is often used because it is readily available and relatively safe. Chloroprocaine may be safer because it also has a fast onset and its plasma half-life is extremely short (23 seconds). Both midazolam and ketamine may lead to some amnesia for the patient which may be advantageous in this emergency situation, however, too much of the IV drugs could obtund the patient and may lead to aspiration of gastric contents. A good coach at the head of the bed may be invaluable for reassuring the patient as to the care (*Chestnut: Obstetric Anesthesia, ed 3 p 438*).

717. (A)   The most common complication after a spinal or epidural anesthetic is placed is systemic hypotension. Treatment is threefold: increasing left uterine displacement (LUD); administering more intravenous fluids; and evaluating the need for vasopressors. Although IV fluids are used to decrease the incidence of hypotension after spinal anesthesia and should be rapidly infused if the parturient has not received prehydration fluids along with left uterine displacement, vasopressors are often needed. Initial studies suggested that ephedrine was a better choice compared with phenylephrine and other α-adrenergic agonists, as noted in animal studies looking at changes in uterine blood flow. More recent human studies looking at ephedrine and phenylephrine use have noted no difference in the prophylactic or treatment use of these drugs for maternal hypotension; maternal bradycardia was more common with phenylephrine whereas maternal tachycardia was more common with ephedrine; and neonatal arterial pH was higher when phenylephrine was used as compared with ephedrine. Why this occurs is unclear but may be related to ephedrine's ability to cross the placenta causing β-adrenergic stimulation in the newborn. In this patient who has LUD, adequate IV hydration and a heart rate of 100 beats/min, phenylephrine would be the preferred vasopressor. Epinephrine is rarely needed but should be available and used when there is severe hypotension not responsive to phenylephrine or ephedrine, especially when there is associated fetal bradycardia. Intravenous fluids with dextrose are used only for maintenance fluids and should not be used to prevent or treat hypotension from regional anesthesia because the fluid load causes significant maternal and fetal hyperglycemia and hyperinsulinemia. After delivery, the sugar supply for the newborn stops but the insulin response continues, often causing fetal hypoglycemia post delivery. Hetastarch solutions are not only expensive but may alter platelet function, producing more bleeding at the time of delivery, and are not recommended for routine use to treat hypotension (*Chestnut: Obstetric Anesthesia, ed 3, pp 422-426; Hughes: Anesthesia for Obstetrics, ed 4, pp 32-33, 204-207*).

718. (D)   A threatened abortion is defined as uterine bleeding without cervical dilation before 20 weeks gestation. Bleeding may be accompanied by cramping or backache. Half of these cases will go on to spontaneously abort. An inevitable abortion has cervical dilation and/or rupture of membranes and will spontaneously abort. A complete abortion occurs when there is complete expulsion of the fetus and the placenta, and in these cases there is no need for a D&C. If there is only partial expulsion of tissue, as in this case, an incomplete abortion has occurred and these require a D&E to remove the remaining fetal or placental tissue. In these cases the cervix has usually dilated some and the patient usually can be managed with some mild sedation, because the most painful part of a D&E is cervical dilation. A habitual or recurrent abortion refers to the occurrence of three of more consecutive spontaneous abortions (*Chestnut: Obstetric Anesthesia, ed 3, pp 244-247*).

719. **(D)** 2-Chloroprocaine administered epidurally appears to decrease the quality and duration of subsequently administered fentanyl or morphine. The exact mechanism is unclear but does not seem to be related to the acid pH of chloroprocaine (because neutralization with bicarbonate has similar antagonistic properties). Butorphanol (a κ-receptor agonist) does not appear to be antagonized (*Chestnut: Obstetric Anesthesia, ed 3, pp 178, 199; Hughes: Anesthesia for Obstetrics, ed 4, p 75*).

720. **(B)** Earlier diagnosis of complete molar pregnancies has decreased the incidence of medical complications. However, excessive uterine size occurs in up to one half of patients with a complete molar pregnancy and is associated with a high incidence of medical complications. Medical complications when the uterine size is greater than 14 to 16 weeks gestational size include ovarian theca-lutein cysts 4% to 50%, hyperemesis gravidarum 15% to 30%, pregnancy induced hypertension 11% to 27%, anemia with hemoglobin less than 10 in 10% to 54%, acute cardiopulmonary distress 6% to 27%, malignant sequelae (metastasis) 4% to 36%, and hyperthyroidism 1% to 7% (*Chestnut: Obstetric Anesthesia, ed 3, pp 249-251*).

721. **(B)** Several cases of maternal cardiac arrest have occurred in pregnant women who were administered bupivacaine (Marcaine, Sensorcaine). Typically, the patients received an unintentional IV bolus of 0.75% bupivacaine intended for the epidural space. They had a brief grand mal seizure followed by cardiovascular collapse. Successful treatment may be prolonged and involves basic resuscitation (intubation, ventilation with 100% oxygen, cardiac compression with left uterine tilt, defibrillation, epinephrine, vasopressin, amiodarone), as well as rapid delivery of the fetus (if possible within 4 to 5 minutes). Delivery of the fetus makes successful resuscitation of the mother more likely. Incremental small injections of local anesthetic looking for toxicity should decrease the chance for cardiovascular collapse. Bupivacaine 0.75% now is considered contraindicated for use in the epidural space of parturients. Recent literature has shown that the IV injection of 20% Intralipid (dose 4 mL/kg followed by 0.5 mL/kg/min) may make resuscitation both easier and more likely. Both levobupivacaine (Chirocaine) and ropivacaine (Naropin) were developed to have a long duration of action, like bupivacaine, but with less cardiac toxicity. Although these compounds have less cardiac toxicity than bupivacaine, they are more cardiac toxic than lidocaine (intermediate duration of action) and chloroprocaine (short duration of action) (*Barash: Clinical Anesthesia, ed 5, pp 464-467; Chestnut: Obstetric Anesthesia, ed 3, pp 194-195; Hughes: Anesthesia for Obstetrics, ed 4, pp 81-87, 436-437*).

722. **(A)** Transient neurologic syndrome (TNS) occurs most commonly after spinal anesthesia with lidocaine (Xylocaine). Symptoms include back pain that develops after the block resolves and radiates to the buttocks and legs. The pain is not associated with motor or sensory loss or electromyographic changes. It can be severe, requiring hospital admission of outpatients and typically resolves within 1 to 4 days. It appears to occur more commonly when patients are operated on when they are in the lithotomy position and appears less likely when patients are pregnant (*Chestnut: Obstetric Anesthesia, ed 3, p 196; Hughes: Anesthesia for Obstetrics, ed 4, pp 79-81*).

723. **(D)** Chloroprocaine undergoes oxidative decomposition and has undergone several different formulations over the years to decrease this decomposition. When EDTA was used, the incidence of severe deep back pain that lasted several hours become noted. This back pain was felt to be related to calcium chelation from the EDTA in the local anesthetic solution that leaked out of the intervertebral foramen and produced hypocalcemic tetany of the paraspinal muscles. Currently, the EDTA has been removed and the chloroprocaine manufactured today is in colored vials to reduce the rate of oxidation (*Chestnut: Obstetric Anesthesia, ed 3, pp 195-196; Hughes: Anesthesia for Obstetrics, ed 4, pp 75-76*).

724. **(C)** The metabolic product of prilocaine (Citanest) is ortho-toluidine, which can produce methemoglobinemia. This occurs when doses of prilocaine greater than 600 mg are used (*Hughes: Anesthesia for Obstetrics, ed 4, p 81*).

725. **(E)** Chloroprocaine (Nesacaine) is an ester-type local anesthetic with a very short half-life in both maternal and fetal blood. The in vitro half-life is 21 seconds for maternal blood and 43 seconds for fetal blood. All the other local anesthetics are amides and require liver metabolism (*Chestnut: Obstetric Anesthesia, ed 3, p 333, Hughes: Anesthesia for Obstetrics, ed 4, p 75*).

Chapter 9

Neurologic Physiology and Anesthesia

726. Following clipping of an anterior communicating artery aneurysm, a 59-year-old man is admitted to the intensive care unit (ICU). Serum sodium is 115 mEq/L, 24 hour urine sodium collection 350 mmol (normal range 40 to 117 mmol/24 h) and central venous pressure (CVP) is 1 cm H_2O. The most likely cause of these findings is:
    A. Tubular necrosis
    B. Diabetes insipidus
    C. Cerebral salt wasting syndrome
    D. Syndrome of inappropriate antidiuretic hormone (SIADH)
    E. Primary hyperaldosteronism

727. Intracranial hypertension is defined as a sustained increase in intracranial pressure (ICP) above
    A. 5 mm Hg
    B. 15 mm Hg
    C. 25 mm Hg
    D. 40 mm Hg
    E. None of the above

728. Calculate cerebral perfusion pressure from the following data:

    Blood pressure (BP) 100/70, heart rate (HR) 65 beats/min, central venous pressure (CVP) 20 mm Hg, ICP 15 mm Hg
    A. 60 mm Hg
    B. 65 mm Hg
    C. 70 mm Hg
    D. 75 mm Hg
    E. Cannot be determined

729. The afferent input for somatosensory evoked potentials (SSEPs) is carried through which spinal cord tract?
    A. Spinocerebellar
    B. Spinothalamic
    C. Dorsal columns
    D. Corticospinal
    E. Vestibulospinal

730. By what percentage does cerebral blood flow (CBF) change for each mm Hg increase in $Paco_2$?
    A. 1%
    B. 2%
    C. 7%
    D. 10%
    E. 25%

731. Which of the following intravenous anesthetics is contraindicated in patients with intracranial hypertension?
- **A.** Propofol
- **B.** Fentanyl
- **C.** Thiopental
- **D.** Midazolam
- **E.** Ketamine

732. The term *luxury perfusion* refers to a situation that occurs in the brain when
- **A.** Blood flow has resumed after a period of ischemia
- **B.** Blood flow is directed from a normal region of the brain to an ischemic region
- **C.** Vasoparalysis exists
- **D.** The Robin Hood phenomenon exists
- **E.** A zone of ischemic penumbra exists

733. A 62-year-old patient is scheduled to undergo resection of a frontal lobe intracranial tumor under general anesthesia. Preoperatively, the patient is alert and oriented, and has no focal neurologic deficits. Within what range should $Paco_2$ be maintained?
- **A.** 15 and 20 mm Hg
- **B.** 20 and 25 mm Hg
- **C.** 25 and 30 mm Hg
- **D.** 40 and 45 mm Hg
- **E.** None of the above

734. A 2-year-old child is anesthetized for resection of a posterior fossa tumor. Preoperatively, the patient is lethargic and disoriented. Which of the following is most likely to adversely alter ICP?
- **A.** 5% dextrose in water
- **B.** Normal saline
- **C.** Lactated Ringer's solution
- **D.** 5% albumin
- **E.** Fresh frozen plasma

735. A 22-year-old patient is anesthetized for resection of a temporal lobe tumor. Preoperatively, he is lethargic and confused. After induction of general anesthesia, which of the following would be the most appropriate drug to control systemic arterial blood pressure during direct laryngoscopy and tracheal intubation?
- **A.** Esmolol
- **B.** Nitroglycerine
- **C.** Hydralazine
- **D.** Isoflurane
- **E.** Nitroprusside

736. Normal global CBF is
- **A.** 25 mL/100 g/min
- **B.** 50 mL/100 g/min
- **C.** 75 mL/100 g/min
- **D.** 100 mL/100 g/min
- **E.** 150 mL/100 g/min

737. The lower and upper mean arterial blood pressure limits of CBF autoregulation are, respectively
- **A.** 25 and 125 mm Hg
- **B.** 25 and 200 mm Hg
- **C.** 40 and 250 mm Hg
- **D.** 60 and 160 mm Hg
- **E.** 50 and 200 mm Hg

738. How much will CBF increase in a patient whose $Paco_2$ is increased from 35 to 45 mm Hg?
  A. There is no relationship between $Paco_2$ and CBF
  B. 10 mL/100 g/min
  C. 25 mL/100 g/min
  D. 40 mL/100 g/min
  E. 50 mL/100 g/min

739. Select the **FALSE** statement concerning autonomic hyperreflexia.
  A. Distention of a hollow viscus below the level of the spinal cord transection can elicit autonomic hyperreflexia
  B. Up to 85% of patients with a spinal cord transection above the T6 dermatome will exhibit autonomic hyperreflexia under general anesthesia
  C. Propranolol is effective in treating hypertension associated with autonomic hyperreflexia
  D. Spinal anesthesia is effective in preventing autonomic hyperreflexia
  E. Cutaneous stimulation below the level of the spinal cord transection can elicit autonomic hyperreflexia

740. What is the normal cerebral metabolic rate for oxygen ($CMRO_2$) per minute?
  A. 0.5 mL/100 g brain tissue
  B. 2.0 mL/100 g brain tissue
  C. 3.5 mL/100 g brain tissue
  D. 7.5 mL/100 g brain tissue
  E. 10 mL/100 g brain tissue

741. A 14-year-old girl with severe scoliosis is to undergo spine surgery. Anesthesia is maintained with fentanyl, N_2O 50% in O_2, vecuronium, and isoflurane. Neurologic function of the spinal cord is monitored by SSEPs. In reference to the SSEP waveform, spinal cord ischemia would be manifested as
  A. Increased amplitude and increased latency
  B. Decreased amplitude and increased latency
  C. Decreased amplitude and decreased latency
  D. Increased amplitude and decreased latency
  E. Increased amplitude and no change in latency

742. For each 1° C decrease in body temperature, how much will $CMRO_2$ be diminished?
  A. 3%
  B. 5%
  C. 6%
  D. 10%
  E. 20%

743. A 24-year-old carpenter is treated for a closed head injury sustained 3 days earlier after falling from a roof. He has been hemodynamically stable, but despite aggressive efforts to pharmacologically reduce ICP, he is now unconscious and unresponsive to painful stimuli. All of the following are clinical criteria consistent with a diagnosis of brain death in this patient **EXCEPT**
  A. Persistent apnea for 10 minutes
  B. Absence of pupillary light reflex
  C. Persistent spinal reflexes
  D. Decorticate posturing
  E. Absence of oropharyngeal reflex

744. Which of the following is the most sensitive means of detecting venous air embolism (VAE)?
  A. Electroencephalography (EEG)
  B. Pulmonary artery catheter
  C. Transesophageal echocardiography
  D. Mass spectrometry
  E. Right atrial catheterization

745. When intracranial hypertension exists, the main compensatory mechanism from the body is
  A. Increased absorption of cerebrospinal fluid (CSF) at the intracranial arachnoid villi
  B. Increased absorption of CSF in the spinal arachnoid villi
  C. Shifting of CSF from intracranial to spinal subarachnoid space
  D. Reduction of cerebral blood volume due to compression of intracranial arteries
  E. Decreased production of CSF at the choroid plexus

746. Select the correct order from greatest to least for the sensitivity of the following neurophysiologic monitoring techniques to volatile anesthetics (SSEP [somatosensory evoked potential]; VEP [visual evoked potential]; BAEP [brainstem auditory evoked potential]).
  A. SSEP > VEP > BAEP
  B. VEP > SSEP > BAEP
  C. BAEP > VEP > SSEP
  D. SSEP > BAEP > VEP
  E. SSEP = VEP > BAEP

747. Patients can be safely imaged in the magnetic resonance imaging (MRI) scanner with conventional versions of which of the following monitors?
  A. Pulmonary artery catheter with cardiac output probe
  B. Foley catheter with temperature probe
  C. Electrocardiogram (ECG) electrodes
  D. Pulse oximeter
  E. Arterial line

748. What is the minimum quantity of intracardiac air that can be detected by a precordial Doppler?
  A. 0.25 mL
  B. 5.0 mL
  C. 10 mL
  D. 25 mL
  E. 50 mL

749. With regard to regulation of blood flow, the correct order of vascular responsiveness to $Paco_2$ from most to least sensitive is
  A. Cerebrum > spinal cord > cerebellum
  B. Cerebrum > cerebellum > spinal cord
  C. Cerebellum > cerebrum > spinal cord
  D. Cerebellum > spinal cord > cerebrum
  E. Spinal cord > cerebrum > cerebellum

750. Select the **TRUE** statement concerning administration of glucose-containing solutions to the patient with a closed head injury versus a patient with a spinal cord injury.
  A. Glucose-containing solutions are contraindicated in both patient groups
  B. Glucose-containing solutions are contraindicated in patients with closed head injury but acceptable in patients with spinal cord injuries
  C. Glucose-containing solutions are acceptable in patients with closed head injuries but contraindicated in patients with spinal cord injuries
  D. Glucose-containing solutions may be given to either patient group if blood glucose concentrations do not exceed 200 mg/dL
  E. Glucose-containing solutions are acceptable in both patient groups.

751. A 67-year-old patient is scheduled to undergo posterior cervical fusion in the sitting position under general anesthesia. A central venous catheter is inserted from the right basilic vein and advanced toward the heart. Intravascular electrocardiography (ECG; with the exploring electrode attached to the V lead) is used to aid in placement of the catheter. After the catheter is advanced 45 cm, the tracing shown in the figure is noted on the ECG. At this time the anesthesiologist should

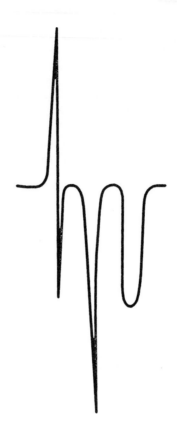

A. Advance the catheter 5 cm
B. Advance the catheter slightly
C. Leave the catheter in the present position
D. Withdraw the catheter 1 cm
E. Remove the catheter and defibrillate the heart

752. Critical CBF in patients anesthetized with isoflurane is
A. 5 mL/100 g/min
B. 10 mL/100 g/min
C. 18 mL/100 g/min
D. 25 mL/100 g/min
E. 32 mL/100 g/min

753. What effect does cerebral ischemia have on CBF autoregulation?
A. CBF autoregulation is ablated
B. CBF autoregulation is ablated at low cerebral perfusion pressures but remains intact at high cerebral perfusion pressures
C. CBF autoregulation is ablated at high cerebral perfusion pressures but remains intact at low cerebral perfusion pressures
D. The CBF autoregulatory curve is shifted to the right
E. The CBF autoregulatory curve is shifted to the left

754. The most rapid maneuver available for lowering ICP in a patient with a large intracranial mass is
A. Mannitol, 1 g/kg IV
B. Ketamine, 1 mg/kg IV
C. Hyperventilation to 25 mm Hg P_{aCO_2}
D. Furosemide, 1 mg/kg IV
E. Methylprednisolone, 30 mg/kg IV

755. What effect does thiopental have on the CO_2 responsiveness of the cerebral vasculature?
    A. Thiopental attenuates the effect of hypocarbia on CBF
    B. Thiopental attenuates the effect of hypercarbia on CBF
    C. Thiopental augments the effect of hypercarbia on CBF
    D. Thiopental augments the effect of hypocarbia on CBF
    E. Thiopental does not affect CO_2 reactivity at a dose used clinically

756. Each of the following is a relative contraindication to the sitting position **EXCEPT**
    A. Ventriculoatrial shunt
    B. Platypnea-orthodeoxia
    C. Right-to-left intracardiac shunt
    D. Ventriculoperitoneal shunt
    E. Patent foramen ovale

757. A 72-year-old patient undergoing resection of an astrocytoma in the sitting position suddenly develops hypotension. Air is heard on the precordial Doppler ultrasound. Each of the following therapeutic maneuvers to treat VAE is appropriate **EXCEPT**
    A. Discontinue N_2O
    B. Apply jugular venous pressure
    C. Implement positive end-expiratory pressure (PEEP)
    D. Administer epinephrine to treat hypotension
    E. Flood the surgical wound with saline

758. Which of the following is the **LEAST** likely sequela of venous air embolism during posterior fossa surgery in the upright position?
    A. Arterial hypoxemia
    B. Bronchoconstriction
    C. Stroke
    D. Hypertension
    E. Increase in pulmonary dead space

759. A 55-year-old business executive is scheduled for colonoscopy and polypectomy under general anesthesia. A bruit is auscultated over the right carotid artery on physical examination. The patient is otherwise healthy. Which of the following would be the most appropriate course of action?
    A. Cancel surgery and obtain coronary angiogram
    B. Cancel surgery and obtain Doppler ultrasound carotid blood flow studies
    C. Cancel surgery and obtain dobutamine stress echocardiogram
    D. Proceed with surgery and obtain a carotid angiogram postoperatively
    E. Proceed with surgery

760. How long after a stroke can anesthesia for surgery be carried out with about the same risk of a perioperative occlusive vascular accident as existed immediately before the previous stroke?
    A. 1 week
    B. 6 weeks
    C. 6 months
    D. 9 months
    E. 1 year

761. A 13-year-old boy is anesthetized with 0.5% isoflurane, 50% N_2O, and fentanyl for scoliosis repair. Somatosensory evoked potentials (SSEP) monitoring is conducted during the procedure. Which of the following structures is **NOT** involved in conveyance of the stimulus from the posterior tibial nerve to the cerebral cortex?
    A. Corticospinal tract
    B. Medial lemniscus
    C. Brain stem
    D. Internal capsule
    E. Dorsal root ganglion

762. A 19-year-old woman is undergoing surgery for a Harrington rod placement. General anesthesia is administered with desflurane, nitrous oxide, and fentanyl. After completion of spinal instrumentation, a wake-up test is undertaken. Four thumb twitches are present when the nerve stimulator attached to the ulnar nerve is activated. The volatile anesthetic and nitrous oxide have been discontinued for 10 minutes when the patient is asked to move her hands and feet. After repeated commands, the patient still does not move her hands or feet. The most appropriate intervention at this time would be
   A. 3 mg neostigmine plus 0.6 mg glycopyrrolate IV
   B. 20 μg naloxone IV
   C. 0.1 mg flumazenil IV
   D. Institute SSEP monitoring
   E. Reduce the distraction on the rods

763. A 75-year-old patient is undergoing craniotomy for resection of a large astrocytoma. During administration of isoflurane anesthesia, arterial blood gas sampling reveals a $Paco_2$ of 30 mm Hg. At this time, this patient's global cerebral blood flow would be approximately
   A. $10 \text{ mL} \times 100 \text{ g brain weight}^{-1} \times \text{min}^{-1}$
   B. $20 \text{ mL} \times 100 \text{ g brain weight}^{-1} \times \text{min}^{-1}$
   C. $30 \text{ mL} \times 100 \text{ g brain weight}^{-1} \times \text{min}^{-1}$
   D. $40 \text{ mL} \times 100 \text{ g brain weight}^{-1} \times \text{min}^{-1}$
   E. $50 \text{ mL} \times 100 \text{ g brain weight}^{-1} \times \text{min}^{-1}$

764. A 24-year-old patient is brought to the intensive care unit after sustaining a closed head injury in a motor vehicle accident. Each of the following would be useful in managing intracranial hypertension in this patient **EXCEPT**
   A. Corticosteroids
   B. Barbiturates
   C. Hyperventilation to a $Paco_2$ of 35 mm Hg
   D. Osmotic diuretics
   E. Placement of the patient in reverse Trendelenburg position

765. Preoperative treatment of subarachnoid hemorrhage (SAH) patients, without concomitant cerebral vasospasm, might include any of the following **EXCEPT**
   A. Induced hypertension (to 20% above baseline)
   B. Administration of nimodipine
   C. Sedation
   D. Analgesic therapy
   E. Administration of antiepileptic drugs

766. Which of the following pharmacologic agents would have the **LEAST** effect on somatosensory evoked potentials?
   A. Isoflurane
   B. Nitrous oxide
   C. Sodium thiopental
   D. Etomidate
   E. Vecuronium

767. A 75-year-old patient with signs and symptoms of a leaking cerebral aneurysm is brought to the emergency room for evaluation. T-wave inversion, a prolongation of the QT interval, and U waves are noted on the preoperative ECG. Appropriate action at this point would be
   A. Begin infusion of nitroglycerin
   B. Check serum calcium and potassium
   C. Administer esmolol
   D. Place a pulmonary artery catheter
   E. Delay surgery until myocardial infarction has been ruled out

768. Which of the following pharmacologic agents would have the **LEAST** effect on transcranial motor evoked potentials (MEPs)?
   A. Isoflurane
   B. Nitrous oxide
   C. Etomidate
   D. Diazepam
   E. Fentanyl

769. Ketamine
   A. Decreases cerebral blood flow (CBF)
   B. Augments the CO_2 responsiveness of the cerebral vasculature
   C. Reduces cerebral metabolic rate (CMR)
   D. Increases cerebral blood volume (CBV)
   E. Blunts cerebral autoregulation

770. CMR is decreased by
   A. Isoflurane
   B. Seizure
   C. Hyperthermia
   D. Ketamine
   E. Corticosteroids

771. Which of the following is **LEAST** likely to impair CBF autoregulation?
   A. Halothane 1 minimum alveolar concentration (MAC)
   B. Intracranical tumors
   C. Nitrous oxide 50%
   D. Cerebral ischemia
   E. Sevoflurane 2 MAC

772. An 18-year-old patient is brought to the intensive care unit after sustaining a cervical spine injury and quadriplegia during a motor vehicle accident. In the first 24 hours after the injury, the patient is at risk for
   A. Hypothermia, hypotension, pulmonary edema
   B. Fever, hypertension
   C. Fever, hypotension, hypoglycemia
   D. Autonomic hyperreflexia
   E. Impaired cerebral autoregulation

773. Signs and symptoms of intracranial hypertension include
   A. Papilledema
   B. Headache
   C. Nausea and vomiting
   D. Decreased mentation
   E. All of the above

774. An 89-year-old man with a history of transient ischemic attacks is scheduled to undergo a carotid endarterectomy under general anesthesia. Which of the following would be appropriate in the anesthetic management of this patient?
   A. Hyperventilation of the lungs to a $Paco_2$ of 30 mm Hg to reduce ICP
   B. Injection of local anesthetic around the carotid body to prevent bradycardia
   C. Initiation of deliberate hypotension (after induction of anesthesia) to reduce bleeding
   D. Induction of anesthesia with sodium thiopental
   E. Permissive hypercapnia to a $Paco_2$ of 50 mm Hg to promote the Robin Hood phenomenon

775. Anesthetics that decrease ICP include
   A. Isoflurane
   B. Nitrous oxide
   C. Propofol
   D. Sevoflurane
   E. Fentanyl

776. Therapy that is useful in the treatment of cerebral vasospasm includes all of the following **EXCEPT**
  A. Blood pressure elevation
  B. Hemodilution
  C. Diuretics
  D. Calcium channel blockers
  E. Avoiding hyperglycemia

777. All of the following are associated with acromegalic patients undergoing transsphenoidal hypophysectomy **EXCEPT**
  A. Enlargement of the tongue and epiglottis
  B. Narrowing of the glottic opening
  C. Nasal turbinate enlargement
  D. 20% to 30% incidence of difficult intubation
  E. Increased need for postop continuous positive airway pressure (CPAP) because obstructive sleep apnea (OSA) is more common

778. The CBF autoregulatory curve is shifted to the right by
  A. Hypoxia
  B. Volatile anesthetics
  C. Hypercarbia
  D. Chronic hypertension
  E. Fentanyl

779. Autoregulation is abolished by
  A. Hyperbaric oxygen
  B. Cardiopulmonary bypass with a core temperature 27° C
  C. Chronic hypertension
  D. 3% isoflurane
  E. Diabetes insipidus

780. Etomidate does all of the following **EXCEPT**
  A. Abolishes CO_2 reactivity
  B. Reduces $CMRO_2$
  C. Produces direct cerebral vasoconstrictor
  D. Reduces CBF
  E. Increases both SSEP amplitude and latency

781. Following a motor vehicle accident, a 25-year-old male patient is brought to the operating room for repair of facial lacerations and fractures, and abdominal exploration. The patient is extremely micrognathic and weighs 150 kg (330 pounds). Acceptable techniques for securing the airway include
  A. Mask technique
  B. Awake fiberoptic intubation
  C. Direct laryngoscopy after rapid sequence induction
  D. Blind nasal intubation
  E. Laryngeal mask airway

782. After resection of a grade II astrocytoma in a 60-year-old patient, the serum sodium is 127 mEq/L. Urine sodium is 25 mEq/L. Therapy could include which of the following?
  A. Intranasal or IV vasopressin (DDAVP)
  B. 500 mL 5% saline over 30 minutes
  C. Chlorpropamide
  D. Leave intubated and hyperventilate
  E. Demeclocycline

783.   A 48-year-old, 110-kg, man with history of meningioma is scheduled for craniotomy for tumor debulking. His
        wife states he has been somnolent and confused. On exam he is noted to be hyperventilating, sleepy, but arousable and
        hypertensive. Useful measures for his anesthetic include
        A. Rapid sequence induction using succinylcholine
        B. Premedication with 2 mg IV morphine to lower BP and slow breathing
        C. 10 cm H_2O PEEP to reduce atelectasis
        D. Esmolol to reduce response to intubation
        E. Hyperventilation to 25 mm Hg

784.   If during an MRI scan a patient were to become pinned by a large (50 kg) metallic object, the appropriate course of
        action would be to
        A. Stop the scan immediately to release the magnet
        B. Summon enough people to pull the object away
        C. Interrupt electrical power for 60 seconds to release the magnetic force
        D. Cut up the metal object and remove piecemeal
        E. None of the above

785.   A 45-year-old man is undergoing a posterior cervical fusion in the sitting position. Induction of anesthesia and tra-
        cheal intubation are uneventful. Anesthesia is maintained with N_2O, 50% in O_2, and sevoflurane. Suddenly, air is
        heard on the precordial Doppler ultrasound. Other observations consistent with venous air embolism include
        A. Decreased Pao_2
        B. Increased end-tidal nitrogen
        C. Decreased arterial blood pressure
        D. Decreased end-tidal CO_2
        E. All of the above

786.   In patients with increased ICP, hyperventilation is typically limited to a $Paco_2$ of 30 to 35 mm Hg because additional
        hyperventilation
        A. Is virtually impossible
        B. Causes brain ischemia due to a rightward shifting of the oxyhemoglobin dissociation curve
        C. May be associated with a worsening of neurologic outcome
        D. Could result in paradoxical cerebral vasodilation
        E. May result in clinically significant hyperkalemia

787.   Of the measures below, which is the **LEAST** useful in response to suspected VAE during a neurosurgical procedure in
        the upright position?
        A. Application 10 cm H_2O PEEP
        B. Discontinuation N_2O
        C. Placement of wax on cut bone edges
        D. Trendelenburg position
        E. Flooding surgical field with saline

Neurologic Physiology and Anesthesia

Answers, References, and Explanations

726. (C) The triad associated with cerebral salt-wasting syndrome consists of hyponatremia, volume contraction, and urine sodium concentrations inappropriately high for the given level of serum sodium. It is mainly seen in patients with subarachnoid hemorrhage (SAH). A possible etiology may be release of brain natriuretic peptide, leading to excess urinary sodium excretion. It is treated with volume replacement, utilizing normal to hypertonic intravenous sodium chloride solution, but avoiding overly rapid serum sodium correction as this may result in central pontine myelinolysis. Cerebral salt wasting syndrome (usually hypovolemic) is difficult to differentiate from SIADH (usually normovolemic or mildly hypervolemic) because patients with SAH can have high antidiuretic hormone (ADH) levels secondary to trauma, pain etc. A definitive diagnosis requires demonstration of a negative sodium balance over several days in the setting of ongoing hypovolemia or obtaining a 24 hour urine sodium sample. Clinically, the former is often not feasible because of competing interests for prophylaxis or treatment of cerebral vasospasm with moderate hypervolemia. In the setting of cerebral salt-wasting syndrome, the 24-hour sodium value is elevated. In contrast, hyponatremia associated with SIADH is due to renal retention of free water (rather than renal loss of sodium). Accordingly, the quantity of sodium collected over the 24-hour period and CVP should be relatively normal in SIADH patients. The patient presented in this question is hyponatremic, has a low CVP, and a 24-hour urine sodium that is clearly elevated. Collectively, this supports the diagnosis of cerebral salt-wasting syndrome. Diabetes insipidus and primary hyperaldosteronism are incorrect responses, as both would be associated with increased plasma concentrations. Tubular necrosis has nothing to do with this pathophysiologic process (*Barash: Clinical Anesthesia, ed 5, pp 190, 1149-1150; Cottrell: Anesthesia and Neurosurgery, ed 4, pp 370, 599, 604; Miller: Anesthesia, ed 6, p 2147*).

727. (B) Elevated ICP frequently is the final stage of a pathologic cerebral insult (e.g., head injury, intracranial tumor, subarachnoid hemorrhage, metabolic encephalopathy, or hydrocephalus). The intracranial contents consist of three components: brain parenchyma (80% to 85%); blood (3% to 6%); and CSF (5% to 15%). None of these components is compressible; accordingly, an increase in the volume of any of these requires a compensatory decrease in the volume of one or both of the other components to avoid the development of intracranial hypertension. Normal ICP is less than 15 mm Hg. As measured in the supine position, intracranial hypertension is defined as a sustained increase in ICP above 15 to 20 mm Hg (*Stoelting: Basics of Anesthesia, ed 5, p 456*).

728. (A) Cerebral perfusion pressure is equal to mean arterial pressure (MAP) minus the greater of CVP or ICP. In the present case, MAP equals 80 mm Hg (diastolic pressure, 70, plus one-third the pulse pressure, 10). Thus, 80 − 20 = 60 (*Stoelting: Basics of Anesthesia, ed 5, p 454*).

729. (C) Somatosensory evoked potentials (SSEPs) are voltage signals that appear in response to electrical stimulation of peripheral nerves. The impulse elicited by electrical stimulation of a peripheral nerve ascends the ipsilateral dorsal column of the spinal cord, decussates in the medulla oblongata, and is ultimately recorded on the contralateral somatosensory cortex of the brain. The signals are composed of negative and positive voltage deflections with specific latencies and amplitudes. In general, the earlier deflections represent impulses and synapses within the spinal cord or brain stem, whereas the later impulses represent thalamic and/or cortical synapses. Intraoperative monitoring of SSEPs provides the ability to assess the integrity of the peripheral nerve (e.g., posterior tibial nerve, dorsal columns, brain stem, medial lemniscus, internal capsule, and contralateral somatosensory cortex) (*Stoelting: Basics of Anesthesia, ed 5, p 313*).

730. (B) Hyperventilation of the lungs causes constriction of cerebral blood vessels, which reduces global cerebral blood flow (CBF) and cerebral blood volume (CBV). This effect is mediated by changes in the pH induced in the extracellular fluid. In contrast to autoregulation, CO_2 reactivity is preserved in most patients with severe brain injury; thus, hyperventilation can rapidly lower ICP through the reduction in CBV. Although the effects of hyperventilation on CBV and ICP are almost immediate, the duration of effect wanes after 6 to 10 hours of hyperventilation and may last up to 24 to 36 hours, because the pH of the extracellular fluid equilibrates to the lower $Paco_2$ level. Generally speaking, CBF increases (or decreases) by approximately 2% for each mm Hg increase (or decrease) in $Paco_2$. Cerebral blood flow (CBF) increases (or decreases) 1 mL/100 g/min per 1 mm Hg increase (or decrease) in $Paco_2$. Because normal global CBF is 50 mL/100 g/min, a 1 mL/100 g/min alteration in CBF represents a 2% change (*Barash: Clinical Anesthesia, ed 5, p 749*).

731. (E) Of the choices listed in this question, ketamine is the only intravenous anesthetic not recommended for patients with intracranial hypertension because it increases cerebral metabolic rate (CMR), CBF, CBV, and ICP. Barbiturates, etomidate, and propofol decrease CMR, CBF, CBV, and ICP. All three of these agents indirectly decrease CBF by their inhibitory effect on CMR. However, unlike thiopental, etomidate also has a direct vasoconstrictor effect on the cerebral vasculature. One potential advantage of etomidate over thiopental is that it does not produce significant cardiovascular depression. Although not as pronounced as the barbiturates, benzodiazepines such as midazolam also reduce CMR and CBF. Flumazenil, a benzodiazepine antagonist, has been reported to reverse the effect of midazolam on CMR, CBF, CBV, and ICP. Consequently, flumazenil should be avoided in midazolam-anesthetized patients known to have intracranial hypertension. Generally speaking, the opioid anesthetics, such as morphine and fentanyl, cause either a minor reduction or have no effect on CBF and CMR. Although many of the these IV drugs reduce ICP, none has been shown to provide neuroprotection to humans with either focal (like stroke) or global (like cardiac arrest) ischemia (*Stoelting: Basics of Anesthesia, ed 5, pp 455-456*).

732. (C) During acute focal cerebral ischemia, regional vasoparalysis results in impaired coupling between CBF and metabolism. Consequently, CBF exceeds CMR and is passively associated with systemic arterial blood pressure. Under these circumstances, autoregulation and the reactivity of the cerebrovasculature to carbon dioxide is also impaired. Thus, tight control of systemic arterial blood pressure is important in managing patients with focal ischemia, because cerebral perfusion is highly dependent on mean arterial blood pressure. Blood flow directed from a normal region of the brain to an ischemic region is known as the "Robin Hood phenomenon," (i.e., robbing from the rich and giving to the poor). Thus, choice B and D are synonymous incorrect responses (*Cottrell: Anesthesia and Neurosurgery, ed 4, p 34*).

733. (C) Cerebral ischemia has been reported in both humans and laboratory animals when the $Paco_2$ is reduced below 20 mm Hg. It is likely that cerebral ischemia is caused by a leftward shift of the oxyhemoglobin dissociation curve (produced by the severe alkalosis) and possibly by intense cerebral vasoconstriction. A leftward shift of the oxyhemoglobin dissociation curve increases the affinity of hemoglobin for O_2, which reduces off-loading of O_2 from hemoglobin at the capillary bed. This effect combined with decreased CBF can result in cerebral ischemia. Combined with the fact that there is very little additional benefit in terms of reducing CBV and ICP, it is recommended to limit acute hyperventilation of the lungs to a $Paco_2$ of 25 to 30 mm Hg. Within this range, reduction in ICP is maximal and risk of cerebral ischemia is minimal. As an aside, hyperventilation-induced respiratory alkalosis can precipitate hypokalemia. Specifically, serum potassium decreases 0.6 mEq/L for each 0.1 unit increase in pH. Thus, overly aggressive hyperventilation should be guarded against to avoid possible hypokalemia-induced cardiac arrhythmias (*Miller: Anesthesia, ed 6, pp 2132-2133*).

734. (A) Five percent dextrose in water (D5W) is contraindicated in neurosurgical patients with intracranial hypertension for two reasons. First, D5W easily passes through the blood-brain barrier. Once in the brain tissue, glucose is rapidly metabolized, leaving only free water, which causes cerebral edema. Second, hyperglycemia is associated with increased severity of neurologic damage in patients with cerebral ischemia. This is thought to result from increased lactate production during anaerobic glycolysis during the period of ischemia (*Miller: Anesthesia, ed 6, pp 841-842*).

735. (A) Except esmolol, all of the drugs listed are potent cerebral vasodilators capable of further increasing ICP, which would be highly undesirable in this patient. In contrast, esmolol is a cardioselective β_1-adrenergic receptor antagonist with rapid onset and short duration of action due to hydrolysis by red blood cell esterases. Plasma cholinesterases and red cell membrane acetylcholinesterase do not play a role in its degradation. Esmolol effectively blunts the sympathetic response to direct laryngoscopy and tracheal intubation, yet is devoid of deleterious effects on CBV or ICP (*Cottrell: Anesthesia and Neurosurgery, ed 4, pp 256, 300; Miller: Anesthesia, ed 6, pp 818-820*).

736. (B) Normal global CBF is approximately 45 to 55 mL/100 g/min. Cortical CBF (gray matter) is approximately 75 to 80 mL/100 g/min and subcortical CBF (mostly white matter) is approximately 20 mL/100 g/min. Factors that regulate CBF include Pa_{CO_2}, Pa_{O_2}, CMR, cerebral perfusion pressure, autoregulation, and the autonomic nervous system (*Hines: Stoelting's Anesthesia and Co-Existing Disease, ed 5, p 200; Miller: Anesthesia, ed 6, pp 813-814*).

737. (D) Cerebral blood flow (CBF) autoregulation is the intrinsic capability of the cerebral vasculature to adjust its resistance to maintain CBF constant over a wide range of mean arterial blood pressures. In normal subjects, the lower limit of CBF autoregulation corresponds to a mean arterial pressure of approximately 50 to 60 mm Hg and the upper limit is a mean arterial pressure of 150 to 160 mm Hg. At mean arterial blood pressures above or below the limits of CBF autoregulation, CBF is pressure dependent. Although the precise mechanism of CBF autoregulation is not known, it is thought to result from an intrinsic characteristic of cerebral vascular smooth muscle that has not yet been identified (*Hines: Stoelting's Anesthesia and Co-Existing Disease, ed 5, p 201*).

738. (B) Cerebral blood flow (CBF) will increase by approximately 1 mL/100 g/min for every 1 mm Hg increase in Pa_{CO_2}, (i.e., approximately 2%). This effect is caused by a CO_2-mediated decrease in the pH of the extracellular fluid surrounding the cerebral vessels, which causes cerebral vasodilatation. The pH changes rapidly because CO_2 diffuses freely across the cerebral vascular endothelium into the extracellular fluid. However, the change in pH wanes after 6 to 10 hours because extracellular fluid pH is gradually normalized by reabsorption of HCO_3^- and excretion of H by the kidneys. An increase in Pa_{CO_2} of 10 mm Hg (from 35 to 45 mm Hg) will result in an increase in CBF of approximately 10 mL/100 g/min (*Hines: Stoelting's Anesthesia and Co-Existing Disease, ed 5, p 200*).

739. (C) Autonomic hyperreflexia is a neurologic disorder that occurs in association with resolution of spinal shock and a return of spinal cord reflexes. Cutaneous or visceral stimulation (such as distention of the urinary bladder or rectum) below the level of the spinal cord transection initiates afferent impulses that are transmitted to the spinal cord at this level, which subsequently elicits reflex sympathetic activity over the splanchnic nerves. Because modulation of this reflex sympathetic activity from higher centers in the central nervous system is lost (as a result of the spinal cord transection), the reflex sympathetic activity below the level of the injury results in intense generalized vasoconstriction and hypertension. Bradycardia occurs secondary to activation of baroreceptor reflexes. The incidence of autonomic hyperreflexia during general anesthesia depends on the level of the spinal cord transection. Approximately 85% of patients with a spinal cord transection above the T6 dermatome will exhibit this reflex during general anesthesia. In contrast, it is difficult to elicit this reflex in patients with a spinal cord transection below the T10 dermatome. Treatment of autonomic hyperreflexia is with ganglionic blocking drugs (e.g., trimethaphan), α-adrenergic receptor antagonists (e.g., phentolamine), direct-acting vasodilators, (e.g., nitroprusside or nitroglycerin), and deep general or regional anesthesia. Patients with autonomic hyperreflexia should not be treated initially with propranolol or other β-adrenergic receptor antagonists for two reasons. First, bradycardia can be potentiated by $β_1$-adrenergic receptor blockade; second, $β_2$-adrenergic receptor blockade in skeletal muscle will leave the α-adrenergic properties of circulating catecholamines unopposed, causing a paradoxical hypertensive response and possible congestive heart failure (*Barash: Clinical Anesthesia, ed 4, pp 1109-1110; Miller: Anesthesia, ed 5, pp 568-569*).

740. (C) The brain is an obligate aerobe, as it cannot store oxygen. Under normal circumstances, there is a substantial safety margin in that the delivery of oxygen is considerably greater than demand. Oxygen consumption is in the range of 3 to 5 mL/100 g of brain tissue/min, whereas the delivery of oxygen is approximately 50 mL blood/100 g brain tissue/min. Whole-brain oxygen consumption represents about 20% of total-body oxygen utilization (*Miller: Anesthesia, ed 6, pp 813-814*).

741. (B) Somatosensory evoked potentials (SSEPs) are composed of negative and positive voltage deflections with specific latencies and amplitudes. Baseline values for latency and amplitude must be determined for each patient at the onset of surgery because the characteristics of SSEP waveforms change with recording circumstances (for example, the latency becomes greater and the amplitude becomes smaller as the distance between the neural generator and the recording electrode is increased). Additionally, anesthetic medications can significantly alter the SSEP recording. A decrease in the amplitude or an increase in the latency in the SSEP waveform from baseline values may suggest ischemia along the sensory pathway in question (*Miller: Anesthesia, ed 6, pp 1532-1537*).

742. (C) The cerebral metabolic rate for oxygen ($CMRO_2$) decreases approximately 6% per 1° C of temperature reduction. Hypothermia has been reported to improve neurologic outcome after focal or global brain ischemia. Historically, the extent of brain protection was thought to be proportional to the magnitude of hypothermia-mediated reduction in $CMRO_2$. However, more recent studies have demonstrated that temperature reductions of a mere 1° C to 2° C significantly improve postischemic neurologic outcome. Proposed mechanisms for temperature modulation of postischemic neurologic outcome include alterations in $CMRO_2$, blood-brain barrier stability, membrane depolarization, ion homeostasis (e.g., calcium fluxes), neurotransmitter release (e.g., glutamate or aspartate), enzyme function (e.g., phospholipase, xanthine oxidase, or nitric oxide synthase), and free radical production or scavenging (*Miller: Anesthesia, ed 5, p 697; Faust: Anesthesiology Review, ed 3, pp 376-378*).

743. (D) Brain death is defined as irreversible cessation of brain function. It is extremely important to identify and reverse any factors that can mimic the clinical or laboratory criteria for brain death, such as hypothermia, drug intoxication (hypnotic sedatives and major tranquilizers), or metabolic encephalopathy. Clinical criteria for brain death can be divided into those that are related to cortical function and those that are related to brain stem function. Absence of cortical function is manifested by lack of spontaneous motor activity, consciousness, and purposeful movement in response to painful stimuli. Absence of brain-stem function is manifested by the inability to elicit reflexes, such as the pupillary response to light and the corneal, oculocephalic, oculovestibular, oropharyngeal, and respiratory reflexes. For example, in patients without brain-stem function there is no increase in heart rate when atropine is administered intravenously, and there is no respiratory effort during apnea even when the $Paco_2$ is greater than 60 mm Hg. Decerebrate and decorticate posturing are not consistent with the diagnosis of brain death (*Miller: Anesthesia, ed 6, pp 2955-2972*).

CRITERIA FOR DETERMINATION OF BRAIN DEATH

1. Absent cerebral and brain stem function
2. Well-defined irreversible etiology
3. Persistent absence of all brain function after observation or treatment
4. Hypothermia, drug intoxication, metabolic encephalopathy, and shock excluded

(*Darby JM, Stein K, Grenvik A, et al: Approach to management of the heart beating "brain dead" organ donor. JAMA 261:2222, 1989. Copyrighted 1989, American Medical Association.*)

CLINICAL TESTS OF BRAIN DEATH

Cerebral unresponsiveness

No spontaneous motor activity

Absent pupillary, corneal, and oculocephalic/oculovestibular reflexes

Absent cough reflex with deep tracheal suctioning

No increase in heart rate in response to intravenous administration of atropine (2 mg)

No respiratory efforts on apnea testing ($Paco_2$ >60 mm Hg)

Electrocerebral silence documented by electroencephalography (desirable)

(*Darby JM, Stein K, Grenvik A, et al: Approach to management of the heart beating "brain dead" organ donor. JAMA 261:2222, 1989. Copyrighted 1989, American Medical Association.*)

744. (C) The most common complications associated with the surgical sitting position include venous air embolism (VAE), paradoxical VAE, cardiovascular instability, pneumocephalus, subdural hematoma, peripheral neuropathy, and quadriplegia (quadriplegia is possibly caused by compression ischemia of the cervical spinal cord in patients with aberrant spinal cord blood supply). Venous air embolism (VAE) occurs when air is entrained into open veins in the presence of negative intraluminal pressures (i.e., negative with respect to atmospheric pressure). Significant VAE can result in reduced cardiac output and profound hypoxia. Current devices used to detect VAE include the transesophageal echocardiograph, Doppler ultrasound, pulmonary artery catheter, mass spectrometer (to monitor changes in $Peco_2$ and Pen_2), right atrial catheter, and esophageal stethoscope (to listen for a "mill wheel" cardiac murmur). The most sensitive means of diagnosing VAE include transesophageal echocardiography or precordial Doppler monitoring (see explanation to question 748) (*Barash: Clinical Anesthesia, ed 5 pp 773-774; Cottrell: Anesthesia and Neurosurgery, ed 4, pp 342-347; Faust: Anesthesiology Review, ed 3, pp 389-391; Miller: Anesthesia, ed 6, pp 1532-1537*).

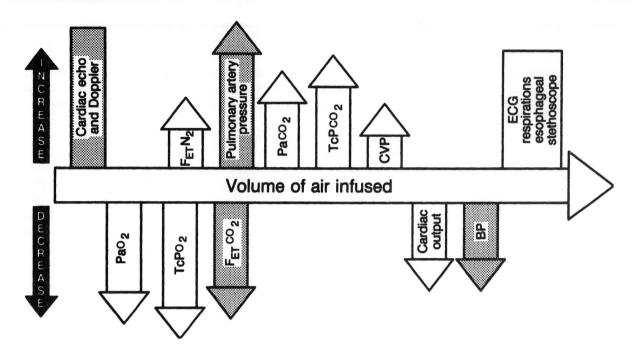

745. **(C)** Intracranial pressure is determined by the pressure contribution of three volume compartments: brain paren-chyma 80%-90%, CSF 5% to 10%, blood 5% to 10%. Under normal circumstances, ICP is maintained within the normal range (i.e., ≤ 15 mm Hg) over a wide range of intracranial volumes (ICV) due to the following three compensatory mechanisms: (1) translocation of CSF from the intracranial to spinal subarachnoid space; (2) translocation of intracranial blood (primarily venous) to systemic circulation; and (3) reabsorption of CSF across arachnoid villi into the dural venous sinus, and ultimately, into systemic circulation.

Once these compensatory mechanisms are exhausted, small increases in ICV result in large increases in ICP (i.e., a situation of increased intracranial elastance) which leaves the brain vulnerable to ischemia and hernia-tion. Cerebrospinal fluid (CSF) production is fairly constant (0.35 to 0.40 mL/min) regardless of ICP (*Faust: Anesthesiology Review, ed 3, pp 376-378; Hines: Stoelting's Anesthesia and Co-Existing Disease, ed 5, pp 202-203; Miller: Anesthesia, ed 6, pp 2127-2130*).

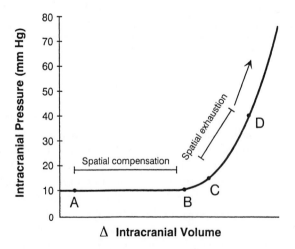

746. **(B)** Many of the commonly used anesthetic agents can alter the characteristics of evoked potential waveforms. In general, volatile anesthetics cause a dose-dependent increase in the latency and decrease in the amplitude of SSEPs. Brain stem auditory evoked potentials (BAEPs) are the most resistant to the depressant effects of volatile anesthetics, whereas VEPs are the most sensitive. In general, up to 1 MAC of isoflurane, enflurane, or halothane is compatible with adequate SSEP monitoring (*Miller: Anesthesia, ed 6, pp 1527-1532*).

747. (E) The MRI scanner is potentially dangerous for several reasons. The most obvious is the risk of projectiles traveling toward the patient. Objects made of iron, nickel, and cobalt are strongly pulled by the constant magnetic force (up to 3 tesla). A more insidious, but equally dangerous hazard is represented by indwelling devices, such as pacemakers, pumps, aneurysm clips and orthopedic prostheses. The interactions between these and the magnetic field can be harmful or even lethal for the patient under some circumstances. Lastly, the antenna effect of the MRI scanner can induce heat in wires that are in close proximity to the patient. For this reason pulmonary artery (PA) catheters and urinary catheters with temperature wires embedded in them cannot be used in patients undergoing MRI scanning. Standard pulse oximeters and ECG wires are also unacceptable, but special MRI compatible probes with fiberoptic "cables" can be safely used as can "wireless" ECG patches. Arterial lines do not pose a problem in the scanner because no wires come into contact with patient. The fluid-filled tubing is not ferromagnetic and the transducer is fixed, away from the patient (*Stoelting: Basics of Anesthesia, ed 5, pp 553-554; Miller: Anesthesia, ed 6, p 2646*).

748. (A) Except for the transesophageal echocardiograph (TEE), the Doppler ultrasound is the most sensitive device for detection of intracardiac air. Under ideal circumstances, as little as 0.25 mL of intra cardiac air can be detected by this device. In contrast, TEE can detect even smaller volumes of intracardiac air (*Barash: Clinical Anesthesia, ed 5, p 773*).

749. (B) Arterial carbon dioxide tension ($Paco_2$) is one of the most important extracerebral biochemical factors regulating CBF. The cerebral vasculature is most sensitive to changes in $Paco_2$ within the physiologic range (i.e., approximately 20 to 80 mm Hg). In general, the regional sensitivity of the cerebral vasculature to changes in $Paco_2$ (i.e., CO_2 responsiveness) is directly proportional to the resting CMR for each region of the brain. Regional CO_2 responsiveness is greatest in the cerebrum, less in the cerebellum, and least in the spinal cord (*Cottrell: Anesthesia and Neurosurgery, ed 4, pp 54-55; Faust: Anesthesiology Review, ed 3, pp 376-378*).

750. (A) Both laboratory and clinical studies have reported that hyperglycemia at the time of either focal (e.g., stroke) or global (e.g., systemic shock or cardiac arrest) ischemia results in a worsening of neurologic outcome (i.e., both histologic and functional). Unfortunately, it is not widely appreciated that the administration of glucose does not need to produce high blood glucose levels to augment postischemic cerebral injury. Thus, glucose-containing solutions should not be administered to patients who are at risk for either cerebral or spinal cord injury (*Cottrell: Anesthesia and Neurosurgery, ed 4, pp 243-244*).

751. (D) The tip of multiorificed right atrial catheters must be accurately placed at the junction of the superior vena cava and right atrium, because air has a tendency to localize at this junction. There are several methods that can be used to ensure that the catheter tip is accurately positioned at this junction. For example, a chest x-ray film can be obtained. However, there may be difficulty in interpreting the position of the tip of the catheter, and the catheter could migrate after the x-ray film is obtained. Cardiovascular pressures could be monitored, but this technique requires that the tip of the catheter first be introduced into the right ventricle and then pulled back into the right atrium. Introduction of the tip of the catheter into the right ventricle could cause dysrhythmias, heart block, or bleeding or rupture of cardiac structures. A technique frequently used to accurately place multiorificed catheters at the junction of the superior vena cava and right atrium is intravascular ECG. The appropriate position of the catheter is confirmed when a large negative P complex is obtained on the ECG. The P complex shown in the figure of this question is biphasic, which indicates that the tip of the catheter is in the midatrial position and should be withdrawn slightly until there is a large negative downward configuration of the P complex. Lastly, transesophageal echocardiography can be used to confirm catheter tip placement (*Miller: Anesthesia, ed 6, p 2141*).

752. (B) Critical CBF is the CBF below which EEG evidence of cerebral ischemia begins to appear. Critical CBF in patients anesthetized with isoflurane, desflurane, or sevoflurane is approximately 10 mL/100 g/min. In contrast, critical CBF in patients anesthetized with halothane is 18 to 20 mL/100 g/min, and critical CBF in patients anesthetized with enflurane is about 15 mL/100 g/min. Based on studies that compared the requirement for shunt placement after carotid artery cross-clamping in patients under isoflurane, enflurane, and halothane anesthesia, it appears that isoflurane might provide some degree of cerebral protection against incomplete regional cerebral ischemia in humans, however, anesthesia-modulated brain protection remains speculative, as outcome-based evidence is lacking in humans (*Faust: Anesthesiology Review, ed 3, p 100*).

753.   **(A)**   It is important to note that CBF autoregulation is easily impaired and modified by numerous factors, such as cerebral vasodilators (including volatile anesthetics), chronic hypertension, and cerebral ischemia. Cerebral ischemia abolishes CBF autoregulation such that CBF becomes passively dependent on the cerebral perfusion pressure (*Hines: Stoelting's Anesthesia and Co-Existing Disease, ed 5, p 201*).

754.   **(C)**   Changes in plasma $Paco_2$ will affect cerebral vascular tone. Hypocarbia (associated with hyperventilation) will rapidly cause vasoconstriction, thereby reducing CBF, CBV, and ICP. Thus, hyperventilation is the technique that will be most rapidly available to decrease ICP in patients with an intracranial mass (*Cottrell: Anesthesia and Neurosurgery, ed 4, pp 300-301; Hines: Stoelting's Anesthesia and Co-Existing Disease, ed 5, pp 203-204*).

755.   **(E)**   In general, the cerebrovascular response to changes in $Paco_2$ is preserved after the administration of intravenous anesthetics. Specifically, in humans, CO_2 reactivity is maintained with barbiturate concentrations sufficient to produce burst suppression on the EEG (*Cottrell: Anesthesia and Neurosurgery, ed 4, pp 138-139; Morgan: Clinical Anesthesiology, ed 4, p 622*).

756.   **(D)**   There are a number of practical reasons for using the sitting position. These include better surgical exposure; less tissue retraction and bleeding; a lower incidence of cranial nerve damage; ready access to the patient's airway, chest, and extremities; and more complete resection of the lesion. Although there are minimal objective data, there are, nonetheless, some conditions considered relative contraindications to the sitting position. These include an open ventriculoatrial shunt, presence of right-to-left intracardiac shunts (because of the potential for paradoxical VAE), presence of platypnea-orthodeoxia (i.e., patients who are well oxygenated in the supine position but become hypoxic when they assume the upright position; these patients have hemodynamic-dependent right-to-left intracardiac shunts), and the tendency to develop cerebral ischemia when the patient assumes the upright position. In contrast to the situation with ventriculoatrial shunts, air cannot be entrained via a ventriculoperitoneal shunt directly into the circulation. Ventriculoperitoneal shunt is not a relative contraindication to surgery in the sitting position (*Barash: Clinical Anesthesia, ed 5, pp 772-773*).

757.   **(C)**   The general approach to treating patients following VAE is to: (1) stop further air entrainment; (2) aspirate entrained air; (3) prevent expansion of existing air; and (4) support cardiovascular function. Cessation of subsequent air entrainment is achieved by flooding the surgical field with irrigation fluid. Additionally, noncollapsible veins can be sealed using electrocautery, vessel ligation, or bone wax. Neck veins can be compressed as a means of increasing jugular venous pressure, which mitigates or prevents further air entry and helps localize the source of air. A multiorificed right atrial catheter, placed before the event, is the most effective means of aspirating VAE. In order to prevent expansion of the VAE, nitrous oxide is immediately discontinued. Cardiovascular function is supported using inotropes, vasopressors, and intravenous fluids as indicated. Of the response options provided, PEEP is the least correct answer. Approximately 20% to 30% of humans have a probe patent foramen ovale. Initiation of PEEP may increase the risk of paradoxical embolism or decrease venous effluent from the calvarium, resulting in increased CBV and ICP (*Miller: Anesthesia, ed 6, 2138-2142*).

758.   **(D)**   The risk of venous air entrainment exists whenever the operative field is above the level of the right atrium. Air enters the venous circulation and travels to the right atrium where it continues into the right ventricle and passes into the lungs or passes right to left through a patent foramen ovale. Passage through the patent foramen may lead to stroke or, if air finds its way into coronary arteries, cardiac arrest. Air in the pulmonary artery can increase pulmonary vascular resistance (PVR) and cause right heart strain and dysrhythmias. Reflex bronchoconstriction may be caused by microvascular bubbles and by the release of inflammatory mediators from endothelial cells resulting in hypoxemia. Venous air embolism causes hypotension, not hypertension and death is usually from cardiovascular collapse (*Stoelting: Basics of Anesthesia, ed 5, p 459*).

759.   **(B)**   Surgical treatment of carotid artery stenosis greatly decreases the risk of stroke, especially in men with a stenosis diameter greater than 70%. Studies show a high rate of stroke in patients with asymptomatic carotid stenosis greater than 75%, and 80% of carotid atherothrombotic strokes occur without warning. The Asymptomatic Carotid Atherosclerosis Study, the largest completed clinical trial, demonstrated that patients with asymptomatic carotid stenosis ($\geq$ 60%) who were treated with carotid endarterectomy and aspirin have a reduced 5-year risk of ipsilateral stroke compared with patients treated with aspirin alone (5.1% versus 11.0%). Doppler studies also show that 70% to 75% stenosis represents the point at which a pressure drop across the stenosis is likely to occur. Thus, if collateral circulation is not adequate, low-flow transient ischemic attacks and infarcts occur. It would be considered most appropriate to further study the patient's carotid artery disease before proceeding with an elective case.

Although ischemic heart disease is a major cause of morbidity and mortality following carotid endarterectomy, dobutamine stress echocardiography or coronary angiogram studies are not routinely obtained. Exceptions to this practice include the following: patients with unstable angina, recent myocardial infarction, with evidence of ongoing ischemia, decompensated congestive heart failure, and significant valvular disease (*Hines: Stoelting's Anesthesia and Co-Existing Disease, ed 5, pp 152-155; Miller: Anesthesia, ed 6, pp 2099-2100*).

760. (B)   In patients who have suffered a cerebral vascular accident as a result of occlusive vascular disease, there is a loss of normal vasomotor responses to changes in $Paco_2$ and arterial blood pressure in the areas of ischemia (i.e., vasomotor paralysis) as well as disruption of the blood-brain barrier. Approximately 4 to 6 weeks is required for these changes to stabilize. Therefore, it is recommended that anesthesia for elective non-neurologic surgical procedures be postponed for at least 4 weeks and preferably 6 weeks after an occlusive vascular accident to minimize the risk of a subsequent perioperative occlusive vascular accident (*Miller: Anesthesia, ed 6, p 842*).

761. (A)   Somatosensory evoked potentials (SSEPs) recorded on the contralateral cerebral cortex are the physiologic response of the nervous system to peripheral nerve stimulation. Extraction of SSEPs from the background EEG is accomplished by computerized signal averaging for summation. Somatosensory evoked potentials (SSEPs) assess the integrity of the peripheral nerve (usually posterior tibial or median), dorsal column, brain stem, medial lemniscus, internal capsule, and contralateral somatosensory cortex. However, they do not evaluate the integrity of the ventral or lateral spinothalamic tracts or the corticospinal tract. The corticospinal tract is readily eliminated from the answer set because it is a motor (rather than sensory) pathway (*Miller: Anesthesia, ed 6, p 842*).

762. (B)   The differential diagnosis for a nonmoving patient during a wake-up test includes presence of neuromuscular blockade, inadequate volatile or nitrous oxide washout, or presence of opiates or sedative hypnotic-type drugs. There are also a few other extremely rare central causes, such as stroke. Because gross neuromuscular blockade has worn off in this patient and the volatile anesthetic and nitrous oxide have largely been washed out, a trial of naloxone would not be unreasonable. An initial small dose (e.g., 20 μg) may be all that is needed to reverse the effects of the morphine. If this dose is not effective, it should be repeated. Reducing distraction on the Harrington rods would only be considered if the patient squeezed her hands, yet failed to move her feet (*Cottrell: Anesthesia and Neurosurgery, ed 4, p 581; Wedel: Orthopedic Anesthesia, p 187*).

763. (D)   Arterial CO_2 tension ($Paco_2$) is the single most potent physiologic determinant of CBF and CBV. Between $Paco_2$ values of 20 and 80 mm Hg, CBF decreases 1 to 1.5 mL $\times$ 100 g brain weight^{-1} $\times$ min^{-1} and CBV decreases approximately 0.05 mL $\times$ 100 g brain weight^{-1} for each 1 mm Hg decrease in $Paco_2$. Decreasing the $Paco_2$ to 25 to 30 mm Hg should provide near-maximal reductions in CBF, CBV, and ICP, lasting up to 24 hours, without adversely affecting acid-base/electrolyte (e.g., decreases in potassium or ionized calcium) status or decreasing cerebral oxygen delivery (i.e., as a result of intense cerebral vasoconstriction and a leftward shift of the oxyhemoglobin dissociation curve). Because this patient's $Paco_2$ is 10 mm Hg below normal, CBF also would be reduced to approximately 35 to 40 mL $\times$ 100 g brain weight^{-1} $\times$ min^{-1} (*Cottrell: Anesthesia and Neurosurgery, ed 4, pp 300-301; Faust: Anesthesiology Review, ed 3, pp 376-378; Hines: Stoelting's Anesthesia and Co-Existing Disease, ed 5, pp 203-204*).

764. (A)   Intracranial pressure (ICP) is determined by the relationship between the intracranial vault (formed by the skull), volume of brain parenchyma, volume of CSF, and CBV. Studies evaluating the effectiveness of corticosteroids in the setting of head injury, or global or focal brain ischemia, have demonstrated either no improvement or a worsening of neurologic outcome. All intravenous anesthetics, except ketamine, cause some degree of reduction in CMR, CBF, CBV, and ICP (provided ventilation is not depressed). Of intravenous anesthetics, barbiturates are thought to be the "gold standard" for anesthetic-mediated brain protective therapy during focal or incomplete global brain ischemia. However, this has yet to be proven in humans. The impact of hyperventilation on ICP is discussed in the explanation to question 763. In the setting of traumatic brain injury, hyperventilation is an acceptable intervention. However, the Brain Trauma Foundation advises against aggressive hyperventilation, because the data suggest worsening of outcome associated with $Paco_2$ values below 35 mm Hg. Both osmotic and loop diuretics are effective in reducing ICP. Elevation of the head above the level of the heart facilitates effluent of blood from the calvarium, which results in decreases in CBV and ICP (*Barash: Clinical Anesthesia, ed 5, pp 782-786; Cottrell: Anesthesia and Neurosurgery, ed 4, pp 676-682*).

765. (A)   After SAH, patients may experience rebleeding, cerebral vasospasm, intracranial hypertension, and seizures. Provided the patient is not experiencing cerebral vasospasm, hypertension should be avoided in order to minimize aneurismal wall tension, thereby mitigating the risk of re-rupture. In contrast, had this patient been in vasospasm, induced hypertension would have been an appropriate therapeutic intervention (also see explanation to question 776). Hypertension is avoided, in part, by the administration of sedative and analgesic medications. Antiepileptic drugs and calcium channel blockers (e.g., nimodipine) often are administered in an attempt to prevent or mitigate seizures and the sequelae of cerebral vasospasm, respectively (*Hines: Stoelting's Anesthesia and Co-Existing Disease, ed 5, pp 217-220*).

766. (E)   Somatosensory evoked potentials (SSEPs) are used to monitor the integrity of sensory pathways in the nervous system during neurosurgical or orthopedic surgery (also see explanation to question 761). Volatile anesthetics (e.g., isoflurane) and barbiturates (e.g., sodium thiopental) decrease the amplitude and increase the latency of SSEP waveforms. Nitrous oxide decreases the amplitude but has no effect on latency. Etomidate increases both the amplitude and latency. In contrast, nondepolarizing muscle relaxants (e.g., vecuronium) have no effect on sensory pathways of the nervous system and, thus, can be used during SSEP monitoring (*Barash: Clinical Anesthesia, ed 5, pp 760-762; Miller: Anesthesia, ed 6, pp 1527-1529*).

767. (B)   In addition to ECG changes (e.g., T-wave inversion, depression of the ST segment, appearance of U waves, prolonged QT interval, and, rarely, Q waves), abnormal thallium scintigraphy, regional wall-motion abnormalities, and elevated creatine kinase-MB isoenzymes have been reported in patients with SAH. Although historically considered a functionally insignificant neurogenic phenomena, there is increasing evidence that these changes may be a sign of underlying myocardial ischemia. However, even if myocardial ischemia is present, it seems to have a minimal impact on patient outcome (i.e., morbidity and mortality). Because electrolyte abnormalities (e.g., hypokalemia or hypocalcemia) may contribute to the etiology of the ECG changes, it would probably be most appropriate to quantify these electrolytes before initiating other therapies or canceling emergency surgery. Nitroglycerine is a potent cerebral vasodilator that could have a deleterious effect on ICP in patients with increased intracranial elastance (see explanation to question 745) (*Barash: Clinical Anesthesia, ed 5, p 779; Cottrell: Anesthesia and Neurosurgery, ed 4, pp 370-371; Hines: Stoelting's Anesthesia and Co-Existing Disease, ed 5, pp 217-220*).

768. (E)   Limitations in SSEP monitoring have prompted interest in monitoring the motor system. Specifically, MEPs are used to monitor the integrity of motor pathways in the nervous system during neurosurgical, orthopedic, or major vascular (e.g., procedures that involve cross-clamping of the thoracic aorta) surgery. Electrical or magnetic stimulation of the motor cortex produces an evoked potential that is propagated via descending motor pathways and can be recorded from the spinal epidural space, spinal cord, peripheral nerve, or the muscle itself. In general, inhalational and intravenous anesthetics decrease the amplitude and increase the latency of the MEP response. Fentanyl is an exception to this rule and has little, if any, effect on MEP monitoring (*Cottrell: Anesthesia and Neurosurgery, ed 4, pp 195-197; Miller: Anesthesia, ed 6, pp 1533, 1539-1540*).

769. (D)   Ketamine is thought to increase CBF and, consequently, CBV and ICP by two mechanisms: (1) there may be a direct effect on cerebral vascular smooth muscle to cause vasodilation, and (2) there may be a "coupled" effect caused by an increase in CMR. There is some controversy regarding the effect of ketamine on CBF/CMR coupling. Animal studies in vivo indicate that CMR and CBF are increased proportionally in structures of the limbic system. In contrast, there is evidence from one human study that although ketamine increased CBF (up to 62%), CMR remained unchanged. Cerebral CO_2 responsiveness and autoregulation are not altered by ketamine (*Cottrell: Anesthesia and Neurosurgery, ed 4, pp 135-136*).

770. (A)   In contrast to ketamine and increased neural activity (e.g., seizures or hyperthermia), which increase CBF and CMR, volatile anesthetics cause a simultaneous, dose-dependent increase in CBF and decrease in CMR (i.e., volatile anesthetics "uncouple" global CBF and CMR) (*Miller: Anesthesia, ed 6, p 821*).

771. (C)   Maintenance of a relatively constant CBF despite changes in systemic mean arterial blood pressure is termed autoregulation. The upper and lower limits of autoregulation, in normotensive adult humans, are cerebral perfusion pressures of 150 and 50 mm Hg, respectively. Autoregulation appears to be impaired by intracranial tumors, and head trauma and volatile anesthetics. In contrast, nitrous oxide, barbiturates, and fentanyl do not appear to disturb autoregulation (*Hines: Stoelting's Anesthesia and Co-Existing Disease, ed 5, pp 201-202*).

772. (A)   Acute spinal cord injury above T4-T6 produces a sympathectomy below the level of injury, which decreases systemic arteriolar and venous vasomotor tone, and abolishes vasopressor reflexes (i.e., spinal shock). This pathophysiologic process may continue for up to 6 weeks after injury. As spinal shock resolves, patients with spinal cord injuries cephalad to T4-T6 may develop autonomic hyperreflexia (i.e., acute generalized sympathetic hyperactivity as a result of stimulation below the level of injury). Neurogenic pulmonary edema may develop during either spinal shock or autonomic hyperreflexia. Thermoregulation is lost, resulting in poikilothermia, because the hypothalamic thermoregulatory center is unable to communicate with the peripheral sympathetic pathways. In the cool environment of the intensive care unit, spinal cord injury patients are unable to vasoconstrict below the level of injury and, thus, may experience hypothermia. Loss of sympathetic-mediated vasomotor tone also results in hypotension (*Hines: Stoelting's Anesthesia and Co-Existing Disease, ed 5, pp 239-240*).

773. (E) Signs and symptoms of intracranial hypertension include nausea and vomiting, systemic hypertension, bradycardia, altered level of consciousness, irregular breathing pattern, papilledema, seizure activity, personality changes, and coma (*Hines: Stoelting's Anesthesia and Co-Existing Disease, ed 5, pp 202-203*).

774. (D) General anesthesia can be induced safely in patients with carotid artery disease using intravenous anesthetics, such as thiopental, midazolam, propofol, or etomidate. Isoflurane, in conjunction with N_2O or opioids, is a good choice for maintenance of anesthesia in these patients, because critical CBF is reduced during isoflurane, sevoflurane, or desflurane anesthesia, which may provide some cerebral protection (also see explanation to question 752). Arterial blood pressure and $Paco_2$ should be maintained in the normal ranges for each patient because the vasculature within ischemic regions of the brain have lost the ability to autoregulate CBF and respond to changes in $Paco_2$. Marked reductions in arterial blood pressure may reduce CBF (especially via collateral channels) to ischemic brain tissue. Theoretically, if $Paco_2$ is increased from normal, cerebral blood vessels surrounding the region of ischemia that retain normal CO_2 responsiveness will dilate, diverting regional cerebral blood flow away from the ischemic brain tissue (i.e., steal phenomenon). Conversely, if the $Paco_2$ is reduced from normal, the cerebral blood vessels surrounding the ischemic brain tissue will constrict, diverting rCBF to ischemic areas of the brain (inverse steal phenomenon or Robin Hood effect). Hyperventilating the lungs in an attempt to produce the inverse steal phenomenon is not recommended because the actual effect may be unpredictable and supportive evidence in humans that this is beneficial is lacking. The carotid sinus (not carotid body) baroreceptor reflex can be blunted by intravenous injection of atropine or by local infiltration of the area of the carotid sinus with a local anesthetic (*Cottrell: Anesthesia and Neurosurgery, ed 4, pp 460-461, 464-465*).

775. (C) In general, all volatile anesthetics (e.g., isoflurane, sevoflurane, and desflurane) are potent direct cerebral vasodilators that produce dose-dependent increases in CBF, CBV and ultimately ICP when concentrations exceed 0.6 MAC. The order of vasodilator potency is approximately halothane >> enflurane > isoflurane = sevoflurane = desflurane. As discussed in the response to question 731, opioids have little, if any, effect on CMR, CBF, or ICP. The effect of N_2O on CBF, CBV, and ICP is controversial. In a number of animal and human studies, N_2O increased CBF by 35% to 103%. Conversely, in other animal studies, N_2O was consistently found to have only minimal effects on CBF. Differences between species may be one factor contributing to these conflicting results. Because N_2O appears to increase CBF and CBV in humans, it seems prudent to discontinue N_2O in patients in whom intracranial hypertension is not responsive to other therapeutic maneuvers propofol and barbiturates are potent cerebral vasoconstrictors and can decrease the ICP. (*Faust: Anesthesiology Review, ed 3, pp 376-378; Hines: Stoelting's Anesthesia and Co-Existing Disease, ed 5, pp 201-202*).

776. (C) After SAH, the incidence and severity of cerebral vasospasm have been reported to correlate with the amount and location of blood in the calvarium. Angiographic evidence of vasospasm has been noted in up to 70% of SAH patients. However, clinically significant vasospasm occurs in only 20% to 30% of SAH patients. The incidence peaks approximately 7 days after SAH. Calcium channel blockers (e.g., nimodipine) decrease the morbidity and mortality associated with vasospasm, but investigators have been unable to demonstrate any significant change in the incidence or severity of vasospasm. This suggests that the beneficial effects of nimodipine may be related to inhibition of primary and secondary ischemic cascades, rather than direct cerebral vasodilation. Treatment of vasospasm also includes "triple H therapy" (*H*ypervolemia, induced *H*ypertension, and *H*emodilution) and cerebral angioplasty. The rationale of induced hypervolemia and hypertension is that ischemic regions of brain have impaired autoregulation and, thus, CBF is perfusion pressure dependent. Hemodilution is thought to increase blood flow through the cerebral microcirculation (because of improved rheology and reactive hyperemia). One argument against hemodilution is that increases in CBF are offset by concomitant decreases in the oxygen-carrying capacity. Taken together, blood pressure reductions and diuretic use are incorrect responses to this condition (*Cottrell: Anesthesia and Neurosurgery, ed 4, pp 373-375*).

777. **(E)** Enlargement of the tongue and epiglottis predisposes the patient to upper airway obstruction and makes visualization of the vocal cords more difficult. The vocal cords are enlarged, making the glottic opening narrower. In addition, subglottic narrowing may be present as well as tracheal compression from an enlarged thyroid (seen in about 25% of acromegalic patients). This often necessitates the use of a narrower endotracheal tube than one might choose based on the facial enlargement. The placement of nasal airways may be more difficult due to the enlarged nasal turbinates. The use of CPAP is contraindicated after transsphenoidal hypophysectomy (*Barash: Clinical Anesthesia, ed 5, pp 776, 1149; Fleisher: Anesthesia and Uncommon Diseases, ed 5, pp 21-22; Hines: Stoelting's Anesthesia and Co-Existing Disease, ed 5, pp 402-403*).

778. **(D)** Chronic hypertension shifts the CBF autoregulatory curve to the right. The clinical significance of this observation is that CBF could decrease and cerebral ischemia could occur at a higher mean systemic arterial blood pressure in patients with chronic hypertension compared with normal patients. Chronic antihypertensive therapy to control systemic blood pressures within the normal range may restore normal CBF autoregulation (*Cottrell: Anesthesia and Neurosurgery, ed 4, p 32; Hines: Stoelting's Anesthesia and Co-Existing Disease, ed 5, p 201*).

779. **(D)** Cerebral autoregulation is disturbed in a number of diseases (e.g., acute cerebral ischemia, mass lesions, trauma, inflammation, prematurity, neonatal asphyxia, and diabetes mellitus). The final common pathway of dysfunction, in its most extreme form, is termed vasomotor paralysis. Hyperoxia has little or no effect on autoregulation. During normothermic and moderate hypothermic (i.e., approximately 27° C), cardiopulmonary bypass with, autoregulation is well preserved. Chronic hypertension causes a rightward shift of the autoregulation curve toward higher upper and lower cerebral perfusion pressure limits (also see explanation to question 778). Autoregulation is impaired by volatile anesthetics (e.g., isoflurane). At greater than 2 MAC, autoregulation is abolished (*Cottrell: Anesthesia and Neurosurgery, ed 4, pp 34-38; Faust: Anesthesiology Review, ed 3, p 57*).

780. **(A)** The cerebral pharmacologic profile of etomidate is similar to that of thiopental in that it produces a dose-related decrease in the CMR and CBF (via direct cerebral vasoconstriction and coupling to decreased CMR). As noted, after barbiturate administration, intravenous etomidate does not disturb cerebral autoregulation or CO_2 reactivity as discussed in the explanation to questions 766 and 783. Etomidate increases both amplitude and latency during SSEP monitoring (*Cottrell: Anesthesia and Neurosurgery, ed 4, p 135; Barash: Clinical Anesthesia, ed 5, pp 760-762 [Table 27-8]*).

781. **(B)** Nasal intubation should be avoided in patients with suspected basal skull (e.g., disruption of the cribriform plate of the ethmoid bone) fractures or sinus injuries. Because approximately 10% of head injury patients have associated cervical spine injuries, it is prudent to assume that all head injury patients have co-existing cervical spine injury until proven otherwise. Additionally, the patient described in this question may have abnormal airway anatomy because of extreme micrognathia, facial injuries, and obesity. Taken together, direct laryngoscopy with rapid sequence induction is probably not an acceptable technique for securing this patient's airway. In contrast, awake intubation by direct or fiberoptic laryngoscopy or performance of tracheostomy are considered appropriate techniques for tracheal intubation of this patient: Mask and laryngeal mask airway (LMA) techniques may provide a patent airway, but do not ensure protection of the airway against aspiration of gastric contents (*Barash: Clinical Anesthesia, ed 5, pp 1263-1266; Cottrell: Anesthesia and Neurosurgery, ed 4, pp 255-257*).

782. **(E)** This patient has mild hyponatremia and is unable to excrete a dilute urine as noted by the urine sodium greater than 20 mEq/L. These are consistent with the syndrome of inappropriate secretion of ADH (SIADH). Antidiuretic hormone (ADH) is also known as vasopressin. Inappropriate secretion of ADH (SIADH) may result from a variety of causes including CNS lesions, pulmonary infections, hypothyroidism and drugs (e.g., chlorpropamide, narcotics). After identifying the cause, treatment is started and usually consists mainly of water restriction. With severe hyponatremia, i.e., Na less than 120 mEq/L and signs of mental confusion, aggressive treatment with hypertonic sodium chloride may be needed, however, too much and too rapid infusion as in B may induce central pontine myelinolysis and may cause permanent brain damage. With severe hyponatremia, the dose of 200 to 300 mL of a 5% solution of sodium chloride is usually administered over several hours. The antibiotic demeclocycline interferes with ADH at the level of the renal tubules to produce dilute urine and is sometimes used for the treatment of SIADH. In the future, the experimental drug, Tolvaptan, (OPC-41061) may replace desmopressin. Tolvaptan is a vasopressin antagonist. Desmopressin acetate (DDAVP) is used to treat patients with complete diabetes insipidus (DI) whereas chlorpropamide is used to treat incomplete DI. Patients with DI have a lack of ADH and have high output of poorly concentrated urine and hypernatremia. Leaving the patient intubated and hyperventilating him or her will not help (*Barash: Clinical Anesthesia, ed 5,* *pp 779, 1149-1150; Fleischer: Anesthesia and Uncommon Diseases, ed 5, pp 430-432; Hines: Stoelting's Anesthesia and Co-Existing Disease, ed 5, pp 403-404; Miller: Anesthesia, ed 6, pp 1052-1053, 1105).*

783. (D) This patient has several signs consistent with elevated intracranial pressure: hypertension, hyperventilation and somnolence. Use of morphine premedication is ill-advised because it would sedate him further, blunt his hyperventilation and thus raise ICP. Furthermore, narcotics in this setting can lower blood pressure sufficiently to alter cerebral perfusion pressure. Use of PEEP can promote impairment of venous drainage as well as raise ICP in patients with intracranial hypertension. Hyperventilation is an effective maneuver for lowering ICP in the short term. $Paco_2$ levels in the 30 to 35 mm Hg range suffice for this and there is no evidence that additional hyperventilation has any added therapeutic benefit. Use of esmolol prior to intubation may blunt the hyperdynamic response to laryngoscopy and prevent ICP elevation (*Stoelting: Basics of Anesthesia, ed 5, p 458*).

784. (E) MRI scanners contain powerful magnets that range from 0.5 to 3 tesla (5000 to 30,000 gauss). By contrast, the Earth's magnetic field is 0.5 gauss. Metal objects brought into the scanner room can become dangerous projectiles that fly toward the middle of the magnet, where the patient is located. Small items can be pulled away but larger items may not be removable even with a winch and thus require a magnet shut-down, the process know as a quench.

MRI magnets are always on. Stopping the scan or cutting the power to magnet for 60 seconds does not release the magnetic force. Quenching is an expensive process that involves making the coil resistive and boiling away the helium (which is vented to the outside). Attempting to pull the object described in this question away from the magnet would be nearly impossible, but even if it could be successfully carried out there would be great risk. For example, if the grip were lost and the object released, it could fly toward the patient inside the scanner. Cutting up metallic objects attached to scanner (if a non-ferromagnetic saw could be found) would be equally if not more dangerous than attempting a pull away (*Stoelting: Basics of Anesthesia, ed 5, pp 553-554*).

785. (E) Progressive entrainment of air into the pulmonary microcirculation reduces lung perfusion and increases pulmonary vascular resistance and alveolar dead-space ventilation. The increase in pulmonary vascular resistance is reflected by increases in pulmonary arterial and central venous pressures. A large air embolus can result in right ventricular outflow obstruction, which will dramatically reduce cardiac output, resulting in systemic hypotension. Increased alveolar dead space results in a decrease in $Peco_2$. In severe VAE, CO_2 cannot be eliminated and $Paco_2$ increases. Pen_2 increases because air diffuses into the pulmonary alveoli. The sensitivity of continuous $Peco_2$ monitoring is similar to that for continuous Pen_2 monitoring (*Barash: Clinical Anesthesia, ed 5, pp 773-774; Cottrell: Anesthesia and Neurosurgery, ed 4, pp 342-347; Faust: Anesthesiology Review, ed 3, pp 389-391*).

786. (C) The cerebrovascular response to hyperventilation was reviewed in the explanations to questions 754, 763 and 764. Hyperventilation, and the resulting respiratory alkalosis, causes a leftward (not rightward) shifting of the oxyhemoglobin dissociation curve. In doing so, hemoglobin undergoes a conformation change, making it more reluctant to release oxygen at the tissue level. As discussed in the explanation to question 733, hyperventilation-induced respiratory alkalosis can precipitate hypokalemia. Specifically, serum potassium decreases 0.6 mEq/L for each 0.1 unit increase in pH. Thus, overly aggressive hyperventilation should be guarded against in order to avoid electrolyte perturbations that may result in cardiac arrhythmias (*Cottrell: Anesthesia and Neurosurgery, ed 4, pp 300-301; Hines: Stoelting: Anesthesia and Co-Existing Disease, ed 5, pp 203-204*).

787. (A) Venous air embolism is a hazard of any operation in which the operative field is located above the heart. Measures to successfully manage VAE include prevention of further air entrainment (Trendelenburg position, flooding surgical field with saline, placement of wax on cut bone edges), removal of air from the right atrium if a catheter is in place, and supporting hemodynamics with calcium, pressors and inotropes and discontinuation of N_2O to prevent bubble expansion. Some neuroanesthesiologists avoid use of N_2O in any instance where there is a chance of VAE (*Stoelting: Basics of Anesthesia, ed 5, p 459*).

Chapter 10

Anatomy, Regional Anesthesia, and Pain Management

DIRECTIONS (Questions 788–897): Each of the questions or incomplete statements in this section is followed by answers or by completions of the statement, respectively. Select the ONE BEST answer or completion for each item.

788. Tachyphylaxis to local anesthetics is most closely related to which of the following?
   A. Speed of injection
   B. Dosing interval
   C. Temperature of local anesthetic
   D. Volume of local anesthetic
   E. pH of solution

789. Which of the following techniques is **LEAST** effective in a treatment of pruritus from administration of neuraxial opiates?
   A. Nalbuphine 5 mg IV
   B. Dexmedetomidine 30 μg IV
   C. Diphenhydramine 50 mg IV
   D. Hydroxyzine 20 mg IM
   E. Propofol 10 mg IV

790. The maximum dose of lidocaine containing 1:200,000 epinephrine that can be administered to a 70-kg patient for regional anesthesia (other than spinal anesthesia) is
   A. 50 mg
   B. 100 mg
   C. 200 mg
   D. 500 mg
   E. 1000 mg

791. Which of the following concentrations of epinephrine corresponds to a 1:200,000 mixture?
   A. 0.5 μg/mL
   B. 5 μg/mL
   C. 50 μg/mL
   D. 0.5 mg/mL
   E. None of the above

792. An anesthesia pain service consult is sought for a 78-year-old patient with a complaint of pain in the distribution of the trigeminal nerve. The patient has no other medical problems except a history of congestive heart failure for which he takes digoxin and thiazide. In addition to his chief complaint, the patient over the last 72 hours has complained of dysesthesia in the feet, difficulty with vision, and emesis times three. The most appropriate step at this time would be
   A. Trigeminal nerve block with bupivacaine
   B. Obtain neurologic workup for multiple sclerosis
   C. Administration of fentanyl and ondansetron
   D. Initiate therapy with carbamazepine
   E. Obtain a digoxin level

793. Which of the following is the earliest sign of lidocaine toxicity?
    A. Shivering
    B. Nystagmus
    C. Lightheadedness and dizziness
    D. Tonic-clonic seizures
    E. Nausea and vomiting

794. An analgesic effect similar to the epidural administration of 10 mg of morphine could be achieved by which dose of intrathecal morphine?
    A. 0.1 mg
    B. 1 mg
    C. 5 mg
    D. 10 mg
    E. There is no correlation

795. Which local anesthetic undergoes the **LEAST** hepatic clearance
    A. Chloroprocaine
    B. Bupivacaine
    C. Etidocaine
    D. Prilocaine
    E. Lidocaine

796. Which of the following is the most important disadvantage of interscalene brachial plexus block compared with other approaches?
    A. Not suitable for operations on the shoulder
    B. Large volumes of local anesthetics required
    C. Frequent sparing of the ulnar nerve
    D. Frequent sparing of the musculocutaneous nerve
    E. High incidence of pneumothorax

797. A 68-year-old woman is to undergo foot surgery under spinal anesthesia. Which of the following statements concerning the immediate physiologic response to the surgical incision is true?
    A. The cardiovascular response to stress will be blocked, but the adrenergic response will not
    B. The adrenergic response to stress will be blocked, but the cardiovascular response will not
    C. Both the adrenergic and cardiovascular responses will be blocked
    D. Neither the adrenergic or cardiovascular response will be blocked
    E. The cardiovascular response will be blocked but the adrenergic response will be augmented

798. The "snap" felt just before entering the epidural space represents passage through which ligament?
    A. Anterior longitudinal ligaments
    B. Posterior longitudinal ligaments
    C. Ligamentum flavum
    D. Supraspinous ligament
    E. Interspinous ligament

799. The common element thought to be present in every case of cauda equina syndrome after continuous spinal anesthesia is
    A. Use of microcatheter
    B. Maldistribution of local anesthetic
    C. Administration of lidocaine
    D. Addition of epinephrine
    E. Hyperbaricity

800. A sciatic nerve block is performed in a healthy 26-year-old male patient for bunion surgery. Fifteen mL of 1.5% mepivacaine is slowly injected after the landmarks are identified and a paresthesia is elicited in the great toe. In what order would the following nerve fibers be blocked?
  A. Sympathetic, proprioception, pain, motor
  B. Sympathetic, pain, proprioception, motor
  C. Motor, pain, proprioception, sympathetic
  D. Pain, proprioception, sympathetic, motor
  E. Pain, proprioception, motor, sympathetic

801. A 95-year-old woman has persistent and prolonged thoracic pain after a herpes zoster infection. Which of the treatments below would be the **LEAST** efficacious in the treatment of her pain?
  A. Oral amitriptyline
  B. Oral clonidine
  C. Topical capsaicin ointment
  D. Transcutaneous electrical nerve stimulation (TENS)
  E. Topical lidocaine patch

802. The deep peroneal nerve innervates the
  A. Lateral aspect of the dorsum of the foot
  B. Entire dorsum of the foot
  C. Web space between the great toe and the second toe
  D. Web space between the third and fourth toes
  E. Medial aspect of the dorsum of the foot

803. The correct arrangement of local anesthetics in order of their ability to produce cardiotoxicity from most to least is
  A. Bupivacaine, lidocaine, ropivacaine
  B. Bupivacaine, ropivacaine, lidocaine
  C. Lidocaine, bupivacaine, ropivacaine
  D. Ropivacaine, bupivacaine, lidocaine
  E. Lidocaine, ropivacaine, bupivacaine

804. Allodynia is defined as
  A. Spontaneous pain in an area or region that is anesthetic
  B. Pain initiated or caused by a primary lesion or dysfunction in the nervous system
  C. An unpleasant abnormal sensation, whether spontaneous or evoked
  D. An increased response to a stimulus that is normally painful
  E. Pain caused by a stimulus that does not normally provoke pain

805. The primary mechanism by which the action of tetracaine is terminated when used for spinal anesthesia is
  A. Systemic absorption
  B. Uptake into neurons
  C. Hydrolysis by pseudocholinesterase
  D. Hydrolysis by nonspecific esterases
  E. Spontaneous degradation at 37° C

806. Complex regional pain syndrome type I (reflex sympathetic dystrophy) is differentiated from complex regional pain syndrome type II (causalgia) by knowledge of its
  A. Etiology
  B. Chronicity
  C. Affected body region
  D. Type of symptoms
  E. Rapidity of onset

807. The primary determinant of local anesthetic potency is
   A. pKa
   B. Molecular weight
   C. Lipid solubility
   D. Concentration
   E. Protein binding

808. Which of the following would have the greatest effect on the level of sensory blockade after a subarachnoid injection of hyperbaric 0.75% bupivacaine?
   A. Coughing during placement of the block
   B. Addition of epinephrine to the local anesthetic solution
   C. Barbotage
   D. Patient weight
   E. Patient position

809. Which of the following local anesthetics would produce the lowest concentration in the fetus relative to the maternal serum concentration during a continuous lumbar epidural?
   A. Etidocaine
   B. Bupivacaine
   C. Lidocaine
   D. Chloroprocaine
   E. Mepivacaine

810. Severe hypotension associated with high spinal anesthesia is caused primarily by
   A. Decreased cardiac output secondary to decreased preload
   B. Decreased systemic vascular resistance
   C. Decreased cardiac output secondary to bradycardia
   D. Decreased cardiac output secondary to decreased myocardial contractility
   E. Increased shunting through metarterioles

811. Select the one true statement concerning phantom limb pain.
   A. Most phantom limb pain becomes more severe with time
   B. Most amputees do not experience phantom limb pain
   C. Nerve blocks may be used to treat phantom limb pain
   D. Trauma amputees have a higher incidence of phantom limb pain than nontrauma amputees
   E. The incidence of phantom limb pain increases with more distal amputations

812. Which of the following local anesthetics used for intravenous regional anesthesia (Bier block) is most rapidly metabolized and thus, least toxic?
   A. Lidocaine
   B. Ropivacaine
   C. Mepivacaine
   D. Prilocaine
   E. Etidocaine

813. Select the **FALSE** statement regarding spinal anatomy and spinal anesthesia.
   A. The addition of phenylephrine to lidocaine will prolong spinal anesthesia
   B. A high thoracic sensory block will result in total sympathetic blockade
   C. The largest vertebral interspace is L5-S1
   D. The dural sac extends to the S4-S5 interspace
   E. Tetracaine provides longer anesthesia than does procaine

814. Four days after a left total hip arthroplasty, an obese 62-year-old woman complains of severe back pain in the region where the epidural was placed. Over the ensuing 72 hours, the back pain gradually worsens and a severe aching pain that radiates down the left leg to the knee develops. The most likely diagnosis is
   A. Epidural abscess
   B. Epidural hematoma
   C. Anterior spinal artery syndrome
   D. Arachnoiditis
   E. Meralgia paresthetica

815. Which of the following choices is **NOT** consistent with a limb affected by complex regional pain syndrome?
   A. Osteoporosis
   B. Allodynia
   C. Dermatomal distribution of pain
   D. Atrophy of the involved extremity
   E. Hyperesthesia

816. The main advantage of neurolytic nerve blockade with phenol versus alcohol is
   A. Denser blockade
   B. Blockade is permanent
   C. The effects of the block can be evaluated immediately
   D. The block is less painful
   E. Phenol is selective for sympathetic fibers

817. How much local anesthetic should be administered per spinal segment to patients between 20 and 40 years of age receiving a lumbar epidural anesthetic?
   A. 0.25 to 0.5 mL
   B. 0.5 to 1.0 mL
   C. 1 to 2 mL
   D. 2 to 3 mL
   E. 3 to 5 mL

818. The artery of Adamkiewicz most frequently arises from the aorta at which spinal level?
   A. T1-T4
   B. T5-T8
   C. T9-T12
   D. L1-L4
   E. L5-S3

819. The anterior and posterior spinal arteries originate from the
   A. Common carotid and vertebral arteries, respectively
   B. Internal carotid and vertebral arteries, respectively
   C. Internal carotid and posterior cerebral arteries, respectively
   D. Vertebral and anterior cerebellar arteries, respectively
   E. Vertebral, radicular arteries and the posterior inferior cerebellar arteries, respectively

820. Important landmarks for performing a sciatic nerve block (classic approach of Labat) include
   A. Iliac crest, sacral hiatus, greater trochanter
   B. Iliac crest, coccyx, and greater trochanter
   C. Posterior superior iliac spine, coccyx, and greater trochanter
   D. Posterior superior iliac spine, greater trochanter and sacral hiatus
   E. Posterior superior iliac spine and greater trochanter

821.   A 36-year-old female patient is undergoing thyroidectomy under a deep cervical plexus nerve block. Which of the following complications would be **LEAST** likely with this block?
   A. Horner's syndrome
   B. Subarachnoid injection
   C. Blockade of the recurrent laryngeal nerve
   D. Blockade of the spinal accessory nerve
   E. Vertebral artery injection

822.   A retrobulbar block anesthetizes each of the following nerves **EXCEPT**
   A. Ciliary nerves
   B. Cranial nerve IV (trochlear nerve)
   C. Cranial nerve III (oculomotor nerve)
   D. Cranial nerve VI (abducens nerve)
   E. Maxillary branch of the trigeminal nerve

823.   Which of the following muscles of the larynx is innervated by the external branch of the superior laryngeal nerve?
   A. Vocalis muscle
   B. Thyroarytenoid muscles
   C. Posterior cricoarytenoid muscle
   D. Oblique arytenoid muscles
   E. Cricothyroid muscle

824.   All the following agents are acceptable for use in a Bier block **EXCEPT**
   A. 0.5% Lidocaine
   B. 0.5% Mepivacaine
   C. 0.5% Procaine
   D. 0.5% Prilocaine
   E. 0.25% Bupivacaine

825.   The stellate ganglion lies in closest proximity to which of the following vascular structures?
   A. Common carotid artery
   B. Internal carotid artery
   C. Vertebral artery
   D. Axillary artery
   E. Aorta

826.   Which of the following structures in the antecubital fossa is the most medial?
   A. Brachial artery
   B. Radial nerve
   C. Tendon of the biceps
   D. Median nerve
   E. Musculocutaneous nerve

827.   During placement of an epidural in a 78-year-old patient scheduled for a total knee arthroplasty, the patient complains of a sharp sustained pain radiating down his left leg as the catheter is inserted to 2 cm. The most appropriate action at this time would be
   A. Leave the catheter at 2 cm, give test dose
   B. Give small dose to relieve pain then advance 1 cm
   C. Withdraw the catheter 1 cm, give test dose
   D. Withdraw needle and catheter, reinsert in a new position
   E. Abandon epidural technique, place long-acting spinal anesthetic

828.   Cutaneous innervation of the plantar surface of the foot is provided by the
   A. Sural nerve
   B. Posterior tibial nerve
   C. Saphenous nerve
   D. Deep peroneal nerve
   E. Superficial peroneal nerve

829. Which of the following local anesthetics has the lowest ratio of dosage required for cardiovascular collapse to dosage required for central nervous system toxicity?
    A. Lidocaine
    B. Etidocaine
    C. Bupivacaine
    D. Prilocaine
    E. Chloroprocaine

830. A 57-year-old patient is scheduled for hemorrhoidectomy. The patient has a history of mild chronic obstructive pulmonary disease, hypertension, and traumatic foot amputation from a tractor accident. His only hospitalizations were for two suicide attempts related to phantom limb sensations 10 years ago. He takes phenelzine (Nardil), thiazide, and potassium. Which of the following anesthetic techniques would be most appropriate for this patient?
    A. Spinal anesthetic with 0.5% hyperbaric bupivacaine
    B. Epidural anesthetic with 0.5% bupivacaine
    C. Local infiltration with lidocaine and epinephrine, sedation with propofol and meperidine
    D. General anesthesia with thiopental sodium (Pentothal), succinylcholine, nitrous oxide, isoflurane, meperidine
    E. General anesthesia with propofol, succinylcholine, nitrous oxide, fentanyl

831. If the recurrent laryngeal nerve were transected bilaterally, the vocal cords would
    A. Be in the open position
    B. Be in the closed position
    C. Be in the intermediate position (i.e., 2-3 mm apart)
    D. Not be affected unless the superior laryngeal nerve were also injured
    E. Appear exactly the same as if an intubating dose of succinylcholine were given

832. A 63-year-old woman undergoes total knee arthroplasty under spinal anesthesia. Two days later she complains of a severe headache on the left side of her head. Pain intensity is not related to posture. The **LEAST** likely cause of this headache is
    A. Caffeine withdrawal
    B. Malingering
    C. Viral illness
    D. Migraine
    E. Postdural puncture headache

833. What is the correct order of structures (from cephalad to caudad) in the intercostal space?
    A. Nerve, artery, vein
    B. Vein, nerve, artery
    C. Vein, artery, nerve
    D. Artery, nerve, vein
    E. Artery, vein, nerve

834. Which of the following types of regional anesthesia is associated with the greatest serum concentration of lidocaine?
    A. Intercostal
    B. Caudal
    C. Epidural
    D. Brachial plexus
    E. Femoral nerve block

835. Differences in which of the following local anesthetic properties account for the fact that the onset of an epidural block with 3% 2-chloroprocaine is more rapid than 2% lidocaine?
    A. Protein binding
    B. pKa
    C. Lipid solubility
    D. Concentration
    E. Ester versus amide structure

836. A 69-year-old man with a history of diabetes mellitus and chronic renal failure is to undergo placement of a dialysis fistula under regional anesthesia. During needle manipulation for a supraclavicular brachial plexus block, the patient begins to cough and complain of chest pain and shortness of breath. The most likely diagnosis is
   A. Angina
   B. Pneumothorax
   C. Phrenic nerve irritation
   D. Intravascular injection of local anesthetic
   E. Intrathecal injection of local anesthetic

837. Which of the following nerves is located immediately lateral to the trachea?
   A. Vagus
   B. Recurrent laryngeal
   C. Phrenic
   D. Long thoracic
   E. Spinal accessory

838. If a needle is introduced 1.5 cm inferior and 1.5 cm lateral to the pubic tubercle, to which nerve will it lie in close proximity?
   A. Obturator nerve
   B. Femoral nerve
   C. Lateral femoral cutaneous nerve
   D. Sciatic nerve
   E. Ilioinguinal nerve

839. The most common complication associated with a supraclavicular brachial plexus block is
   A. Blockade of the phrenic nerve
   B. Intravascular injection into the vertebral artery
   C. Spinal blockade
   D. Blockade of the recurrent laryngeal nerve
   E. Pneumothorax

840. Which portion of the upper extremity is not innervated by the brachial plexus?
   A. Posterior medial portion of the arm
   B. Elbow
   C. Lateral portion of the forearm
   D. Medial portion of the forearm
   E. Anterolateral portion of the arm

841. Which section of the brachial plexus is blocked with a supraclavicular block?
   A. Roots
   B. Trunks
   C. Divisions
   D. Cords
   E. Branches

842. A celiac-plexus block would **NOT** effectively treat pain resulting from a malignancy involving which of the following organs?
   A. Uterus
   B. Adrenal gland
   C. Stomach
   D. Pancreas
   E. Gallbladder

843.   A healthy 27-year-old female stepped on a nail and is to undergo débridement of a wound on her right great toe. She is anxious about general anesthesia but agrees to an ankle block with mild sedation. Which nerves must be adequately blocked in order to perform the surgery?
   A.   Deep peroneal, posterior tibial, saphenous, sural
   B.   Deep peroneal, saphenous, superficial peroneal, sural
   C.   Deep peroneal, posterior tibial, superficial peroneal, sural
   D.   Deep peroneal, posterior tibial, saphenous, superficial peroneal
   E.   Deep peroneal, posterior tibial, saphenous

844.   A 54-year-old man is administered morphine via patient-controlled analgesia (PCA) pump after a left total hip arthro-plasty. The pump is programmed to deliver a maximum dose of 2 mg every 15 minutes (lockout time) as needed for patient comfort. The total maximum dose that can be delivered in 4 hours is 30 mg. On the first day the patient receives 15 doses every 4 hours by pressing the delivery button every 15 to 18 minutes. How should his pain control be further managed?
   A.   Discontinue the PCA pump and administer intramuscular morphine
   B.   Increase the lockout time from 15 to 25 minutes
   C.   Change the analgesic from morphine to fentanyl
   D.   Increase the dose to 3 mg every 15 minutes as needed up to a total maximum dose of 40 mg every 4 hours
   E.   Make no changes

845.   The mechanism of the TENS unit in relieving pain is
   A.   Direct electrical inhibition of type A-delta and C fibers
   B.   Depletion of neurotransmitter in nociceptors
   C.   Hyperpolarization of spinothalamic tract neurons
   D.   Activation of inhibitory neurons
   E.   Distortion of nociceptors

846.   Epidural use of which of the following opioids would result in the greatest incidence of delayed respiratory depression?
   A.   Sufentanil
   B.   Fentanyl
   C.   Morphine sulfate
   D.   Hydromorphone
   E.   Methadone

847.   A 21-year-old patient reports tingling in her thumb during cesarean section under epidural anesthesia. To which der-matomal level would this correspond?
   A.   C4
   B.   C5
   C.   C6
   D.   C7
   E.   C8

848.   Which of the following would hasten the onset and increase the clinical duration of action of a local anesthetic, and provide the greatest depth of motor and sensory blockade when used for epidural anesthesia?
   A.   Addition to 1:200,000 epinephrine
   B.   Increasing the volume of local anesthetic
   C.   Increasing the concentration of local anesthetic
   D.   Increasing the dose
   E.   Placing the patient in the head-down position

849.   Select the **FALSE** statement concerning neurolytic nerve blocks.
   A.   There is little difference in the efficacy between alcohol and phenol
   B.   Destruction of peripheral nerves can be followed by a denervation hypersensitivity that is worse than the original pain
   C.   Neurolytic blocks should be reserved for patients with short life expectancies
   D.   Neurolytic blockade with phenol is permanent
   E.   Intrathecal neurolysis may be an effective management for certain pain conditions

850. The addition of epinephrine to epidural bupivacaine will
- **A.** Prolong motor blockade only
- **B.** Prolong sensory blockade only
- **C.** Prolong motor and sensory blockade
- **D.** Shorten duration of sensory blockade
- **E.** Have no effect on either duration of motor or sensory blockade

851. The epidural administration of a mixture of chloroprocaine and bupivacaine would have
- **A.** A latency similar to chloroprocaine with a duration of action similar to bupivacaine
- **B.** A latency shorter than chloroprocaine with a duration of action longer than bupivacaine
- **C.** A latency shorter than chloroprocaine with a duration of action similar to bupivacaine
- **D.** A latency longer than chloroprocaine with a duration of action similar to chloroprocaine
- **E.** A latency longer than chloroprocaine with a duration of action shorter than bupivacaine

852. Each of the following is associated with an increased incidence postdural puncture headaches (PDPH) **EXCEPT**
- **A.** Young age
- **B.** Female gender
- **C.** Early ambulation
- **D.** Pregnancy
- **E.** Large needle size

853. Each of the following items describes pain in the abdominal viscera **EXCEPT**
- **A.** Pain is transmitted via the vagus nerve
- **B.** The nerve fibers are type C
- **C.** Pain is not in a dermatomal distribution
- **D.** Pain is characterized by a dull aching or burning sensation
- **E.** Distention of the transverse colon causes more pain than surgical transection

854. A 24-year-old man undergoes repair of a right anterior shoulder dislocation under interscalene brachial plexus block. Anesthesia is produced with 30 mL of 0.5% bupivacaine with 5 µg/mL of epinephrine. The next morning, the patient complains of numbness in his right arm and hand. The most likely cause of these complaints is
- **A.** Excessive retraction by the surgeon
- **B.** Prolonged pressure on the brachial plexus from malpositioning
- **C.** Pressure on the right medial epicondyle from malpositioning
- **D.** Pressure on the right posterior humerus from malpositioning
- **E.** Residual anesthesia

855. Which of the following patients would be **LEAST** likely to develop a decrease in heart rate with a high (C8) level spinal anesthesia?
- **A.** A 15-year-old female patient with history of Wolff-Parkinson-White syndrome
- **B.** A 73-year-old patient with glaucoma treated with pilocarpine eye drops
- **C.** A 33 year old with a T6 paraplegia
- **D.** A 45-year-old diabetic man with a history orthostatic hypotension
- **E.** A 47-year-old patient who had a myocardial infarction 1 month ago, now taking procainamide

856. A 35-year-old woman receives a popliteal block for ankle and foot surgery. Which other nerve must be blocked in order to have complete anesthesia of the foot?
- **A.** Deep peroneal nerve
- **B.** Superficial peroneal nerve
- **C.** Sural nerve
- **D.** Saphenous nerve
- **E.** Posterior tibial nerve

857.   The most common complication of a celiac plexus block is
       A. Hypotension
       B. Seizure
       C. Subarachnoid injection
       D. Retroperitoneal hematoma
       E. Constipation

858.   The occipital portion of the skull receives sensory innervation from
       A. Spinal accessory nerve (nerve XI)
       B. Facial nerve (nerve VII)
       C. Ophthalmic branch of trigeminal nerve (nerve V)
       D. Maxillary branch of trigeminal nerve (nerve V)
       E. None of the above

859.   Each of the following is a potential complication of lumbar sympathetic blocks **EXCEPT**
       A. Puncture of the renal pelvis
       B. Intravascular injection (aorta)
       C. Seizure
       D. S1 nerve block
       E. Accidental subarachnoid injection

860.   After placement of an epidural catheter in a 55-year-old patient for total hip arthroplasty, an entire epidural dose is
       administered into the subarachnoid space. Physiologic effects consistent with subarachnoid injection of large volumes
       of local anesthetic include all of the following **EXCEPT**
       A. Hypotension
       B. Bradycardia
       C. Respiratory depression
       D. Constricted pupils
       E. Possible cauda equina syndrome

861.   A 49-year-old type I diabetic patient with a long history of burning pain in the right lower extremity receives a spinal
       anesthetic with 100 mg of procaine with 5% dextrose. The patient reports no relief in symptoms but has complete
       bilateral motor blockade. What diagnosis is consistent with this differential blockade examination?
       A. Diabetic neuropathy
       B. Central pain
       C. Myofascial pain
       D. Meralgia paresthetica
       E. Complex regional pain syndrome I (reflex sympathetic dystrophy)

862.   An 18-year-old man has a seizure during placement of an interscalene brachial plexus block with 2% lidocaine. The
       anesthesiologist begins to hyperventilate the patient's lungs with 100% O_2 using an anesthesia bag and mask. The
       rationale for this therapy includes all of the following **EXCEPT**
       A. Helps to prevent and treat hypoxia
       B. Hyperventilation decreases blood flow and delivery of lidocaine to the brain
       C. Hyperventilation induces hypokalemia which elevates the seizure threshold
       D. Hyperventilation induces alkalosis which elevates the seizure threshold
       E. Hyperventilation induces alkalosis which converts lidocaine to the protonated (ionized) form

863.   Para-aminobenzoic acid is a metabolite of
       A. Mepivacaine
       B. Ropivacaine
       C. Bupivacaine
       D. Procaine
       E. Prilocaine

864. Which statement concerning peripheral nerve structure and function is **FALSE?**
   A. Both nonmyelinated and myelinated nerves are surrounded by Schwann cells
   B. The speed of propagation of an action potential along a nerve axon is greatly enhanced by myelin
   C. Generation of an action potential is an "all-or-nothing" phenomenon
   D. Propagation of an action potential along myelinated nerve axons occurs by saltatory conduction via the nodes of Ranvier
   E. Myelination renders nerves less sensitive to local anesthetic blockade

865. A 42-year-old woman with a morbid fear of general anesthesia receives an interscalene block for shoulder arthroscopy consisting of 20 mL 0.5% ropivacaine. Much of her arm, shoulder and hand are numb, but the patient complains of pain as the incision is made at the upper portion of the shoulder. The most appropriate next step is
   A. Repeat block
   B. Perform intercostobrachial block
   C. Perform superficial cervical plexus block
   D. Perform a deep cervical plexus block
   E. Induce general anesthesia

866. According to the 2004 American Society of Regional Anesthesia and Pain Medicine (ASRA) practice advisory on infectious complications of regional anesthesia and pain medicine, the most important action to maintain aseptic technique and prevent cross-contamination during regional anesthesia techniques is
   A. Wearing surgical gown
   B. Hand washing
   C. Using soap and water instead of alcohol-based antiseptics
   D. Keeping fingernails short
   E. Using povidone iodine (e.g., Betadine) instead of alcohol-based chlorhexidine to scrub

867. A 75-year-old woman with a history of pulmonary embolism is scheduled for a right lower lobectomy for lung cancer. She is receiving dalteparin (Fragmin) for deep vein thrombosis (DVT) prophylaxis. How long after her last dose should one wait prior to placement of a thoracic epidural?
   A. 12 hours
   B. 24 hours
   C. 30 hours
   D. 72 hours
   E. No waiting necessary

868. How long should a patient be off clopidogrel (Plavix) before performing a central neuraxial block?
   A. 1 day
   B. 2 days
   C. 7 days
   D. 14 days
   E. No waiting necessary

869. Addition of bicarbonate to local anesthetics results in
   A. Delayed onset of action
   B. Reduced toxicity
   C. Increased duration of action
   D. Increased anesthetic potency
   E. Reduced pain with skin infiltration

870. Through which of the following would a spinal needle **NOT** pass during a midline placement of a subarachnoid block in the L3-L4 lumbar space?
   A. Supraspinous ligament
   B. Interspinous ligament
   C. Ligamentum flavum
   D. Posterior longitudinal ligament
   E. Dura mater

871. What epidural dose of bupivacaine will give similar sensory analgesia as 10 mL of 2% lidocaine?
      A. 5 mL of 0.25%
      B. 10 mL of 0.25%
      C. 5 mL of 0.5%
      D. 10 mL of 0.5%
      E. 5 mL of 0.75%

872. Each of the following additives to a spinal anesthetic possesses analgesic properties **EXCEPT**
      A. Clonidine
      B. Neostigmine
      C. Epinephrine
      D. Fentanyl
      E. All of the above posses analgesic activity

873. Which of the following local anesthetics is inappropriately paired with a clinical application because of its properties or toxicity?
      A. Tetracaine, topical anesthesia
      B. Bupivacaine, intravenous anesthesia
      C. Prilocaine, infiltrative anesthesia
      D. Chloroprocaine, epidural anesthesia
      E. Ropivacaine, epidural anesthesia

874. Discharge criteria from the post-anesthesia care unit (PACU) would be reached fastest after a 20 to 30 mL volume of which of the following epidurally administered local anesthetics?
      A. 3% 2-chloroprocaine
      B. 2% lidocaine
      C. 1% etidocaine
      D. 0.75% ropivacaine
      E. 0.5% levobupivacaine

875. A caudal block with 0.25% bupivacaine and 1:200,000 epinephrine is planned for postoperative analgesia after bilateral inguinal hernia repair in a 5 month old. Each of the following would be consistent with an intravascular injection **EXCEPT**
      A. Systolic blood pressure increase by 15 mm Hg
      B. Heart rate decrease by 10 bpm
      C. Ventricular extrasystoles
      D. Seizure
      E. T-wave amplitude of 25 percent over baseline

876. Which is **NOT** a potential complication of a stellate ganglion block
      A. Recurrent laryngeal nerve paralysis
      B. Subarachnoid block
      C. Brachial plexus block
      D. Pneumothorax
      E. Increased heart rate

877. An axillary block utilizing the transarterial approach with 0.5% bupivacaine and epinephrine (1:200,000) is performed in a 70-kg patient. Thirty mL is injected posterior to the axillary artery and 30 mL anterior to it. How many mg have been injected and was the maximum recommended dose exceeded?
      A. 150 mg bupivacaine, 150 µg epinephrine did not exceed maximum dose
      B. 150 mg bupivacaine, 150 µg epinephrine exceeded maximum dose
      C. 300 mg bupivacaine, 300 µg epinephrine did not exceed maximum dose
      D. 300 mg bupivacaine, 300 µg epinephrine exceeded maximum dose
      E. Transarterial blocks should never contain epinephrine and the block should not be done

878. Five days after knee arthroscopy under spinal anesthesia, a 55 year old complains of double vision and difficulty hearing. The other likely finding would be
A. Headache
B. Fever
C. Weakness in legs
D. Mental status changes
E. Backache

879. Administration of an interscalene block is associated virtually 100% of the time with
A. Hoarseness
B. Ulnar nerve blockade
C. Ipsilateral Horner's syndrome
D. Diaphragmatic hemiparalysis
E. Bradycardia

880. Which of the following nerves can be electrically stimulated at the ankle to produce flexion of the toes?
A. Posterior tibial nerve
B. Saphenous nerve
C. Deep peroneal nerve
D. Superficial peroneal nerve
E. Sural nerve

881. Which of the following observations, after nerve injury, is correctly paired with the appropriate nerve?
A. Inability to flex the forearm—ulnar nerve
B. Numbness in the thumb—radial nerve
C. Inability to extend the forearm—musculocutaneous nerve
D. Numbness in the little finger—median nerve
E. All are correctly paired

882. During an airway exam, a 53-year-old patient mentions that his right thumb tingles and then becomes numb if he extends his head for more than a few seconds. This symptom most likely represents a (an)
A. Unstable c-spine
B. Lhermitte's phenomenon
C. C6 nerve root irritation
D. C8 radiculopathy
E. Carpal tunnel syndrome

883. When performing an interscalene block with a peripheral nerve stimulator you note diaphragmatic movement. You should now
A. Inject the local anesthetic as the needle is in an appropriate location
B. Redirect the needle in an anterior direction
C. Redirect the needle in a more cephalad direction
D. Redirect the needle in a posterior direction
E. Advance the needle about 0.5 cm more and inject

884. During placement of an interscalene block the patient becomes hypotensive, bradycardic and cyanotic. Most likely cause is
A. Vertebral artery injection
B. Carotid artery injection
C. Phrenic nerve blockade
D. Total spinal
E. Stellate ganglion block

885. The reason that ropivacaine is marketed as pure S enantiomers is because the S form is associated with
  A. More rapid onset
  B. Longer duration
  C. Reduced cardiac toxicity
  D. Reduced incidence of anaphylaxis
  E. Less motor blockade

886. Nerves that originate from the sacral plexus include each of the following **EXCEPT**
  A. Femoral nerve
  B. Tibial nerve
  C. Superficial peroneal nerve
  D. Deep peroneal nerve
  E. Sural nerve

887. The only technique shown to prevent anesthetic-related nerve injury (ARNI) during placement of peripheral nerve blocks is
  A. Ultrasound guided regional technique
  B. Transarterial technique
  C. Nerve stimulator
  D. Paresthesia technique
  E. None of the above

888. An axillary block is performed on a healthy 19-year-old athlete. Thirty mL of 0.75% bupivacaine is injected incrementally. Fifteen minutes after the bupivacaine injection, the patient has a seizure and experiences a ventricular fibrillation arrest. Which of the measures below is **NOT** indicated.
  A. Begin chest compressions at 100 per minute
  B. Ventilate with 100% oxygen
  C. Bolus propofol to bind local anesthetic
  D. Infuse 20% lipid emulsion
  E. Repeat emulsion infusion if fibrillation continues

889. The structure **LEAST** likely to be encountered during placement of interscalene block is
  A. Phrenic nerve
  B. Vertebral artery
  C. Recurrent laryngeal nerve
  D. Subarachnoid space
  E. Vagus nerve

890. All of the following are symptoms of a developing epidural hematoma **EXCEPT**
  A. Radicular back pain
  B. Bowel and bladder dysfunction
  C. Sensory deficits
  D. Motor deficits
  E. Fever and chills

891. In addition to C nerve fibers, which nerve fibers carry pain impulses?
  A. A-α
  B. A-β
  C. A-γ
  D. A-δ
  E. B

892. An intradural mass lesion at the tip of a drug infusion catheter is **LEAST** likely to present as
  A. Piloerection, rhinorrhea, sweating, and more pain
  B. Development of numbness in T8 dermatomal pattern
  C. Hypopnea
  D. Perianal numbness
  E. Unilateral hip flexor weakness

893. Benzocaine is unique among the local anesthetics for which of the following reasons?
   A. It is a weak acid
   B. It can be used topically
   C. It is metabolized by same enzyme as succinylcholine
   D. It can promote formation of methemoglobin
   E. Is a vasoconstrictor

894. Which statement concerning local anesthetics is **CORRECT?**
   A. The un-ionized form of a local anesthetic binds to the nerve membrane to actually block conduction
   B. If one node of Ranvier is blocked, conduction will be reliably interrupted
   C. The ability of a local anesthetic to block nerve conduction is directly proportional to the diameter of the fiber
   D. The presence of myelin enhances the ability of a local anesthetic to block nerve conduction
   E. Local anesthetics block transmission by inhibiting the voltage-gated potassium ion channels

895. Postdural puncture headaches
   A. Usually occur immediately following dural puncture
   B. Are relieved 8 to 12 hours after an epidural blood patch is performed
   C. Occur more frequently in nonpregnant patients compared with pregnant patients
   D. Can be associated with neurologic deficits
   E. Are more frequent in the elderly compared with younger adults

896. Which of the following procedures for treatment of chronic pain requires localization of the epidural space with an epidural needle as part of technique?
   A. Transcutaneous electrical nerve stimulation
   B. Nucleoplasty
   C. Spinal cord stimulation
   D. Intradiskal electrothermal therapy
   E. Annuloplasty

897. Each of the following drugs has been used to treat neuropathic pain. Selective inhibition of serotonin and norepinephrine reuptake is the mechanism of which drug?
   A. Duloxetine
   B. Mexiletine
   C. Gabapentin
   D. Tramadol
   E. Carbamazepine

DIRECTIONS (Questions 898 through 901): Please match the structure below with the letter that corresponds to it in the ultrasound image.

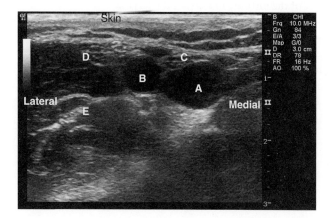

898. Musculocutaneous nerve

899. Axillary artery

900. Axillary vein

901. Ulnar nerve

DIRECTIONS (Questions 902 through 914): Each group of questions consists of several numbered statements followed by lettered headings. For each numbered statement, select the ONE lettered heading that is most closely associated with it. Each lettered heading may be selected once, more than once, or not at all.

902. Phrenic nerve

903. Cardiac accelerator fibers

904. Pudendal nerve

905. Pain fibers to the uterus

906. Inhibitory presynaptic fibers to the gastrointestinal tract
  A. C3-C5
  B. T1-T4
  C. T5-T12
  D. T10-L1
  E. S2-S4

907. Sensory innervation to the posterior one third of the tongue

908. Motor innervation to the cricothyroid muscle

909. Sensory innervation below the vocal cords to the carina

910. Sensory innervation to the mucous membranes of the false cords

911. Motor innervation to the tonsils

912. Sensory innervation to the posterior pharynx

913. Motor innervation to most of the intrinsic muscles of the larynx

914. Motor innervation to the superior and middle constrictor muscles
  A. Glossopharyngeal nerve
  B. Internal branch of the superior laryngeal nerve
  C. External branch of the superior laryngeal nerve
  D. Recurrent laryngeal nerve
  E. Cranial nerve XI

Anatomy, Regional Anesthesia, and Pain Management

Answers, References, and Explanations

788. (B) Tachyphylaxis is a well-known phenomenon associated with repeated injections of local anesthetics leading to decreased effectiveness. Interestingly, the dosing interval seems most important in the development of tachyphylaxis. If the dosing interval is short (and no pain between injections) tachyphylaxis does not develop. However, with longer dosing intervals (and pain between injections) tachyphylaxis develops (*Barash: Clinical Anesthesia, ed 5, pp 458-459*).

789. (B) The treatment of pruritus, the most common side effect of neuraxial opiates, is primarily with opioid antagonists, mixed opioid agonist-antagonist, and antihistamine drugs (by their sedating effects). Nalbuphine is a mixed opioid agonist-antagonist; diphenhydramine and hydroxyzine have antihistamine properties. Propofol at very low doses (e.g., 10 mg) has been useful to treat pruritus not only induced by neuraxial opiates but also the pruritus associated with cholestatic liver disease. Propofol does not affect analgesia, whereas opioid antagonists and mixed agonist-antagonist may reverse some or all of the analgesia, depending upon dose. Dexmedetomidine is a highly selective α_2-receptor agonist that has a faster onset and shorter duration of action compared with clonidine. Dexmedetomidine has analgesic properties, can potentiate neuraxial analgesia when injected spinally, and can perhaps decrease the incidence of pruritus by reducing the narcotic dose is used. It does not treat pruritus (*Miller: Anesthesia, ed 6, p 2740; Stoelting: Pharmacology and Physiology in Anesthetic Practice, ed 4, pp 91, 158, 434*).

790. (D) The maximum dose of local anesthetics containing 1:200,000 epinephrine that can be used for major nerve blocks is lidocaine, 500 mg; mepivacaine, 500 mg; prilocaine, 600 mg; bupivacaine, 225 mg; etidocaine, 400 mg; and tetracaine, 200 mg (*Miller: Anesthesia, ed 6, pp 584-589*).

791. (B) 1:200,000 means 1 g = 1000 mg = 1,000,000 μg per 200,000 mL
1,000,000 μg/200,000 mL = 5 μg/mL

792. (E) The early signs of digitalis toxicity include loss of appetite and nausea and vomiting. In some patients there may be pain that is similar to trigeminal neuralgia. Pain or discomfort in the feet and pain and discomfort in the extremities may be a feature of digitalis toxicity. Transient visual disturbances (e.g., amblyopia, scotomata) have been reported in patients with digitalis toxicity. In this patient, it would be prudent to obtain a digoxin level as an early part of the workup for these complaints. He may also have true trigeminal neuralgia, and workup for this condition can be undertaken after digitalis toxicity has been ruled out (*Stoelting: Pharmacology and Physiology in Anesthetic Practice, ed 4, pp 314-315*).

793. (C) Toxic reactions to local anesthetics are usually due to intravascular or intrathecal injection or to an excessive dosage. The initial symptoms of local anesthetic toxicity are lightheadedness and dizziness. Patients also may note perioral numbness and tinnitus. Progressive central nervous system (CNS) excitatory effects include visual and auditory disturbances, shivering, muscular twitching, and ultimately, generalized tonic-clonic seizures. CNS depression can ensue, leading to respiratory depression or arrest (*Miller: Anesthesia, ed 6, pp 592-598*).

794. (B) The site of action of spinally administered opiates is the substantia gelatinosa of the spinal cord. Epidural administration is complicated by factors related to dural penetration, absorption in fat, and systemic uptake; therefore, the quantity of intrathecally administered opioid required to achieve effective analgesia is typically much smaller. The ratio of epidural to intrathecal dose of morphine is approximately 10:1. Morphine is typically given in doses of 3 to 10 mg in the lumbar epidural space. Intrathecal morphine dosage is 0.2 to 1.0 mg. Onset time for epidural administration is 30 to 60 minutes with a peak effect in 90 to 120 minutes. Onset time for intrathecal administration is shorter than epidural administration. Duration of 12 to 24 hours of analgesic effect can be expected by either route (*Barash: Clinical Anesthesia, ed 5, pp 1422-1423*).

795. **(A)** Commonly injected local anesthetics are divided chemically into two groups: the aminoesters (esters) and the aminoamides (amides). The esters include procaine, chloroprocaine and tetracaine (all have one letter i in the name). The amides are lidocaine, mepivacaine, prilocaine, bupivacaine, levobupivacaine, etidocaine and ropivacaine (all have two i's in the name). The esters undergo plasma clearance by cholinesterases and have relatively short half-lives, whereas the amides undergo hepatic clearance and have longer half-lives (*Barash: Clinical Anesthesia, ed 5, p 462*).

796. **(C)** The major disadvantage of the interscalene block for hand and forearm surgery is that blockade of the inferior trunk (C8-T1) is often incomplete. Supplementation of the ulnar nerve often is required. The risk of pneumothorax is quite low, but blockade of the ipsilateral phrenic nerve occurs in up to 100% of blocks. This can cause respiratory compromise in patients with significant lung disease (*Miller: Anesthesia, ed 6, pp 1686-1689*).

797. **(C)** Surgical trauma includes a wide variety of physiologic responses. General anesthesia has no or only a slight inhibitory effect on endocrine and metabolic responses to surgery. Regional anesthesia inhibits the nociceptive signal from reaching the CNS and, therefore, has a significant inhibitory effect on the stress response, including adrenergic, cardiovascular, metabolic, immunologic, and pituitary. This effect is most pronounced with procedures on the lower part of the body and less with major abdominal and thoracic procedures. The variable effect is probably due to unblocked afferents, i.e., vagal, phrenic, or sympathetic (*Barash: Clinical Anesthesia, ed 5, p 1150*).

798. **(C)** The structures that are traversed by a needle placed in the midline prior to the epidural space are as follows: skin, subcutaneous tissue, supraspinous ligament, interspinous ligament, and ligamentum flavum. The ligamentum flavum is tough and dense and a change in the resistance to advancing the needle is often perceived and to many feels like a "snap." The anterior and posterior longitudinal ligaments bind the vertebral bodies together. See also explanation and diagram in question 870 (*Barash: Clinical Anesthesia, ed 5, pp 698-699*).

799. **(B)** The symptoms of cauda equina syndrome include low back pain, bilateral lower extremity weakness, saddle anesthesia and loss of bowel and bladder control. Pooling of local anesthetics in dependent areas of the spine within the subarachnoid space has been identified as the causative factor in cases of cauda equina syndrome. Microlumen catheters may enhance the nonuniform distribution of solutions within the intrathecal space, but cauda equina syndrome has been associated with the use of larger catheters, 5% lidocaine with dextrose, and 2% lidocaine, as well as 0.5% tetracaine (*Barash: Clinical Anesthesia, ed 5, p 712; Stoelting: Basics of Anesthesia, ed 5, pp 132, 631-632*).

800. **(B)** Differential nerve blockade is a complex process where anatomic and chemical factors determine the susceptibility of fibers to blockade by local anesthetics. Diameter, myelinization, and location within the nerve trunk affect the onset and regression time. In general, the small unmyelinated sympathetic fibers are blocked first, followed by unmyelinated C fibers (pain and temp), then small myelinated fibers (proprioception, touch, pressure), and finally the large myelinated fibers (motor) (*Barash: Clinical Anesthesia, ed 5, pp 456-457, 708; Cousins: Neural Blockade in Clinical Anesthesia and Management of Pain, ed 3, pp 45-46*).

801. **(B)** Acute herpes zoster is due to the reactivation of the varicella-zoster virus. Acute treatment includes symptomatic pain treatment and antiviral drugs (e.g., acyclovir). It is typically a benign and self-limiting disease in patients younger than 50 years of age. As one gets older, the incidence of postherpetic neuralgia (PHN) defined as pain persisting beyond the healing of the herpes zoster lesions increases. The incidence of PHN is about 50% in patients older than 50 years. Treatment of established PHN has been shown to be resistant to interventions and, thus, can be difficult. However, proven therapies include tricyclic antidepressants, anticonvulsants, topical local anesthetics (e.g., 5% lidocaine patch), topical capsaicin and TENS. Sympathetic blocks can provide excellent analgesia but are most useful during the more acute stages of the disease rather than during the late chronic stages. Sympathetic blocks in the acute stages may decrease the incidence of PHN. Oral clonidine, which is used to treat hypertension and opioid withdrawal, has not been shown to be an effective treatment for postherpetic neuralgia (*Morgan: Clinical Anesthesiology, ed 4, p 407; Raj: Practical Management of Pain, ed 3, pp 187-189*).

802. **(C)** The deep peroneal nerve innervates the short extensors of the toes and the skin of the web space between the great and second toe. The deep peroneal nerve is blocked at the ankle by infiltration between the tendons of the anterior tibial and extensor hallucis longus muscle (*Brown: Atlas of Regional Anesthesia, ed 3, pp 141-143; Miller: Anesthesia, ed 6, pp 1703-1704*).

803. **(B)** Central nervous system (CNS) toxicity from local anesthetics generally parallels anesthetic potency (e.g., bupivacaine is four times as potent as lidocaine, ropivacaine is three times as potent as lidocaine). Cardiovascular (CV) toxicity occurs at a higher blood level than CNS toxicity. For bupivacaine and ropivacaine, CV toxicity occurs at two times the CNS dose, whereas for lidocaine the CV toxicity occurs at seven times the CNS toxicity levels, making lidocaine the least cardiotoxic, and bupivacaine the most cardiotoxic of the listed local anesthetics (*Barash: Clinical Anesthesia, ed 5, pp 459-467; Stoelting: Basics of Anesthesia, ed 5, pp 127-131*).

804. **(E)** The International Association for the Study of Pain (IASP) has defined several pain terms. Anesthesia dolorosa refers to spontaneous pain in an area or region that is anesthetic. Neuropathic pain is pain initiated or caused by a primary lesion or dysfunction in the nervous system. Dysesthesia is an unpleasant abnormal sensation, whether spontaneous or evoked. Hyperalgesia is an increased response to a stimulus that is normally painful. Allodynia is pain caused by a stimulus that does not normally provoke pain (*Morgan: Clinical Anesthesia ed 4, p 361; Loeser: Bonica's Management of Pain, ed 3, pp 17-20*).

805. **(A)** Ester local anesthetics are hydrolyzed by cholinesterase enzymes that are present mainly in plasma and, in a smaller amount, in the liver. Because there are no cholinesterase enzymes present in cerebrospinal fluid (CSF), the anesthetic effect of tetracaine will persist until it is absorbed into systemic circulation. The rate of hydrolysis varies, with chloroprocaine being fastest, procaine intermediate, and tetracaine the slowest. Toxicity is inversely related to the rate of hydrolysis; tetracaine is, therefore, the most toxic (*Miller: Anesthesia, ed 6, p 589; Morgan: Clinical Anesthesiology, ed 4, p 309; Stoelting: Pharmacology and Physiology in Anesthetic Practice, ed 4, pp 186-187*).

806. **(A)** Complex regional pain syndrome type I or CRPS type I also called reflex sympathetic dystrophy (RSD) is a clinical syndrome of continuous burning pain, usually occurring after minor trauma. Patients present with variable sensory, motor, autonomic, and trophic changes. Complex regional pain syndrome type II or CRPS type II (causalgia) exhibits the same features of reflex sympathetic dystrophy, but the etiology is usually major traumatic damage to large nerves (e.g., median nerve of the upper extremity or tibial division of the sciatic nerve in the lower extremity) (*Barash: Clinical Anesthesia, ed 5, pp 1456-1458; Morgan: Clinical Anesthesia, ed 4, p 406; Raj: Practical Management of Pain, ed 3, p 306*).

807. **(C)** The potency of local anesthetics is directly related to their lipid solubility. In general, the speed or onset of action of local anesthetics is related to the pKa of the drug. Drugs with lower pKa values have a higher amount of non-ionized molecules at physiologic pH and penetrate the lipid portion of nerves faster (an exception is chloroprocaine, which has a fast onset of action that may be related to the higher concentration of drug used). The amount of protein binding seems related to the duration of action of local anesthetics (more protein binding has longer duration of action) (*Raj: Practical Management of Pain, ed 3, pp 560-561; Stoelting: Pharmacology and Physiology in Anesthetic Practice, ed 4, pp 180-181*).

808. **(E)** Many factors have an effect on the sensory level after a subarachnoid injection. The baricity of the solution and the patient position are the most important determinants of sensory level. The other listed options have little to no effect on sensory level. Patient height also has little effect on sensory level (*Miller: Anesthesia, ed 6, p 1668*).

809. **(D)** Chloroprocaine is an ester local anesthetic that is rapidly metabolized by pseudocholinesterase. With the epidural injection of chloroprocaine, very little drug is available to cross the placenta, because the half-life is about 45 seconds (and that which crosses is also rapidly metabolized making fetal effects essentially non-significant). The amide local anesthetics undergo liver metabolism and have relatively long half-lives, but with prolonged epidural administration may accumulate in the fetus (*Barash: Clinical Anesthesia, ed 5, pp 1154-1155; Miller: Anesthesia, ed 6, p 2323*).

810. **(A)** Hypotension with a high spinal anesthesia is related to sympathetic blockade; venodilation (decreases preload), arterial dilation (decreases afterload) and a decrease in heart rate (cardioaccelerator fibers T1-T4 blockade and a fall in right atrial filling that affects the intrinsic chronotropic stretch receptors). With a high spinal, the decrease in venous dilation is the predominant cause of hypotension (*Barash: Clinical Anesthesia, ed 5, pp 708-709; Miller: Anesthesia, ed 6, pp 1658-1659; Stoelting: Basics of Anesthesia, ed 5, pp 259-262*).

811. (C)   The incidence of phantom limb pain is estimated to be 60% to 85%. The incidence of phantom limb pain does not differ between traumatic and nontraumatic amputees. The incidence of phantom pain increases with more proximal amputation. Although very difficult to treat, nerve blocks are commonly used in an attempt to treat phantom pain. These include trigger point injections, peripheral and central nerve blocks, and sympathetic blocks (*Raj: Practical Management of Pain, ed 3, pp 213-218*).

812. (D)   Prilocaine is the most rapidly metabolized of the amide local anesthetics and therefore least toxic. 2-Chloroprocaine is hydrolyzed rapidly in the blood and, therefore, would appear to be ideal, but it has been associated with a high incidence of thrombophlebitis and is therefore not recommended. To avoid toxicity, maximum doses are as follows: prilocaine, 3 to 4 mg/kg; lidocaine, 1.5 to 3 mg/kg; ropivacaine, 1.2 to 1.8 mg/kg. Bupivacaine is not recommended for Bier blocks because of reports of cardiovascular toxicity and death that have occurred (*Cousins: Neural Blockade in Clinical Anesthesia and Management of Pain, ed 3, p 400; Miller: Anesthesia, ed 6, pp 586-588, 1695*).

813. (D)   Both phenylephrine and epinephrine will prolong a spinal anesthetic when administering lidocaine. The Taylor approach for spinal anesthesia uses a paramedian approach to the L5-S1 interspace—the largest interspace of the vertebral column. The sympathetic nervous system originates in the thoracic and lumbar spinal cord T1-L3; therefore, a high thoracic sensory level can cause a complete sympathetic block. The dural sac extends to S2-S3, not S4-S5. The spinal cord extends to L3 in the infant and L1-L2 in adults (*Barash: Clinical Anesthesia, ed 5, pp 693-694, 708; Miller: Anesthesia, ed 6, pp 585, 589, 1654-1656*).

814. (A)   Development of an epidural abscess is fortunately an exceedingly rare complication of spinal and epidural anesthesia. Most anesthetic related epidural abscesses are associated with epidural catheters. When an epidural abscess is developing, prompt recognition and treatment are essential if permanent sequelae are to be avoided. Symptoms from an epidural abscess may not become apparent until several days (mean 5 days) after placement of the block. There are four clinical stages of epidural abscess symptom progression. Initially, localized back pain develops. Second stage includes nerve root or radicular pain. The third stage involves motor and sensory deficits followed by the last stage of paraplegia. Unlike an epidural hematoma, in which severe back pain is the key feature, patients with epidural abscesses will complain of radicular pain approximately 3 days after development of the back pain. Anterior spinal artery syndrome is characterized predominantly by motor weakness or paralysis of the lower extremities. Meralgia paresthetica is related to entrapment of the lateral femoral cutaneous nerve as it courses below the inguinal ligament and is associated with burning pain over the lateral aspect of the thigh. It is not a complication of epidural anesthesia (*Morgan: Clinical Anesthesia, ed 4, pp 320-321; Raj: Practical Management of Pain, ed 3, p 649*).

815. (C)   Complex regional pain syndromes are associated with trauma. The main feature is burning and continuous pain that is exacerbated by normal movement, cutaneous stimulation, or stress, usually weeks after the injury. The pain is not anatomically distributed. Other associated features include cool, red, clammy skin and hair loss in the involved extremity. Chronic cases may be associated with atrophy and osteoporosis (*Barash: Clinical Anesthesia, ed 5, pp 1456-1458; Miller: Anesthesia, ed 6, pp 2774-2775*).

816. (D)   Neurolytic blockade with phenol (6% to 10% in glycerine) is painless because phenol has a dual action as both a local anesthetic and a neurolytic agent. The initial block wears off over a 24-hour period, during which time neurolysis occurs. For this reason you must wait a day to determine effectiveness of the neurolytic block. Alcohol (100% ethanol) is painful on injection and should be preceded by local anesthetic injection. Unfortunately, there is no neurolytic agent that affects only sympathetic fibers (*Barash: Clinical Anesthesia, ed 5, p 1464*).

817. (C)   In general, each 1-2 mL of local anesthetic will anesthetize about one spinal segment in the 20 to 40-year-old patient. Because of the negative intrathoracic pressure transmitted to the epidural space with breathing, about two thirds of the segments are blocked above the level of the lumbar placement and one third of segments are blocked below the injection. For example, to achieve a T4 block when an epidural is placed at the L2-L3 space about 10 segments above and 5 segments below the epidural would be needed (15 segments) or about 20-25 mL. As one gets older, the dose of local anesthetic mL/segment decreases (e.g., 80 year old may need 0.75-1.5 mL/segment). Also, pregnant patients are more sensitive to local anesthetics and reduced doses are needed (*Barash: Clinical Anesthesia, ed 5, pp 705-706; Morgan: Clinical Anesthesiology, ed 4, p 312; Stoelting: Basics of Anesthesia, ed 5, p 266*).

818. (C)

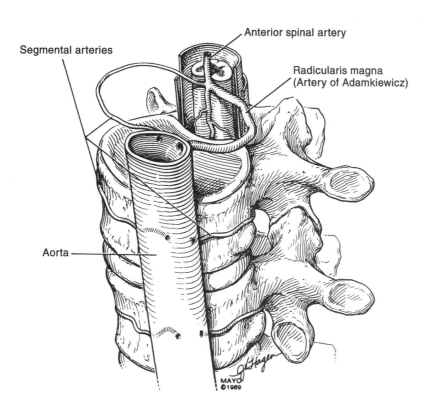

Segmental arteries

Anterior spinal artery

Radicularis magna
(Artery of Adamkiewicz)

Aorta

MAYO
©1989

The artery of Adamkiewicz is also called the *arteria radicularis magna* and is one of the "feeder" arteries for the anterior spinal artery. Damage to this artery can lead to ischemia in the thoracolumbar region and may result in paraplegia. The origin of this artery is variable (e.g., T9-T12 in 75% of cases, L1-L2 in 10% of cases) (*Barash: Clinical Anesthesia, ed 5, p 958; Miller: Anesthesia, ed 6, p 2087*).

819. (E) The one anterior spinal artery supplies about 75% of the blood flow to the spinal cord (motor tracts) and arises from the vertebral arteries and radicular arteries from the aorta. It descends in front of the anterior longitudinal sulcus of the spinal cord. The two posterior spinal arteries supply about 25% of the blood flow to the spinal cord (sensory tracts) and arise from the posterior and inferior cerebellar arteries, the vertebral arteries, and the radicular arteries (*Barash: Clinical Anesthesia, ed 5, p 958; Miller: Anesthesia, ed 6, pp 2086-2087*).

820. (D) To perform a sciatic nerve block, first draw a line from the posterior superior iliac spine to the greater trochanter, then draw a 5-cm line perpendicular from the midpoint of this line caudally and a second line from the sacral hiatus to the greater trochanter. The intersection of the second line with the perpendicular line marks the point of entry (*Brown: Atlas of Regional Anesthesia, ed 3, pp 105-110; Miller: Anesthesia, ed 6, p 1700*).

821. (D) Complications of deep cervical plexus block include injection of the local anesthetic into the vertebral artery, subarachnoid space, or epidural space. Other nerves that may be anesthetized include the phrenic nerve (which is why bilateral deep cervical plexus blocks should be performed with caution, if at all), and the recurrent laryngeal nerve (*Barash: Clinical Anesthesia, ed 5, p 723; Brown: Atlas of Regional Anesthesia, ed 3, pp 191-195; Miller: Anesthesia, ed 6, p 1707*).

822. (E) A retrobulbar block anesthetizes the three cranial nerves responsible for movement of the eye. The ciliary nerves are also blocked, providing anesthesia to the conjunctiva, cornea, and uvea. The ophthalmic branch of the trigeminal nerve provides sensory innervation to the skin of the forehead, cornea, and eyelid. This branch of the trigeminal nerve may be blocked, but the maxillary branch would be spared (*Barash: Clinical Anesthesia, ed 5, pp 984-986; Brown: Atlas of Regional Anesthesia, ed 3, pp 185-188*).

823. (E) The vagus nerve innervates the airway by two branches: the superior laryngeal nerves and the recurrent laryngeal nerves. All the muscles of the larynx are innervated by the recurrent laryngeal nerve except for the cricothyroid muscle. The superior laryngeal nerve divides into the internal and external laryngeal branches. The external

laryngeal branch innervates the cricothyroid muscle. The internal laryngeal branch provides sensory fibers to the cords, epiglottis and the arytenoids (*Barash: Clinical Anesthesia, ed 5, p 724; Brown: Atlas of Regional Anesthesia, ed 3, pp 207-211*).

824. (E)   Because of the potential for cardiotoxicity and because bupivacaine has no advantages over other local anesthetics in this setting, it is no longer recommended for use in intravenous regional anesthesia (*Miller: Anesthesia, ed 6, p 1695*).

825. (C)

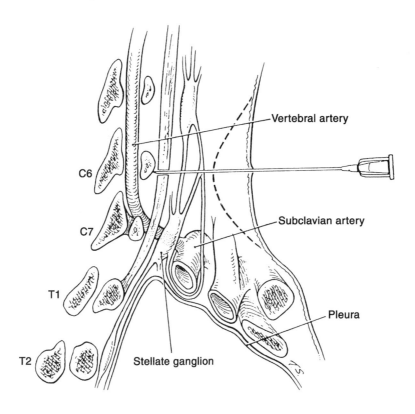

The stellate ganglion usually lies in front of the neck of the first rib. The vertebral artery lies anterior to the ganglion as it has just originated from the subclavian artery. After passing over the ganglion, it enters the vertebral foramen and lies posterior to the anterior tubercle of C6 (*Barash: Clinical Anesthesia, ed 5, pp 736-737; Brown: Atlas of Regional Anesthesia, ed 3, pp 199-203; Raj: Practical Management of Pain, ed 3, pp 655-657*).

826. (D)   The median nerve is the most medial structure in the antecubital fossa. To block this nerve, first the brachial artery is palpated at the level of the intercondylar line between the medial and lateral epicondyles, and then a needle is inserted just medial to the artery and directed perpendicularly to the skin (*Brown: Atlas of Regional Anesthesia, ed 3, pp 73-74; Morgan: Clinical Anesthesia, ed 4, pp 338-339*).

827. (D)   When an epidural catheter is placed without fluoroscopic guidance, the exact location of the needle tip relative to the anatomic structures of the back can only be surmised. If malposition of either the needle or the catheter is suspected, it is prudent to withdraw the entire apparatus and reinsert a second time. In this case, it is possible that the catheter tip has found its way into a nerve root. Under these circumstances, injection of a local anesthetic or narcotic could produce pressure that would lead to ischemia and possible neurologic damage. During placement or injection of an epidural catheter, a paresthesia is always a warning sign that should be heeded (*Raj: Practical Management of Pain, ed 3, p 650*).

828. (B)   There are five nerves that supply the ankle and foot: the posterior tibial, sural, superficial and deep peroneal, and saphenous nerves. These nerves are superficial at the level of the ankle and are easy to block. The posterior branch of the tibial nerve gives rise to the medial and lateral plantar nerves, which supply the plantar surface of the foot (*Barash: Clinical Anesthesia, ed 5, pp 743-744; Brown: Atlas of Regional Anesthesia, ed 3, pp 141-143*).

829. (C) In general, in both in vivo and in vitro studies there is an overall direct correlation between anesthetic's potency and its direct depressant effect on myocardial contractility. The ratio of dosage required for cardiovascular collapse in animal models compared with that required to produce neurologic symptoms is the lowest for bupivacaine, levo-bupivacaine and ropivacaine (2.0). Ratios for other local anesthetics are as follows: prilocaine, 3.1; procaine and chloroprocaine, 3.7; etidocaine, 4.4; lidocaine and mepivacaine, 7.1 (*Barash: Clinical Anesthesia, ed 5, pp 462-466*).

830. (E) Reactivation of phantom limb sensations has been reported in patients who have received both spinal and epidural anesthetics (90% in some series). In the majority of these cases (80%), phantom limb sensation persisted until the block receded. With a history of a phantom limb sensations that drove this patient to attempt suicide, it is probably wise to avoid spinal and epidural anesthetics. Phenelzine (Nardil) is a monoamine oxidase (MAO) inhibitor that is occasionally used for the treatment of depression. Any anesthetic or combination of techniques that involves meperidine is contraindicated in patients receiving MAO inhibitors. The combination of meperidine and MAO inhibitors has been associated with hyperthermia, hypotension, hypertension, ventilatory depression, skeletal muscle rigidity, seizures, and coma. Because of this unfavorable drug interaction, meperidine should be avoided in patients receiving MAO inhibitors. Accordingly, the only acceptable choice in this question would be general anesthesia with propofol, succinylcholine, nitrous oxide, and fentanyl. As an interesting side point, the drug phenelzine prolongs the duration of action of succinylcholine by decreasing plasma cholinesterase activity (*Miller: Anesthesia, ed 6, pp 423-424; Morgan: Clinical Anesthesiology, ed 4, p 657; Raj: Practical Management of Pain, ed 3, p 212*).

831. (C) The recurrent laryngeal nerve innervates all the muscles of the larynx except the cricothyroid muscle, which tenses the vocal cords and is innervated by the external branch of the superior laryngeal nerve. With bilateral transections of the recurrent laryngeal nerve, the vocal cords lie within 2 to 3 mm of the midline. The airway maybe inadequate and a tracheostomy may be needed (*Miller: Anesthesia, ed 6, p 2538*).

832. (E) Postdural puncture headache (PDPH) will have a postural component. When supine, the headache is usually gone but may be mild in some cases. When the head is elevated the headache may be severe, is bilateral and may be associated with diplopia, nausea and vomiting. The headache pain is typically frontal and/or occipital in location (*Barash: Clinical Anesthesia, ed 5, p 711; Stoelting: Basics of Anesthesia, ed 5, p 260*).

833. (C) VAN (*Vein, Artery, Nerve*) describes the anatomical relationship of the intercostal structures deep to the lower border of the ribs from cephalad to caudal direction. The block is performed by walking off the inferior edge of the rib typically about 5 to 7 cm from midline. The two principle risks are pneumothorax and intravascular injection of local anesthetics. Because of the close proximity of the vein and artery to the nerve, intercostal blocks have relatively high blood levels as compared to other blocks (e.g., epidural, brachial plexus, infiltration) and caution with dose is needed if many levels are blocked (*Morgan: Clinical Anesthesiology, ed 4, pp 353-354; Stoelting: Basics of Anesthesia, ed 5, pp 282-283*).

834. (A) The site of injection of the local anesthetic is one of the most important factors influencing systemic local anesthetic absorption and toxicity. The degree of absorption from the site of injection depends on the blood supply to that site. Areas that have the greatest blood supply have the greatest systemic absorption. For this reason, the greatest plasma concentration of local anesthetic occurs after an intercostal block, followed by caudal epidural, lumbar epidural, brachial plexus, sciatic/femoral nerve block, and subcutaneous (*Barash: Clinical Anesthesia, ed 5, pp 460-461; Miller: Anesthesia, ed 6, p 591; Stoelting: Basics of Anesthesia, ed 5, p 130*).

835. (D) Local anesthetics are weak bases. The neutral (non-ionized) form of the molecule is able to pass through the lipid nerve cell membrane, whereas the ionized (protonated) form actually produces anesthesia. Chloroprocaine has the highest pKa of local anesthetics, meaning that a greater percentage of it will exist in the ionized form at any given pH than any of the other local anesthetics. Despite this fact, 3% chloroprocaine has a more rapid onset than 2% lidocaine, presumably because of the greater number of molecules (concentration). If one compares onset time for 1.5% lidocaine against 1.5% chloroprocaine, the former will have a more rapid onset (*Miller: Anesthesia, ed 6, p 584*).

836. (B) The risk of pneumothorax is a significant limitation for supraclavicular brachial plexus blocks (incidence 0.5%-6% depending upon experience). Furthermore, the technique is difficult to teach and describe. For these reasons, this block should not be performed in patients in whom a pneumothorax or phrenic nerve block (40%-60%

of patients) would result in significant dyspnea or respiratory distress. A pneumothorax should be considered if the patient begins to complain of chest pain or shortness of breath or begins to cough during placement of supraclavicular brachial plexus block (*Barash: Clinical Anesthesia, ed 5, p 728; Miller: Anesthesia, ed 6, p 1690*).

837. (B) The structures in the neck from medial to lateral are the recurrent laryngeal nerve, carotid artery, vagus nerve, internal jugular vein, and phrenic nerve (*Brown: Atlas of Regional Anesthesia, ed 3, pp 28, 33, 208-209; Clemente: Anatomy: Regional Atlas of the Human Body, ed 3, p 586*).

838. (A) The obturator nerve provides variable cutaneous innervation of the thigh. An obturator nerve block is achieved by placement of the needle 1 to 2 cm lateral to and 1 to 2 cm below the pubic tubercle. After contact with the pubic bone, the needle is withdrawn and walked cephalad to identify the obturator canal. Between 10 and 15 mL of local anesthetic should be placed in the canal. If a nerve stimulator is used, contraction of the adductor muscles with nerve stimulation indicates proximity to the nerve (*Stoelting: Basics of Anesthesia, ed 5, p 285*).

839. (A) The most serious complication associated with a supraclavicular brachial plexus block is pneumothorax. The most common complication is a phrenic nerve block which is usually mild and relatively common (40%-60% of blocks). Bilateral supraclavicular blocks however, are not recommended due to the possibility of bilateral phrenic nerve paralysis or pneumothoraces. Other potential complications include Horner's syndrome, nerve damage or neuritis, or intravascular injection (*Miller: Anesthesia, ed 6, p 1690; Stoelting: Basics of Anesthesia, ed 5, p 278*).

840. (A) The arm receives sensory innervation from the brachial plexus except for the shoulder, which is innervated by the cervical plexus, and the posterior medial aspect of the arm, which is supplied by the intercostobrachial nerve (*Brown: Atlas of Regional Anesthesia, ed 3, pp 27-31; Stoelting: Basics of Anesthesia, ed 5, p 277*).

841. (B) The brachial plexus starts out at the root level from the ventral rami of C5-T1 with a small amount from C4 and T2. These roots at the level of the scalene muscle become the 3 trunks: superior, middle and inferior. The trunks then divide into the dorsal and ventral divisions at the lateral edge of the first rib. When the divisions enter the axilla, they become the cords: posterior, lateral and medial. At the lateral border of the pectoralis muscle they become the five peripheral nerves: radial, musculocutaneous, median, ulnar and axillary. The plexus is blocked at the distal level of the trunks just before they become divisions. Here a small volume of anesthetic is required and no part of the plexus is spared, as with axillary or interscalene block. The block can be performed with the arm in any position (*Brown: Atlas of Regional Anesthesia, ed 3, pp 27-35, 47-54; Cousins: Neural Blockade in Clinical Anesthesia and Management of Pain, ed 3, p 352; Miller: Anesthesia, ed 6, p 1689*).

842. (A) The celiac plexus innervates most of the abdominal viscera, including the lower esophagus, stomach, all of the small intestine and the large intestine up to the splenic flexure as well as the pancreas, liver, biliary tract, spleen, kidneys, adrenal glands and omentum. The pelvic organs (e.g., uterus, ovaries, prostate, distal colon) are supplied by the hypogastric plexus (*Brown: Atlas of Regional Anesthesia, ed 3, pp 313, 325*).

843. (D) The great toe is innervated by the deep peroneal, posterior tibial, superficial peroneal, and occasionally the saphenous nerve. All four of these nerves should be blocked for surgery on the great toe (*Miller: Anesthesia, ed 6, pp 1703-1704; Stoelting: Basics of Anesthesia, ed 5, p 288*).

844. (D) Frequent dosing by a patient receiving postoperative analgesia through a PCA pump suggests the need to increase the magnitude of the dose. It is important to keep in mind that a patient should be given a sufficient loading dose of narcotic before initiative therapy with a PCA pump. Otherwise, the patient will be playing the frustrating game of "catch up" (*Barash: Clinical Anesthesia, ed 5, p 1421*).

845. (D) Transcutaneous electrical nerve stimulation (TENS) is low-intensity electrical stimuli (2 and 100 Hz,) that produces a tingling or vibratory sensation. It is thought that TENS units produce analgesia by releasing endogenous endorphins. These endorphins have an inhibitory effect at the spinal cord level and augment descending inhibitory pathways (*Miller: Anesthesia, ed 6, pp 2776-2777; Stoelting: Basics of Anesthesia, ed 5, p 591*).

846. (C) Although the more hydrophilic drugs such as morphine have a longer duration of action of analgesia, they also have a higher potential for inducing delayed respiratory depression through cephalad migration in the CNS, as compared with the more lipid-soluble drugs listed in this question (*Barash: Clinical Anesthesia, ed 5, pp 1426-1428; Miller: Anesthesia, ed 6, pp 1472-1474*).

847. (C)   The thumb corresponds to dermatome C6, the second and middle fingers correspond to dermatome C7, and the fourth and little fingers correspond to dermatome C8 (*Stoelting: Basics of Anesthesia, ed 5, p 249*).

848. (D)   Increasing the total dose (mass) of local anesthetic is more efficacious in hastening the onset and increasing the duration of an epidural anesthetic than increasing the volume or increasing the concentration (while holding the total dose constant) (*Barash: Clinical Anesthesia, ed 5, p 707*).

849. (D)   Alcohol and phenol are similar in their ability to cause nonselective damage to neural tissues. Alcohol causes pain when injected and sometimes is mixed with bupivacaine, whereas phenol is relatively painless. Neural tissue will regenerate; therefore, neurolytic blocks are never "permanent" and neurolysis can lead to a denervation hypersensitivity, which can be extremely painful (*Barash: Clinical Anesthesia, ed 5, p 1464; Morgan: Clinical Anesthesiology, ed 4, pp 388-389*).

850. (B)   Epinephrine's effect on the duration of anesthesia depends on the local anesthetic and the site. Infiltration and peripheral block duration with most agents will be prolonged with epinephrine. The addition of epinephrine to epidural 0.5% or 0.75% bupivacaine has not been shown to increase the duration of the motor blockade but does extend the duration of the sensory block. The effect of epinephrine is greater for the intermediate duration local anesthetics lidocaine and mepivacaine (*Barash: Clinical Anesthesia, ed 5, p 707; Miller: Anesthesia, ed 6, pp 1674-1675*).

851. (E)   Mixtures of local anesthetics have been used to take advantage of the short latency of certain agents (chloroprocaine) and the long duration of other agents (bupivacaine). Duration of epidural anesthesia by mixtures of chloroprocaine and bupivacaine has been shown to be shorter than bupivacaine alone and onset time longer than chloroprocaine alone (*Miller: Anesthesia, ed 6, pp 585-586*).

852. (C)   Younger adults have a higher incidence of PDPH than older adults. Women have a slightly higher incidence than men. Pregnant women have a higher incidence than nonpregnant women. Since the incidence and severity of PDPH relates to the amount of CSF leakage through the dural hole, it makes sense that the larger the needle and the more holes in the dura the greater incidence of PDPH. In addition, the shape of the tip of the needle is important; a cutting needle (e.g.. Quincke) has a greater incidence of PDPH than noncutting needles (e.g., Whitacre, Sprotte). The incidence of headache has been shown to be less when the dural fibers are split longitudinally rather than when they are cut while the needle is held in a transverse direction. The timing of ambulation relative to dural puncture has not been shown to affect the incidence of postspinal headache. The block should wear off before ambulation is attempted (*Barash: Clinical Anesthesia, ed 5, p 711; Miller: Anesthesia, ed 6, p 1669*).

853. (A)   Virtually all pain arising in the thoracic or abdominal viscera is transmitted via the sympathetic nervous system in unmyelinated type C fibers. Visceral pain is dull, aching, burning, and nonspecific. Visceral pain is caused by any stimulus that excites nociceptive nerve endings in diffuse areas. In this regard, distention of a hollow viscus causes a greater sensation of pain than does the highly localized damage produced by transecting the gut (*Raj: Practical Management of Pain, ed 3, pp 223-225*).

854. (E)   The brachial plexus is not normally retracted during repair of an anterior shoulder dislocation. Prolonged pressure on the brachial plexus will result in hand or arm numbness. This may occur if this structure becomes pinched between the clavicle and the head of the humerus, as seen in patients placed in steep Trendelenburg position with the shoulders resting against shoulder braces. Prolonged pressure on the medial epicondyle may produce an ulnar neuropathy, whereas prolonged pressure against the posterior surface of the humerus may produce a radial neuropathy. Bupivacaine is a long-acting local anesthetic and may cause numbness for 8 to 12 hours (*Brown: Atlas of Regional Anesthesia, ed 3, p 39*).

855. (D)   The cardiac accelerator fibers originate in the T1-T4 segments. A high spinal, above T1, can cause bradycardia by anesthetizing these fibers. Diabetic patients who display orthostatic hypotension have an autonomic neuropathy. The cardiac accelerator fibers are essentially ablated in these patients and therefore, the slowing of heart rate does not ordinarily develop with high spinals. Pilocarpine, a parasympathomimetic agent, will not prevent bradycardia with spinal anesthesia. Patients with Wolff-Parkinson-White syndrome will become bradycardic when the autonomic accelerator fibers are interrupted, as will patients with a spinal cord transection below T4. Recent myocardial infarction does not eliminate susceptibility to bradycardia with sympatholysis unless the patient has a complete heart block (*Hines: Stoelting's Anesthesia and Co-Existing Disease, ed 5, pp 72, 242-243, 374-375*).

856. **(D)** All of the nerves of the foot with the exception of the saphenous are derived from the sciatic nerve. The sciatic nerve distally becomes the tibial and peroneal nerves which can be blocked at the popliteal fossa for surgery below the knee. The saphenous nerve is a branch of the femoral nerve and provides sensory innervation along the medial aspect of the lower leg between the knee and the medial malleolus and must also be blocked for surgery below the knee (*Brown: Atlas of Regional Anesthesia, ed 3, pp 135-138, 142; Morgan: Clinical Anesthesiology, ed 4, pp 350-352*).

857. **(A)** The sympathectomy produced by a celiac plexus block causes hypotension by decreasing preload to the heart. This complication can be avoided by volume loading the patient with lactated Ringer's solution. Subarachnoid injection is the most serious complication of celiac plexus block. Seizure is possible with an intravascular injection. Retroperitoneal hematoma is also possible, but extremely rare. This block frequently relieves constipation by interrupting the sympathetic fibers and leaving the parasympathetic fibers unopposed (*Barash: Clinical Anesthesia, ed 5, pp 737-738*).

858. **(E)** The occiput receives sensory innervation from the greater and lesser occipital nerves, which are terminal branches of the cervical plexus. Blockade of these nerves is usually carried out as a diagnostic step in the evaluation of head and neck pain (*Barash: Clinical Anesthesia, ed 5, p 724; Brown: Atlas of Regional Anesthesia, ed 3, p 155*).

859. **(D)** Potential complications from lumbar sympathetic block include subarachnoid injection, puncture of a major vessel (e.g., aorta) or renal pelvis, neuralgia, somatic nerve damage, perforation of a disk, infection, ejaculatory failure, and chronic back pain. Blockade of nerves arising from the lumbar plexus is possible, but given the anatomic location of the sacral plexus, blockade of an S1 nerve would be extremely unlikely if not impossible (*Brown: Atlas of Regional Anesthesia, ed 3, p 309; Raj: Practical Management of Pain, ed 3, p 678*).

860. **(D)** With the unintentional injection of an epidural dose of local anesthetic into the subarachnoid space, spinal anesthesia develops rapidly. Blockade of the sympathetic fibers (T1-L2) produces hypotension, particularly if the patient is hypovolemic. Bradycardia is produced by blocking the cardiac accelerator fibers (T1-T4). Respiratory arrest is due to hypoperfusion of the respiratory centers as well as paralysis of the phrenic nerve (C3-C5). The pupils become dilated after intrathecal injection of large quantities of local anesthetics; they will return to normal size after the block recedes. Cauda equina syndrome has occasionally developed when the epidural dose was unintentionally administered into the subarachnoid space (most commonly with chloroprocaine). If one suspects an unintentional placement of the epidural dose subarachnoid, supportive methods are initially done (the basic ABC's of resuscitation). One can also aspirate CSF from the epidural catheter (if it was inserted) to help remove some of the drug as well as reducing the pressure in the subarachnoid space, which might help better perfuse the spinal cord and decrease the chance of cauda equina syndrome developing (*Barash: Clinical Anesthesia, ed 5, p 712; Miller: Anesthesia, ed 6, pp 1660, 1676; Southorn: Reducing the potential morbidity of an unintentional spinal anaesthetic by aspirating cerebrospinal fluid, Br J Anaesth 76:467-469, 1996*).

861. **(B)** Somatic pain in the extremities is relieved with spinal anesthesia. If a patient fails to obtain pain relief despite complete sympathetic, sensory, and motor blockade, a "central" mechanism for the pain is likely or the lesion causing the pain is higher in the CNS than the level of blockade achieved by the spinal. Central pain states may include encephalization, psychogenic pain, or malingering. Persistence of pain in the lower extremities after successful spinal blockade suggests a central source or psychological source of pain (*Miller: Anesthesia, ed 6, pp 2763-2772*).

862. **(E)** During a seizure, administration of 100% O_2 helps to prevent and treat hypoxia in a patient who otherwise might not be breathing. Hyperventilation also causes cerebral vasoconstriction and decreased delivery of local anesthetic to the brain. Hyperventilation induces hypokalemia and respiratory alkalosis, both of which result in hyperpolarization of nerve membranes and elevation of the seizure threshold. Hyperventilation also raises the patient's pH (respiratory alkalosis) and converts lidocaine into the non-ionized (nonprotonated) form, which crosses the membrane more easily than the ionized form, which is detrimental (*Stoelting: Basics of Anesthesia, ed 5, p 130*).

863. **(D)** Para-aminobenzoic acid is a metabolite of the ester-type local anesthetics. Local anesthetics may be placed into two distinct categories based on their chemical structure: ester or amide. The amides, which are ropivacaine lidocaine, etidocaine, prilocaine, mepivacaine and bupivacaine, are metabolized in the liver. The ester local anesthetics are cocaine, procaine, chloroprocaine, tetracaine, and benzocaine. These drugs are metabolized by the enzyme pseudocholinesterase found in the blood. Para-aminobenzoic acid is a metabolic breakdown product of ester anesthetic and is responsible for allergic reactions in some individuals (*Stoelting: Pharmacology and Physiology in Anesthetic Practice, ed 4, pp 180-189*).

864. (E) Peripheral nerve axons are always enveloped by a Schwann cell. The myelinated nerves may be enveloped many times by the same Schwann cell. Transmission of nerve impulses (i.e., action potentials) along nonmyelinated nerves occurs in a continuous fashion, whereas transmission along myelinated nerves occurs by saltatory conduction from one node of Ranvier to the next. Myelination speeds transmission of neurological impulses; it also renders nerves more susceptible to local anesthetic blockade. An action potential is associated with an inward flux of sodium that occurs after a certain membrane threshold has been exceeded (*Miller: Anesthesia, ed 6, pp 576-579*).

865. (C) The needle insertion site for an interscalene block is C6. Local anesthetics usually spread to C5, C6 and C7 which supply much, but not all, of the cutaneous innervation to the shoulder. With low-to-moderate volume blocks there will be sparing of the (C3-C4) nerve roots, which supply some of the innervation to the anterior shoulder. Of note, C8 and T1 may also be spared, often resulting in the need for ulnar nerve supplementation if this block were used for a hand operation. Complete anesthesia for shoulder arthroscopy may require a supplemental superficial cervical plexus with use of low to moderate volumes of a local anesthetic (*Hebl: Mayo Clinic Atlas of Regional Anesthesia and Ultrasound Guided Peripheral Nerve Blockade, Chapter 9, in press*).

866. (B) Hand washing is one of the most important techniques to prevent infections especially when alcohol-based antiseptic solutions are used with sterile gloves. Although soap and water remove bacteria, they do not effectively kill organisms. Antiseptic solutions with alcohol appear better than nonalcoholic antiseptics (e.g., povidone iodine). Nail length does not appear to be a risk factor for infections, because the majority of bacterial growth occurs along the proximal 1 mm of nail adjacent to the subungual skin. Universal use of gowns and gloves does not appear to be better than gloves alone in preventing infections in ICUs and presumably is less important than adequate hand washing and use of sterile gloves (*Hebl JR: Infections complications: A new practice advisory - The importance and implications of aseptic techniques during regional anesthesia. Reg Anesth Pain Med, 31:289-290, 311-323, 2006*).

867. (A) In patients taking low-molecular weight heparin, or LMWH (e.g., enoxaparin, dalteparin, tinzaparin), caution should be exercised before proceeding with an epidural or spinal anesthetic because of the risk of producing an epidural or spinal hematoma. The amount of time between the last dose of the LMWH and the relative safety of starting a central neuraxial block depends on the dose of the LMWH. At the lower doses, used for thromboprophylaxis, the LMWH should be held at least 10 to 12 hours prior to the block. At the higher doses, used to treat an established DVT, one should wait at least 24 hours after the last dose of LMWH prior to the block (*Barash: Clinical Anesthesia, ed 5, p 713; Miller: Anesthesia, ed 6, pp 1677, 2742-2743; Second Consensus Conference on Neuraxial Anesthesia and Anticoagulation, April 25-28, 2002, www.asra.com/consensus-statements/2.html*).

868. (C) Patients taking nonsteroidal anti-inflammatory drugs (NSAIDs), ticlopidine and clopidogrel, exert effects on platelet function. Nonsteroidal anti-inflammatory drugs (NSAIDs) are not a problem if given alone before epidural or spinal anesthesia. But patients taking ticlopidine should wait 14 days and patients taking clopidogrel should wait 7 days before having a neuraxial block placed, because of the increased risk of spinal hematoma formation. Keep in mind that caution is always needed and the ASRA statement of "Careful preoperative assessment of the patient to identify alterations of health that might contribute to bleeding is crucial" is important (*Barash: Clinical Anesthesia, ed 5, p 713; Second Consensus Conference on Neuraxial Anesthesia and Anticoagulation, April 25-28, 2002, www.asra.com/consensus-statements/2.html*).

869. (E) Adding sodium bicarbonate to local anesthetic solutions hastens the onset of action of the local anesthetics, especially when the local anesthetic solution contains epinephrine (which is produced at a lower pH). By raising the pH, more of the local anesthetic is in the non-ionized, more lipid-soluble state. Raising the pH too much (i.e., >6.05-8) would cause precipitation of the local anesthetic. It also seems to decrease pain with skin infiltration. Pain on injection can also be decreased by a slow injection of the local anesthetic (*Barash: Clinical Anesthesia, ed 5, p 460; Miller: Anesthesia, ed 6, p 585*).

870.   **(D)**

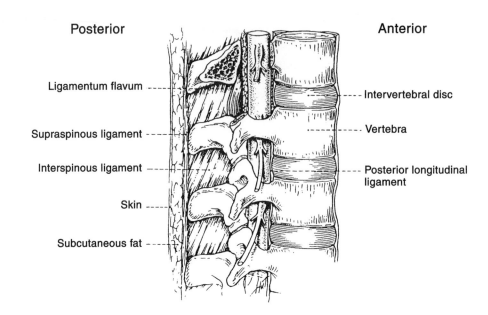

Posterior — Anterior

Ligamentum flavum

Supraspinous ligament

Interspinous ligament

Skin

Subcutaneous fat

Intervertebral disc

Vertebra

Posterior longitudinal ligament

This figure shows the anatomic structures that must be traversed by the spinal needle during performance of a subarachnoid block. The structures include the skin, subcutaneous tissue, supraspinous ligament, interspinous ligament, the ligamentum flavum, and finally the dura (posterior). If you were to continue to advance the spinal needle, you would encounter the dura (anteriorly) while exiting the subarachnoid space, the posterior longitudinal ligament, the periosteum of the vertebral body, and finally, bone (*Cousins: Neural Blockade in Clinical Anesthesia and Management of Pain, ed 3, p 205*).

871.   **(D)**   In the epidural space, bupivacaine is four times more potent than lidocaine, so 0.5% bupivacaine is similar to 2% lidocaine. The duration of the bupivacaine block will be longer because bupivacaine has a long duration of action and lidocaine has an intermediate duration of action (*Barash: Clinical Anesthesia, ed 5, pp 459-463*).

872.   **(E)**   Drugs with α-agonist activity (phenylephrine/epinephrine) possess some analgesic activity but less than narcotics and local anesthetics. In addition, intrathecal epinephrine will reduce systemic/vascular uptake of local anesthetics, thereby enhancing their effects, including hypotension. Clonidine alone, when administered neuraxially, is an effective analgesic. Neostigmine has some mild analgesia properties but experience is limited. Opioids added to the spinal solution enhance surgical anesthesia and provide postoperative pain. Fentanyl 25 μg is commonly added for short surgical procedures (outpatient) whereas morphine can be used when longer postoperative analgesia is desired for inpatients (*Morgan: Clinical Anesthesiology, ed 4, p 309; Stoelting: Basics of Anesthesia, ed 5, p 256*).

873.   **(B)**   For topical anesthesia, lidocaine, tetracaine, dibucaine and benzocaine are effective, as well as the combination of lidocaine and prilocaine or EMLA cream. For intravenous regional anesthesia or Bier blocks, many drugs have been used. Ester local anesthetics are not used for IV regional blocks because they can be broken down in the blood stream (by plasma ester hydrolysis) which can shorten the drug's duration of action and can also cause thrombophlebitis of the vein (reported with chloroprocaine). Because cardiovascular collapse has been reported with bupivacaine, and would likely also occur with etidocaine and ropivacaine, if the tourniquet unintentionally is released while the block is setting up, they are not used for intravenous regional anesthesia. Lidocaine and prilocaine are used for Bier blocks because of their relative safety. For infiltrative anesthesia, all local anesthetics can be used. All local anesthetics can be used in the epidural space, although procaine and tetracaine are rarely used (procaine has a slow onset and tetracaine has marked motor block) (*Miller: Anesthesia, ed 6, pp 586-591; Stoelting: Basics of Anesthesia, ed 5, p 127*).

874.   **(A)**   Procaine and 2-chloroprocaine have a short duration of action; lidocaine, mepivacaine and prilocaine have an intermediate duration of action; etidocaine, bupivacaine, levobupivacaine, tetracaine and ropivacaine have a long duration of action. For similar sensory anesthesia, a higher concentration of local anesthetic is needed for the short duration of local anesthetics compared with both the intermediate and long duration agents, because they are less potent (*Barash: Clinical Anesthesia, ed 5, pp 705-707; Miller: Anesthesia, ed 6, pp 1674-1675*).

875. **(B)** A change in the T-wave amplitude of 25 percent, an increase in heart rate of 10 beats per minutes, or systolic blood pressure greater than 15 mm Hg is considered a positive response to an epinephrine containing local anesthetic solution. A slight drop in heart rate may result if the block is properly performed and no intravascular injection occurs (*Motoyama: Smith's Anesthesia for Infants and Children, ed 7, p 464*).

876. **(E)** All of the choices listed are potential complications of stellate ganglion blockade except an increase in heart rate. The stellate ganglion supplies sympathetic fibers to the upper extremity and head and some to the heart. Loss of the cardiac acceleratory fibers may slow the heart rate, not speed it up. Other potential complications of stellate ganglion blockade include accidental injection of the local anesthetic into a vertebral artery resulting in seizure and inadvertent cervical epidural (*Barash: Clinical Anesthesia, ed 5, pp 736-737*).

877. **(D)** A total of 60 mL of 0.5% bupivacaine with epinephrine (1:200,000) was used. A 0.5% solution = 0.5 g in 100 mL of fluid = 500 mg/100 mL = 5 mg/mL. A 1:200,000 solution means 1 gram in 200,000 mL = 1000 mg/200,000 mL = 1 mg/200 mL = 1000 µg/200 mL = 5 µg/mL. Therefore 60 mL of 0.5% bupivacaine with 1:200,000 epinephrine contains 60 mL × 5 mg/mL or 300 mg bupivacaine and 60 mL × 5 µg/mL or 300 µg of epinephrine. For a major nerve block the maximum recommended dose with epinephrine (1:200,000) is 500 mg for lidocaine and mepivacaine, 600 mg with prilocaine, and 225 mg with bupivacaine. Epinephrine is used in the local anesthetic to check for intravascular injection of the incremental doses and is not contraindicated but should be used for this block (*Miller: Anesthesia, ed 6, p 588*).

878. **(A)** Post dural puncture headaches (spinal headaches) usually develop within 12 to 48 hours after a dural puncture, but may develop immediately or take months to develop. The most characteristic symptom is a postural component where the headache occurs in the upright position and is usually completely gone when the patient is in the supine position. The headache is typically frontal and/or occipital in location. Other symptoms include nausea, vomiting, anorexia, visual disturbances (blurred vision, double vision, photophobia) and occasionally hearing loss (routinely found with auditory testing) (*Stoelting: Basics of Anesthesia, ed 5, p 878*).

879. **(D)** Ipsilateral phrenic nerve block with diaphragmatic paralysis occurs is virtually 100% of patients receiving an interscalene block. This produces a 25% reduction in pulmonary function, making this block a contraindication in patients with borderline pulmonary function. Blockage of the recurrent laryngeal nerve can occur but is rare; however, if the patient has contralateral vocal cord palsy and develops a recurrent laryngeal nerve block, complete airway obstruction can occur. With this block, the inferior trunk of the brachial plexus where the ulnar nerve is derived may be spared (*Miller: Anesthesia, ed 6, p 1688; Stoelting: Basics of Anesthesia, ed 5, pp 276-278*).

880. **(A)** Five nerves are blocked when performing an ankle block. The saphenous, superficial peroneal, and sural nerves are all sensory below the ankle and electrical stimulation would have no effect. Stimulation of the posterior tibial nerve causes flexion of the toes by stimulating the flexor digitorum brevis muscles and abduction of the first toe by stimulating the abductor hallucis muscles. The posterior tibial nerve also is sensory to most of the plantar part of the foot. Stimulation of the deep peroneal nerve causes extension of the toes by stimulating the extensor digitorum brevis muscles. The deep peroneal nerve has a small sensory branch for the first interdigital cleft. From the practical standpoint, many anesthesiologists perform a purely infiltration block of these nerves. If a nerve stimulator is used, it is mainly used to find the posterior tibial nerve, which can be hard to anesthetize if small volumes of local anesthetic are administered. The posterior tibial nerve can be difficult to stimulate in diabetics with diabetic neuropathy (*Loeser: Bonica's Management of Pain, ed 3, pp 1614-1627*).

881. **(B)** The motor responses include: arm flexion at the elbow (musculocutaneous nerve), arm extension at the elbow (radial nerve), forearm pronation, wrist flexion and thumb opposition (median nerve), ulnar deviation of the wrist, little finger flexion, thumb adduction and flaring of the fingers (ulnar nerve), wrist and finger extension (radial nerve). The sensory response (includes some variations) is: back of the arm, forearm and radial side dorsal side of the hand (radial nerve), skin of the lateral forearm (musculocutaneous nerve), ulnar side of the hand and both surfaces of the ulnar one and one-half fingers (ulnar nerve), the radial side of the palm of the hand as well as the dorsal aspect of the radial three and one-half fingers (median nerve). To evaluate the setup of a brachial plexus block, a common technique is to perform the four P's (*Push, Pull, Pinch, Pinch*). Have the patient push or extend the forearm (radial), pull or flex the forearm (musculocutaneous nerve), pinch the index or second finger (median nerve), pinch the little finger (ulnar nerve) (*Brown: Atlas of Regional Anesthesia, ed 3, pp 27-35; Neal JM, et al. Upper Extremity Regional Anesthesia - Essentials of Our Current Understanding, 2008. Reg Anesth Pain Med 34:134-170, 2009*).

882. **(C)** Unilateral numbness or paresthesia in the upper extremity during extension of the neck usually represents nerve root impingement at the vertebral foramina. Specifically, unilateral degenerative changes restrict the foramen to such a degree that it compresses and irritates the nerve root traversing the vertebral foramen when the head is extended. Treatment ranges from NSAIDs, to steroids and may require surgical intervention if there is muscle weakness (*Stoelting: Basics of Anesthesia, ed 5, p 249; Miller: Anesthesia, ed 6, p 1687*).

883. **(D)** Although a successful interscalene block causes ipsilateral phrenic nerve paralysis in almost 100% of patients, identifying the phrenic nerve means you are anterior to the brachial plexus and you should reposition your needle. You should redirect the needle in a posterior direction (*Barash: Clinical Anesthesia, ed 5, pp 726-728; Miller: Anesthesia, ed 6, pp 1686-1689*).

884. **(D)** With an intravascular injection, the main symptoms would most likely be CNS toxicity (e.g., seizures) as blood flow is directly to the brain. The Bezold-Jarish reflex (hypotension and bradycardia) has been reported in awake, sitting patients undergoing shoulder surgery with an interscalene block. This maybe related to intra-cardiac mechanoreceptors being stimulated by the decreased venous return in the sitting position. This leads to decreased sympathetic tone and increased parasympathetic tone. Breathing is still present with this reflex. Block of the stellate ganglion would produce a Horner's syndrome, which is not associated with breathing abnormalities. Injection into the intrathecal space is uncommon, but possible, especially if the needle is not pointed in the caudal direction, and would lead to a total spinal block with little local anesthetic injected (e.g., hypotension, bradycardia respiratory paralysis that would lead to cyanosis) (*Barash: Clinical Anesthesia, ed 5, pp 726-728; Miller: Anesthesia, ed 6, pp 1686-1689*).

885. **(C)** The pipecoloxylidide local anesthetics (mepivacaine, bupivacaine, ropivacaine and levobupivacaine) are chiral drugs, which means they have an asymmetric carbon atom (i.e., have a left- or S and a right- or R hand configuration). Mepivacaine and bupivacaine are racemic mixtures (50% S: 50% R mixture). The pure S forms show reduced neurotoxicity and reduced cardiotoxicity (e.g., ropivacaine and levobupivacaine). Lidocaine is an achiral compound (i.e., has no chiral carbon atom) (*Barash: Clinical Anesthesia, ed 5, p 458; Stoelting: Pharmacology and Physiology in Anesthetic Practice, ed 4, pp 180-181*).

886. **(A)** Nerves to the lower extremity emerge from the L2 to S3 nerve roots. The upper roots (mainly L2-L4) form the lumbar plexus which gives rise to the femoral, obturator, and lateral femoral cutaneous nerves. A branch from the lumbar plexus along with the sacral plexus gives rise to the sciatic nerve. Branches of the sciatic nerve include the common peroneal (branches to make the superficial and deep) and the tibial, and the sural nerves (*Barash: Clinical Anesthesia, ed 5, pp 739-740; Miller: Anesthesia, ed 6, pp 1695-1696*).

887. **(E)** Anesthetic-related nerve injuries to the brachial plexus are rare and poorly understood. The only way to minimize nerve injury is to minimize trauma to neural fibers. Although ultrasound-guided technique is promising, currently there is no clinical evidence for this (*Neal JM, et al. Upper extremity regional anesthesia - Essentials of our current understanding, 2008. Reg Anesth Pain Med, 34:134-170, 2009*).

888. **(C)** Local anesthetic toxicity is a multisystem phenomenon, but the most crucial manifestation involves the heart (atrioventricular conduction block, arrhythmias, myocardial depression, and cardiac arrest). In isolated cardiac tissue hypercarbia, acidosis and hypoxia will augment the negative inotropic and chronotropic effects of bupivacaine. In the event of seizure and ventricular fibrillation, hypercarbia and hypotension would cause a severe acidosis and hypoxia, which would potentiate the toxicity of bupivacaine. To reduce these cardiotoxic effects, the initial resuscitation efforts are aimed at maximizing oxygen delivery, increasing tissue perfusion and ventilation. This is accomplished through chest compressions, assisted ventilation with oxygen, intravenous sodium bicarbonate, and inotropic and chronotropic support with pharmacological agents such as atropine, epinephrine, dopamine, and dobutamine. Standard cardiopulmonary resuscitation may not be successful in some cases, and placement of the patient on cardiopulmonary bypass may be necessary. Recently, lipid infusions have been shown to reduce the toxicity of intravascularly injected bupivacaine. Propofol is formulated as a lipid emulsion, and as such would bind bupivacaine to some degree, but this effect would be overshadowed by the substantial cardiac depressant of the anesthetic (*Miller: Anesthesia, ed 5, pp 592-596, 1731-1732*).

889. **(E)** When performing an interscalene block, the needle is usually placed at the line extending lateral to the cricoid cartilage that intersects the interscalene groove at the C6 level. The needle in inserted in a slightly posterior and a 45° caudad direction. The caudad direction is used to decrease the chance of injecting the local anesthetic into the vertebral artery, or obtaining a spinal or epidural block. The phrenic nerve is routinely blocked (100% of the time) and occasionally the recurrent laryngeal nerve is blocked (*Stoelting: Basics of Anesthesia, ed 5, pp 276-278; Miller: Anesthesia, ed 6, pp 1686-1689*).

890. (E) Epidural hematomas are rare complications of spinal anesthesia (1:200,000) and epidural anesthesia (1:150,000). However, in the presence of LMWH the incidence is much higher: 1:40,000 with spinal anesthesia and 1:3000 with continuous epidural catheter. Clinical symptoms include radicular back pain, bowel and bladder dysfunction, sensory or motor deficits. An MRI is the diagnostic test of choice and prompt decompressive laminectomy is the treatment of choice (*Fleischer: Anesthesia and Uncommon Diseases, ed 5, p 573*).

891. (D) Peripheral nerves are classified according to the fiber size and physiologic properties such as the presence or absence of myelin, conduction velocity, location, and function. Type A fibers range in diameter from 1 to 22 μm, are myelinated, and have moderate-to-fast conduction velocities. These fibers are subclassified into four groups based on their location and function. Type A-alpha and A-beta fibers provide motor and proprioception function to muscles and joints; type A-gamma fibers innervate muscle spindles and provide for muscle tone; and type A-delta fibers provide pain, temperature and touch sensation. Type B fibers are preganglionic sympathetic nerves that are less than 3 μm in diameter, myelinated, and have medium conduction velocities. Type C fibers are postganglionic sympathetic nerves that are very small in diameter, are not myelinated, and have slow conduction velocities. Type C fibers are also afferent sensory nerves involved in pain, temperature, and touch (*Miller: Anesthesia, ed 6, p 577*).

892. (C) Overdose of intrathecal opiates would not be a sign of an intradural mass lesion. Granulomas at the tip of intrathecal catheters used with intrathecal drug delivery systems are gaining increased attention. Granulomas are more frequently associated with high concentrations and doses of either morphine (>10 mg/day) or hydromorphone (>10 mg/day). Most patients who will develop granulomas receive the intrathecal medications for more than 6 months. Presenting symptoms may include loss of drug effect, new pain or paresthesias or neurologic deficits. Patients should be routinely screened for signs and symptoms of granuloma formation at scheduled intrathecal pump refill appointments. Suspicious cases should undergo prompt diagnostic imaging and consideration of neurosurgical consultation (*Barash: Clinical Anesthesia, ed 5, p 1468*).

893. (A). In addition to benzocaine, tetracaine and lidocaine can also be used as topical anesthetics. Pseudocholinesterase, the enzyme responsible for the metabolism of succinylcholine, metabolizes all of the ester local anesthetics, benzocaine, procaine, chloroprocaine and tetracaine. Benzocaine does promote the formation of methemoglobin, but is not alone in that regard since prilocaine also causes formation of methemoglobin. The pKa of benzocaine is 3.5, which qualifies it as a weak acid and as such exists in uncharged at physiologic pH. All other local anesthetic pKa's are higher than 7.4, meaning that some fraction of them exists in the protonated form (*Stoelting: Basics of Anesthesia, ed 5, p 127; Stoelting: Pharmacology and Physiology in Anesthetic Practice, ed 4, p 187*).

894. (D) The un-ionized form of the local anesthetic traverses the nerve membrane whereas the ionized form actually blocks conduction. About three nodes of Ranvier must be blocked to achieve anesthesia. The ability of a local anesthetic to block conduction is inversely proportional to the diameter of the fiber. The presence of myelin enhances the ability of a local anesthetic to block conduction, as does rapid firing. The local anesthetic blocks nerve transmission by inhibiting the voltage-gated sodium ion channels (*Stoelting: Basics of Anesthesia, ed 5, pp 124-128*).

895. (D) Postdural puncture headaches (PDPHs) typically appear within 12 to 48 hours of a dural puncture but may be immediate and occasionally have become delayed for several days or months after a dural puncture. The headaches are characterized by dull or throbbing frontal or occipital pain, which worsens with sitting and improves with reclining. Postspinal headaches may be associated with neurologic symptoms such as diplopia, tinnitus, and reduced hearing acuity. Very rarely, a subdural hematoma will develop. The etiology of postspinal headaches is believed to be caused by a reduction in CSF pressure and resulting tension on meningeal vessels and nerves (which results from leakage of CSF through the needle hole in the dura mater). Factors associated with an increased incidence of postspinal headaches include pregnancy, size and type of needle used to perform the block (larger needles and Quincke more common than smaller needles and Whitacre or Sprotte), and the number of dural punctures. They occur more frequently in young adults compared with children and the elderly. Conservative therapy for a postspinal headache includes bed rest, analgesics, and oral and intravenous hydration. If conservative therapy is not successful after 24 to 48 hours, an epidural "blood patch" with 10 to 20 mL of the patient's blood can be performed. An epidural "blood patch" usually provides prompt relief of the postspinal headache (*Stoelting: Basics of Anesthesia, ed 5, pp 260-261*).

896. (C)   When inserting a spinal cord stimulator, a 15 gauge needle is advanced into the epidural space via the paramedian approach. After confirmation of proper needle placement with AP and lateral fluoroscopic views, the stimulation electrode is passed through the needle and threaded to the desired vertebral level. The needle is then removed and the leads attached to the external programmer. Transcutaneous electrical nerve stimulation (TENS) unit electrodes are applied to the skin. With nucleoplasty, intradiskal electro-thermal therapy and annuloplasty, the needle is inserted to access the intervertebral disk (*Stoelting: Basics of Anesthesia, ed 5, pp 633-637*).

897. (A)   Many drugs have been used to treat neuropathic pain, including analgesics (NSAIDs and opioids), first-generation antiepileptic drugs (e.g., carbamazepine and phenytoin), second-generation antiepileptic drugs (e.g., gabapentin, pregabalin), topical agents (e.g., lidocaine, capsaicin), antiarrhythmics (e.g., mexiletine), tricyclic antidepressants (e.g., amitriptyline, nortriptyline, desipramine) as well as other antidepressants (e.g., duloxetine, venlafaxine). Duloxetine (Cymbalta) is a selective serotonin and norepinephrine reuptake inhibitor (SNRI) that is used for major depressive disorders, generalized anxiety disorders, fibromyalgia and diabetic peripheral neuropathic pain. Mexiletine is an orally effective amine analogue of lidocaine and may be effective in decreasing neuropathic pain when other drugs have failed. Gabapentin, a structural analogue of GABA, works by increasing the synthesis of the inhibitory neurotransmitter GABA. Tramadol is an opioid agonist that has moderate activity at the μ receptor and weak activity at the ϰ and δ opioid receptors. In addition, tramadol enhances the spinal inhibitory pathways by inhibiting the neuronal uptake of norepinephrine and serotonin as well as presynaptic stimulation of serotonin release. Carbamazepine (Tegretol) is an anticonvulsant with specific analgesic properties for trigeminal neuralgia. Carbamazepine seems to reduce polysynaptic responses by an unknown mechanism (*Cousins: Neural Blockade in Clinical Anesthesia and Pain Medicine, ed 4, p 1065; Morgan: Clinical Anesthesiology, ed 4, pp 405-406; Physicians Desk Reference 2009, ed 63, pp 1801-1810, 3019-3022; Stoelting: Pharmacology and Physiology in Anesthetic Practice, ed 4, pp 117, 378-379, 575*).

898. (E)   899. (B)   900. (A)   901. (C)

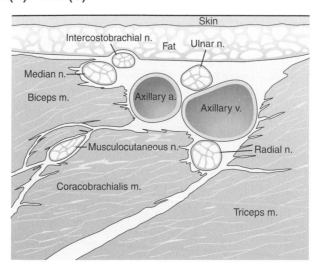

902. (A)   903. (B)   904 (E)   905. (D)   906. (C)

In the normal adult, breathing and coughing can be done exclusively by the diaphragm, which is innervated by the phrenic nerve (C3-C5). The heart rate is dependent upon intrinsic pacemaker activity of the SA node, which can be affected by the autonomic nervous systems sympathetic nervous systems cardiac accelerator fibers (T1-T4) as well as the parasympathetic nervous systems vagus nerve (cranial nerve 10). The first stage of labor pain is related to uterine contractions and dilation of the cervix (T10-L1). The second stage of labor is related to both uterine pain (T10-L1), as well as birth canal pain which is supplied by the pudendal nerves (S2-S4). The greater splanchnic (T5-T9) and the lesser splanchnic (T10-T12) nerves supply sympathetic fibers to the celiac plexus which inhibits much of the gastrointestinal tract (*Barash: Clinical Anesthesia, ed 5, pp 278-279, 790, 1158*).

907. (E)   908. (C)   909. (D)   910. (B)   911. (A)   912. (A)   913. (D)   914. (E)

When an awake intubation is needed, local anesthetics can be applied topically or by injection. Innervation of the airway includes the glossopharyngeal nerve, cranial nerve XI, and branches of the vagus nerve (internal and external branches of the superior laryngeal nerve and the recurrent laryngeal nerve). The glossopharyngeal nerve provides sensory innervation of the posterior one third of the tongue, the vallecula and the anterior surface of the epiglottis (lingual branch), the pharyngeal walls (pharyngeal branch) and the tonsils (tonsillar branch). With the exception of the cricothyroid muscle, the recurrent laryngeal nerve of the vagus provides motor innervation of all the intrinsic muscles of the larynx. The cricothyroid muscle is supplied by the external branch of the superior laryngeal nerve of the vagus. The sensory innervation of the mucosa of the larynx down to the vocal folds comes from the internal branch of the superior laryngeal nerve of the vagus, and the sensory innervation of the mucosa of the larynx below the vocal folds comes from the recurrent laryngeal nerve of the vagus. The muscles of the pharynx are supplied through the pharyngeal plexus from motor fibers from the eleventh cranial nerve (accessory nerve) (*Barash: Clinical Anesthesia, ed 5, pp 622-623; Brown: Atlas of Regional Anesthesia, ed 3, pp 207-222*).

Chapter 11

Cardiovascular Physiology and Anesthesia

915. A 67-year-old man is to undergo a radical retropubic prostatectomy. He has aortic stenosis with a gradient of 37 mm Hg at rest. He has an allergy to penicillin. Which of the following is the best regimen for subacute bacterial endocarditis (SBE) prophylaxis in this patient?
   A. Ampicillin and gentamicin
   B. Vancomycin and gentamicin
   C. Clindamycin and gentamicin
   D. Clindamycin alone
   E. None of the above

916. A 68-year-old patient is undergoing elective coronary revascularization. Just before cardiopulmonary bypass, the hemoglobin concentration is 8.3 g/dL and platelet count is 253,000/mm^3. After cardiopulmonary bypass is initiated, the patient is cooled to 20° C and 2 units of packed red blood cells (RBCs) are transfused because of bleeding. During bypass, the anesthesiologist notices that the platelet count is 10,000/mm^3 and the hemoglobin concentration is 8 g/dL. The most likely cause of thrombocytopenia is
   A. Sequestration
   B. Hemolytic transfusion reaction
   C. Dilutional thrombocytopenia
   D. Disseminated intravascular coagulation
   E. Heparin-induced thrombocytopenia

917. Which of the following is the most sensitive indicator of left ventricular myocardial ischemia?
   A. Wall-motion abnormalities on the echocardiogram
   B. ST-segment changes in lead V5 of the electrocardiogram (ECG)
   C. Appearance of V waves on the pulmonary capillary wedge pressure tracing
   D. Elevation of the pulmonary capillary wedge pressure
   E. Decrease in cardiac output as measured by the thermodilution technique

918. Oxygen consumption (VO_2) is measured in a 70-kg subject on a treadmill at 2500 mL per minute. This corresponds to:
   A. 1 metabolic equivalent (MET)
   B. 5 METs
   C. 10 METs
   D. 15 METs
   E. 20 METs

919. Accidental injection of air into a peripheral vein would be **LEAST** likely to result in arterial air embolism in a patient with which of the following anatomic cardiac defects?

A. Patent ductus arteriosus
B. Eisenmenger's syndrome
C. Teratology of Fallot
D. Pulmonary atresia with ventricular septal defect
E. Tricuspid atresia

920. Each of the following could be placed on the x-axis of the curve shown in the figure **EXCEPT**

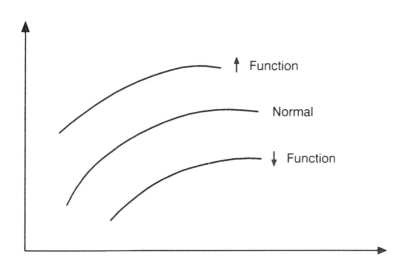

A. Stroke volume
B. Left ventricular end-diastolic pressure
C. Left ventricular end-diastolic volume
D. Left atrial pressure
E. Pulmonary artery occlusion pressure

921. The ECG rhythm strip below represents

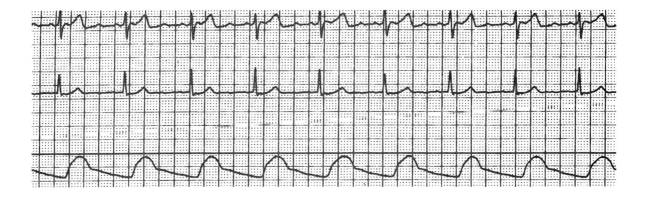

A. Atrial flutter
B. Third-degree heart block
C. Sinus tachycardia second-degree heart block
D. Malfunctioning DDD pacemaker
E. Junctional rhythm

922. A 71-year-old man is undergoing revascularization of three coronary vessels on cardiopulmonary bypass at 28° C. After the first graft is sewn into the aorta, the arterial pressure measured from a left radial artery is 47 mm Hg and the pulmonary artery pressure is 6 mm Hg. Thirty minutes later, the arterial pressure is 52 mm Hg and pulmonary artery pressure is 31 mm Hg. The most likely explanation for this is
   A. Malposition of the aortic cannula
   B. Malposition of the venous cannula
   C. Faulty ventricular venting
   D. Bypass associated sympathetic nervous system stimulation
   E. Pulmonary artery catheter migration

923. A 78-year-old patient is anesthetized for right hemicolectomy with isoflurane and nitrous oxide. Vecuronium is administered to facilitate muscle relaxation. At the end of the operation, the neuromuscular blockade is reversed with neostigmine 4 mg and glycopyrrolate 0.8 mg. The rhythm below is noted shortly after administration of these drugs. The patient's blood pressure is 90/60. The most appropriate course of action at this point is

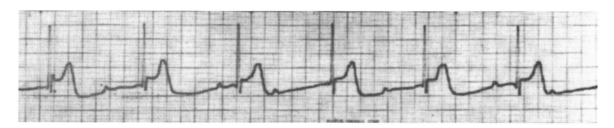

   A. DC cardioversion
   B. Isoproterenol drip
   C. Atropine
   D. Transcutaneous pacemaker
   E. Begin chest compressions

924. While on cardiopulmonary bypass during elective coronary artery revascularization, the patient is noted to have bulging sclerae. Mean arterial pressure is 50 mm Hg, temperature is 28° C, and there is no ECG activity. The most appropriate action to take at this time is to
   A. Administer mannitol, 50 gm IV
   B. Administer furosemide, 20 mg IV
   C. Decrease the cardiac index
   D. Check the position of the aortic cannula
   E. Check the position of the venous return cannula

925. Which of the following correctly describes the effect of transposition of the great vessels on the rate of induction of anesthesia?
   A. Inhalation induction is faster than normal; intravenous induction is slower than normal
   B. Inhalation induction is slower than normal; intravenous induction is faster than normal
   C. Both inhalation and intravenous induction are faster than normal
   D. Both inhalation and intravenous induction are slower than normal
   E. Inhalation induction is normal; intravenous induction is faster than normal

926. Anastomosis of the right atrium to the pulmonary artery (Fontan procedure) is a useful surgical treatment for each of the following congenital cardiac defects **EXCEPT**
   A. Tricuspid atresia
   B. Hypoplastic left heart syndrome
   C. Pulmonary valve stenosis
   D. Truncus arteriosus
   E. Pulmonary artery atresia

927. By what percentage is tissue metabolic rate reduced during cardiopulmonary bypass at 30° C?
   A. 10%
   B. 25%
   C. 50%
   D. 75%
   E. 90%

928. Effective inflation of an intra-aortic balloon catheter should occur at which of the following times?
   A. Immediately after P wave on ECG
   B. Immediately after closure of aortic valve
   C. During opening of the aortic valve
   D. During systolic upstroke on arterial tracing
   E. At midpoint of QRS complex

929. Afterload reduction is beneficial during anesthesia for noncardiac surgery in patients with each of the following conditions **EXCEPT**
   A. Aortic insufficiency
   B. Mitral regurgitation
   C. Tetralogy of Fallot
   D. Congestive heart failure
   E. Patent ductus arteriosus

930. Administration of protamine to a patient who has not received heparin can result in
   A. Anticoagulation
   B. Hypercoagulation
   C. Profound bradycardia
   D. Seizure
   E. Hypertension

931. The primary determinants of myocardial O_2 consumption, from most to least important, are
   A. Preload > afterload > heart rate
   B. Heart rate > preload > afterload
   C. Afterload > preload > heart rate
   D. Heart rate > afterload > preload
   E. Afterload > heart rate > preload

932. Cardiac tamponade is associated with
   A. Pulsus alternans
   B. Pulsus tardus
   C. Pulsus parvus
   D. Pulsus paradoxus
   E. Bisferiens pulse

933. Which of the following drugs should **NOT** be administered via an endotracheal tube?
   A. Lidocaine
   B. $NaHCO_3$
   C. Atropine
   D. Naloxone
   E. Epinephrine

934. The mean arterial pressure in a patient with a blood pressure of 180/60 mm Hg is
   A. 90 mm Hg
   B. 100 mm Hg
   C. 110 mm Hg
   D. 120 mm Hg
   E. 130 mm Hg

935. Hypothyroidism and hyperthyroidism could develop in patients receiving which of the following antidysrhythmic drugs?
- **A.** Amiodarone
- **B.** Verapamil
- **C.** Phenytoin
- **D.** Lidocaine
- **E.** Procainamide

936. Calculate the systemic vascular resistance (in dynes/sec/cm^{-5}) from the following data: cardiac output 5.0 L/min, central venous pressure 8 mm Hg, mean arterial blood pressure 86 mm Hg, mean pulmonary arterial blood pressure 20 mm Hg, pulmonary capillary wedge pressure 9 mm Hg, heart rate 85 beats/min, patient weight 100 kg.
- **A.** 750
- **B.** 1000
- **C.** 1250
- **D.** 1500
- **E.** Cannot be calculated

937. Which of the following is **NOT** included in tetralogy of Fallot?
- **A.** Patent ductus arteriosus
- **B.** Right ventricular hypertrophy
- **C.** Ventricular septal defect
- **D.** Overriding aorta
- **E.** Pulmonic stenosis

938. A 65-year-old female patient with sepsis is undergoing an emergency exploratory laparotomy. After induction of anesthesia and tracheal intubation, the patient's blood pressure is noted to be 65 systolic with a heart rate of 120 beats/min. Cardiac output determined by a thermodilution pulmonary artery catheter is 13 L/min. Of the following vasopressors the **LEAST** appropriate choice would be
- **A.** Dobutamine
- **B.** Dopamine
- **C.** Norepinephrine
- **D.** Epinephrine
- **E.** Phenylephrine

939. Characteristics of ß$_2$ stimulation include each of the following **EXCEPT**
- **A.** Inhibition of insulin secretion
- **B.** Glycogenolysis
- **C.** Gluconeogenesis
- **D.** Renin secretion
- **E.** Uterine relaxation

940. A 61-year-old male patient with hypertropic cardiomyopathy is scheduled for left ventricular myectomy under general anesthesia. Which of the following anesthetics would provide the most stable hemodynamics in this patient?
- **A.** N$_2$O-narcotic
- **B.** Ketamine
- **C.** Halothane
- **D.** Sevoflurane
- **E.** Isoflurane

941. A healthy 59-year-old, 60-kg woman with a normal preoperative ECG develops wide complex tachycardia under general anesthesia for breast biopsy. Blood pressure is 81/47 mm Hg and heart rate is 220 beats/min and regular. The most appropriate therapy would be
- **A.** Electrical cardioversion
- **B.** Administration of lidocaine, 60 mg IV
- **C.** Administration of procainamide, 20 mg/min IV
- **D.** Administration of amiodarone, 300 mg IV
- **E.** Adenosine, 6 mg IV

942. Although ß-adrenergic receptor blockade is the best treatment for reentrant tachydysrhythmia associated with Romano-Ward syndrome, these dysrhythmias can also be effectively treated with
   A. Lidocaine
   B. Procainamide
   C. Quinidine
   D. Left stellate ganglion blockade
   E. Right stellate ganglion blockade

943. A 64-year-old patient with an axial flow left ventricular assist device (HeartMate II, Jarvik 2000) is scheduled for laparoscopic cholecystectomy under general anesthesia. Monitoring which of the following parameters is likely to be difficult in this patient?
   A. Blood pressure with blood pressure cuff
   B. Blood pressure with arterial line
   C. Pulmonary artery pressure with pulmonary artery (PA) catheter
   D. Temperature with esophageal temperature probe
   E. End tidal isoflurane concentration with mass spectrometer

944. In a normal person, what percentage of the cardiac output is dependent on the "atrial kick"?
   A. 25%
   B. 35%
   C. 45%
   D. 55%
   E. 65%

945. This arterial waveform is consistent with

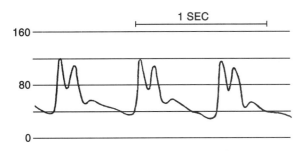

   A. Aortic regurgitation
   B. Aortic stenosis
   C. Cardiac tamponade
   D. Hypovolemia
   E. Severe diastolic dysfunction

946. A 1-year-old child with tetralogy of Fallot is to undergo elective repair of a left inguinal hernia under general anesthesia. Which of the following anesthetics would provide the most stable hemodynamics in this patient?
   A. Sevoflurane and N_2O
   B. Isoflurane and N_2O
   C. Desflurane and oxygen
   D. Fentanyl and N_2O
   E. Ketamine

947.   The left ventricular pressure-volume loop shown in the figure depicts

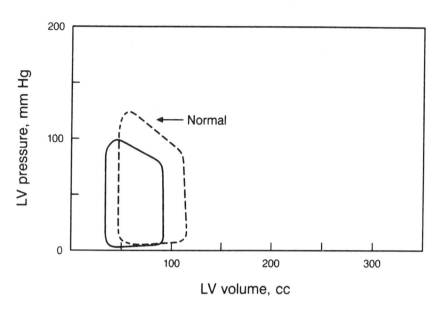

A. Mitral stenosis
B. Mitral regurgitation
C. Aortic stenosis
D. Acute aortic insufficiency
E. Chronic aortic insufficiency

948.   A 54-year-old patient is undergoing a three-vessel coronary artery bypass graft under general anesthesia. After induction, the pulmonary capillary wedge pressure is 15 mm Hg and pulmonary artery pressures are 26/13 mm Hg. Suddenly, new 30-mm Hg V waves appear on the monitor screen. Systemic blood pressure is 120/70 mm Hg, heart rate is 75 beats/min, and pulmonary artery pressure is 50/35 mm Hg. Which of the following drugs should be administered to the patient?
A. Nitroglycerin
B. Nitroprusside
C. Esmolol
D. Phenylephrine
E. Dobutamine

949.   A 62-year-old patient scheduled for elective repair of an abdominal aortic aneurysm develops a wide complex regular tachycardia (heart rate 150) during induction of anesthesia. Blood pressure is 110/78. Which of the following drugs would be most useful in the management of this dysrhythmia?
A. Lidocaine, 100 mg IV
B. Amiodarone, 150 mg IV over 10 minutes
C. Adenosine, 6 mg rapidly over 3 seconds
D. Verapamil, 5 to 10 mg IV
E. Esmolol, 35 mg IV

950.   Under maximum stress, how much cortisol is produced per day?
A. 50 mg
B. 150 mg
C. 250 mg
D. 350 mg
E. Up to 1000 mg

951. A VVI pacemaker programmed to pace at a rate of 70 beats/min is noted on the preoperative ECG to pace at 61 beats/min. The most likely reason for this decrease in the pacing heart rate is
   A. Decreased atrial rate
   B. Third-degree heart block
   C. Trifascicular heart block
   D. Battery failure
   E. Normal variation

952. Calculate the cardiac output from the following data: patient weight 70 kg, hemoglobin concentration 10 mg/dL, arterial blood gases on 100% O_2: Pao_2 450 mm Hg, $Paco_2$ 32 mm Hg, pH 7.46, Sao_2 99%. Mixed venous blood gases are: Pvo_2 30 mm Hg, $Paco_2$ 45 mm Hg, pH 7.32, Svo_2 60%.
   A. 2.5 L/min
   B. 3.0 L/min
   C. 3.5 L/min
   D. 4.0 L/min
   E. 4.5 L/min

953. Normal resting myocardial O_2 consumption is
   A. 2.0 mL/100 g/min
   B. 3.5 mL/100 g/min
   C. 10 mL/100 g/min
   D. 15 mL/100 g/min
   E. 25 mL/100 g/min

954. A 22-year-old man with hypertrophic cardiomyopathy (HOCM) is undergoing an elective cholecystectomy under general anesthesia. Immediately after induction with thiopental, 5 mg/kg IV, the arterial blood pressure decreases from 140/82 to 70/40 mm Hg. What would be the most appropriate drug for treatment of hypotension in this patient?
   A. Ephedrine
   B. Mephentermine
   C. Isoproterenol
   D. Phenylephrine
   E. Epinephrine

955. A 65-year-old patient with moderate aortic stenosis develops a sudden increase in heart rate during an appendectomy under general anesthesia. The ventricular rate is 190 beats/min and is irregularly irregular, arterial blood pressure is 70/45 mm Hg, and there is 2 mm ST-segment depression in lead V5 of the ECG. Which of the following would be the most appropriate treatment for myocardial ischemia in this patient?
   A. Electrical cardioversion
   B. Esmolol
   C. Nitroglycerin
   D. Verapamil
   E. Phenylephrine

956. After emergency repair of a ruptured abdominal aortic aneurysm, a 68-year-old patient is mechanically ventilated in the intensive care unit with 20 cm H_2O of positive end-expiratory pressure (PEEP) for 3 days. Sodium nitroprusside has been infused at a rate of 1.5 μg/kg/min for 48 hours to control hypertension. Suddenly, the systemic blood pressure falls from 130/70 to 50 mm Hg systolic and the Sao_2 drops to 75%. The most likely cause of this scenario is
   A. Cyanide toxicity
   B. Acute myocardial infarction
   C. Tension pneumothorax
   D. Hyperventilation
   E. Methemoglobinemia

957. Normal resting coronary artery blood flow is
      A. 10 mL/100 g/min
      B. 40 mL/100 g/min
      C. 75 mL/100 g/min
      D. 120 mL/100 g/min
      E. 160 mL/100 g/min

958. Each of the following is associated with an increased incidence of pulmonary artery rupture in patients with pulmonary artery catheters **EXCEPT**
      A. Hypothermia
      B. Presence of pulmonary artery atheromas
      C. Old age
      D. Anticoagulation
      E. Pulmonary artery catheter migration

959. Allergic reactions to protamine can occur with each of the following **EXCEPT?**
      A. Diabetes treated with NPH insulin
      B. Diabetes treated with regular insulin
      C. Diabetics treated with PZI insulin
      D. Previous vasectomy
      E. Allergy to seafood

960. A 66-year-old patient is undergoing a three-vessel coronary artery bypass operation. Anticoagulation is achieved with 20,000 units of heparin. How much protamine should be administered to this patient to completely reverse the heparin after cardiopulmonary bypass?
      A. 150 mg
      B. 250 mg
      C. 350 mg
      D. 450 mg
      E. 550 mg

961. The graph below represents

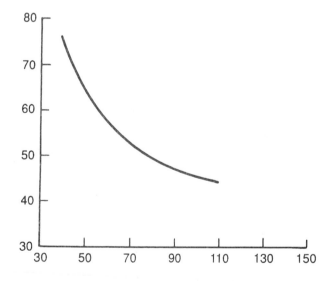

      A. Ventricular end-diastolic pressure as a function of ventricular end-diastolic volume
      B. Stroke volume as a function of end-diastolic pressure
      C. Cardiac index as a function of end-diastolic pressure
      D. Cardiac output as a function of ventricular end-diastolic volume
      E. Diastolic time (as percentage of cardiac cycle) as a function of heart rate

962. A 72-year-old woman is undergoing cardiopulmonary bypass for aortic and mitral valve replacement. The surgery is uneventful; however, in the intensive care unit, blood is noted to ooze from the pulmonary artery catheter and venous access sites. Mediastinal chest tube output is 500 mL/hour. A thromboelastogram is obtained and shown in the figure. What is the most likely cause of profuse bleeding in this patient?

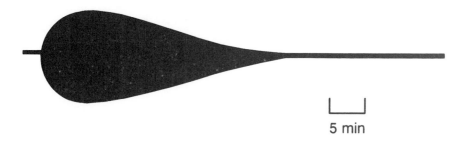

5 min

    A. Fibrinolysis
    B. Excess heparin
    C. Thrombocytopenia
    D. Factor VIII deficiency
    E. Poor surgical hemostasis

963. A 170-micrometer filter must be used for administration of each of the following **EXCEPT**
    A. Fresh frozen plasma
    B. Cryoprecipitate
    C. Platelets
    D. Packed red cells
    E. Albumin

964. The dose of adenosine necessary to convert paroxysmal supraventricular tachycardia to normal sinus rhythm should be initially reduced
    A. In patients receiving theophylline for chronic asthma
    B. In patients with a history of arterial thrombotic disease taking dipyridamole
    C. In patients with a history of chronic renal failure
    D. In patients with hepatic dysfunction
    E. In chronic alcoholics

965. A 56-year-old male patient is anesthetized for elective coronary revascularization. A urinary catheter is placed after induction and coupled to a temperature transducer. A pulmonary artery catheter is inserted, and the temperature probe on the distal portion of the catheter is also connected to a transducer. The reason for measuring the temperature of both the bladder and the blood in the pulmonary vasculature is
    A. Both are necessary for determining cardiac output by the thermodilution technique
    B. Bladder temperature is more accurate prebypass; pulmonary artery catheter temperature is more accurate postbypass
    C. Pulmonary artery catheter temperature is more accurate prebypass; bladder temperature is more accurate postbypass
    D. It is helpful in determining the likelihood of recooling after discontinuation of cardiopulmonary bypass
    E. It is the average of these two temperatures, which is important in determining patient body warmth

966. Which of the following would be the best intraoperative transesophageal echocardiograph (TEE) view to monitor for myocardial ischemia?
    A. Mid-esophageal 4 chamber view
    B. Transgastric mid-papillary left ventricular short axis view
    C. Mid-esophageal long axis view
    D. Mid-esophageal 2 chamber view
    E. Transgastric 2 chamber view

967. Select the true statement regarding CPR and defibrillation by a health care provider in patients experiencing sudden cardiac arrest
   A. Defibrillation times one should always precede CPR
   B. CPR should always be carried out for 2 minutes prior to defibrillation
   C. Two minutes of chest compressions alone (no ventilation) should be carried out prior to first shock
   D. If arrest less than 1 minute (witnessed) one biphasic shock then 5 cycles of CPR
   E. If arrest less than 1 minute (witnessed) three biphasic shocks then 5 cycles of CPR

968. Which of the following medications blocks angiotensin at the receptor?
   A. Losartan (*Cozaar*)
   B. Terazosin (*Hytrin*)
   C. Lisinopril (*Prinivil, Zestril*)
   D. Spironolactone (*Aldactone*)
   E. Amlodipine (*Norvasc*)

969. Untoward effects associated with administration of sodium bicarbonate during massive blood transfusion include each of the following **EXCEPT**
   A. Hyperosmolality
   B. Paradoxical cerebrospinal fluid acidosis
   C. Hypercarbia
   D. Hypernatremia
   E. Hyperkalemia

970. Useful therapy for hypercyanotic "tet spells" in patients with tetralogy of Fallot might include any of the following **EXCEPT**
   A. Esmolol
   B. Lactated Ringer's solution bolus (5 mL/kg)
   C. Phenylephrine
   D. Isoproterenol
   E. Morphine

971. Sildenafil (Viagra) belongs to the same class of drugs as which of the following?
   A. Yohimbine
   B. Nitroglycerin
   C. Enalapril
   D. Milrinone
   E. Hydralazine

972. What is the minimal time after angioplasty and placement of a drug eluting stent that dual antiplatelet therapy should be continued before considering stopping it for elective surgery?
   A. 3 months
   B. 6 months
   C. 1 year
   D. 18 months
   E. Never

973. Hirudin is used in patients with
   A. Heparin resistance
   B. Protamine allergy
   C. Heparin induced thrombocytopenia type I
   D. Heparin induced thrombocytopenia type II
   E. Antithrombin deficiency

974. Which of the following anatomical sites is associated with the **LEAST** incidence of central line infection?
   A. Internal jugular vein
   B. External jugular vein
   C. Subclavian vein
   D. Femoral vein
   E. The incidence is roughly equal for all sites

975. The effects of clopidogrel (Plavix) can be reversed with
   A. Fresh frozen plasma
   B. Protamine
   C. Aprotinin
   D. Factor VIII concentrate
   E. None of the above

976. A disadvantage of port access coronary artery bypass surgery utilizing the da Vinci Robot versus "standard" coronary artery revascularization with cardiopulmonary bypass is
   A. Need for hypothermic cardiac arrest
   B. Greater incidence of intraoperative hypoxia
   C. Greater incidence of trauma to sternum
   D. Increased transfusion requirements
   E. Increased risk of neuropsychiatric deficits

977. A right sided double lumen tube will be used to separate ventilation of the right and left lungs for a left pneumonectomy. The plan for placement is to insert the distal tube into the trachea with a laryngoscope and then to advance the distal tube into the right mainstem bronchus under bronchoscopic guidance. After insertion of the tube with the laryngoscope, CO_2 is seen on mass spectrometer and the scope is passed through bronchial port until it exits the tube inside the lumen of the patient's airway. A structure is seen which appears to be the carina. The scope is then passed into the right branch and the structure in the picture below is visualized. The scope is located in the

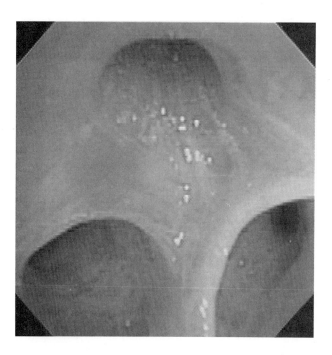

   A. Right mainstem bronchus
   B. Left mainstem bronchus
   C. Lingular segment
   D. Right upper lobe
   E. Left upper lobe

978. Which of the following maneuvers (after assuring proper tube placement) is **LEAST** likely to raise the PaO_2 during one-lung ventilation with a double lumen endotracheal tube?
   A. Continuous positive airway pressure (CPAP) to the non-dependent lung
   B. Positive end-expiratory pressure (PEEP) to the dependent lung
   C. Clamping the pulmonary artery by surgeon during pneumonectomy
   D. Raising mean arterial pressure from 60 to 85 mm Hg
   E. Continuous infusion of epoprostenol (Flolan) via central line

979. Which of the following drugs or interventions will cause the **LEAST** increase in heart rate in the transplanted denervated heart?
   A. Glucagon
   B. Atropine
   C. Isoproterenol
   D. Norepinephrine
   E. Pacemaker

980. A patient with known Wolff-Parkinson-White syndrome develops a wide complex tachycardia during a hernia operation under general anesthesia. Vital signs are stable and pharmacologic treatment is desired. Which of the following drugs is most likely to be successful in controlling heart rate in this patient?
   A. Verapamil
   B. Esmolol
   C. Adenosine
   D. Digoxin
   E. Procainamide

981. A 63-year-old patient with a DDD-R pacemaker is scheduled for right hemicolectomy. The indication for pacemaker implantation was sick sinus syndrome and the pacemaker has been reprogrammed to the asynchronous (DOO) mode at a rate of 70 for surgery. After induction, the patient's native heart rate rises to 85 beats/min with blood pressure 130/90 mm Hg. Which of the following actions would be most appropriate?
   A. Turn off pacemaker for duration of case
   B. Administer lidocaine
   C. Administer esmolol
   D. Change volatile from isoflurane to desflurane and deepen anesthetic
   E. Observe

982. The main advantage of milrinone is that it lacks which side effect, compared with amrinone for long term use?
   A. Tachycardia
   B. Hypothyroidism
   C. Thrombocytopenia
   D. Hyperglycemia
   E. Pulmonary toxicity

983. Systemic inflammatory response syndrome (SIRS) differs from sepsis in that patients with SIRS have
   A. A normal temperature
   B. A heart rate less than 90 beats/min
   C. A normal white blood cell (WBC) count
   D. A normal $Paco_2$ level
   E. No documented infection

984. Arrange the percutaneous insertion sites from nearest to farthest for placement of a pulmonary artery catheter.
   A. Left internal jugular, right internal jugular, antecubital, femoral
   B. Right internal jugular, left internal jugular, antecubital, femoral
   C. Right internal jugular, left internal jugular, femoral, antecubital
   D. Left internal jugular, right internal jugular, femoral, antecubital
   E. Right internal jugular, femoral, left internal jugular, antecubital

985. A pulmonary artery catheter capable of continuously monitoring $S\bar{v}O_2$ is placed in a patient for coronary artery bypass surgery. Just before instituting cardiopulmonary bypass, the $S\bar{v}O_2$ falls from 85% to 71%. Which of the following could account for this change in $S\bar{v}O_2$?
    A. Cooling the patient to 27° C
    B. Transfusion of 2 units packed RBCs
    C. Epinephrine, 25 μg IV
    D. Myocardial ischemia
    E. Administration 1 g $CaCl_2$

986. Which of the following terms refers to myocardial relaxation or diastole
    A. Inotropy
    B. Chronotropy
    C. Dromotropy
    D. Bathmotropy
    E. Lusitropy

987. A 31-year-old female with primary pulmonary hypertension is scheduled for a mastectomy. Pharmacologic agents that might be useful in reducing pulmonary vascular resistance include each of the following **EXCEPT**
    A. Prostaglandin I_2 (epoprostenol)
    B. Oxygen
    C. Nitric oxide
    D. Milrinone
    E. Nitrous oxide

988. Pulmonary vascular resistance as a function of lung volume is the **LEAST** at which volume?
    A. Total lung volume
    B. Residual volume
    C. Functional residual capacity (FRC)
    D. Expiratory reserve volume
    E. Depends on the fluid volume status of the patient

989. A 45-year-old patient with hypertrophic cardiomyopathy is anesthetized for skin grafting after suffering third degree burns on his legs. As skin is being harvested from his back, his heart rate rises and his systolic blood pressure falls to 85 mm Hg. Which of the following interventions is **LEAST** likely to improve this patient's hemodynamics?
    A. Administration of esmolol
    B. Fluid bolus
    C. Dobutamine infusion
    D. Administration of sufentanil
    E. Phenylephrine infusion

990. A 59-year-old patient is scheduled for right knee replacement. The patient has a long history of congestive heart failure (CHF) with room air O_2 saturation of 87% in the holding area. Rales are audible throughout both lung fields with the patient upright. The most appropriate plan would be
    A. Arterial line and spinal with isobaric bupivacaine
    B. Arterial line, etomidate induction, sevoflurane, intraoperative TEE
    C. Arterial line, propofol induction, N_2O, isoflurane, pulmonary artery catheter
    D. Arterial line, central venous pressure line (CVP) ketamine induction, N_2O narcotic anesthetic, furosemide, milrinone
    E. Cancel the case

991. Which of the following drugs is **LEAST** likely to cause unfavorable hemodynamic changes in patients with severe mitral stenosis?
    A. Ketamine
    B. Remifentanil
    C. Pancuronium
    D. Desflurane
    E. Nitrous oxide

992. You made an infusion of dopamine by mixing 200 mg of dopamine in 250 mL of sodium chloride (NS) or 5% dextrose injection (D5W). What is the infusion pump rate when infusing dopamine at a rate of 5 µg/kg/min for this 70-kg patient?
- **A.** 6 mL/hr
- **B.** 10 mL/hr
- **C.** 16 mL/hr
- **D.** 20 mL/hr
- **E.** 26 mL/hr

993. The following are ideal parameters for the anesthetic management of high filling pressures, high systemic vascular resistance (SVR) and fast heart rate?
- **A.** Aortic stenosis
- **B.** Mitral stenosis
- **C.** Aortic insufficiency
- **D.** Cardiac tamponade
- **E.** Hypertrophic cardiomyopathy (HOCM)

994. Which of the following treatments would be the LEAST useful in treatment of the rhythm shown below?

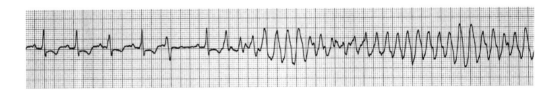

- **A.** Procainamide
- **B.** Magnesium
- **C.** Overdrive pacing
- **D.** Unsynchronized cardioversion
- **E.** Isoproterenol infusion

DIRECTIONS: (Questions 995 through 997) each group of questions consists of several numbered statements followed by lettered headings. For each numbered statement select the ONE lettered heading that is most closely associated with it. Each letter heading may be selected once, more than once or not at all.

995. P wave flattening, widening of the QRS complex, peaked T wave

996. Depressed ST segments, flat T wave, U wave present

997. Normal or increased PR interval, short QT interval
- **A.** Hypokalemia
- **B.** Hyperkalemia
- **C.** Hyponatremia
- **D.** Hypernatremia
- **E.** Hypercalcemia

Cardiovascular Physiology and Anesthesia

Answers, References, and Explanations

915. (E) In 2007, the American Heart Association revised the guidelines for prevention of infective endocarditis (IE). Presently, only patients with underlying cardiac conditions with the highest risk for an adverse outcome from IE should receive antibiotic prophylaxis for selected dental procedures. Prophylaxis is not recommended for patients undergoing elective genitourinary (GU) or gastrointestinal (GI) procedures. The cardiac conditions with the highest risk include: prosthetic cardiac valves, previous IE, several types of congenital heart disease (CHD), and cardiac transplantation recipients who develop cardiac valvulopathy. Any of the antibiotics listed in the question or cephalexin 2 g orally (or other first or second generation oral cephalosporin in equivalent dosage) or clindamycin 600 mg orally, IM or IV should be administered 30 to 60 minutes before the procedure. This patient has aortic stenosis and does not need any prophylaxis (*Wilson W, Taubert KA, Gewitz, et al.: Prevention of infective endocarditis—Guidelines from the American Heart Association. Circulation, 115:1736-1754, 2007. http://circ.ahajournals.org*).

916. (A) The effects of hypothermia on cardiovascular physiology are related in part to changes in blood viscosity and rheology, fluid and electrolyte balance, and coagulation. The overall effect of hypothermia on the coagulation system is to reduce hemostasis. For example, platelets are readily sequestered reversibly in the portal circulation, and at 20° C there is almost complete sequestration of platelets. However, upon rewarming to 35° C, the platelet count returns to normal within approximately 1 hour. These platelets function normally (as measured by bleeding time) and have a normal life span (*Kaplan: Cardiac Anesthesia, ed 4, p 1139*).

917. (A) All of the choices listed in this question occur during myocardial ischemia. However, of the choices listed, presence of left ventricular wall-motion abnormalities is the most sensitive indicator (*Barash: Clinical Anesthesia, ed 5, p 943; Miller: Anesthesia, ed 6, pp 1378-1379, 2066-2068*).

918. (C) One MET is equal to the amount of energy expended during 1 minute at rest, which is roughly 3.5 mL of oxygen per kg of bodyweight per minute (3.5 mL/kg/min). For a 70-kg (150 lb.) person one MET would equal 250 mL O_2 per minute. So 2500 mL would correspond to 10 METs.
Recall that 4 METs are the equivalent of climbing two flights of stairs at a reasonable rate without stopping, or walking on level ground at 4 mph; and 10 METs are equivalent to participating in strenuous activity such as swimming, skiing, playing basketball or jogging at about 6 mph (*Barash: Clinical Anesthesia, ed 5, p 481; Miller: Anesthesia, ed 6, pp 702, 933-934*).

919. (A) The anesthetic management of patients with congenital heart disease (CHD) requires thorough knowledge of the pathophysiology of the defect. In general, congenital heart defects can be categorized into those that result in left-to-right intracardiac shunting and into those that result in right-to-left shunting. The main feature in congenital heart defects, which result in right-to-left intracardiac shunting, is a reduction in pulmonary blood flow and arterial hypoxemia. The more common congenital heart defects that result in right-to-left intracardiac shunting include tetralogy of Fallot, Eisenmenger's syndrome, Ebstein's malformation of the tricuspid valve, pulmonary atresia with a ventricular septal defect, tricuspid atresia, and patent foramen ovale. Meticulous care must be taken to avoid infusion of air via intravenous solutions, because this can lead to arterial air embolism. Patients with congenital cardiac defects that result in left-to-right intracardiac shunting, such as patent ductus arteriosus, are at minimal risk for arterial air embolism, because blood flow through the shunt is primarily from the systemic vascular system to the pulmonary vascular system (*Barash: Clinical Anesthesia, ed 5, pp 926-928; Miller: Anesthesia, ed 6, pp 2008-2012*).

920. **(A)** The Frank-Starling curve relates left ventricular filling pressure to left ventricular work. Left ventricular end-diastolic volume, left ventricular end-diastolic pressure, left atrial pressure, pulmonary artery occlusion pressure, and in some instances, central venous pressure, can reflect left ventricular filling pressure. Left ventricular work can be represented on the y-axis by left ventricular stroke work index, stroke volume, cardiac output, cardiac index, and arterial blood pressure (*Miller: Anesthesia, ed 6, pp 724-728*).

921. **(A)** The rhythm strip in the question depicts atrial flutter. The importance of examining more than one lead is emphasized in this question. The lower tracing looks like a junctional rhythm, but upon examination of the upper tracing, discrete P waves (actually F waves) corresponding to a rate of about 300/min are easily discerned. An atrial rate of 300 is common, often with 2:1 conduction, yielding a ventricular rate of 150/min. In the rhythm presented here, the ventricular rate is around 75/min, corresponding to a 4:1 conduction (*Miller: Anesthesia, ed 6, p 1401*).

922. **(E)** During cardiopulmonary bypass, it is common for a pulmonary artery catheter to migrate distally 3 to 5 cm into the pulmonary artery. In fact, pulmonary artery catheter migration during cardiopulmonary bypass is so common that withdrawing the catheter 3 to 5 cm before the initiation of cardiopulmonary bypass may be routinely indicated. Distal catheter migration into a wedge position is often detected by noting an increase in the measured pulmonary artery pressure. Pulmonary artery catheter migration during cardiopulmonary bypass has been implicated in cases of pulmonary artery rupture. Although catheter migration is the most likely explanation for a rise in pulmonary artery pressure during cardiopulmonary bypass, the anesthesiologist must also consider inadequate ventricular venting as a potential cause of increasing pulmonary artery pressures during cardiopulmonary bypass, particularly if the pulmonary artery pressure does not decline after withdrawal of the pulmonary artery catheter from a presumed wedge position. Ventricular distention during cardiopulmonary bypass is detrimental because it can increase myocardial oxygen demand at a time when there is no coronary blood flow. Malposition of the aortic cannula may result in unilateral facial blanching. Malposition of the venous cannula may result in facial or scleral edema or may manifest as poor blood return to the cardiopulmonary bypass circuit (*Barash: Clinical Anesthesia, ed 5, pp 915-916; Miller: Anesthesia, ed 6, pp 1306, 1312*).

923. **(C)** Anticholinesterase drugs may have significant cholinergic side effects, including sinoatrial and atrioventricular node slowing, bronchoconstriction, and peristalsis. There is a high incidence of transient cardiac dysrhythmias after administration of these drugs. The cardiac effects vary from clinically unimportant atrial and junctional bradydysrhythmias, ectopic ventricular foci, to clinically important dysrhythmias such as high-grade heart block, including complete heart block and cardiac arrest. The rhythm strip in this question is that of a low-grade heart block with a junctional rhythm. The most appropriate treatment of this rhythm is administration of atropine (*Miller: Anesthesia, ed 6, p 523; Morgan: Clinical Anesthesiology, ed 4, pp 229-230*).

924. **(E)** Incorrect positioning of the aortic perfusion and venous return cannulae are possible complications associated with cardiopulmonary bypass. Improper positioning of the aortic cannula would tend to result in unilateral facial blanching, whereas facial edema (e.g., bulging sclerae) reflects venous congestion and may be caused by improper positioning of the venous return canula. Incorrect positioning of the venous return cannula can occur when the cannula is inserted too far into the superior vena cava, which causes obstruction of the right innominate vein. If the venous cannula is inserted too far into the inferior vena cava, venous return from the lower regions of the body can be impaired and abdominal distention can occur. If this happens, the vena caval cannula should be withdrawn to a more proximal position and the adequacy of the venous return from the patient to the cardiopulmonary bypass machine should be confirmed. A properly positioned venous return cannula will bleed back with nonpulsatile flow when the proximal end is lowered below the patient (*Hensley: Cardiac Anesthesia, ed 4, pp 208-209; Stoelting: Basics of Anesthesia, ed 5, p 387*).

925. **(B)** Transposition of the great vessels is a congenital cardiac defect that results from failure of the truncus arteriosus to rotate during organogenesis such that the aorta arises from the right ventricle and the pulmonary artery arises from the left ventricle. As a result, the left and right ventricles are not connected in series and the pulmonary and systemic circulations function independently. This results in profound arterial hypoxemia; survival is not possible unless there is a concomitant defect that allows for intermixing of blood between the two circulations. Induction of anesthesia with volatile anesthetics will be delayed because minimal portions of inhaled drugs will reach the systemic circulation. In contrast, anesthetic drugs that are administered intravenously will be distributed with minimal dilution to the brain; therefore, doses and rates of injection should be reduced in these patients (*Hensley: Cardiac Anesthesia, ed 4, p 389; Hines: Stoelting's Anesthesia and Co-Existing Disease, ed 5, pp 56-57*).

926. **(D)** The Fontan procedure (usually modified Fontan) is an anastomosis of the right atrial appendage to the pulmonary artery. This procedure is most frequently performed to treat congenital cardiac defects, which decrease pulmonary artery blood flow (e.g., pulmonary atresia and stenosis, and tricuspid atresia). The Fontan procedure is also used to increase pulmonary blood flow when it is necessary to surgically convert the right ventricle to a systemic ventricle (e.g., hypoplastic left heart syndrome). Truncus arteriosus occurs when a single arterial trunk, which overrides both ventricles (which are connected via a ventricular septal defect), gives rise to both the aorta and pulmonary artery. Surgical treatment of this defect includes banding of the right and left pulmonary arteries and enclosure of the associated ventricular septal defect (*Hines: Stoelting's Anesthesia and Co-Existing Disease, ed 5, pp 55, 58; Miller: Anesthesia, ed 6, pp 2010-2014*).

927. **(C)** For each degree Celsius body temperature is lowered, tissue metabolic rate declines approximately 5% to 8%. A core temperature of 28° C to 30° C would correspond roughly to a 50% reduction in metabolic rate (*Barash: Clinical Anesthesia, ed 5, p 911; Miller: Anesthesia, ed 6, p 1978*).

928. **(B)** By deflating just before ventricular systole, an intra-aortic balloon pump (IABP) is designed to reduce aortic pressure and afterload, thereby enhancing left ventricular ejection and reducing wall tension and oxygen consumption. By inflating in diastole, just after closure of the aortic valve, diastolic aortic pressure and coronary blood flow are increased. Thus proper timing of inflation and deflation is crucial to correct functioning of an IABP. The P wave on the ECG is a late diastolic event and inflating the IABP just after the P wave would minimize augmentation of diastolic coronary blood flow. In addition, inflation of the device that late in diastolic would risk having the balloon inflated during ventricular systole, which would dramatically increase ventricular afterload and worsen the myocardial oxygen supply and demand balance. Similarly, the midpoint of the QRS complex represents the electrical activation of the ventricles, which heralds the end of ventricular diastole, a time when the balloon should be deflating before ventricular ejection (*Miller: Anesthesia, ed 6, p 1991; Stoelting: Basics of Anesthesia, ed 5, pp 389-390*).

929. **(C)** Afterload reduction during anesthesia is beneficial in all of the conditions listed in this question except tetralogy of Fallot. In tetralogy of Fallot, blood is shunted through a ventricular septal defect from the pulmonary circulation to the systemic circulation because of right ventricular outflow obstruction. A decrease in systemic vascular resistance would augment this right-to-left shunt through the ventricular septal defect, which would reduce pulmonary vascular blood flow and exacerbate systemic hypoxemia (*Fleischer: Anesthesia and Uncommon Diseases, ed 5, pp 108-110; Hines: Stoelting's Anesthesia and Co-Existing Disease, ed 5, pp 50-53*).

930. **(A)** Protamine is a basic compound isolated from the sperm of certain fish species and is a specific antagonist of heparin. The dose of protamine is 1.3 mg for each 100 units of heparin. If protamine is administered to a patient who has not received heparin, it can bind to platelets and soluble coagulation factors, producing an anticoagulant effect. There is no evidence that protamine has negative inotropic or chronotropic properties. Some persons (e.g., diabetics taking NPH insulin) may be allergic to protamine. Hypotension may occur when protamine is administered rapidly because it induces histamine release from mast cells (*Hensley: Cardiac Anesthesia, ed 4, p 505*).

931. **(D)** The primary goal in the anesthetic management of patients with coronary artery disease is to maintain the balance between myocardial O_2 supply and demand. Myocardial O_2 consumption (i.e., myocardial O_2 demand) is determined by three factors: myocardial wall tension, heart rate, and myocardial contractile state. Myocardial wall tension is directly related to the end-diastolic ventricular pressure or volume (preload) and systemic vascular resistance (afterload). In general, myocardial work in the form of increased heart rate results in the greatest increase in myocardial O_2 consumption. Also, for a given increase in myocardial work, the increase in myocardial O_2 consumption is much less with volume work (preload) than with pressure work (afterload) (*Barash Clinical Anesthesia, ed 5, pp 868, 876-877; Miller: Anesthesia, ed 6, pp 1946-1948; Stoelting: Pharmacology and Physiology in Anesthetic Practice, ed 4, p 754*).

932. **(D)** Pulsus paradoxus describes an inspiratory fall in systolic arterial blood pressure of greater than 10 mm Hg often seen in cardiac tamponade. This inspiratory decline in systolic blood pressure represents an exaggeration of the normal small drop in blood pressure seen with inspiration in spontaneously breathing patients. In cardiac tamponade, ventricular filling is limited by the presence of blood, thrombus, or other material in the pericardial space. During inspiration in the spontaneously breathing patient, negative intrathoracic pressure enhances filling of the right ventricle. Because total cardiac volume is limited by the pressurized pericardium in tamponade cases, as the right ventricle fills with inspiration, left ventricular preload and blood pressure decline. Pulsus paradoxus is occasionally seen in cases of severe airway obstruction and right ventricular infarction. Pulsus parvus and pulsus tardus describe, respectively, the diminished pulse wave and delayed upstroke in patients with aortic stenosis. Pulsus alternans describes alternating smaller and larger pulse waves, a condition sometimes seen in patients with severe left ventricular dysfunction. A bisferiens pulse is a pulse waveform with two systolic peaks seen in cases of significant aortic valvular regurgitation (*Miller: Anesthesia, ed 6, pp 1285-1286*).

933.   **(B)**   The word ALONE gives 5 drugs that can be administered down the endotracheal tube (ETT)—*A*tropine, *L*idocaine, *O*xygen, *N*aloxone, *E*pinephrine. In addition, vasopressin may be administered down the ETT. Although preoperatively clear antacids (e.g., Bicitra) have been administered orally to raise gastric pH in patients at high risk for aspiration with induction of general anesthesia to decrease the severity of acid aspiration, should aspiration occur, bicarbonate should not be instilled down the endotracheal tube, because it would worsen the aspiration and might produce an alkaline burn to the lung (*Barash: Clinical Anesthesia, ed 5, pp 1393-1395*).

934.   **(B)**   Mean arterial pressure can be calculated using the following formula:

$$MAP = BP_D + \frac{1}{3}(BP_S - BP_D)$$

where MAP (mm Hg) is the mean arterial pressure, BP_D (mm Hg) is the diastolic blood pressure, and BP_S (mm Hg) is the systolic blood pressure (*Morgan: Clinical Anesthesiology, ed 4, p 118*).

935.   **(A)**   Amiodarone is a benzofurane derivative with a chemical structure similar to that of thyroxine, which accounts for its ability to cause either hypothyroidism or hyperthyroidism. Altered thyroid function occurs in 2% to 4% of patients when amiodarone is administered over a long period. Amiodarone prolongs the duration of the action potential of both atrial and ventricular muscle without altering the resting membrane potential. This accounts for its ability to depress sinoatrial and atrioventricular node function. Thus, amiodarone is effective pharmacologic therapy for both recurrent supraventricular and ventricular tachydysrhythmias. In patients with Wolff-Parkinson-White syndrome, amiodarone increases the refractory period of the accessory pathway. Atropine-resistant bradycardia and hypotension may occur during general anesthesia because of the significant anti-adrenergic effect of amiodarone. Should this occur, isoproterenol should be administered or a temporary artificial cardiac pacemaker should be inserted (*Hensley: Cardiac Anesthesia, ed 4, p 93*).

936.   **(C)**   Systemic vascular resistance can be calculated using the following formula:

$$SVR = (MAP - CVP)/CO \times 80$$

where SVR is the systemic vascular resistance, MAP (mm Hg) is the mean arterial pressure, CVP (mm Hg) is the central venous pressure, CO (L/min) is the cardiac output, and 80 is a factor to convert Wood units to dynes/sec/cm^{-5}. Calculation of SVR from the data in this question is as follows:

$$SVR = (86 - 8)/5 \times 80 = 1248 \text{ dynes/sec/cm}^{-5}$$

(*Morgan: Clinical Anesthesiology, ed 4, p 424*).

937.   **(A)**   Tetralogy of Fallot is the most common congenital heart defect associated with a right-to-left intracardiac shunt. This congenital defect is characterized by a tetrad of congenital cardiac anomalies, including a ventricular septal defect, an aorta that overrides the ventricular septal defect, obstruction of the pulmonary artery outflow tract, and right ventricular hypertrophy. The ventricular septal defect is typically large and single, an infundibular pulmonary artery stenosis is usually prominent, and the distal pulmonary artery may be hypoplastic or even absent. Although many patients with tetralogy of Fallot have a patent ductus arteriosus, this is not included in the definition (*Hines: Stoelting's Anesthesia and Co-Existing Disease, ed 5, pp 50-51*).

938.   **(A)**   The etiology of hypotension can be placed into two broad categories: decreased cardiac output and decreased systemic vascular resistance, or both. In this case, cardiac output is greater than normal, as one often sees in early sepsis. Treatment of this hypotension should be carried out with pharmacologic agents with strong α-agonist properties. Of the choices in this question, phenylephrine is the only drug that is a pure α-agonist. Dopamine in high doses has strong activity but significant ß$_1$ activity and some ß$_2$ activity as well. Norepinephrine likewise possesses strong α activity with some ß$_1$ activity. Vasopressin is a potent vasoconstrictor useful in the management of septic shock. Any of the aforementioned pharmacologic agents could be used to support pressure in patients with sepsis in conjunction with definitive treatment for the septic source. Because dobutamine is predominantly a ß$_1$-agonist, it would be an extremely poor choice for a patient with a high cardiac output in the face of a low systemic vascular resistance (*Miller: Anesthesia, ed 6, pp 646-652, 806-807; Morgan: Clinical Anesthesia, ed 4, pp 1055-1057*).

939. (A) β-Adrenergic receptors are responsible for mediating activation of the cardiovascular system, vascular and respiratory smooth muscle relaxation, renin secretion by the kidneys, and several metabolic functions, such as lipolysis, glycogenolysis, and insulin secretion. ß$_1$-Adrenergic receptors primarily mediate the cardiac effects (i.e., heart rate, contractility, and conduction velocity) and the release of fatty acids from adipose tissue, whereas ß$_2$-receptors primarily mediate vascular airway and uterine smooth muscle tone, and glycogenolysis. α-Adrenergic receptors mediate intestinal and urinary bladder-sphincter tone (*Morgan: Clinical Anesthesia, ed 4, pp 243, 246; Stoelting: Basics of Anesthesia, ed 5, pp 65-71*).

940. (C) The primary goal in the anesthetic management of patients with hypertropic cardiomyopathy (formerly called idiopathic hypertrophic subaortic stenosis) is to reduce the gradient across the left ventricular outflow obstruction. In general, drugs that increase myocardial contractility or reduce preload or afterload increase the magnitude of this obstruction. Halothane (less available now in the United States, but used extensively in other countries) is an ideal volatile anesthetic agent for maintaining anesthesia in these patients because it is a direct myocardial depressant, but it does not decrease systemic vascular resistance. Both of these characteristics are beneficial for these patients, because they do not increase the magnitude of left ventricular outflow obstruction. Should hypotension develop, phenylephrine, a pure α-adrenergic receptor agonist, should be administered to increase arterial blood pressure because it increases systemic vascular resistance, thereby reducing left ventricular outflow obstruction (*Stoelting: Basics of Anesthesia, ed 5, pp 382-383*).

941. (A) An unstable patient with a wide complex tachycardia is presumed to be ventricular tachycardia (VT) and this rythm represents a medical emergency which requires immediate synchronized cardioversion (*2005 American Heart Association guidelines for cardiopulmonary resuscitation and emergency cardiovascular care. Circulation, 112:IV69-IV73, 2005; Miller: Anesthesia, ed 6, p 1404*).

942. (D) Romano-Ward syndrome is a rare congenital abnormality characterized by prolonged QT intervals on the ECG. Jervell-Lange-Nielsen syndrome is a congenital syndrome characterized by prolonged QT intervals on the ECG in association with congenital deafness. An imbalance between the right and left sides of the sympathetic nervous system may play a role in the etiology of these syndromes. This imbalance can be temporarily abolished with a left stellate ganglion block, which shortens the QT intervals. If this is successful, surgical ganglionectomy may be performed as permanent treatment (*Kaplan: Cardiac Anesthesia, ed 4, pp 186-187*).

943. (A) The use of mechanical circulatory support is becoming more frequent because of advances in technology and a relative scarcity of organs available for transplant. Mechanical circulatory support can be used as bridge therapy for patients awaiting cardiac transplantation, or a bridge to recovery for those recovering from a viral cardiomyopathy or patients recovering from cardiogenic shock after myocardial infarction. In other patients, it can be destination therapy. Currently, the HeartMate VE is the only mechanical device approved for destination therapy in the United States. Various versions of these devices can be used to support the right (not approved for destination therapy), the left, or both ventricles. Axial (continuous) flow is non-pulsatile and non-physiologic. These pumps are connected in parallel to the heart. Specifically, on the left side, blood is taken from the apex of the heart and returned to circulation via the aorta. In this configuration, little or no blood exits the aortic valve during systole. Measuring blood pressure with a cuff is not accurate in most patients and may be impossible. Pulse oximeters do work with some patients, but this, too, requires pulsatile flow. Measurement of blood pressure with an arterial line is easily done, just as it is in patients on cardiopulmonary bypass undergoing open heart operations (*Miller: Anesthesia, ed 7, p 1941*).

944. (A) In a normal heart, approximately 20% to 30% of the cardiac output is produced by the "atrial kick." In pathologic conditions, such as aortic stenosis, the "atrial kick" may contribute more substantially to cardiac output (*Morgan: Clinical Anesthesiology, ed 4, p 423*).

945. **(A)**   The figure in this case shows a bisferiens pulse, recognized by its two systolic peaks. A bisferiens pulse can be seen in patients with significant aortic regurgitation. In aortic regurgitation, the left ventricle ejects a large volume of blood in systole with a rapid diastolic runoff as blood flows both to the periphery and back into the left ventricle. The first systolic peak of the bisferiens pulse represents the wave of blood ejected from the left ventricle. The second systolic peak represents a reflected pressure wave from the periphery. In contrast, patients with aortic stenosis display a delayed pulse wave with a diminished upstroke (pulses tardus and pulses parvus), whereas patients with cardiac tamponade show an exaggerated inspiratory decline in systolic blood pressure (pulsus paradoxus). Patients with hypovolemia may demonstrate systolic blood pressure variation, particularly during mechanical ventilation (*Miller: Anesthesia, ed 6, p 1285*).

946. **(E)**   In patients with tetralogy of Fallot, it is important to maintain systemic vascular resistance to reduce the magnitude of the right-to-left intracardiac shunt. Therefore, induction of anesthesia in these patients is best accomplished with ketamine 3 to 4 mg/kg IM or 1 to 2 mg/kg IV. Remember that with right to left shunts, IV medications work more rapidly. Induction of anesthesia with a volatile anesthetic such as sevoflurane may be used, but careful monitoring of systemic oxygenation is needed because any decrease in systemic blood pressure would increase the right to left shunt (and would decrease the oxygen saturation). Ketamine will usually improve arterial oxygenation, which reflects increased pulmonary blood flow due to ketamine-induced increases in systemic vascular resistance (*Hines: Stoelting's Anesthesia & Co-Existing Disease, ed 5, pp 50-53; Morgan: Clinical Anesthesiology, ed 4, p 482*).

947. **(A)**   Mitral stenosis in adults occurs almost exclusively in individuals who had rheumatic fever during childhood. Mitral stenosis causes pathophysiologic changes both proximal and distal to the abnormal valve. In general, the left ventricle is "protected" or unloaded, that is, it is not exposed to excessive volume or pressure loads and therefore rarely associated with abnormalities in left-sided myocardial contractility. In contrast, proximal to the valve, a diastolic pressure gradient develops between the left atrium and left ventricle in order to force blood across the stenotic valve orifice, which results in elevated left atrial pressures and decreased left atrial compliance and function. The elevated left atrial pressures are reflected back into the pulmonary vascular system, causing an increase in pulmonary vascular resistance and eventually poor right ventricular function. The left ventricular pressure-volume loop in patients with mitral stenosis demonstrates low-to-normal left ventricular end-diastolic volumes and pressures and a corresponding reduction in stroke volume (*Morgan: Clinical Anesthesiology, ed 4, p 467*).

948. **(A)**   Ischemia of the posterior wall of the left ventricle and posterior leaflet of the mitral valve can cause prolapse of the posterior leaflet and retrograde blood flow into the left atrium during systole. This can be manifested as V (ventricular) waves on the pulmonary capillary wedge pressure tracing even before ST-segment depression can be seen on the ECG (*Miller: Anesthesia, ed 6, pp 1312-1313; Morgan: Clinical Anesthesiology, ed 4, pp 469-471*).

949. **(B)**   The patient described in this question has a wide complex tachycardia of undetermined origin. As this patient appears to be hemodynamically stable and has an uncertain rhythm, amiodarone 150 mg IV over 10 minutes, repeated as needed to a maximum dose of 2.2 g IV over 24 hours is recommended. (*2005 American Heart Association guidelines for cardiopulmonary resuscitation and emergency cardiovascular care. Circulation. 112: IV69-IV76, 2005; Miller: Anesthesia, ed 6, p 1404; Hensley: Cardiac Anesthesia, ed 4, p 92*).

950. **(B)**   The daily production of cortisol under normal circumstances is approximately 15 to 20 mg. Under maximum stress, daily cortisol production can increase to 75 to 150 mg/day yielding a plasma cortisol level of 30 to 50 μg/dL (*Hines: Stoelting's Anesthesia & Co-Existing Disease, ed 5, p 396*).

951. **(D)**   The anesthetic management of patients with artificial cardiac pacemakers should include ECG monitoring to confirm continued function of the pulse generators as well as emergency equipment (e.g., electrical defibrillator, external converter magnet) and drugs (atropine, isoproterenol) to maintain an acceptable intrinsic heart rate if the artificial pacemaker malfunctions. Inadvertent displacement of the endocardial electrodes by catheters has not been reported when the electrodes have been in place for 4 weeks or more. In general, anesthetic drugs will not alter the function of artificial cardiac pacemakers. However, the stimulation thresholds for ventricular capture are not static values and can be altered by a number of physiologic events. For example, acute hypokalemia and respiratory alkalosis will increase the threshold for ventricular capture, which could result in a loss of pacing. In contrast, acute hyperkalemia and acidosis will decrease the threshold for ventricular capture, which may make the patient vulnerable to ventricular fibrillation (VF). A decrease in the programmed rate of the pacemaker greater than 10% is a sign of battery failure. Should this occur, elective surgery should be canceled and a thorough evaluation of the pacemaker should be undertaken (*Hensley: Cardiac Anesthesia, ed 4, p 482; Miller: Anesthesia, ed 6, pp 1416-1427*).

952. **(E)** The Fick equation can be used to calculate cardiac output ($\dot{Q}$) if the patient's O_2 consumption ($\dot{V}o_2$), arterial O_2 content (Cao_2), and mixed venous O_2 content ($C\bar{v}o_2$) are determined. The downfalls of this type of $\dot{Q}$ measurement are threefold: (1) sampling and analysis errors in $\bar{v}o_2$, (2) changes in Q while samples are being taken, and (3) accurate determination of $\bar{v}o_2$ may be difficult because of cumbersome equipment. The Fick equation is as follows:

$$\dot{Q} = \frac{\dot{V}o_2}{(Cao_2 - C\bar{v}o_2) \times 10}$$

$$\dot{V}o_2 = 250 \text{ mL/min } (\approx 4\text{mL/kg})$$

$$Cao_2 = 1.36 \times \text{hemoglobin concentration} \times Sao_2 + (0.003 \times Pao_2)$$

$$1.36 \times 10 \text{ mg/dL} \times 0.99$$
$$13.5 \text{ mL } O_2/\text{dL of blood}$$

$$C\bar{v}o_2 = 1.36 \times \text{hemoglobin concentration} \times S\bar{v}o_2 + (0.003 \times Pvo_2)$$

$$1.36 \times 10 \text{ mg/dL} \times 0.60$$
$$8.16 \text{ mL } O_2/\text{dL of blood}$$

$$\dot{Q} = \frac{250\text{mL/min}}{(13.5\text{mL/dL} - 8.16\text{mL/dL}) \times 10\,{}^*} = 250/53.4 = 4.68 \text{ L/min}$$

*The factor 10 converts O_2 content to mL O_2/L of blood (instead of mL O_2/dL of blood) (*Hensley: Cardiac Anesthesia, ed 4, pp 128-130; Miller: Anesthesia, ed 6, p 1331*).

953. **(C)** Myocardial preservation is achieved during cardiopulmonary bypass primarily by infusing cold (4° C) cardioplegia solutions containing potassium chloride 20 mEq/L. This rapidly produces hypothermia of the cardiac muscle and a flaccid myocardium. In the normal contracting muscle at 37° C, myocardial O_2 consumption is approximately 8 to 10 mL/100 g/min. This is reduced in the fibrillating heart at 22° C to approximately 2 mL/100 g/min. Myocardial O_2 consumption of the electromechanically quiescent heart at 22° C is less than 0.3 mL/100 g/min (*Miller: Anesthesia, ed 6, pp 1976-1978; Stoelting: Basics of Anesthesia, ed 5, p 388*).

954. **(D)** All of the drugs listed in this question except phenylephrine will increase the inotropic state of the myocardium, which can increase left ventricular outflow obstruction and decrease cardiac output. Phenylephrine, because it is a pure α-adrenergic receptor agonist, has minimal direct effects on myocardial contractility (*Hines: Stoelting's Anesthesia and Co-Existing Disease, ed 5, p 119*).

955. **(A)** The classic signs and symptoms of critical aortic stenosis (angina, syncope, and congestive heart failure) are related primarily to an increase in left ventricular systolic pressure, which is necessary to maintain forward stroke volume. These elevated pressures cause concentric left ventricular hypertrophy. With severe disease, the left ventricular chamber becomes dilated and myocardial contractility diminishes. The primary goals in the anesthetic management of such patients undergoing noncardiac surgery are to maintain normal sinus rhythm and avoid prolonged alterations in heart rate (especially tachycardia), systemic vascular resistance, and intravascular fluid volume. Supraventricular tachycardia (especially new onset atrial fibrillation) should be terminated promptly by electrical cardioversion in this patient because of concomitant hypotension and myocardial ischemia (*Hines: Stoelting's Anesthesia and Co-Existing Disease, ed 5, pp 36-38, 68*).

956. **(C)** Positive end-expiratory pressure (PEEP) is produced by the application of positive pressure to the exhalation valve of the mechanical ventilator at the conclusion of the expiratory phase. It is often used to increase arterial oxygenation when F_{IO_2} exceeds 0.50 to reduce the hazard of O_2 toxicity. Positive end-expiratory pressure (PEEP) increases lung compliance and functional residual capacity by expanding previously collapsed but

perfused alveoli, thus improving ventilation/perfusion matching and reducing the magnitude of the right to left transpulmonary shunt. There are, however, a number of potential hazards associated with the use of PEEP. These include decreased cardiac output, pulmonary barotrauma (i.e., tension pneumothorax), increased extravascular lung water, and redistribution of pulmonary blood flow. Barotrauma, such as pneumothorax, pneumomediastinum, and subcutaneous emphysema, occurs as a result of overdistention of alveoli by PEEP. Pulmonary barotrauma should be suspected when there is abrupt deterioration of arterial oxygenation and cardiovascular function during mechanical ventilation with PEEP. If barotrauma is suspected, a chest x-ray film should be obtained and if a tension pneumothorax is present, a chest tube should be placed in the involved chest cavity (*Morgan: Clinical Anesthesiology, ed 4, pp 1038-1039*).

957.   **(C)**   Resting coronary artery blood flow is approximately 225 to 250 mL/min or about 75 mL/100 g/min, or approximately 4% to 5% of the cardiac output. Resting myocardial O_2 consumption is 8 to 10 mL/100 g/min, or approximately 10% of the total body consumption of O_2 (*Barash: Clinical Anesthesia, ed 5, p 868; Stoelting: Pharmacology and Physiology in Anesthetic Practice, ed 4, pp 752-753*).

958.   **(B)**   Pulmonary artery rupture is a disastrous but fortunately rare complication associated with the use of pulmonary artery catheters. The hallmark of pulmonary artery rupture is hemoptysis, which may be minimal or copious. Efforts should be made to separate the lungs. This can be achieved by endobronchial intubation with a double-lumen endotracheal tube. The presence of atheromas in the pulmonary artery is not associated with an increased risk of pulmonary artery rupture. Atheromatous changes are usually minimal or absent in the middle and distal portions of the pulmonary artery (i.e., in the segments where the tip of the pulmonary artery catheter typically resides) (*Miller: Anesthesia, ed 6, pp 1306-1307*).

959.   **(B)**   Anaphylactic and anaphylactoid reactions to protamine occur in less than 5% of all allergic reactions during anesthesia and when they occur, usually do so within 5 to 10 minutes of exposure. These reactions can occur in patients who have been exposed to protamine (e.g., diabetics taking NPH or PZI insulin, both of which contain protamine as a protein modifier; regular insulin does not contain protamine). Since protamine in derived from salmon sperm, patients with seafood allergies as well as men who have had a vasectomy (who may develop circulating antibodies to spermatozoa) may also develop a reaction. The likelihood of reactions may be reduced with prior administration of H_1 blockers, H_2 blockers and corticosteroids. Protamine should be avoided in patients who have a history of previous anaphylactic reactions to protamine (*Hines: Stoelting's Anesthesia and Co-Existing Disease, ed 5, pp 527-529; Stoelting: Basics of Anesthesia, ed 5, p 390*).

960.   **(B)**   Twenty thousand units of heparin is equal to 200 mg. Heparin is commonly neutralized by administration of 1.3 mg of protamine for each milligram of heparin. Protamine is a basic protein that combines to the acidic heparin molecule to produce an inactive complex that has no anticoagulant properties. The half-life of heparin is 1.5 hours at 37° C. At 25° C, metabolism of heparin is minimal (*Hensley: Cardiac Anesthesia, ed 4, p 504; Miller: Anesthesia, ed 6, p 1982*).

961.   **(E)**   Unlike most organs of the body where perfusion is continuous, coronary perfusion is somewhat intermittent. It is determined by the difference between aortic diastolic pressure and left and right ventricular end diastolic pressures. During systole, left ventricular pressure increases to or above systemic arterial pressure, resulting in almost complete occlusion of the intramyocardial portions of the coronary arteries. Thus, perfusion of the left ventricular myocardium occurs almost entirely during diastole, resulting in a decrease in left ventricular coronary perfusion as heart rate increases. In contrast, the right ventricle is perfused during both systole and diastole, because right ventricular pressures remain less than that of the aorta. An increase in heart rate results in a relatively shorter diastolic period (*Morgan: Clinical Anesthesiology, ed 4, p 432*).

962.   **(A)**   The thromboelastograph is a viscoelastometer that measures the viscoelastic properties of blood during clot formation. The coagulation variables measured from a thromboelastogram are: (1) the R value (reaction time; normal value 7.5 to 15 minutes) and K value (normal 3 to 6 minutes), which reflects clot formation time; (2) MA (maximum amplitude; normal value 50 to 60 mm), which represents maximum clot strength; and (3) A_{60} (amplitude 60 minutes after the MA; normal value MA – 5 mm), which represents the rate of clot destruction (i.e., fibrinolysis). The MA is determined by fibrinogen concentration, platelet count, and platelet function. The thromboelastogram depicted in the figure of this question is consistent with fibrinolysis (*Barash: Clinical Anesthesia, ed 5, pp 229-230; Miller: Anesthesiology, ed 6, pp 1341-1342*).

963. **(E)** At the time of collection, an anticoagulant is added to donor blood. Nonetheless, small clots will occasionally form in the units, requiring filtration at the time of transfusion. A 170-μm filter is present in standard blood administration sets for this purpose. Those filters permit rapid transfusion and should be used for infusions of platelets, fresh frozen plasma, cryoprecipitate, red blood cells, and granulocyte concentrates. Albumin does not need to be administered through a 170-mm filter because it does not contain blood clots (*Miller: Anesthesiology, ed 6, p 1815*).

964. **(B)** Adenosine in doses of 6 mg IV (repeated if needed 1-2 minutes later with 12 mg) can be very effective in the treatment of supraventricular tachycardias, including those associated with Wolff-Parkinson-White (WPW) syndrome (unless atrial fibrillation [AF] with a wide complex WPW occurs, where adenosine may increase the heart rate [HR]). The drug is rapidly metabolized such that it is not influenced by liver or renal dysfunction. Its effects, however, can be markedly enhanced by drugs that interfere with nucleotide metabolism such as dipyridamole. Administration of the usual dose of adenosine to a patient receiving dipyridamole may result in asystole. If adenosine is used in patients receiving dipyridamole, or the patient has a central line, the initial dose is 3 mg. Methylxanthines, such as caffeine, theophylline, and amrinone, are competitive antagonists of this drug, and doses may need to be adjusted accordingly (*2005 American Heart Association guidelines for cardiopulmonary resuscitation and emergency cardiovascular care. Circulation; 112:IV70-IV73, 2005; Barash: Clinical Anesthesia, ed 5, pp 316-317; Fleisher: Anesthesia and Uncommon Diseases, ed 5, p 69; Morgan: Clinical Anesthesiology, ed 4, p 260*).

965. **(D)** Temperature of the thermal compartment can be measured accurately in the pulmonary artery, distal esophagus, tympanic membrane, or nasopharynx. These temperature monitoring sites are reliable, even during rapid thermal perturbations such as cardiopulmonary bypass. Other temperature sites, such as oral, axillary, rectal, and urinary bladder, will estimate core temperature reasonably accurately except during extreme thermal perturbations. During cardiac surgery, the temperature of the urinary bladder is usually equal to the pulmonary artery when urine flow is high. However, it may be difficult to interpret urinary bladder temperature because it is strongly influenced by urine flow. The adequacy of rewarming after coronary artery bypass is thus best evaluated by considering both the core and urinary bladder temperatures (*Stoelting: Pharmacology and Physiology in Anesthetic Practice, ed 4, p 694; Morgan: Clinical Anesthesiology, ed 4, p 499; Stoelting: Basics of Anesthesia, ed 5, pp 387-388*).

966. **(B)** The transgastric mid-papillary short axis view images myocardium supplied by all three major coronary arteries: left anterior descending (LAD), left circumflex (CX), and right coronary (RCA) arteries. Thus, this view is preferred for the purpose of ischemia monitoring. The mid-esophageal 4 chamber view displays the antero-lateral (LAD or CX) and inferoseptal (LAD or RCA) walls only, while the long axis view displays the anterior septal (LAD) and inferolateral (CX or RCA) walls. Two chamber views display the anterior (LAD) and inferior (RCA) walls. (*Kahn RA, Shernan SK, Konstadt SN, et al: Intraoperative Echocardiography. In: Essentials of Cardiac Anesthesia, Kaplan, ed, Philadelphia, W.B. Saunders, 2008, p 206*).

967. **(D)** The most frequent initial rhythm in a witnessed sudden cardiac arrest (SCA) is ventricular fibrillation (VF). Delays in either starting CPR or defibrillation reduce survival from SCA. Current recommendations for health care providers in any facility with an automated external defibrillator (AED) readily available is AED use within moments of the cardiac arrest. If an AED is not readily available then CPR is started until the AED arrives at the scene. Recall 1 cycle of CPR is 30 compressions and 2 breaths. It is no longer recommended to do a 3 shock sequence with biphasic defibrillators, because it is unlikely for the second or third shock to work after a failed first shock, and the second and third shocks may be harmful. After the shock continue CPR for 5 cycles, check for a pulse. Then if VF persists, repeat 1 shock and add epinephrine or vasopressin before or after a shock when an IV or IO line is available. With monophasic defibrillators it may be OK to do 3 shock sequences, but all adult shocks should be 360 joules. With out-of-hospital unwitnessed cardiac arrest by EMS personnel, 5 cycles of CPR (about 2 minutes) should be performed before checking the ECG and attempting defibrillation, especially when the response interval is greater than 4 minutes because shock effectiveness appears more successful after CPR (*2005 American Heart Association guidelines for cardiopulmonary resuscitation and emergency cardiovascular care. Circulation, 112:IV35-41, IV58-61, 2005*).

968. **(A)** The renin-angiotensin-aldosterone system is important in controlling blood pressure and blood volume. Renin helps to convert angiotensinogen to Angiotensin I. Angiotensin converting enzyme (ACE) helps to convert Angiotensin I to Angiotensin II. Angiotensin II has many pharmacologic actions including potent vasoconstriction action as well as stimulating aldosterone release from the adrenal gland. Losartan is an angiotensin receptor blocker (ARB) and is commonly used to treat hypertension. Patients taking ARBs, as well as patients who are on ACE inhibitors, are more prone to develop hypotension during anesthesia. In addition, the hypotension that develops may be more difficult to treat. That is why ARBs are commonly discontinued the day before surgery. Terazosin is an α_1 blocker, lisinopril is an ACE inhibitor, spironolactone is a competitive antagonist to aldosterone and amlodipine is a calcium channel blocker. Note: If you look at the endings of many generic drug names you can know the drug class, ARBs end in *-sartan*, α_1 blockers end in *-osin*, ACE inhibitors end in *-pril*, and calcium channel blockers end in *-dipine* (*Hines: Stoelting's Anesthesia and Co-Existing Diseases, ed 5, pp 92-97*).

969. **(E)**   Hemodynamically unstable cardiac dysrhythmias can result in hypoperfusion and metabolic acidosis. If severe metabolic acidosis is confirmed on arterial blood gases, intravenous sodium bicarbonate should be administered. Adverse effects associated with administration of sodium bicarbonate are well documented and include severe plasma hyperosmolality, paradoxic cerebral spinal fluid acidosis, hypernatremia, and hypercarbia, particularly in patients who are not adequately ventilated. Bicarbonate lowers potassium by lowering the extracellular hydrogen ion concentration, which results in lowering, not raising the potassium concentration (*Miller: Anesthesia, ed 6, pp 1770, 1781, 2938*).

970. **(D)**   Hypercyanotic attacks primarily occur in infants 2 to 3 months of age and are frequently absent after 2 to 3 years of age. These attacks usually occur without provocation but can be associated with episodes of excitement, such as crying or exercise. The mechanism for these attacks is not known. It is believed, however, that hypercyanotic attacks occur as a result of spasm of the infundibular cardiac muscle or a decrease in systemic vascular resistance; both will exacerbate the right-to-left intracardiac shunt. Phenylephrine, an α-adrenergic receptor agonist, is the drug of choice for treatment of hypercyanotic attacks, because presumably phenylephrine increases systemic vascular resistance, which reduces the intracardiac right-to-left shunt and improves arterial oxygenation. Esmolol is also effective, presumably because it reduces spasm of the infundibular cardiac muscle. Isoproterenol with its betamimetic effects reduces afterload and therefore increases right to left shunting and may exacerbate infundibular spasm. Because hypovolemia may increase sympathetic stimulation, adequate hydration with IV fluids may be helpful (*Fleisher: Anesthesia and Uncommon Diseases, ed 5, pp 108-110; Hines: Stoelting's Anesthesia and Co-Existing Disease, ed 5, p 51*).

971. **(D)**   Sildenafil (Viagra) is used for erectile dysfunction. Erection of the penis involves the local release of nitric oxide (NO) which increases cyclic guanine monophosphate or cGMP in the corpus cavernosum. Sildenafil has no direct effects but inhibits phosphodiesterase type 5 (PDE5) which breaks down cGMP. The net effect is increasing cGMP. Yohimbine is an α-adrenergic blocker. Nitroglycerin and hydralazine are both direct acting smooth muscle relaxants. Enalapril is an ACE inhibitor. Milrinone is an inhibitor of phosphodiesterase type 3 (PDE3) (*Barash: Clinical Anesthesia, ed 5, pp 320, 329-330; Physicians Desk Reference-2008, ed 62, pp 2562, 2986*).

972. **(C)**   After a drug eluting stent (DES) is placed, dual antiplatelet therapy (ASA + clopidogrel) is started to decrease the chance of stent thrombosis. Because stent thrombosis may develop months after a DES is placed, a minimum of 1 year of dual antiplatelet therapy is recommended before stopping the drugs prior to elective surgery. If surgery is planned within one year of angioplasty and stent placement, consideration for using a bare metal stent is recommended (where a minimum of 1 month of antiplatelet therapy is recommended) (*AHA/ACC/SCAI/ACS/ADA Science advisory: Prevention of premature discontinuation of dual antiplatelet therapy in patients with coronary artery stents. J Am Coll Cardiol, 49:734-739, 2007*).

973. **(D)**   Heparin induced thrombocytopenia (HIT) can be either nonimmune (type I) or immune (type II). HIT type I is a transient and clinically insignificant condition where heparin binds to platelets causing a shortening of the platelet's left span and a modest decrease in the platelet count. However, HIT type II can be a serious condition where antibodies are formed (in 6% to 15% of patients who are receiving unfractionated heparin for >5 days) to a complex of heparin and a platelet protein factor 4. This heparin-platelet factor 4 antibody complex binds to endothelial cells, which then stimulates thrombin production with a net result of both thrombocytopenia (>50% reduction in the platelet count) and venous and/or arterial thrombosis (<10% of cases). In patients with HIT, heparin should be avoided. In the setting of a thrombotic event or a patient with HIT needing anticoagulation (e.g., coronary artery bypass graft [CABG]) a direct thrombin inhibitor such as hirudin, lepirudin, bivalirudin or argatroban should be used. (See also answer 411) (*Barash: Clinical Anesthesia, ed 5, pp 236-237; Hines: Anesthesia and Co-Existing Disease, ed 5, pp 425-426*).

974. **(C)** Density of bacterial skin contamination and propensity to develop thrombosis in a cannulated vein are risk factors for the development of catheter-related bloodstream infections (CRBSI). These risk factors are likely highest for femoral lines. In mostly observational studies the risk of CRBSI was found to be lowest for subclavian central venous access. The Centers for Disease Control and Prevention recommends use of subclavian central lines when clinically possible (*Miller: Anesthesia, ed 6, pp 1289-1296*).

975. **(E)** Clopidogrel exerts its antithrombotic action by noncompetitively and irreversibly inhibiting the specific platelet adenosine diphosphate (ADP) receptor named P2Y12. Because the P2Y12 receptor is permanently affected, the duration of action of clopidogrel is for the life of the platelets. No drug reverses these effects and only platelet transfusion can reverse the effects of clopidogrel. (*Barash: Clinical Anesthesia, ed 5, p 235; Fleisher: Anesthesia and Uncommon Diseases, ed 5, pp 370-371*).

976. **(B)** Port access robotic surgery is a less invasive technique for coronary artery revascularization in selected patients. Access is gained to the heart through a left sided mini-thoracotomy. This obviates the need for a sternotomy, but does require one-lung ventilation and may result in hypoxia prior to initiation of cardiopulmonary bypass and after cessation. Hypothermic cardiac arrest is not required for robotic surgery (*Miller: Anesthesia, ed 6, p 1995*).

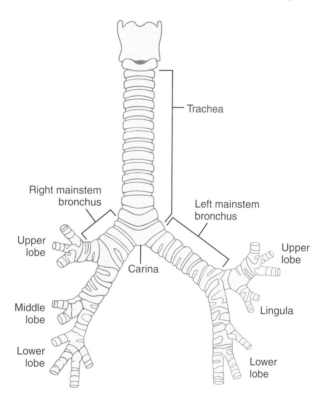

977. **(D)** One technique for placement of double lumen tubes is to simply advance the tube such that the tip of the distal lumen is just above the carina, and then to place it exactly (the distal tube including cuff) into the right mainstem bronchus under direct vision using the bronchoscope. If the tube is initially advanced too far into the right mainstem bronchus (as was it was in this question) a structure resembling the carina will be visualized. The "real" carina separates the left and right lungs and if the bronchoscope is pushed into either the right or the left mainstem bronchi, a secondary "carina" will be visualized. In both cases, the secondary carina has only two branch points. On the left, the branches lead to the left upper lobe and left lower lobe. On the right, the branches lead to the right upper lobe and the right middle lobe. If the three lumens are seen after branching right from the "carina", the "carina" in question is not the true carina, but is, in fact, the branching point for the right upper and right middle lobes (see figure) (*Stoelting: Basics of Anesthesia, ed 5, pp 415-417*).

978. **(E)** During one-lung ventilation $\dot{V}/\dot{Q}$ abnormalities increase. After a few minutes of one lung ventilation, hypoxic pulmonary vasoconstriction (HPV) develops, which helps decrease blood flow to the non-dependent lung. Most patients will have adequate PaO_2 when the dependent lung is ventilated with 100% oxygen, using a tidal volume (V_T) of 8 to 10 mL/kg, and adjusting the respiratory rate to achieve a $PaCO_2$ of 40 mm Hg. In patients who develop hypoxemia with these settings, correction of poor hemodynamics as well as checking the position of the double lumen tube is done first, then adding CPAP to the non-dependent lung, adding PEEP to the dependent lung or having the surgeon clamp the pulmonary artery to the lung about to be removed, will help decrease the $\dot{V}/\dot{Q}$ mismatch. Occasionally, intermittent inflation of the non-dependent lung with 100% oxygen will be needed. Epoprostenol and nitric oxide (NO) would inhibit HPV and might lead to an increase in shunt and a decrease in Pao_2 (*Miller: Anesthesia, ed 6, pp 1890-1900*).

979. (B)   The transplanted heart is essentially denervated and initially has an intrinsic rate of about 110 beats/min. About 25% of patients eventually develop a bradycardia that will require implantation of a permanent cardiac pacemaker. If bradycardia does develop, drugs that exert their effect by blocking the parasympathetic branches of the autonomic nervous system (e.g., atropine) will have no effect. Direct-acting drugs such as glucagon, isoproterenol, epinephrine, norepinephrine will still be effective. Isoproterenol is commonly used for increasing heart rate in cardiac transplant recipients. Epinephrine and norepinephrine may have exaggerated ß-mimetic effects on the heart rate because the increase in blood pressure will not lead to a reflex slowing of the heart rate via the baroreceptor reflexes (i.e., efferent vagus nerve). Drugs with both direct and indirect effects such as ephedrine evoke a less intense response. Implanted mechanical pacemakers work normally in heart transplant recipients since the cardiac leads are placed directly into the myocardium (*Barash: Clinical Anesthesia, ed 5, pp 311, 318, 1373; Hines: Stoelting's Anesthesia and Co-Existing Disease, ed 5, pp 21-22*).

980. (E)   Patients with Wolff-Parkinson-White syndrome have an accessory pathway known as the bundle of Kent, which connects the atria with ventricles without passing through the atrioventricular node. AV nodal reentrant tachycardia (AVNRT) is the most common tachydysrhythmia associated with WPW Syndrome and comprises 95% of arrhythmias associated with this syndrome. Greater than 90% of the time, conduction is orthodromic. That is, conduction passes through the AV node and the His-Purkinje system. Such conduction results in narrow complex tachycardia and any of the drugs mentioned in this question could be used to control rate. AVNRTs that travel through the accessory pathway (fewer than 10% of AVNRTs) are manifested as wide complex tachycardias (antidromic conduction) and are not amenable to treatment with β blockers, calcium channel blockers, adenosine or digoxin, and can, in fact, be made worse with these drugs. Intravenous procainamide, a class Ia antidysrhythmic agent, is the only useful pharmacologic agent among the drugs listed in the question. If pharmacologic therapy fails, electrical cardioversion is indicated to control rate (*Hines: Stoelting's Anesthesia and Co-Existing Disease, ed 5, p 72*).

981. (C)   The DOO setting is the simplest dual chamber pacing mode. Because of concerns about electromagnetic interference from an ESU (electrical surgical unit), i.e., the Bovie, pacemakers may be temporarily programmed into the asynchronous mode for surgery and then reprogrammed to the presurgical mode in the recovery room. With the VOO or DOO modes, the possibility of an R on T phenomenon exists if the native heart rate exceeds the programmed rate or when there are frequent premature ventricular contractions or premature atrial contractions. In the latter case, repolarization (from a PAC or PVC) may occur at the precise moment that the pacemaker is discharging (R wave). Turning off an implanted pacemaker would be extremely difficult in the middle of an operation. Furthermore, a slow rhythm could occur wherein pacing were again necessary. Intravenous lidocaine would be useless in this setting, as would switching the volatile agent from isoflurane to desflurane. At concentrations greater than one minimum alveolar concentration (MAC), desflurane can actually increase heart rate further. Administration of esmolol would slow the heart rate down below 70 so that the pacemaker could again "lead" (*Miller: Anesthesia, ed 6, p 1422*).

982. (C)   Milrinone and amrinone (inamrinone) are phosphodiesterase III inhibitors that increase cyclic adenosine monophosphate (cAMP) levels in cardiac and smooth muscle cells. They both produce positive inotropic effects and vasodilation (arterial and venous). Unlike milrinone, amrinone rapidly produces clinically significant thrombocytopenia especially after prolonged use (*Evers: Anesthetic Pharmacology, pp 664, 698*).

983. (E)   Systemic inflammatory response syndrome (SIRS) can result from a variety of severe clinical insults including cardiopulmonary bypass (CPB). The diagnosis of SIRS requires the presence of two or more of the following four conditions; temperature greater than 38° C or less than 36° C, heart rate greater than 90 beats/min, respiratory rate more than 20 breaths/min or a $Paco_2$ of less than 32 mm Hg, a leukocyte count greater than 12,000 or less than 4000/mm^3 or greater than 10% immature (band) forms. Sepsis is SIRS plus a documented infection (*Barash: Clinical Anesthesia, ed 5, pp 1481-1482; Miller: Anesthesia, ed 6, pp 1975-1976*).

984. (C) When a pulmonary artery catheter is placed from the right internal jugular vein, the right atrium typically is reached at 20 to 25 cm, the right ventricle at 30 to 35 cm, the pulmonary artery at about 40 to 45 cm and the wedge position at 45 to 55 cm. Add about 5 to 10 cm from the left internal jugular vein and the left and right external jugular veins, 15 cm from the femoral veins and 30 to 35 cm from the antecubital veins (*Miller: Anesthesia, ed 6, p 1303*).

985. (D) The $S\bar{v}o_2$ reflects the overall ability of cardiac output to adequately meet metabolic needs, and is thus a comprehensive measure of cardiac performance. There are several factors that can influence $S\bar{v}o_2$. These factors are easily understood by rearranging the Fick equation as follows:

$$S\bar{v}o_2 = Sao_2 \frac{\dot{V}o_2}{CO \times O_2\ Content}$$

See explanation to question 106 for complete definition of O_2 content. Thus, $S\bar{v}o_2$ can be reduced by a decrease in Sao_2, CO, and hemoglobin and an increase in $\dot{V}o_2$. In the present case, labetalol reduces cardiac output through its negative inotropic effect. These factors must be accounted for when interpreting $S\bar{v}o_2$ measurements (*Miller: Anesthesia, ed 6, pp 1331-1332*).

986. (E) Inotropy refers to the force and velocity of ventricular contractions when preload and afterload are held constant. Chronotrophy refers to the heart rate. Dromotropy refers to the conduction of impulses along conductive tissue. Bathmotropy refers to muscular excitation in response to a stimulus. Lusitropy refers myocardial relaxation or diastole. A decrease in lusitropy is seen with the aging myocardium (*Barash: Clinical Anesthesia, ed 5, pp 301-304*).

987. (E) Pulmonary artery hypertension is defined as a mean PA pressure of greater than 25 mm Hg at rest or greater than 30 mm Hg with exercise. Epoprostenol, also called prostacyclin (PGI2), as well as alprostadil (PGE1) is usually administered by a continuous IV infusion centrally and produces both pulmonary and systemic vasodilation but because systemic hypotension is common, its use is limited. Recently inhaled epoprostenol and alprostadil have been described to reduce the systemic side effects. Because hypoxia produces pulmonary vasoconstriction, oxygen therapy is often administered to reduce the magnitude of pulmonary vasoconstriction that may develop. Inhaled nitric oxide (NO) in concentrations from 1 to 80 ppm (typically 20-40 ppm) produces smooth muscle relaxation and reduces PA pressures. Because NO is so rapidly metabolized, it has minimal systemic effects. Milrinone is a phosphodiesterase inhibitor that reduces pulmonary vascular resistance while having some inotropic effects. (If right ventricle failure is severe, norepinephrine or epinephrine may be preferred as an inotrope even though PA pressures will increase). Milrinone is usually administered IV but recently inhaled milrinone has been described to reduce systemic side effects.

Inhaled volatile anesthetics tend to decrease pulmonary artery resistance. On the other hand, nitrous oxide tends to increase pulmonary vascular resistance and is not recommended to be used in patients with pulmonary hypertension (*Fleisher: Anesthesia and Uncommon Diseases, ed 5, pp 51-53, 131-133; Hines: Stoelting's Anesthesia and Co-Existing Disease, ed 5, pp 97-101*).

988. (C) Pulmonary vascular resistance (PVR) is the sum of the resistance of small and large blood vessels and is least at the FRC. When the lung volume increases above FRC, PVR increases due to alveolar compression of the small intra-alveolar blood vessels. When the lung volume decreases below FRC, PVR increases due to the mechanical tortuosity or kinking of the large extra-alveolar blood vessels. Pulmonary vascular resistance (PVR) also increases in areas of atelectasis when hypoxia causes pulmonary vasoconstriction (HPV) (*Miller: Anesthesia, ed 6, pp 684-685*).

989. (C) Hypertrophic cardiomyopathy is characterized by left ventricular outflow tract (LVOT) obstruction and is caused by asymmetric hypertrophy of the intraventricular septal muscle. The compensatory mechanism to maintain cardiac output is left ventricular hypertrophy. Events that increase outflow obstruction include increased myocardial contractility (e.g., β stimulation), decreased ventricular preload (e.g., hypovolemia, venodilation, tachycardia with reduced time to fill the ventricle, positive pressure ventilation), and decreased afterload (e.g., vasodilation). Perioperative management is aimed at preventing an increase in outflow obstruction. Hypotension often responds by increasing preload (fluid administration) and/or increasing afterload (α adrenergic stimulation with phenylephrine). β-Blockade (e.g., esmolol) can help slow a fast heart rate and allow more time for ventricular filling as well as decreasing contractility. If the patient has a painful catecholamine response to surgery, narcotics may be helpful. Drugs with β-adrenergic activity such as ephedrine, dopamine and dobutamine are contraindicated, because they increase myocardial contractility and heart rate which causes more LVOT obstruction (*Stoelting: Basics of Anesthesia, ed 5, pp 382-383; Hines: Stoelting's Anesthesia and Co-Existing Disease, ed 5, pp 115-119*).

990. (E) Congestive heart failure is one of the six major risk factors for patients undergoing elective major noncardiac surgery. The other major risk factors are high risk surgery, ischemic heart disease, cerebrovascular disease, insulin-dependent diabetes mellitus, and preoperative serum creatinine of greater than 2 mg/dL. As this is an elective case, patients with CHF need to be optimally managed prior to surgery. This patient does not appear to be optimally managed and surgery should be canceled (*Hines: Stoelting's Anesthesia and Co-Existing Disease, ed 5, pp 13-15; Stoelting: Basics of Anesthesia, ed 5, p 382*).

991. (B) Symptoms of mitral stenosis develop when the mitral valve orifice (normally 4-6 cm²) is reduced 50% or more. Goals in management revolve around four main areas: preventing tachycardia (which decreases the diastolic time needed for LV filling); avoiding a marked increase in central blood volume (which may cause atrial fibrillation or CHF); preventing sudden drug-induced decreases in systemic vascular resistance (which may cause hypotension and reflex tachycardia); and avoiding hypoxia and hypercarbia (which may exacerbate pulmonary hypertension and cause RV failure). Ketamine, pancuronium, and a rapid increase in the concentration of desflurane may all cause tachycardia, which results in a decrease in cardiac output. Nitrous oxide can be used in most cases, however, in severe cases where there is an increase in pulmonary artery pressure, avoiding nitrous oxide may be beneficial. Remifentanil as well as fentanyl and sufentanil give good analgesia without increasing HR (*Hines: Stoelting's Anesthesia and Co-Existing Disease, ed 5, pp 31-33; Stoelting: Basics of Anesthesia, ed 5, pp 373-374*).

992. (E) Dopamine can be mixed in either D5W or normal saline NS solution. A mixture of 200 mg of dopamine in 250 mL of D5W would yield a concentration of 800 μg/mL (200 mg / 250 mL = 0.8 mg/mL = 800 μg/mL). At an infusion rate of 5 μg/70 kg/60 min, you would need 5 μg × 70 kg × 60 min = 21,000 μg/hr. 21,000 μg/hr divided by 800 μg/mL = 26 mL/hr.

993. (D) Patients with stenotic heart valves (MS, AS) tend to do better with slow normal heart rates because it takes time for the heart chambers to fill during diastole (MS) or empty during systole (AS). Tachycardia in patients with AS may be especially harmful, because tachycardia leads to myocardial ischemia and ventricular dysfunction due to the thick ventricular walls. With cardiac valves that are insufficient (AI) faster heart rates are helpful, because regurgitation occurs during diastole and faster rates decrease diastolic time. Patients with AI also benefit from a lower SVR, which promotes a better cardiac output (high SVR increases the amount of regurgitation during diastole). Too low of a SVR in these patients may lead to decreased coronary artery filling, because filling occurs during diastole. With hypertrophic cardiomyopathy, a high SVR helps to decrease the outflow obstruction, but a fast heart rate increases outflow obstruction. Patients with cardiac tamponade have a fixed ejection fraction that is very dependent upon high filling pressures, and the cardiac output is very much dependent upon the heart rate. A high SVR helps to maintain blood pressure in the face of the decreased cardiac output (*Stoelting; Basics of Anesthesia, ed 5, pp 372-376, 382-384*).

994. (A) The figure shows torsades de pointes ("twisting of the points") in a patient who had a QTc interval of 450 msec and was having an acute myocardial infarction (MI). This condition can be induced by drugs (e.g., quinidine, procainamide, and phenothiazines such as droperidol), electrolyte abnormalities (e.g., hypokalemia, hypomagnesemia) as well as acute cardiac ischemia or infarction. If a prolonged QT interval is present, the shortening of the QT interval is performed as time permits (e.g., correction of electrolyte abnormalities). In the past isoproterenol was used (shortens QT interval) but overdrive atrial or ventricular pacing is the more definitive treatment. Magnesium sulfate has also been used and is recommended by many as the first line emergency drug. If the patient does not have a prolonged QT interval, standard drugs used for ventricular tachycardia can be used. If the patient becomes hemodynamically unstable, unsynchronized shocks (defibrillation doses) should be delivered. (*AHA: 2005 American Heart Association guidelines for cardiopulmonary resuscitation and emergency cardiovascular care. Circulation, 112:IV63-64, 73, 2005; Miller: Anesthesia, ed 6, pp 360, 2934*).

995. (B) 996. (A) 997. (E)
The ECG recording is a reflection of cardiac muscle electrical activity and although it is primarily used to diagnose arrhythmias or cardiac ischemia, the changes that occur may be related to electrolyte disturbances. Both hyperkalemia and hypokalemia are associated with impaired myocardial contractility, conduction disturbances and cardiac arrhythmias. With hyperkalemia, the earliest changes are narrowing and peaking of the T wave (7-9 mEq/L). More severe degrees of hyperkalemia (>7 mEq/L) produce widening of the QRS complex that can merge with the T wave producing a sine wave pattern, decrease in P wave amplitude, and an increase in the PR interval. The terminal event would be VF or asystole.

The earliest changes with hypokalemia include T wave flattening or inversion, appearance of U waves and ST segment depression. With severe hypokalemia the PR interval may become prolonged and the QRS complex may widen, then arrhythmias develop.

Hypocalcemia prolongs the QT interval (ST portion) while hypercalcemia shortens the QT interval. Hypernatremia and hyponatremia do not produce characteristic changes in the ECG (*Barash: Clinical Anesthesia, ed 5, p 1542; Kasper: Harrison's Principle of Internal Medicine, ed 16, pp 260, 262, 1318-1319; Miller: Anesthesia, ed 6, pp 1049-1050, 1106-1107*).

Bibliography

ACC/AHA 2007 Guidelines on Perioperative Cardiovascular Evaluation and Care for Noncardiac Surgery: Executive Summary, *Anesth and Analg* 106:685–712, 2008.

AHA/ACC/SCAI/ACS/ADA Science Advisory: Prevention of premature discontinuation of dual antiplatelet therapy in patients with coronary artery stents, *J Am Coll Cardiol* 49:734–739, 2007.

2005 American Heart Association guidelines for cardiopulmonary resuscitation and emergency cardiovascular care, *Circulation* 112(Suppl. I):IV67–IV77, 2005.

ASA task force on preoperative fasting: Practice guidelines for preoperative fasting and the use of pharmacologic agents to reduce the risk of pulmonary aspiration: Application to healthy patients undergoing elective procedures, *Anesthesiology* 90:896–905, 1999.

Barash PG, Cullen BF, Stoelting RK: *Clinical Anesthesia*, ed 5, Philadelphia, Lippincott Williams & Wilkins, 2006.

Baum VC, O'Flaherty JE: *Anesthesia for Genetic, Metabolic, and Dysmorphic Syndromes of Childhood*, ed 2, Philadelphia, Lippincott Williams & Wilkins, 2007.

Brown DL: *Atlas of Regional Anesthesia*, ed 3, Philadelphia, Lippincott Williams & Wilkins, 2008.

Brunner JMR, Leonard PF: *Electricity, Safety, and the Patient*, Chicago, Year Book Medical Publishers, 1989.

Chestnut DH: *Obstetric Anesthesia: Principles and Practice*, ed 3, Philadelphia, Mosby, 2004.

Chestnut DH, Polley LS, Tsen LC, Wong CA: *Chestnut's Obstetric Anesthesia: Principles and Practice*, ed 4, Philadelphia, Mosby, 2009.

Clemente CD: *Anatomy: A Regional Atlas of the Human Body*, ed 3, Baltimore, Urban and Schwarzenberg, 1987.

Coté CJ, Todres ID, Ryan JF, Goudsouzian NG: *A Practice of Anesthesia for Infants and Children*, ed 3, Philadelphia, W.B. Saunders, 2001.

Cottrell JE, Smith DS: *Anesthesia and Neurosurgery*, ed 4, Mosby, 2001.

Cousins MJ, Bridenbaugh PO: *Neural Blockade in Clinical Anesthesia and Management of Pain*, ed 3, Philadelphia, Lippincott-Raven, 1998.

Cunningham FG, Levano KJ, Bloom SL, et al: *Williams Obstetrics*, ed 22, New York, McGraw-Hill, 2005.

Eger EI II: *Anesthetic Uptake and Action*, Baltimore, Lippincott Williams & Wilkins, 1974.

Ehrenwerth J, Eisenkraft JB: *Anesthesia Equipment: Principles and Applications*, St. Louis, Mosby-Year Book, 1993.

Eisenkraft JB: Potential for barotrauma or hypoventilation with the Drager AV-E ventilator, *J Clin Anesth* 1:452–456, 1989.

Evers AS, Maze M: *Anesthetic Pharmacology – Physiologic Principles and Clinical Practice*, Philadelphia, Churchill Livingstone, 2004.

Faust RJ, Cucchiara RF, Rose SH: *Anesthesiology Review*, ed 3, New York, Churchill Livingstone, 2001.

Fleisher LA: *Anesthesia and Uncommon Diseases*, ed 5, Philadelphia, W.B. Saunders, 2006.

Flick RP, et al: Perioperative cardiac arrests in children between 1988 and 2005 at a tertiary referral center. A study of 92,881 patients, *Anesthesiology* 106:226–237, 2007.

Flick RP, et al: Risk factors for laryngospasm in children during general anesthesia, *Paediatr Anaesth* 18:289–296, 2008.

Groudine SB, et al: New York state guidelines on the topical use of phenylephrine in the operating room, *Anesthesiology* 92:859–864, 2000.

Harmening DM: *Modern Blood Banking and Transfusion Practices*, ed 5, Philadelphia, F.A. Davis, 2005.

Hardman JG, Limbird LE, Gimman AG: *Goodman & Gilman's The Pharmacological Basis of Therapeutics*, ed 10, New York, McGraw-Hill, 2001.

Hebl JR: *Mayo Clinic Atlas of Regional Anesthesia and Ultrasound Guided Nerve Blockade*, In press, 2009.

Hebl JR, Neal JM: Infections complications: A new practice advisory - The importance and implications of aseptic techniques during regional anesthesia, *Reg Anesth Pain Med* 31:289–290, 311–323, 2006.

Hensley FA Jr, Martin DE, Gravlee GP: *A Practical Approach to Cardiac Anesthesia*, ed 4, Philadelphia, Lippincott Williams & Wilkins, 2007.

Hines RL, Marschall KE: *Stoelting's Anesthesia and Co-Existing Disease*, ed 5, Philadelphia, Churchill Livingstone, 2008.

Hughes SC, Levinson G, Rosen MA: *Shnider and Levinson's Anesthesia for Obstetrics*, ed 4, Philadelphia, Lippincott Williams & Wilkins, 2002.

Johnston RR, Eger EI II, Wilson C: A comparative interaction of epinephrine with enflurane, isoflurane and halothane in man, *Anesth Analg* 55:709–712, 1976.

Kahn RA, Shernan SK, Konstadt SN, et al: Intraoperative Echocardiography, In Kaplan JA, ed: *Essentials of Cardiac Anesthesia*, Philadelphia, W.B. Saunders, 2008.

Kaplan JA: *Kaplan's Cardiac Anesthesia*, ed 4, Philadelphia, W.B. Saunders, 1999.

Kasper DL, Braunwald E, Fauci AS, et al: *Harrison's Principles of Internal Medicine*, ed 16, New York, McGraw-Hill, 2005.

Kattwinkel J, et al: *Textbook of Neonatal Resuscitation*, ed 5, American Academy of Pediatrics and American Heart Association, 2006.

Lobato EB, Gravenstein N, Kirby RR: *Complications in Anesthesiology*, Philadelphia, Lippincott Williams & Wilkins, 2008.

Loeser JD: *Bonica's Management of Pain*, ed 3, Philadelphia, Lippincott Williams & Wilkins, 2001.

Longnecker DE, Tinker JH, Morgan GE Jr: *Principles and Practice of Anesthesiology*, ed 2, St. Louis, Mosby, 1998.

Miller RD, et al: *Miller's Anesthesia*, ed 6, Philadelphia, Churchill Livingstone, 2005.

Miller RD, et al: *Miller's Anesthesia*, ed 7, Philadelphia, Churchill Livingstone, 2009.

Morgan GE Jr, Mikhail MS, Murray MJ: *Clincal Anesthesiology*, ed 4, New York, Lange Medical Books/McGraw-Hill, 2006.

Motoyama EK, Davis PJ: *Smith's Anesthesia for Infants and Children*, ed 7, Philadelphia, Mosby, 2006.

Navarro R, et al: Humans anesthetized with sevoflurane or isoflurane have similar arrhythmic response to epinephrine, *Anesthesiology* 80:545–549, 1994.

Neal JM, et al: Upper extremity regional anesthesia—Essentials of our current understanding, 2008, *Regl Anesth Pain Med.* 34:134–170, 2009.

Netter FH: *Atlas of Human Anatomy, Summit*, CIBA-Geigy Corporation, 1989.

O'Grady NP, Alexander M, Dellinger EP, et al: Guidelines for the prevention of intravascular catheter-related infections. Centers for Disease Control and Prevention, *MMWR Recomm Rep* 51(RR10):1–29, 2002.

Physicians' Desk Reference, ed 63, Montvale, Physicians Desk Reference Inc. / Thomson Healthcare, 2008.

Physicians' Desk Reference, ed 62, Montvale, Physicians Desk Reference Inc. / Thomson Healthcare, 2007.

Raj PP: *Practical Management of Pain*, ed 3, St. Louis, Mosby, 2000.

Second Consensus Conference on Neuraxial Anesthesia and Anticoagulation, April 25-28, 2002. www.asra.com/consensus-statements/2.html

Shott SR: Down syndrome: Analysis of airway size and a guide for appropriate intubation, *Laryngoscope* 110:585–592, 2000.

Southorn P, et al: Reducing the potential morbidity of an unintentional spinal anaesthetic by aspirating cerebrospinal fluid, *Br J Anaesth* 76:467–469, 1996.

Stoelting RK, Miller RD: *Basics of Anesthesia*, ed 5, Philadelphia, Churchill Livingstone, 2007.

Stoelting RK, Hillier SC: *Pharmacology and Physiology in Anesthetic Practice*, ed 4, Philadelphia, Lippincott Williams & Wilkins, 2006.

Stoelting RK, Dierdorf SF: *Anesthesia and Co-Existing Disease*, ed 4, New York, Churchill Livingstone, 2002.

Thomas SJ, Kramer JL: *Manual of Cardiac Anesthesia*, ed 2, Philadelphia, Churchill Livingstone, 1993.

Wedel DJ: *Orthopedic Anesthesia*, New York, Churchill Livingstone, 1993.

West JB: *Respiratory Physiology:* ed 6, Philadelphia, Lippincott Williams & Wilkins, 1999.

Wilson W, Taubert KA, Gewitz M, et al: Prevention of Infective Endocarditis—Guidelines from the American Heart Association, *Circulation* 115:1736–1754, 2007: (http://circ.ahajournals.org).

Index

Page numbers followed by f indicate figures, and t indicate tables.

Methohexital, elimination half life, 87
Methoxyflurane
    nephrogenic diabetes insipidus from, 161
    vapor pressure and minimum alveolar concentration by drug, 23t
Meyer-Overton theory, 164
MG (Myasthenia gravis)
    anticholinesterase drugs, 224
    edrophonium for, 170
MH. *See* malignant hyperthermia (MH)
Microshock, macroshock compared with, 29
Midazolam
    as benzodiazepine drug, 95
    reducing unpleasant dreams associated with ketamine, 83
    treating carotid artery disease, 253
    water solubility of, 79
Middle constrictor muscles, innervation of, 289
Minoxidil, side effects of, 100
Minute ventilation (VE)
    CO_2 inhalation increasing, 48
    relationship to VD and $PaCO_2$, 47, 47f
Miosis, eye drops causing, 163
Mitral valve prolapse (MVP), 174
Molar pregnancies, 233
Montelukast (Singulair), 166
Morphine
    abuse of, 223
    epidural vs. intrathecal doses, 273
    as obstetric anesthetic, 227
    onset/duration compared with fentanyl, 85–86
    reasons for not using as labor epidural, 225
    treating postoperative pain, 90
Morphine sulfate
    opioids resulting in delayed respiratory depression, 280
    parenteral to oral conversion of, 177
Motor evoked potentials (MEPs), pharmacological agents effecting, 252
Motor nerves, blocking, 274
MRI (Magnetic resonance imaging)
    appropriate course of action if patient pinned by large metallic object, 255
    potential dangers of, 178, 249
Mucous membranes, innervation of false cords, 289
Multifocal atrial tachycardia (MAT), 46
Multiple endocrine neoplasia, 162
Muscle relaxants
    allergic reactions to, 168
    chemical classes of, 82
    dantrolene, 176
    histamine stimulating, 169
    for intubation, 90–91, 93–94
    nondepolarizing. *See* Nondepolarizing muscle relaxants
    polarizing. *See* Depolarizing muscle relaxants
    rocuronium, 86
Musculocutaneous nerve, identifying on ultrasound, 288
MVP (mitral valve prolapse), 174
MVV (maximum voluntary ventilation), 165–166
Myasthenia gravis (MG)
    anticholinesterase drugs, 224
    edrophonium for, 170
Mydriasis
    atropine and scopolamine causing ocular effects, 103
    from phenylephrine, 171
    from scopolamine, 170
Myocardial contractility, narcotic causing decrease in, 81
Myocardial depression
    anesthetics most likely to cause, 81
    from ketamine, 167

Myocardial infarction, risks for, 45
Myocardial ischemia, 30
Myocardial potassium homeostasis, cardiac dysrhythmias and, 53
Myoglobinemia, as indicator of rhabdomyolysis, 195

N
Nalmefene (Revex), 161
Naloxone
    reversing effects of analgesics, 91
    reversing narcotic induced toxicity, 91
    treating nonmoving patient following wake up test, 251
Naltrexone (Narcan), for treatment of heroin addicts, 161
Narcan (naltrexone), for treatment of heroin addicts, 161
Narcotic drugs. *See also* Opioids
    causing decrease in myocardial contractility, 81
    chloroprocaine as antagonistic to action of, 233
    meperidine, 226
    pruritus as side effect of intraspinal, 227
Nasal cannula, maximum Fio_2 delivery, 25
National Institute of Occupational Safety and Health (NIOSH), 18, 20
Nausea. *See also* Postoperative nausea and vomiting (PONV)
    as side effect of etomidate, 91
    treating in Parkinson's patients, 79
Neck, structures of, 280
Necrotizing enterocolitis (NEH), 206
Neonates
    alveolar ventilation in, 46
    anesthetic requirement for, 117
    blood volume of, 132
    bradycardia in, 196
    cardiovascular system of, 195t
    development of apnea in, 171
    echocardiogram for assessing abnormalities, 196
    estimated blood volume (EBV) in, 198
    hemodynamic indices of, 195
    MAC with sevoflurane in, 114
    oxygen consumption in, 201
    physiologic variables, 201t
    post-operative ventilatory depression in, 198
    risk period for retinopathy of prematurity (ROP), 194
    side effects of succinylcholine in, 198
    spinal anesthesia requirements for, 178
    succinylcholine dose, 196
    thermoregulation in, 200
Neostigmine
    comparing with Sugammadex (ORG 25969), 96
    as reversal agent in surgery with pregnant patients, 176
    time of onset, 84
Nephrogenic diabetes insipidus, from methoxyflurane, 161
Nerve disorders, autonomic hyperreflexia as, 246
Nerve gas poisoning
    atropine for treating, 92
    signs of (DUMBELS), 54
Nerve root irritation, 286
Nerves fibers, C nerve fibers as pain carriers, 287
Neurofibromatosis (von Recklinghausen's disease), 201
Neuroleptic malignant syndrome
    symptoms, 170
    treating, 94
Neurologic injury, use of glucose-containing solutions and, 249
Neurolytic nerve blockade
    characteristics of, 281
    with phenol vs. alcohol, 276
Neuromuscular blockade
    bilateral motor block, 282
    celiac-plexus blocks, 280, 282
    central neuraxial block, 283

Spinal fusion, NSAIDS contraindicated for, 176
Splitting ratio
    comparing anesthetic gases, 28t
    in variable-bypass vaporizers, 19
SSEPs. *See* Somatosensory evoked potentials (SSEPs)
SSRIs (Serotonin uptake inhibitors), for mental depression, 97
Status asthmaticus, medications for treating, 93
Stellate ganglion
    potential complications of blockade, 285
    proximity to vertebral artery, 278
Streptomycin, for plague, 179
Stroke
    carotid artery stenosis increasing risk of, 250
    waiting period for operative procedures following occlusive vascular accident, 251
Subarachnoid bleed, cerebral vasospasm and, 177
Subarachnoid block, structures traversed when performing, 284
Subarachnoid hemorrhage (SAH), 244, 251–252
Subarachnoid injection
    factors impacting sensory level following, 275
    physiologic effects of injecting large volumes of local anesthetic, 282
Succinylcholine
    attenuating side effects of, 84
    bradycardia due to administration of, 88
    care in combining with echothiophate for glaucoma, 81
    causing apnea, 165
    dose for neonates and infants, 196
    drug substitutions for, 90–91
    duration of neuromuscular-blocking action, 95
    Huntington's chorea and, 168
    hyperkalemia as side effect of, 84–85, 89
    increased sensitivity with thermal injuries, 168
    increasing serum [K+], 83
    as muscle relaxant for rapid intubation, 93–94
    resistance to neuromuscular blockage with, 79
    side effects when used to paralyze neonates, 198
    tachycardia induced by, 88
    terminating action of, 92
    treating chest wall stiffness with, 94
    trismus following administration of, 166–167
    uterine blood flow reduction, 220
Sudden infant death syndrome (SIDS), 206
Sufentanil, as obstetric anesthetic, 227
Sugammadex (ORG 25969), 96
Sulfhemoglobinemia, central cyanosis from, 169
Sulfur hexafluoride, 167
Superficial cervical plexus block, for shoulder arthroscopy, 283
Superficial peroneal nerve, innervation of great toe, 280
Superior constrictor muscles, innervation of, 289
Superior laryngeal nerve
    cricothyroid muscle innervated by, 277
    results of bilateral damage to, 165
Supraclavicular brachial plexus blocks
    blocking trunks of brachial plexus, 280
    pneumothorax as complication of, 280
    risk factors related to, 279–280
Supraglottitis, causing airway obstruction, 199
Supraspinal analgesia, 101
Surface tension, in Laplace's law, 15
Surgical trauma, physiologic responses, 274
SVO₂ (mixed venous hemoglobin saturation)
    calculating factors effecting, 48, 48f
    improving, 54–55
Sympathetic nerves
    order of nerve blockade, 274
    pain in abdominal viscera transmitted by, 281

Sympathomimetics, 81t
Synchronized intermittent mandatory ventilation (SIMV), 49, 50f
Syndrome X, insulin resistance and, 177
Systemic absorption, terminating action of tetracaine, 275
Systemic vascular resistance
    decreased by isoflurane, 119
    decreasing at term pregnancy, 222
    reduction by volatile anesthetics, 115, 120
Systolic blood pressure (SBP), 207

T

Tachyarrhythmias, preventing in patients with Wolff-Parkinson-White (WPW) syndrome, 87
Tachycardia
    adrenergic blockers for, 98
    desflurane and isoflurane causing, 117
    succinylcholine induced, 88
    treating with electrical defibrillation, 196
Tachyphylaxis, to local anesthetics, 273
TBW (Total body water)
    comparing physiology of newborns with adults, 203
    in infants, 193
TEE (Transesophageal echocardiograph), 247, 249
TEFs. *See* Tracheoesophageal fistulas (TEFs)
Temperature monitoring, site options for, 24
TENS (Transcutaneous electrical nerve stimulation), 280
Teratogenic agents, susceptibility of fetus to, 222
Terbutaline, side effects of, 221
Testicular innervation, 173
Tetanic stimulation, amplitude of muscle response, 101
Tetanus, post-tetanic facilitation, 101
Tetracaine
    duration of anesthetic effect in infants, 202
    terminating action of, 275
Tetracycline, for plague, 179
Thermal injuries, massive potassium release with, 168
Thermoregulation
    for infants under anesthesia, 198
    in neonates, 200
Thigh
    innervation of, 280
    medial thigh sensation diminished with obturator nerve injury, 180
Thiobarbiturates, 84
Thiocyanate toxicity, 45
Thiopental
    cerebral pharmacologic profile of, 254
    contraindications for use of, 85
    half time for elimination of, 87
    impact on CO₂ responsiveness of cerebral vasculature, 250
    myocardial depression and, 81
    pain at IV site rare, 98
    pH of, 84
    for reducing uterine blood flow, 220
    treating accidental intra-arterial injection, 96
    treating carotid artery disease with, 253
Thoracoabdominal muscles, succinylcholine for treating chest wall stiffness, 94
Thorpe tube, in rotameters, 25
Thromboembolism, causes of maternal death, 221
Thromboprophylaxis, low molecular weight heparin (LMWH) for, 220
Thumb
    corresponding to dermatome C6, 281
    numbness indicating C6 nerve root irritation, 286
    numbness resulting from injury to radial nerve, 285
Thymol, in halothane, 121